Geriatric Nursing

Geriatric Nursing

Charlotte Eliopoulos

Harper & Row, Publishers
London

Cambridge
Mexico City
New York
Philadelphia

San Francisco
São Paulo
Singapore
Sydney

First published in the UK 1980
Reprinted 1982, 1985, 1987

Harper & Row Ltd
28 Tavistock Street
London WC2E 7PN

British Library Cataloguing in Publication Data
Eliopoulos, Charlotte
Geriatric nursing.–(Lippincott nursing series)
1. Geriatric nursing
I. Title
610.73'65 RC954
ISBN 0 06 318132 0

Printed and bound by Butler and Tanner Ltd

CONTENTS

Foreword to the British Edition

Due to the lack of enlightened direction in the first half of this century, geriatric nursing has, for many years, been less attractive to student nurses than other branches of the profession. Seen as a caring without curing operation, it was thought to be dull and dismal, lacking the interest and perhaps the drama of other fields of nursing practice. The abolition of the Poor Law Institution and subsequent legislation provided the framework for change, but the treatment of, and attitudes toward, the aged sick were slow to improve.

In the last thirty to forty years, changes have taken place more rapidly. A more scientific approach has led to higher standards of professional training in geriatric medicine, and has attracted the interest of increasing numbers of doctors. Nurses, too, are finding the subject more rewarding and challenging. The number of old people has quadrupled in the last seventy years, and this must surely be a factor in the change of emphasis.

With these developments in mind, I found it a pleasure to read this new book on the subject. It is a comprehensive textbook, full of heart and wisdom, as well as instruction. It should prove invaluable to the student nurse, or indeed to anyone working with elderly people. As it was written for American nurses, the historical background in Chapter 1 and the social services information in Chapter 25 were not applicable to nursing in the UK. I have rewritten these chapters to include our own history and social service arrangements.

Doris Edmondson S.R.N., Q.I.D.N.
1979

Preface

The growing number of elderly persons in the population, and the more active role they are assuming, have increased society's awareness of the qualities, rights, and needs of its older members. Popular literature that dispels myths concerning the aging process, proliferates. Government is demonstrating greater sensitivity to the problems of old age, as evidenced by legislation promoting increased security and care for the aged. The media exposes the public to the often overlooked pleasures and problems of growing old in America. Society thus has a new concern for the aging population.

The increased numbers of the aged have influenced the helping professions to become more closely involved in the fields of gerontology and geriatrics. During the past few decades alone, tremendous strides have been made in conducting research, preparing specialists, developing educational programs, increasing literature, and providing clinical services in gerontology and geriatrics. Because of the complexities and challenges of working with the aged, greater numbers of professionals are entering this area of specialization.

The nursing profession is experiencing an outstanding attitudinal shift in its view of caring for the aged. Once viewed as the bottom rung of the nursing ladder—a stepchild speciality—gerontological nursing has blossomed into one of the most popular and expanding fields of practice. The sophisticated blend of knowledge and skill required to deliver appropriate gerontological care supports the fact that gerontological nurses must have special cognitive and clinical capabilities.

An introduction to the nursing care of aging persons is offered in this book. Characteristics of the older population are presented to help the reader differentiate myths from realities. There is a review of aging theories, emphasizing their strengths and weaknesses. Characteristics of the normal aging process will be identified and transferred into implications for the aged individual's daily life and the nursing care he or she may require. The unique knowledge and skill utilized in applying the nursing process to the aged will be discussed.

In addition to information pertaining to normal aging and health promotion in old age, it is important for gerontological nurse to understand the special features of the aged's illnesses. A portion of this book reviews major problems that affect each body system, and outlines differences in symptomatology, diagnosis, management, and related nursing care.

Currently popular issues in aging and geriatric care have special chapters devoted to them. Included among these topics are: geriatric pharmacology, sexuality, the dying process, surgical care, sensory deficits, services for the aged, and mental health and illness.

This book is designed as an introduction to gerontology, geriatrics, and nursing care of the aged. It provides a basic framework upon which gerontological nursing practice can be developed. Rather than being all inclusive, this book is a stepping-stone to assist the reader into a deeper exploration of gerontology literature.

The reader should note that the words *old, aged,* and *geriatric* are used throughout the text to describe older persons. Although a negative connotation is often associated with these words, it is the author's belief that the attitudes and behaviors demonstrated to older persons are far more significant than the labels they are given.

C. E.

Acknowledgements

No author writes a book alone; the ideas, support, and efforts of persons too numerous to mention go into the birth of a book.

There are many persons to whom I'd like to express my gratitude. From Jim Kopelke and Sandy Orem I received the encouragement and support that only very special friends can provide as I experienced the many peaks and valleys in the process of writing this book. Praise must go to Gladys Spiller who performed the vital task of transferring hundreds of handwritten pages into typewritten form.

Last, but not least, I am deeply indebted to the many older persons who taught me the wisdom, strength, and beauty of old age.

1

NURSING THE AGED: THE BACKGROUND

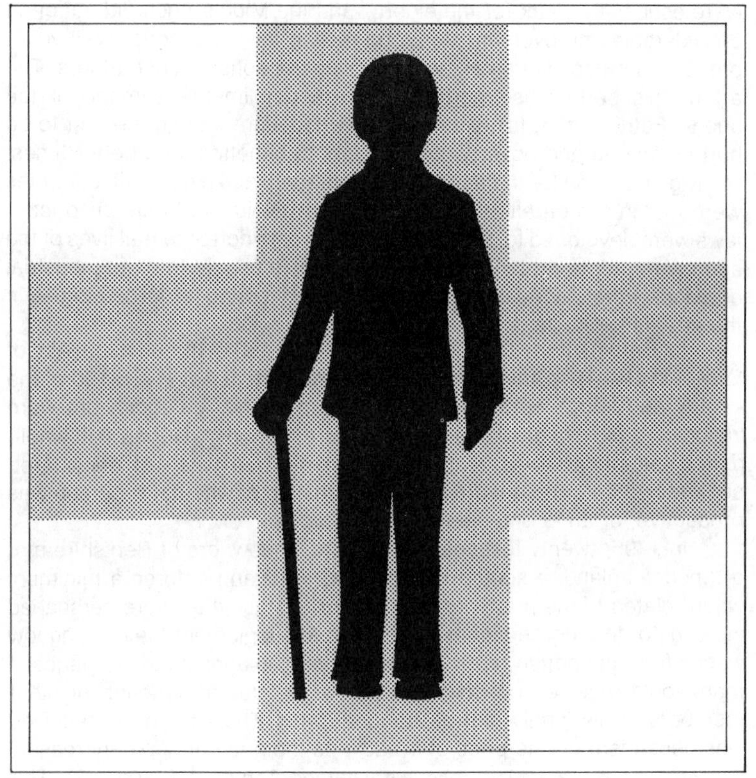

Older members of a society have always received some degree of attention, and many historical writings depict both the positive and negative aspects of growing old. Confucius' time expressed a direct correlation between one's age and the degree of respect to which one was entitled. Taoism viewed old age as the epitome of life, and the ancient Chinese believed that to attain old age was an accomplishment deserving the greatest honor. The early Egyptians, on the other hand, dreaded old age and experimented with a variety of potions and schemes to avoid it. Greek views were divided—the myths portrayed many struggles between old and young, quests for immortality and fountains of youth; Plato saw the aged as society's best leaders, while Aristotle felt they should be denied any role in government matters. The ancient Romans apparently had limited respect for their elders; in the nations which Rome conquered, the sick and old were customarily the first to be killed.

The Bible is laced with a theme of respect for the aged, although early Christian writings did little to elevate their status. The Dark Ages were especially bleak for the elderly, and the Middle Ages did not bring considerable improvement. A strong feeling for the superiority of youth prevailed in medieval times, with uprisings of sons against fathers. The art of this period also portrayed an uncomplimentary image of the aged—Father Time, for example. The aged were among the first to be hurt by famine and poverty, and the last to benefit during better times. Many gains made for the aged in the eighteenth and nineteenth centuries were lost in the cruelties of the industrial revolution. While child labor laws were developed to guard the frail lives of minors, the frail lives of the aged were left unprotected, and those people unable to meet industrial demands were placed at the mercy of their offspring, or forced to beg in the streets for sustenance.

In Britain, from the Poor Law of 1597-1601, through the Act of Elizabeth (1601), to the Old Poor Law Amendment Act (1795-1905), the elderly and infirm were not regarded as a special category, but were included in the general categorization of "the poor". During this whole period, pauperism was recognized, but old age was not considered separately; the criteria were largely a question of whether a person was productive, or an economic liability.

In 1795, twenty justices, clergy, and landowners of Berkshire met at Speenhamland, a suburb of Newbury, to fix and enforce a minimum wage related to the price of bread. Unfortunately, they were persuaded instead not to enforce higher wages, but to supplement the existing low wages from the parish rates. This meant that, in addition to his wages, a man would receive a certain sum per week, plus an amount for other members of his family, out of the local rates. The amount he received was dependent on the price of bread—as the price of a loaf increased, the amount he received rose with it (see Tables 1.1 and 1.2). This

TABLE 1:1

		Income should be for a man.	For a single woman.	For a man and his wife.	With one child.	With two children.	With three children.	With four children.	With five children.	With six children.	With seven children.
When the gallon loaf is	s. d.	s. d.	s. d.	s. d.	s. d.	s. d.	s. d.	s. d.	s. d.	s. d.	s. d.
" "	1 0	3 0	2 0	4 6	6 0	7 6	9 0	10 6	12 0	13 6	15 0
" "	1 1	3 3	2 1	4 10	6 5	8 0	9 7	11 2	12 9	14 4	15 11
" "	1 2	3 6	2 2	5 2	6 10	8 6	10 2	11 10	13 6	15 2	16 10
" "	1 3	3 9	2 3	5 6	7 3	9 0	10 9	12 6	14 3	16 0	17 9
" "	1 4	4 0	2 4	5 10	7 8	9 6	11 4	13 2	15 0	16 10	18 8
" "	1 5	4 0	2 5	5 11	7 10	9 9	11 8	13 7	15 6	17 5	19 4
" "	1 6	4 3	2 6	6 3	8 3	10 3	12 3	14 3	16 3	18 3	20 3
" "	1 7	4 3	2 7	6 4	8 5	10 6	12 7	14 8	16 9	18 10	20 11
" "	1 8	4 6	2 8	6 8	8 10	11 0	13 2	15 4	17 6	19 8	21 10
" "	1 9	4 6	2 9	6 9	9 0	11 3	13 6	15 9	18 0	20 3	22 6
" "	1 10	4 9	2 10	7 1	9 5	11 9	14 1	16 5	18 9	21 1	23 5
" "	1 11	4 9	2 11	7 2	9 7	12 0	14 5	16 10	19 3	21 8	24 1
" "	2 0	5 0	3 0	7 6	10 0	12 6	15 0	17 6	20 0	22 6	25 0

This table was drawn up by the Speenhamland magistrates in 1795, to show what the weekly income of the "industrious poor" should be, linked to the price of the gallon loaf.

From: ***The Poor Law Report of 1834*** by S.G. and E.O. Checkland (eds.), Penguin Books, 1974, p. 209.

scheme—the Speenhamland Act—was adopted by other counties until eventually it was established in about half of rural England. As an automatic subsidy of wages, it removed the incentive for the worker to ask for, or for the employer to provide, a living wage. It soon proved very expensive, as more and more people received relief.

Eventually, the local authorities began to stop offering out-relief. The workhouse became the only place to offer food and shelter. In an effort to cut the cost of poor relief, and in order to deter too many people from seeking it, the discomfort and unpleasantness of life in the workhouse was intensified. In the parish councils' haste to contain the demands of adult working men, the plight of old people, children, and invalids (all classified as "impotents") was completely overlooked. People were faced with a choice between starvation wages or the privations of the workhouse—a comparable contemporary dilemma is whether to opt for social security or a low-paid job.

In 1832 a Royal Commission was appointed to inquire into the practical operation of the laws for the relief of the poor in England and Wales. This led to the Poor Law Amendment Act, passed in 1834. This act restricted out-relief to the old and other "impotent" poor; the workhouse was to be the sole source of relief for the able-bodied. In practice, applications for out-relief were often refused by the workhouse

TABLE 1:2

Price of FLOUR per gallon.	Amount weekly per head	One.	Two.	Three.	Four.	Five.	Six.
s. d.	s. d.	s. d.	s. d.	s. d.	s. d.	s. d.	£ s. d.
1 5	0 0¾	0 3	0 6	0 9	1 0	1 3	0 1 6
1 6	0 1½	0 6	1 0	1 6	2 0	2 6	0 3 0
1 7	0 2¼	0 9	1 6	2 3	3 0	3 9	0 4 6
1 8	0 3	1 0	2 0	3 0	4 0	5 0	0 6 0
1 9	0 3¾	1 3	2 6	3 9	5 0	6 3	0 7 6
1 10	0 4½	1 6	3 0	4 6	6 0	7 6	0 9 0
1 11	0 5¼	1 9	3 6	5 3	7 0	8 9	0 10 6
2 0	0 6	2 0	4 0	6 0	8 0	10 0	0 12 0
2 1	0 6¾	2 3	4 6	6 9	9 0	11 3	0 13 6
2 2	0 7½	2 6	5 0	7 6	10 0	12 6	0 15 0
2 3	0 8¼	2 9	5 6	8 3	11 0	13 9	0 16 6
2 4	0 9	3 0	6 0	9 0	12 0	15 0	0 18 0
2 5	0 9¾	3 3	6 6	9 9	13 0	16 3	0 19 6
2 6	0 10½	3 6	7 0	10 6	14 0	17 6	1 1 0

		Seven.	Eight.	Nine.	Ten.	Eleven.	Twelve.
s. d.	s. d.	£ s. d.	£ s. d.	£ s. d.	£ s. d.	£ s. d.	£ s. d.
1 5	0 0¾	0 1 9	0 2 0	0 2 3	0 2 6	0 2 9	0 3 0
1 6	0 1½	0 3 6	0 4 0	0 4 6	0 5 0	0 5 6	0 6 0
1 7	0 2¼	0 5 3	0 6 0	0 6 9	0 7 6	0 8 3	0 9 0
1 8	0 3	0 7 0	0 8 0	0 9 0	0 10 0	0 11 0	0 12 0
1 9	0 3¾	0 8 9	0 10 0	0 11 3	0 12 6	0 13 9	0 15 0
1 10	0 4½	0 10 6	0 12 0	0 13 6	0 15 0	0 16 6	0 18 0
1 11	0 5¼	0 12 3	0 14 0	0 16 9	0 17 6	0 19 3	1 1 0
2 0	0 6	0 14 0	0 16 0	0 18 0	1 0 0	1 2 0	1 4 0
2 1	0 6¾	0 15 9	0 18 0	1 0 3	1 2 6	1 4 9	1 7 0
2 2	0 7½	0 17 6	1 0 0	1 2 6	1 5 0	1 7 6	1 10 0
2 3	0 8¼	0 19 3	1 2 0	1 4 9	1 7 6	1 10 3	1 13 0
2 4	0 9	1 1 0	1 4 0	1 7 0	1 10 0	1 13 0	1 16 0
2 5	0 9¾	1 2 9	1 6 0	1 9 3	1 12 6	1 15 9	1 19 0
2 6	0 10½	1 4 6	1 8 0	1 11 6	1 15 0	1 18 6	2 2 0

This table was drawn up in 1804-1805, a time of sharply rising food prices, in order to show the increasing amount required to subsidize the price of flour when it exceeded 1s 4d per gallon, so that the poor might always have it at that price.

From: ***The Poor Law Report of 1834*** by S.G. and E.O. Checkland (eds.), Penguin Books, 1974, p. 211.

boards of guardians, and the only alternative was the workhouse. At the same time, conditions in the workhouses were made prisonlike, with hard labor, uniforms and discipline, in order to deter people from seeking relief at all. A further consequence of the act was that the

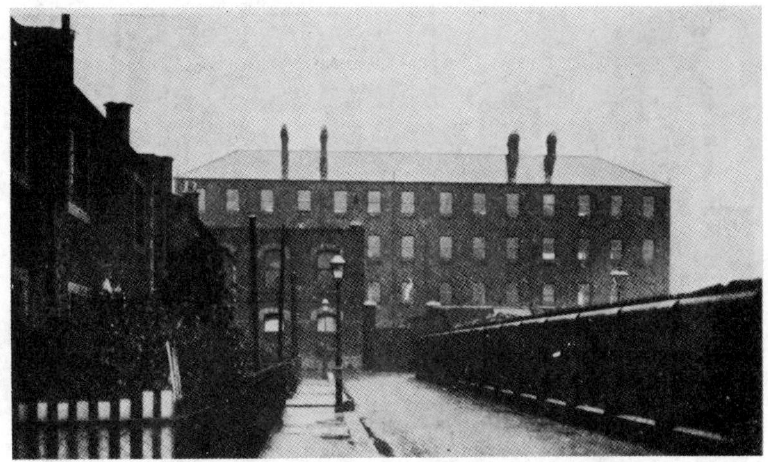

The Poplar workhouse

From the *People of the Abyss,* by J. London   Journeyman Press 1978

workhouse system became a national organization, out of the control of the local councils.

In 1838, the popular writer William Hewitt wrote of "the tearing asunder of husband from wife, parent from children, brother from sister, as . . . in the lands of slavery" under the workhouse system. Old people sent to workhouses were separated from their families; inside the workhouse, men and women were segregated. The separation of elderly couples no longer able to care for themselves persisted until recently, when "double-room" accommodation was provided for them in old people's homes. The reformed Poor Law was extremely harsh, but it continued, with few major changes, until a further Royal Commission was appointed in 1905.

The advent of the Royal Commission of 1905 was an important step. Brought about by the radical influence inside the government of the day, and led by Lloyd George, this inquiry was to lay the foundations of the present welfare state.

One of the most important findings of the commission, which completed its report in 1909, was that poverty had many causes, not the least of which were old age and sickness. Although, in these more enlightened times, such conclusions are quite obvious, this was nevertheless the first time that the needs of the aged had been considered separately from the needs of the poor. Even before the publication of the commission's report, a budget was presented in 1908, introducing, for the first time in our history, an old age pension scheme. The pension was for 5/- (25p) per week maximum, or 7/6 (37½p) per

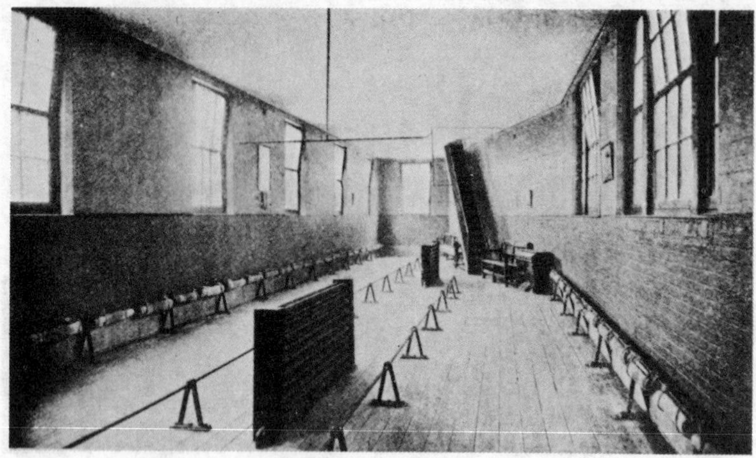

Casual ward, Whitechapel workhouse

From the *People of the Abyss,* by J. London Journeyman Press 1978

week for a married couple on reaching the age of 70. This was the very modest beginning of state help, the costs of which were borne entirely by the government out of taxation, as the pensions were noncontributory. In 1911, a National Insurance Act was passed. This was a contributory scheme, the costs of which were borne by the employee, the employer, and the state, to build up a fund for the support of workers during ill-health, and for free medical attention. This scheme, while a considerable step forward in welfare history, made no allowances for children or for aged dependents. A further reform act, the fifth since 1832, was passed in 1929. This was the Local Government Act, part of which transferred the work of the Board of Guardians (created in 1834 to look after the poor and manage the workhouses) to county and borough councils.

The next important step in the welfare of the aged came with the Beveridge Report of 1942. Sir William Beveridge, a civil servant with considerable experience in social services, recommended a free National Health Service and a Ministry of Social Security to supervise the benefits and allowances. No progress was made on this scheme until the end of World War II, when the National Insurance Act was passed in 1946. The new act followed closely the recommendations of the Beveridge Report: unifying the administration of retirement pensions with other benefits, such as sickness, maternity and unemployment.

The National Health Service, as we know it, came into operation in 1948. In the same year the National Assistance Act came into force, transferring the responsibility for the distribution of money to needy persons from the local authorities to the central government. The central government supervised the distribution of benefits through the National

TABLE 1:3

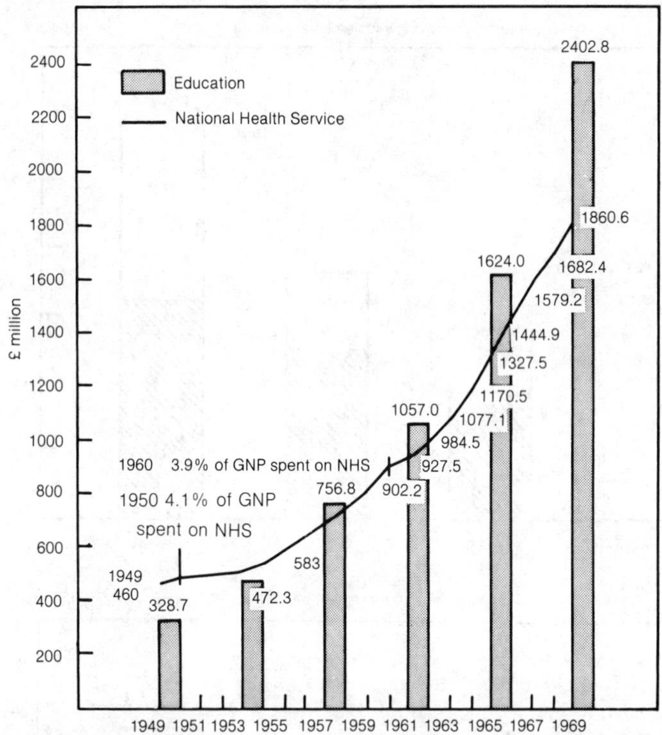

Rising costs of the welfare state – consolidated current and capital expenditure by public sector (central and local).

From: ***Britain 1945-1970***, by L.A. Monk, G. Bell & Sons, 1976, p.57.

Assistance Boards set up in the localities. The local authorities were required by the act to provide accommodation for the aged, infirm, and destitute; this finally ended the Old Poor Law system, and with it the indignity of charity and patronage for circumstances over which the aged had no control.

When all these new and necessary reforms were implemented, they added to the costs of the National Health Service, which were already rising rapidly. (See Table 1.3.)

The 1946 Act raised retirement pensions from 10/- (50p) a week to 26/- (£1.30) a week for a single person, and to 42/- (£2.10) a week for a married couple. Unfortunately, due to the constantly rising cost of living, these sums were totally inadequate for large numbers of old people. Therefore, the National Assistance Scheme of 1948, intended to apply to only a small section of the population, became an indispensable source

TABLE 1.4

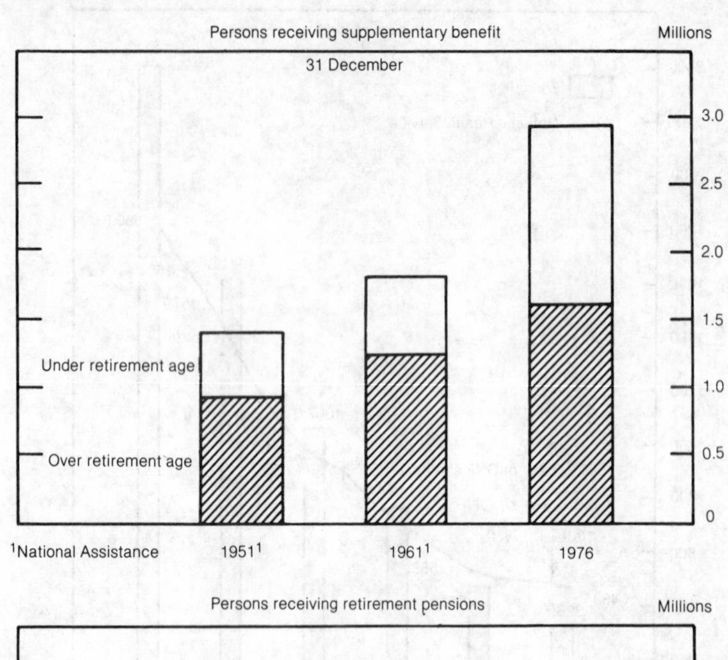

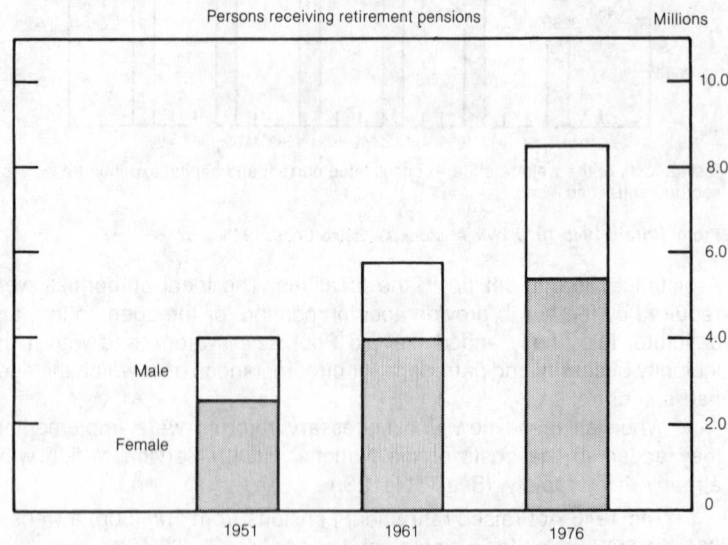

Number of people receiving supplementary benefit and retirement pensions in Great Britain, 1951-1976

From *Facts in Focus*, Crown Copyright © 1972, 1974, 1975, 1978, ***Penguin Reference Books*** in Association with HMSO, p.49.

of income for the majority by 1950. This trend has continued, as can be seen in Table 1.4. When the latest figures are available, they will undoubtedly show a continuing similar pattern.

In 1950, retirement pensions, payable at the age of 60 for a woman and 65 for a man, were increased according to the upward trend in the cost of living, and have subsequently been increased regularly without ever catching up and obviating the need for National Assistance. Nevertheless, the State Retirement Pension has done much to eliminate the indignity of pauperism.

THE AGED SICK IN HOSPITALS

When the 1948 Health Service Act came into operation, there were no purpose-built hospitals for the elderly. At the time, many venerable buildings, previously Poor Law Institutions (workhouses), were pressed into service as geriatric hospitals in their original state. These dismal, dreary, and ill-equipped hospitals, still carrying the stigma "workhouse", were staffed by a few trained nurses and a very high proportion of unqualified staff. The objectives were, at best, to keep the patient clean and fed and free from bedsores. This careful but unimaginative and monotonous treatment was administered until the end. Few of the patients were encouraged, or even allowed, out of bed; and the ones who were would be unlikely to dress. They were all treated as terminally sick, even though many were to remain in these conditions for several years. Often rejected by their families, sometimes outliving their contemporaries, without hope of improvement (or even a little privacy), many patients, not surprisingly, became apathetic and characterless, and were then considered to be mentally ill. Dr. Russell Barton's book *Institutional Neurosis*, published in 1959, investigated automaton behavior seen in the mental and chronic sick (geriatric) hospitals, and came to the conclusion that the symptoms were not necessarily the result of illness, but were caused by the institutional regime foisted on the patients. This reinforced the view of some dedicated geriatricians and nurses who had realized that hope was being abandoned prematurely. New programs of treatment were adopted, and steps were taken to change the demoralized attitude of the staff. The transition for which they worked was by no means easy to accomplish; but with the increasing need for hospital accommodation for the aged sick, the old institutions were upgraded, refitted, and refurbished to meet the standards of modern hospitals. Brighter surroundings and the implementation of rehabilitation programs resulted in a change of attitude to what had been considered a hopeless task. Physical nursing replaced unnecessary sedatives; and the team of nurse, physiotherapist, and occupational therapist encouraged reasonable activity and provided continuing care. From this team effort, a highly specialized branch of nursing has evolved. Multi-disciplinary meetings enable staff to concentrate their professional expertise for the maximum benefit to the patient. This kind of positive, optimistic approach to geriatric care is to be commended. It is a far cry from the old days when the old were automatically committed to the workhouse or lunatic asylum with no hope of discharge.

TABLE 1:5
THE INCREASE IN THE POPULATION OVER 65 FROM 1851-1971, FOR MEN AND WOMEN.

Women over 65 years (thousands)

Age	1851	1861	1871	1881	1891	1901
65-69 years	205.1	233.9	274.2	312.5	357.8	397.1
70-74 years	159.5	178.7	205.7	224.1	268.5	288.5
75-79 years	94.7	104.2	116.9	131.5	152.4	173.9
80-84 years	50.9	54.7	60.9	65.9	73.7	189.3
85 years-over	19.5	25.0	27.9	28.1	33.0	36.1
Age	**1911**	**1921**	**1931**	**1951**	**1961**	**1971**
65-69 years	499.4	603.2	773.4	1130.8	1281.0	1477.0
70-74 years	364.9	425.0	554.5	922.2	1035.8	1197.5
75-79 years	208.6	264.4	331.4	706.8	745.5	851.7
80-84 years	100.8	128.8	158.9	301.1	436.8	535.2
85 years-over	47.6	58.3	73.5	150.4	231.8	342.1

Men over 65 years (thousands)

Age	1851	1861	1871	1881	1891	1901
65-69 years	173.7	200.1	234.6	262.8	293.4	319.3
70-74 years	132.3	146.2	172.6	181.2	210.0	221.8
75-79 years	74.9	82.5	94.0	103.4	115.9	127.8
80-84 years	39.5	40.2	44.7	48.2	50.9	594
85 years-over	15.8	15.5	17.1	17.2	19.3	20.8
Age	**1911**	**1921**	**1931**	**1951**	**1961**	**1971**
65-69 years	412.0	506.3	531.1	863.9	902.4	1170.1
70-74 years	269.0	315.3	422.4	656.9	659.0	759.8
75-79 years	143.9	178.0	228.0	416.1	429.3	449.1
80-84 years	63.8	75.7	93.4	182.6	226.4	237.5
85 years-over	25.8	28.1	34.1	67.2	99.3	120.2

Compiled from: *Census 1971* Age, Marital Condition, and General Tables, Crown Copyright.

The Joint Board of Clinical Nursing Studies has been active since 1970 in standardizing post-basic courses for specialties in nursing and midwifery. The 20-week course for geriatric nursing provides a comprehensive training for SRNs and SENs, in caring for the aged within the hospital and the community. From July 1979, to comply with the EEC directives, student nurses in training for the general register must have planned experience in geriatric, psychiatric, maternity, and community nursing. The gerontological nurse must be aware that aging is a highly individual process in each person. The nurse should be acquainted with the psycho-social factors associated with aging, and must be willing to work with professionals in other disciplines.

An astonishing growth of the population over 60 is shown in Table 1.5. There are many factors, but in general, the improved care of the elderly has played a large part in the survival of many older people. The chart shows that this age group has quadrupled in the past 75 years. If this trend continues, as it seems likely to, a further sociological problem will have to be faced in the caring professions. (See Table 1.6.)·

Empathy, sensitivity, and sincerity are very important qualities in caring for the elderly. It is necessary for nurses to understand and accept their own aging process, and to recognize their own mortality. Today, a growing number of nurses are accepting the challenge of geriatric nursing. Few other specialties provide the opportunity for the nurse to blend the knowledge and skills of so many disciplines. The broad scope allows nurses to contribute to the care of the aged in the community, in acute and chronic conditions, through direct clinical practice and research. Geriatric nursing is a career that is unique, challenging, and rewarding to its practitioners. The elderly, who have been rejected by society, sometimes tend to reject themselves. They wonder why they should become active. Physical recovery is not the complete answer for people without caring families. Loneliness is probably a more serious problem than any physical defect. Age Concern, a registered charity, exists for the welfare of the elderly, and brings together major national organizations. Working with other groups and volunteers they provide visitors for the lonely, lunch clubs, and transport schemes. They are able to advise the government on legislation affecting the elderly and to campaign on their behalf. Small local groups, such as the over-sixties' club, exist in many areas, and provide a meeting place for many social occasions.

It must be clearly understood that old people only differ from the rest of the population in that they have lived longer. They have the same emotional needs and desires as any other age group; the feeling of uselessness is destructive to them. The goal of the care of the aged should be the continuation, as near as physically possible, of their normal lifestyle. There can be no doubt that the elderly can be of value to

TABLE 1:6

THE AGING WORLD

Falling fertility and rising life expectancy means that the average age of the world's population is going up. This aging process is one of the most important social and economic forces at work in the world. 1979 'State of World Population' from the UN Fund for Population Activities.

WORLD AGE BOOM

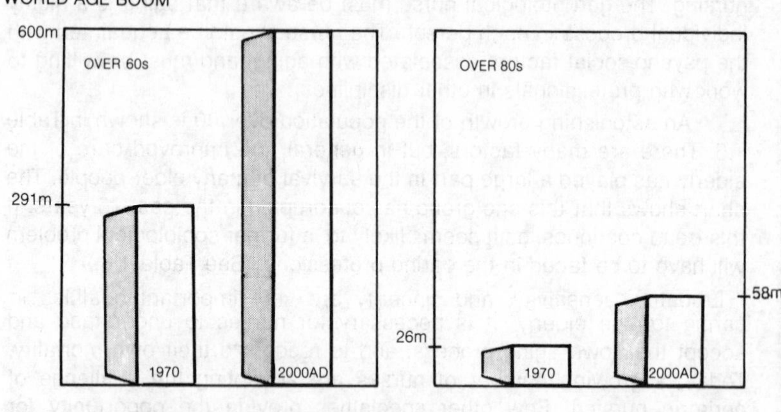

THE THREE AGES OF MAN % population increase 1970-80

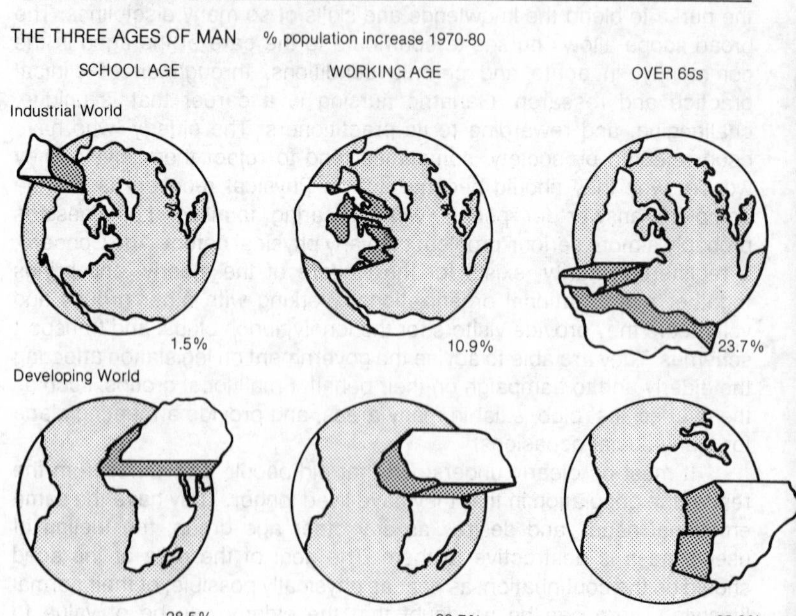

THE GRAYING OF AMERICA

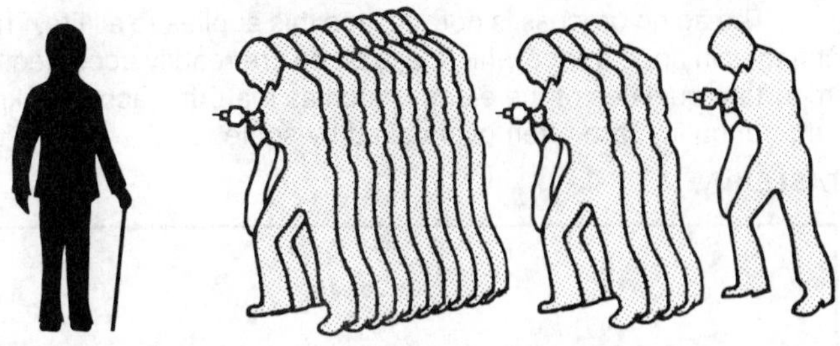

AND OF EUROPE . . .

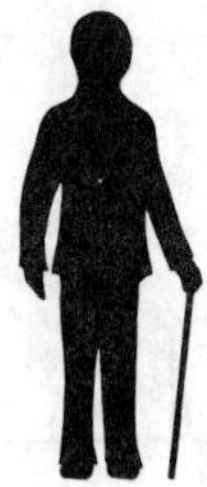

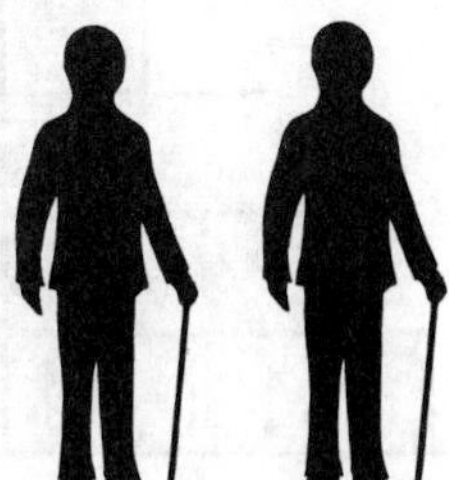

Proportion of pensioners will almost double in 50 years

PROBLEMS FOR WORKERS

Pension contributions up 300%

More older workers means career promotion twice as difficult

AND OF THE THIRD WORLD . . .

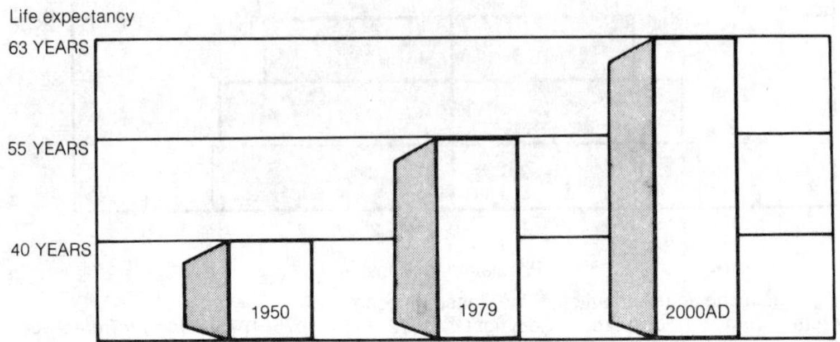

society, for they carry with them a rich culture which they can readily pass on in talking to an interested listener. Traditions will be lost unless we are prepared to listen to the people who hold this valuable link with our heritage, and ensure their dignified position in society.

The aging process is normal, and this applies to all life. The obvious changes in appearance which take place are readily accepted. The more important qualities of the elderly, such as maturity, acquired knowledge, and tranquility, are often overlooked by society.

TABLE 1:7

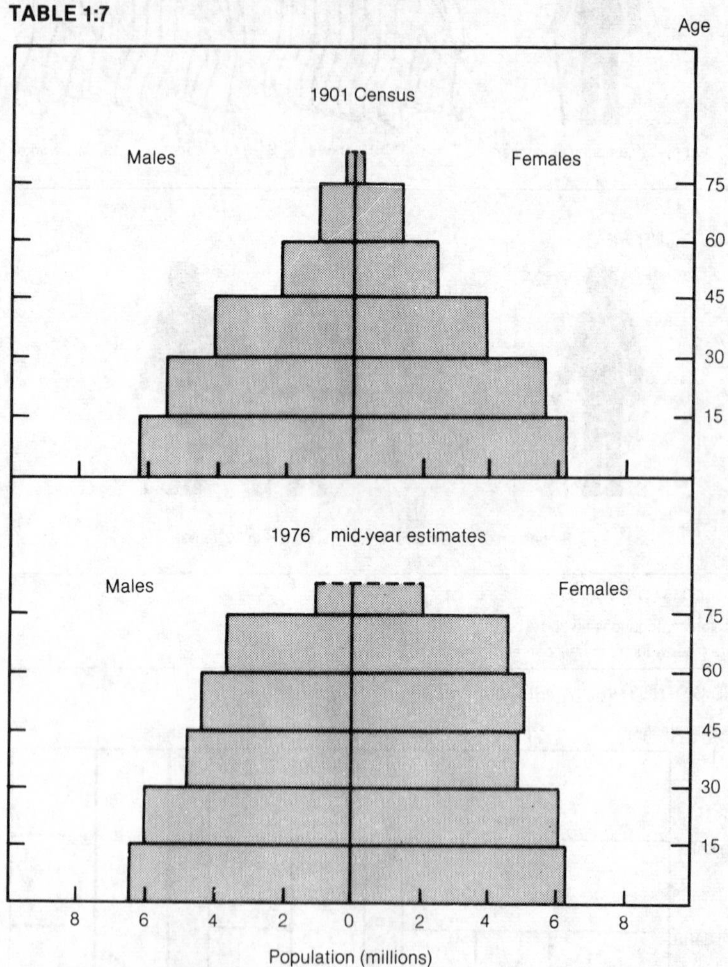

Population and age distribution of the United Kingdom.
From: *Facts in Focus* Crown Copyright © 1972, 1974, 1975, 1978, ***Penguin Reference Books*** in Association with HMSO, p.18.

There are many fit and active older people who remain vital and creative in their later years. Dame Edith Evans appeared in a film in which she acted and sang at the age of 87; George Bernard Shaw was writing plays well into his 80s; Albert Schweitzer lectured until his death at 90. At the age of 89, Arthur Rubenstein gave a recital at New York's Carnegie Hall – unable to see a note of music and relying entirely on his memory. Many people remain active until very late in life, while others have their activities curtailed by compulsory retirement which they are neither ready for nor want. In rural communities it is not uncomon to find people well past retirement age working farms and smallholdings. These people are self-employed, and the restriction of compulsory retirement does not apply. It is society which imposes the arbitrary definition of "pensionable age".

REFERENCES

Barton, R. *Institutional Neurosis* John Wright, 1959.
Brady, R.A. *Crisis in Britain*. Cambridge University Press, 1950.
Checkland, S.G. and E.O. (eds.) *The Poor Law Report on 1834.*Penguin Books, 1974.
Gladden, E.N. *British Public Service Administration.* Staples Press 1961.
Jackson, W.E. *Local Government in England and Wales.* Penguin Books, 1977.
London, J. *The People of the Abyss*. Journeyman Press, 1978,
Marshall, J.D. *The Old Poor Law 1795-1834.* Macmillan, 1968.
Monk, L.A. *Britain 1945-1970*, G. Bell & Sons, 1976.
Trevelyan, G.M. *English Social History*. Penguin Books, 1970.
Brian Watkin. *The National Health Service: The first phase 1948-1974 and after.* Allen & Unwin, 1978.
H.M.S.O. *Age, marital conditions and general tables.* Census 1971. Great Britain.
H.M.S.O. *Persons of Pensionable Age.* Census 1971. Great Britain.

2

THEORIES OF AGING

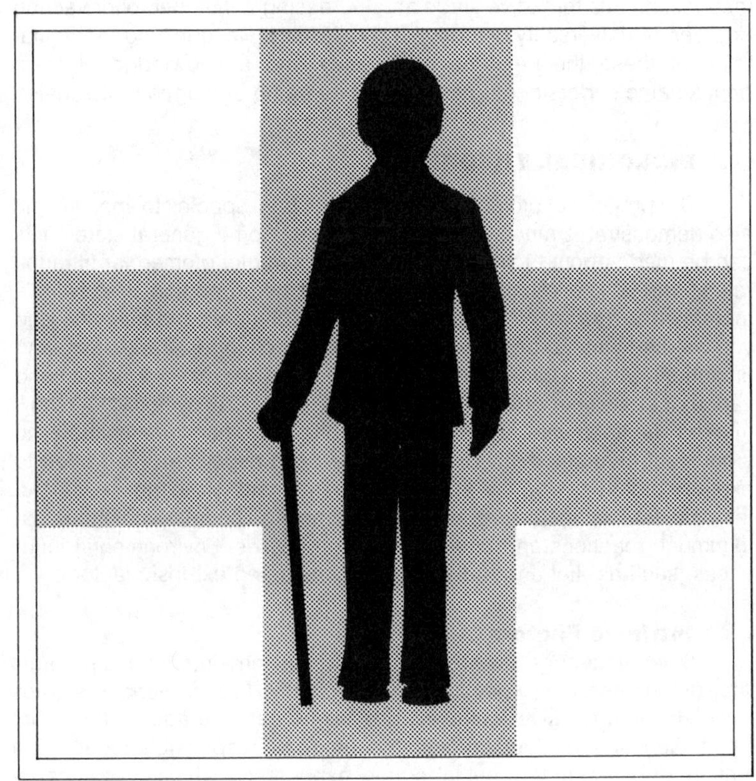

For centuries humanity has explored the mystery of aging, trying to discover a way to lengthen the lifespan and conducting numerous searches for a fountain of youth, the most famous being that of Ponce de Leon. Ancient Egyptian and Chinese relics show evidence of concoctions designed to prolong life or achieve immortality, and various other cultural practices throughout history include specific dietary regimens and the ingestion of herbal preparations. Ancient chemical life expanders prepared from the testicles of tigers may seem ludicrous until compared with modern day injections of embryonic tissue and novocaine, for example. Yoghurt, vitamins, cosmetic creams, and youth spas are some of the many items currently used to maintain youth and prolong the onset of old age.

There is no single factor which causes or prevents aging; the complexities of aging cannot be explained by one theory. Explorations into biological, psychological, and social aging continue, and although some activities focus on a "cure" for aging, most research efforts are aimed toward a better scientific understanding of this process. Aging theories, all in a formative stage and increasing in number, offer varying degrees of universality, validity, and reliability. Recognizing the limitations of these theories, the nurse may find a knowledge of them beneficial to understanding and caring for aging and aged individuals.

BIOLOGICAL THEORIES

The process of biological aging differs from species to species and also demonstrates much diversity in humans. Some general statements can be made about biological aging—for example, glomerular filtration rate at age 90 is one-half that at age 20, and the proportion of body fat is increased with age. However, no two individuals age identically, and you will find varying degrees of physiological changes, capacities, and limitations within a given age group. In addition, the rate of aging among various cells within one individual differs; one body system may show marked declines with advanced age while the others demonstrate no significant changes. Many theories have been espoused in an effort to explain biological aging according to intrinsic or extrinsic factors. Intrinsic factors include genetic programming, cellular mutation, autoimmune reactions and other inherent processes. Environmental influences, such as diet and radiation, are considered extrinsic factors.

Intrinsic Factors

Several theories assume that individuals inherit a genetic program that determines their specific life expectancy. In fact, various studies have shown a positive relationship between parental age and filial life span. Genetic mutations are also thought to be responsible for aging, a pattern depicted below; but laboratory experiments which have accelerated mutation rates have not produced proportionate increases in the rate of aging, thus reducing support of this theory. Some theorists believe that a growth substance fails to be produced causing the cessation of cell growth and reproduction, whereas others hypothesize that an aging factor responsible for development and cellular maturity throughout life is excessively produced. Cross-linkage of DNA strands may impair the cell's ability to function and divide, and the continued occurrence of this process may lead to the manifestations of aging. Although minimal research has been done to support this theory, aging may be a result of a decreased ability of RNA to synthesize and translate messages.

The accumulation of lipofuscin "age pigments" has been considered a biochemical basis for aging. Lipofuscin, a lipoprotein byproduct of metabolism, can be seen under a fluorescent microscope. This insoluble, nonfunctional material is known to accumulate with age as a result of some unplanned, rare metabolic accident. The liver, heart, ovaries, and neurons are the sites in which lipofuscin tends to accumulate. Although the function and significance of this age pigment is not clear at this point, there is a positive relationship between the age of the individual and the number of lipofuscins (Strehler, 1962). Investigators have discovered the presence of lipofuscin in other species at amounts proportionate to the life span of the species, that is, an animal with one-tenth the life span of humans accumulates lipofuscin at a rate approximately ten times greater (Few and Getly, 1967). The existence of well-documented laboratory findings gives popularity to this theory.

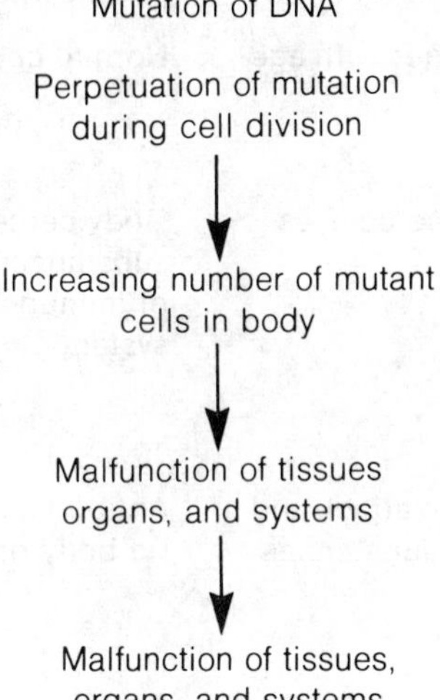

Another fascinating group of theories postulates autoimmune reactions as being responsible for aging. Simply stated, the host attacks its own kind, either because of the presence of foreign cells or substances to which there has been no exposure, or because of a breakdown in the body's immunochemical memory, which makes it sensitive to its own constituents. This is shown diagramatically below. Diseases associated with normal aging and caused by autoimmune reactions, such as rheumatoid arthritis, could be explained by this theory.

One theory used to explain biological aging links collagen to the aging process. There is thought to be an increase in the amount of collagen and a loss of ground substance with age. Collagen may become cross-linked, rigid, and less permeable. The great density of the connective tissue may reduce the rate at which nutrients are deposited and wastes removed, leading to a deterioration of collagen and consequent slowing down of bodily processes. Excess collagen has been found in old tissue, but investigators are not able to determine if this is a causative factor or a result of the aging process.

Another theory attributes aging to the wear and tear of the cells of the body as they perform their highly specific functions over time. Insults and stresses to the body take their toll, and the result is less efficient functioning of the cells. Proponents of this theory point to the shortened life span caused by a life of overexertion and stress. Since each individual reacts differently to life's stresses, it is difficult for this theory to be universally valid.

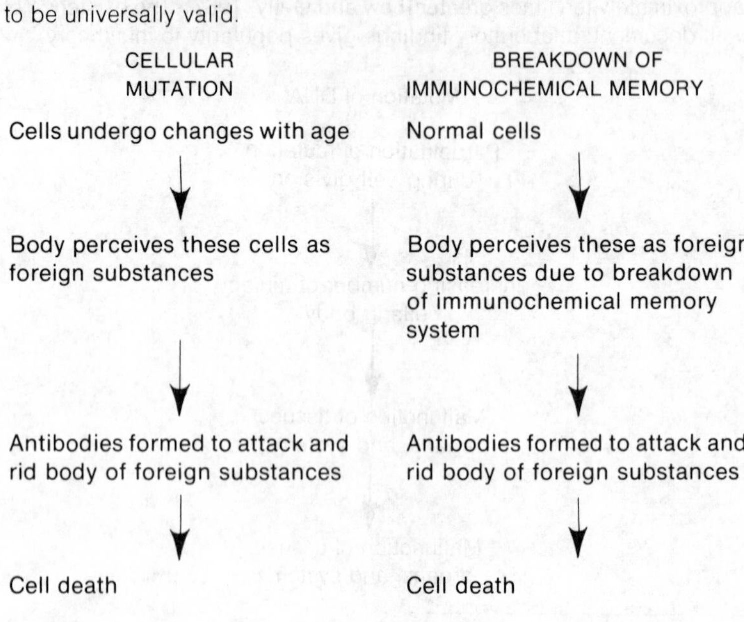

Extrinsic Factors

Disease-producing organisms are often associated with biological aging. Bacteria, fungi, viruses, and other organisms are thought to be responsible for certain physiological changes during the aging process. Although no conclusive evidence presently exists to link these pathogens with the aging process, interest in this theory has been stimulated by the fact that humans and animals have been shown to live longer with the control or elimination of certain pathogens via immunization and the use of antimicrobial drugs.

The relationship of radiation and age changes has been, and continues to be, explored. Research in rats, mice, and dogs has shown a decreased life span resulting from exposures to nonlethal doses of radiation (Strehler, 1962). Repeated exposure to ultraviolet light is known to cause solar elastosis, "old age" type of skin wrinkling resulting from the replacement of collagen by elastin, and also to cause skin cancer in humans. There is some thought that radiation may induce cellular mutations which promote aging.

Nutrition is considered to have a significant influence on the aging process. Experiments with underfed fish have shown their growth rate to be retarded and their life span to be unusually longer (Hershey, 1974). Underfed rats have also proven to live longer than their overfed cohorts, who aged at a faster rate. Obesity in people is said to shorten life, a view supported by insurance statistics. Quality as well as quantity of diet is thought to influence aging. Deficiencies of vitamins and other nutrients and excesses of nutrients such as cholesterol may cause malfunction. Although the full relationship of diet and aging is not understood, there is enough confidence in what is known to suggest that certain dietary habits may minimize or eliminate some ill effects of the aging process.

Several environmental factors known to threaten health are often associated with the aging process. Ingested mercury, lead, arsenic, radioactive isotopes, certain pesticides, and other substances are known to produce pathological changes in the human organism. Smoking and breathing tobacco smoke and other air pollutants have known adverse effects. Emotional stress, crowded living conditions, excessive alcohol intake, and "coping" ability are among the factors thought to influence the aging process.

No single biological theory completely explains the multifarious phenomenon of aging. Some populations are known to have a high proportion of aged individuals, such as in the Caucasus in southern Russia, where there are 12,000 people over age 90 and almost 5,000 who are centenarians (Leaf, 1975). But even extensive investigations have not been able to attribute the longevity in such people to any one factor. Nursing practice can utilize these theories, however, by identifying the elements known to influence aging and then discouraging the exposure to adverse factors and encouraging those which promote health and proper function.

PSYCHOSOCIAL THEORIES

Psychological and social changes during the aging process are closely united, and they have a significant impact on each other. It is difficult to explain mental processes, behavior, and feelings without the perspective of social roles, positions, and norms. A theory of aging that is purely social or psychological would be most unusual, and it is more appropriate to approach these aging factors as *psychosocial* theories. Probably the most controversial and widely discussed is the *disengagement theory*, developed by Elaine Cumming and William Henry (Cumming and Henry, 1961; Cumming, 1964). This theory views aging as a process whereby society and the individual gradually withdraw, or disengage, from each other, to the mutual satisfaction and benefit of both. The benefit to individuals is that they can reflect and be centered on themselves, having been freed from societal roles. The value of disengagement for society is that some orderly means is established for the transfer of power from the old to the young, making it possible for society to continue functioning after its individual members have died.

The theory does not indicate whether it is society or the individual who is responsible for initating the disengagement process, but one may readily detect several difficulties with the premise. Many older persons are highly satisfied to remain engaged and do not want their primary satisfaction to be derived from reflection on younger years. Senators, supreme court judges, and college professors are among those who commonly derive satisfaction and provide a valuable service for society by not disengaging. Since the health of the individual, cultural practices, societal norms, and other factors influence the degree to which a person will participate in society during the later years, some critics of this theory claim that disengagement would not be necessary if society improved the health care and financial means of the aged and increased the acceptance, opportunities, and respect afforded them.

A careful examination of the population studied in the development of the disengagement theory indicates certain of its limitations. The disengagement pattern which Cumming and Henry described was based on a study of 172 middle-class persons between the ages of 48 and 68. This group was wealthier, better educated, and of higher occupational and residential prestige than the general aged population. No blacks or chronically ill persons were involved in the study. Caution is advisable in generalizing for the entire aged population findings based on less than 200 persons who are not representative of the average aged person. While nurses should appreciate that some older individuals may wish to disengage from the mainstream of society, this is not necessarily a process to be expected from all aged persons.

At the opposite pole from the disengagement theory, the *activity theory* (Havighurst, 1963) proclaims that an older person should continue a middle-aged life-style, denying the existence of old age as long as possible, and that society should apply the same norms to old age as it does to middle age and not advocate diminishing activity, interest, and involvement as its members grow old. This theory suggests ways of maintaining activity in the presence of multiple losses associated with the aging process—including substituting intellectual activities for physical activities when physical capacity is reduced, replacing the work role with other roles when retirement occurs, and establishing new friendships when old ones are lost. Declining health, loss of roles, reduced income, a shrinking circle of friends, and other obstacles to maintaining an active life are to be resisted and overcome instead of being accepted.

This theory is not without merit. Activity is generally assumed to be more desirable than inactivity as it facilitates physical, mental, and social well-being. Like a self-fulfilling prophecy, the expectation of a continued active state during old age may be realized. Because of society's currently negative view of inactivity and "acting old," it is probably best to encourage an active live-style among the aged, consistent with society's values. Also supportive of the activity theory is the reluctance of many older persons to accept themselves as old, although one of its problems is the assumption that most older people desire and are able to maintain a middle-aged life-style. Some want their world to shrink to accommodate their decreasing capacities or their preference for less active roles. Many lack the physical, emotional, social, or economic resources to continue active roles in society. Aged people who are expected to maintain an active middle-aged life-style on a retirement income of less than half that of middle-aged people may wonder if society isn't giving them conflicting messages. The results and consequences of multiple expectations to remain active that cannot be fulfilled by the aging individual still need to be researched.

The *developmental theory* of aging, also referred to as the *continuity theory*, (Neugarten, 1964) relates the factors of personality and predisposition toward certain actions in old age to similar factors during other phases of the life cycle. Personality and basic patterns of behavior are said to be unchanged as the individual ages. The activist at age 20 will most likely be an activist at age 70. On the other hand, the young recluse will probably not be active in the mainstream of society when he or she ages. Concepts and patterns developed over a lifetime will determine whether an individual remains engaged and active or becomes disengaged and inactive. The recognition that the unique features of each individual allow for multiple adaptations to aging and that the potential exists for a variety of reactions gives this theory reality and support. Aging is a complex process, and the developmental theory considers these complexities to a greater extent than most other theories. While the implications and impact of this promising theory are uncertain, since it is in an early stage of research, it should be closely followed.

Several other theories, although less developed, need mentioning. One theory (Rose, 1965) views the aged as a subculture whose members are typically forced to interact primarily with each other, due to their negative treatment by society. One problem with this theory is that it is not valid for all social classes of aged people. A similar theory (Streib, 1965) views the aged as a minority group which, like the handicapped and certain racial groups, has visible characteristics that are discriminated against—the signs of being old. Aged persons who do not display such characteristics and are able to maintain a youthful appearance are less discriminated against. This is not valid in all circumstances, however, since older individuals possessing great wealth, status, or fame are often the subjects of admiration rather than discrimination.

To an extent, the biological, psychological, and social processes of aging are interrelated and interdependent. Frequently, loss of a social role alters an individual's drives and speeds physical decline, and poor health forces retirement from work, promoting social isolation and the development of a weakened self-concept. While certain changes occur independently, as separate events, most are closely associated with other age-related factors. It is impractical, therefore, to subscribe solely to one theory of aging. Wise nurses will be eclectic in choosing the aging theories they will utilize in the care of older adults; they will also be cognizant of the limitations of these theories.

REFERENCES

Cumming, Elaine. "New Thoughts on the Theory of Disengagement." In Kastenbaum, Robert, *New Thoughts on Old Age*. Springer, New York, 1964.

——— and **Henry, William E.** *Growing Old: The Process of Disengagement.* Basic Books, New York, 1961.

Few, A., and **Getty, R.** "Occurrence of Lipofuscin as Related to Aging in the Canine and Porcine Nervous System." *Journal of Gerontology*, 22:357–367, 1967.

Havighurst, Robert J. "Successful Aging." In Williams, Richard H., Tibbitts, Clark, and Donahue, Wilma (eds.), *Processes of Aging*, Vol. I. Atherton Press, New York, 1963, pp. 299–320.

Hershey, Daniel. *Lifespan: And Factors Affecting It.* Thomas, Springfield, Ill, 1974.

Leaf, Alexander. *Youth in Old Age.* McGraw-Hill, New York, 1975.

Neugarten, Bernice L. *Personality in Middle and Late Life.* Atherton Press, New York, 1964.

Rose, Arnold. "The Subculture of the Aging: A Framework for Research in Social Gerontology." In Rose, A., and Peterson, W. (eds.), *Older People and Their Social World.* Davis, Philadelphia, 1965, pp. 3–16.

Strehler, Bernard L. *Time, Cells, and Aging.* Academic Press, New York, 1962.

Streib, Gordon F. "Are the Aged a Minority Group?" In Gouldner, A. W., and Miller, S. M. (eds.), *Applied Sociology.* Free Press, New York, 1965.

3

ADJUSTMENTS IN AGING

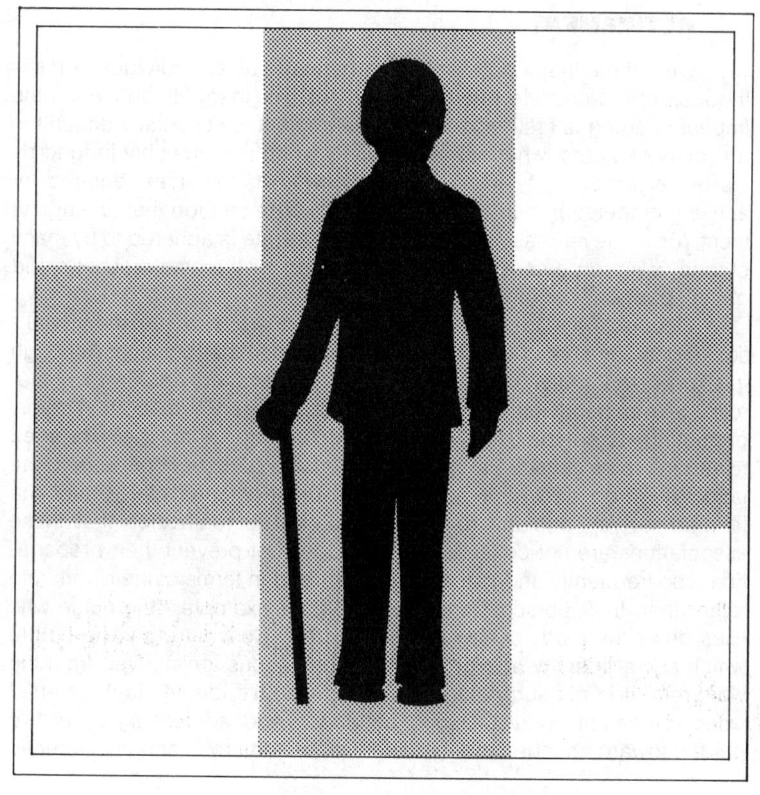

Growing old is not easy. Various changes and losses during the aging process demand multiple adjustments requiring much stamina, ability, and flexibility. Frequently, there are more simultaneous changes than experienced during any other period of life although in "coping" ability, it appears that the old surpass their younger counterparts by far. Many adults find it exhausting enough to keep pace with technological advancements, societal changes, cost-of-living fluctuations, and labor market trends. Imagine how complex and complicated life can be for older individuals, who must also face retirement, reduced income, possible housing changes, frequent losses through death of significant persons, and declining ability to function. To promote an awareness and appreciation of the complex and arduous adjustments involved, the sections below consider some of the factors which affect the successful management of the multiple changes associated with aging and the achievement of satisfaction and well-being during the later years.

RETIREMENT

One of the major adjustments to be made as an individual ages is the loss of a work role through retirement. For many, this is when the impact of aging is first experienced. Retirement is especially difficult in a society like ours, where an individual's worth is commonly judged by his or her productivity. Work is often viewed as the dues required for active membership in a productive society. The attitude that unemployment, for whatever reason, is an undesirable state is adhered to by many of today's aged persons, who were raised under the omnipresent cloud of the "puritan work ethic."

Occupational identity is largely responsible for an individual's social position and for the social role attached to that position. Although it is known that individuals function differently and individually in similar roles, some behaviors continue to be associated with certain roles, promoting stereotypes. How frequently do certain stereotypes assigned to various roles continue to be heard: the tough construction worker; the immoral go-go dancer; the fair judge; the righteous clergyman; the learned lawyer; and the doctor as healer. The realization that these associations are not consistently valid does not prevent their propagation. Too frequently, individuals are described in terms of their work role rather than their personal characteristics, for example, "the nurse who lives down the road" or "my son the doctor." Considering the extent to which social identity and behavioral expectations are derived from the work role, it is not surprising that an individual's identity is threatened when retirement occurs. During childhood and adolescence, we are guided toward an independent, responsible adult role, and in academic settings, we are prepared for our professional roles; but where and when are we prepared for the role of retiree?

Gerontological nursing is concerned with the welfare of both the current aged population and future aged populations. A lifetime of poor health care practices is a handicap that cannot be remedied in old age. Assisting aging individuals with their retirement preparations is preventive intervention, maximizing the potential for health and well-being in old age. As a part of such intervention, aging individuals should be encouraged to establish and practice good health habits, such as proper diet, the avoidance of alcohol, drug, and tobacco abuse, and regular physical examinations.

When one's work is one's primary interest, activity, and source of social contacts, separation from work leaves a significant void in one's life. Aging individuals should be urged to develop interests that are not related to work. Retirement is facilitated by learning how to use, appreciate, and gain satisfaction from leisure time throughout an employed lifetime. In addition, enjoying leisure time is a therapeutic outlet for life stresses throughout the aging process.

Gerontological nurses must understand the realities and reactions encountered when working with retired persons. Insight into this complicated process may be gained by considering the phases of retirement developed by Robert Atchley (1975). Not all retirees go through all phases.

Remote phase: Early in the occupational career, future retirement is anticipated, but rational preparation is seldom done.

Near phase: When the reality of retirement is evident, preparation for leaving one's job begins, as does fantasy regarding the retirement role.

Honeymoon phase: Following the retirement event, a somewhat euphoric period begins whereby fantasies from the preretirement phase are tested. Retirees attempt to do everything they never had time for simultaneously. A variety of factors (finances, health, etc.) limit this, leading to the development of a stable life-style.

Disenchantment phase: As life begins to stabilize, a letdown, sometimes a depression, is experienced. The more unrealistic the preretirement fantasy, the greater the degree of disenchantment.

Reorientation phase: As realistic choices and alternative sources of satisfaction are considered, the disenchantment with the new retirement routine can be replaced by developing a life-style that provides some satisfaction.

Stability phase: An understanding of the retirement role is achieved, and this provides a framework for concern, involvement, and action in one's life. Some enter this phase directly after the honeymoon phase, and some never reach it at all.

Termination phase: The retirement role is lost as a result of either the resumption of a work role or dependency due to illness or disability.

It is obvious that different nursing interventions may be required during each phase. Some of the preretirement planning recommendations discussed earlier can be employed during the remote phase. Counseling regarding the realities of retirement may be part of the near phase, whereas helping retirees place their new found freedom into proper perspective may be warranted during the honeymoon phase. Being supportive of retirees during the disenchantment phase without fostering self-pity and helping them identify new sources of satisfaction may facilitate the reorientation process. Appreciating and promoting the strengths of the stability phase may reinforce an adjustment to retirement. For general nursing there are many considerations related to the phases of retirement. For example, when the retirement phase is terminated due to disease or disability, the tactful management of dependency and the respectful appreciation of losses are most important.

Nurses' self-evaluation of their own attitudes toward retirement are an essential part of their role in the retirement process. Does the nurse see retirement as a period of freedom, opportunity, and growth? or of loneliness, dependency, and meaninglessness? Is the nurse intelligently planning for her own retirement? or denying it, by avoiding encounters with retirement realities? Nurses' views of retirement have an impact of the retiree-nurse relationship, and gerontological nurses can be especially good models of constructive retirement practices and attitudes.

FAMILY CHANGES

The family unit is the major source of satisfaction for many older people and contrary to the belief of many persons, most of the aged have regular, frequent contact with family members. The love and companionship of a spouse, the rewards and pride derived as offspring develop into independent adults, the deepened—and often renewed—relationships with siblings, and the joy of grandchildren and great-grandchildren can be essential ingredients for a satisfying old age. The family can be a key source of support, as well, cushioning the multiple losses and changes associated with aging while instilling hope and interest for a meaningful future.

The parental role is a dynamic one which frequently changes to meet the growth and development needs of both parent and child. During middle and late life, parents must adjust to the independence of their children as they become responsible adult citizens and leave home. Today, the first child usually leaves home and establishes an independent unit 22 to 25 years after the parents were married. For persons who have invested most of their adult lives nurturing and providing for their offspring, a child's independence may have significant impact. Although parents freed from the responsibilities and worries of rearing children have greater time to pursue their own interests, they are also freed from the meaningful, purposeful, and satisfying activities associated with child rearing, and this frequently results in a profound sense of loss.

A woman in late middle age or old age today was influenced by a historical period that emphasized the role of wife and mother. For instance, to provide job opportunities for men returning from World War II, women were encouraged to focus their interests on raising a family and to forfeit the scarce jobs to men. Unlike many of today's younger women, who combine (and in some situations equally value) employment and motherhood, these women centered their lives on their families, from which they derived their sense of fulfillment. Having developed few roles from which to achieve satisfaction other than that of wife and mother, many of today's older women feel a definite void when their children are grown and gone. To compound this problem, the highly mobile life-style of many young persons limits the degree of direct contact she has with her children, who are now adults, and with her grandchildren.

The older man shares many of the same feelings as his wife. Throughout the years, he feels he has performed useful functions, which made him a valuable member of society. He may have fought for his country in undisputably honorable wars. Most likely, he worked hard to support his wife and children, and his masculinity was reinforced with proof of his ability to beget and provide for offspring. With his children grown, he is no longer required to provide—a mixed blessing in which he may sense relief and purposelessness. In addition, he learns that the rules have changed; his pride at being a war hero may have been shattered by antiwar advocates; his ability to support a family without the need for this wife to work is now viewed as oppressive by feminists; his efforts to replenish the earth are scorned by today's zero population proponents; and his attempt to fill the masculine role for which he was socialized is considered "macho" or inane by today's standards.

Although the extended family was not as widespread or perfect as many thought, it was more prevalent in days gone by. It provided immediate support systems, shared responsibilities, economic benefits, and other advantages to both the young and old family member. Grandparenting was an active role which provided a sense of usefulness and satisfaction for the aged, who, in turn, could feel secure that the family unit would be responsible for their growing needs and increased requirements for assistance.

The emergence of today's nuclear family units changed the roles and functions of the individuals in a family. The aged are expected to have limited input into the lives of their adult children. Children are not required to meet the needs of their aging parents for financial support, health services, or housing. Moreover, parents increasingly do not depend on their children for their needs, and the belief that children are the best old-age insurance is a fading one. In addition, grandparenting, although very satisfying, is not usually an active role, especially since grandchildren may be scattered throughout the country. These changes in family structure and function are not necessarily negative. Most children do not abandon or neglect their aging parents, but maintain regular contact. Separate family units may help the parent-child relationship develop on a more adult-to-adult basis—to the mutual satisfaction of young and old. Although the advantages of nuclear family living are often seen primarily as a benefit to younger adults, older adults also enjoy the independence and freedom from responsibilities nuclear family life offers.

A common event that alters family life for the aged is the death of a spouse. The loss of that individual who has shared more love and life experiences, more joys and sorrows, may be intolerable. How, after many decades of living with another human being, does one adjust to the sudden absence of that person? How does one adjust to setting the table for one, to coming home to an empty house, or to not touching that warm, familiar body beside him or her in bed? Adjustment to this significant loss is coupled with the demand to learn the new task of living alone.

Death of a spouse affects more women than men since most older men are married and most older women are widowed—a situation which is projected to continue in the future. Unlike many of today's younger women, who have greater independence through careers and changed norms, most of today's older women have lived family-oriented lives and been dependent on their husbands. Their age, limited education, lack of skills, or long period of unemployment while raising their families are handicaps in a competitive job market. If these women can find employment, adjusting to the new demands of a work role may be difficult and stressful. On the other hand, the unemployed widow may learn that pensions or other sources of income may be reduced or discontinued when the husband dies, necessitating an adjustment to an extremely limited budget. In addition to financial dependence, the woman may have depended on her husband's achievements to provide her with gratification and identity. (Frequently, the achievements of

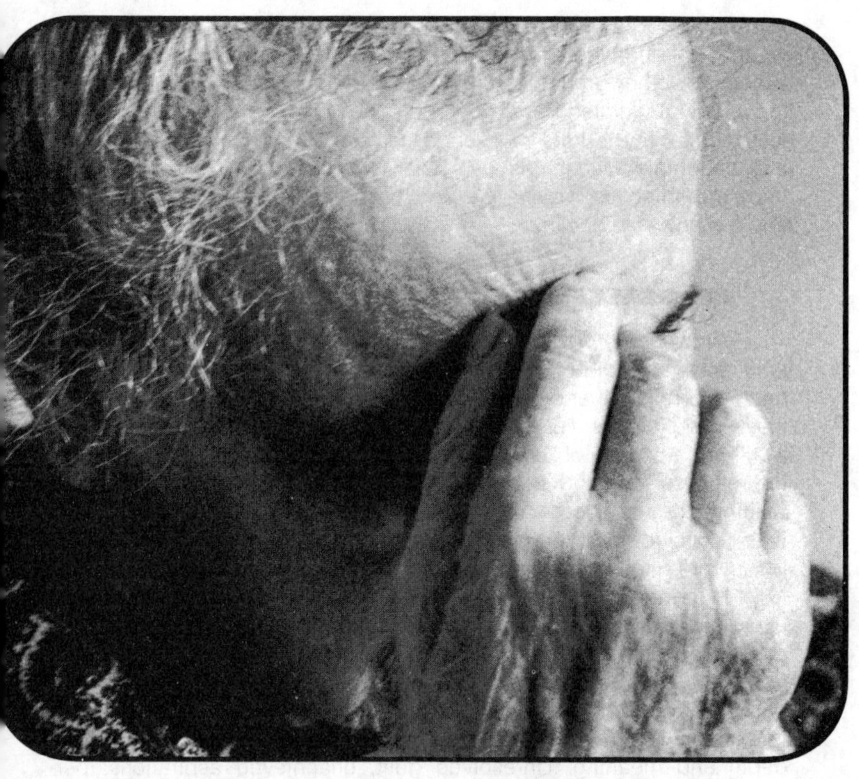

children serve this same purpose.) Sexual desires may be unfulfilled due to lack of opportunity, fear of repercussions from children and society, or residual attitudes from early learnings about sexual mores. If a woman's marriage promoted friendships with other married couples and only inactive relationships with single friends, the new widow may find that her pool of single female friends is scarce.

For the most part, when the initial grief of the husband's death passes, most widows adjust quite well. The high proportion of older women who are widowed provides the availability of friends who share similar problems and life-styles; this is especially true in urban areas. Old friendships may be revived to provide sources of activity and enjoyment. Some widows may discover that the loss of certain responsibilities associated with their partner's death, such as cooking, laundering, and cleaning for a husband, brings them a new and pleasant freedom. With alternative roles to develop, sufficient income, and choice over lifestyle, many women are able to make a successful adjustment to widowhood. The nurse may facilitate this adjustment by identifying sources of friendships and activities—such as clubs, volunteer organizations, or other groups of widows in the community—and by helping the widow understand and obtain all the benefits to which she is entitled. This may require reassuring her that enjoying her new freedom and desiring relationships with other men is no reason to feel guilty, and supporting her as she learns to adjust to the loss of her husband and the new role of widow.

AWARENESS OF MORTALITY

Widowhood, death of friends, and the recognition of declining functions make older persons more aware of the reality of their own death. During their early years, individuals intellectually understand that they will not live forever, but their behaviors deny this reality. The lack of a will and absence of burial plans may be indications of this denial. As the reality of mortality becomes acute with advancing age, interest in fulfilling dreams, deepening religious convictions, strengthening family ties, providing for the ongoing welfare of one's family, and leaving a legacy are often apparent signs.

The significance of a life review in interpreting and refining our past experiences as they relate to our self-concept and help us understand and accept our life history has been well discussed by Robert Butler (1963; 1971). Rather than being a pathological behavior, discussing the past may be quite therapeutic and necessary for the aged. The thought of impending death may be more tolerable if people feel that their life had depth and meaning. Unresolved guilt, unachieved aspirations, perceived failures, and other multitudinous aspects of "unfinished business" may be better understood and perhaps resolved. Although the condition of old age may provide limited opportunities for excitement and achievement, there may be satisfaction in knowing that there *were* achievements, and many excitements as well, in other periods of life. The old woman may be frail and wrinkled, but she can still delight in remembering how she once drove the young men insane. The retired old man may feel that he is useless to society now, but he realizes his worth through the memory of wars he fought to protect his country and the pride he feels in knowing he supported his family through a depression.

The young can benefit from the reminiscences of the aged, growing in depth and gaining a new perspective on life as they learn about their ancestry. Imagine the impact of hearing about slavery or immigration or epidemics or industrialization or wars from an older relative who has been part of making that history. What history book's description of the Great Depression can compare with hearing one's grandparents describe events one's own family experienced—such as going to bed hungry at night? In addition to their place in the future, the young can fully realize their link with the past when the desire of the aged to reminisce is appreciated and fostered.

Older persons should be encouraged to discuss and analyze the dynamics of their lives, and listeners should be receptive and accepting. Poems and autobiographies, as unsophisticated as they may be, should be recognized as significant legacies from the old to the young. I am reminded of my own father-in-law, who at age 71 started a family scrapbook for each of his children. Any photograph, newspaper article, or announcement pertaining to any family member was reproduced and included in every album. The family patiently tolerated this activity—reluctantly sending him copies of graduation programs and photographs for every scrapbook. The family viewed the main value of this activity as providing something benign to keep this old man occupied. It was not until years after his death that the significance of this great task was appreciated as a priceless gift. Such tangible items may serve as an assurance to both young and old that the impact of an aged relative's life will not cease upon death.

DECLINING FUNCTION

The obvious changes in appearance and bodily function which occur during the aging process make it necessary for the aging individual to adjust to a new body image. Colorful soft hair turns gray and dry; flexible straight fingers become bent and painful; body contours are altered and height decreases. Stairs which were once climbed several times daily demand more time and energy to negotiate as the years accumulate. As subtle, gradual, and natural as these changes may be, they are recognized and, consequently, body image and self-concept is affected.

The manner in which individuals perceive themselves and function can determine the roles they play. A construction worker who has less strength and energy may forfeit his work role; a club member who cannot hear speech may forfeit his or her role; fashion models may forfeit that role when they perceive themselves as old. Interestingly, some persons well into their sixth and seventh decades refuse to join a senior citizen club and accept the role associated with being a member of such a club because they do not perceive themselves as being old. The nurse will gain insight into the self-concept of older persons by evaluating what roles they are willing to accept and what roles they reject.

It is sometimes difficult for the aging person to accept the declining efficiency of the body. Poor memory, slow response, easy fatigue, and altered appearance are among the many frustrating results of declining function, and they are dealt with in a variety of ways. Some older people deny them and often demonstrate poor judgment in an attempt to make the same demands on their bodies as they did when younger. Others try to resist these changes by investing in cosmetic surgery, beauty treatments, miracle drugs, and other expensive endeavors that diminish the budget but not the normal aging process. Still others exaggerate these effects and impose an unnecesarily restricted life-style on themselves. Societal expectations frequently determine the adjustment individuals make to declining function.

Common results of declining function are illness and disability. Most older people have one or more chronic diseases (Brody, 1974) and more than a third have some disability which is serious enough to limit major activities, such as work and housekeeping (Riley and Foner, 1968). A fear that the aged have is that their illness or disability may cause them to lose their independence. Becoming a burden to one's family, being unable to meet the demands of daily living and having to enter a nursing home are some of the fears associated with dependency. Children and parents may have difficulty exchanging dependent-independent roles. The physical pain which an illness produces may not be nearly as intolerable as the dependency it causes.

Nurses should help aging persons understand and accept the normal physical decline associated with advanced age. Factors which can promote optimum function should be encouraged, including proper diet, paced activity, regular physical examination, early correction of health problems, and avoidance of alcohol, tobacco, and drug abuse. Assistance should be offered with attention to preserving as much of the individual's independence and dignity as possible.

REDUCED INCOME

Financial resources are important at any age since they affect our diet, health, housing, safety, and independence and influence many of the choices we face in life. The economic profile of many aged persons is dim. Retirement income is less than half the income earned while fully employed. For a majority of the aged, social security income, originally intended as a *supplement*, is actually the *primary source* of retirement income—and it has not even kept pace with inflation. Less than one-fifth of the aged have income from a private pension plan, and those who do often discover that the fixed benefits established when the plan was subscribed to have almost no value because of inflation. (Of the workers who are currently active in the labor force, more than one-half will not have pension plans when they retire.) More than one-fourth of the aged live in poverty; only a minority are fully employed or financially comfortable. Few olderly persons have accumulated enough assets during their lifetime to provide financial security in old age.

TABLE 3-1: RETIREMENT BUDGET: INCOME SOURCES

Income Sources	Current Monthly Income	Income After Retirement
1. Salary	______	______
2. Pension	______	______
3. Other (savings, rents, investments, etc.)	______	______
4. Second job	______	______
5. Social security	______	______
6. Spouse's income	______	______
7.		
8.		
Total		

A reduction in income is a significant adjustment for many older persons, as it triggers off a whole series of other adjustments that must be made. An active social life and leisure pursuits may have to be markedly reduced or eliminated. Relocation to less expensive housing may be necessary, possibly forcing the aged to leave many family and community ties. Dietary practices may be severely altered and health care may be viewed as a luxury over which other basic expenses, such as food and rent, take priority. If the older parent has to depend on children for supplemental income, an additional adjustment in thinking may be needed.

The importance of making financial preparations for old age many years prior to retirement is clear. Nurses should encourage aging working people to determine whether their retirement income plans are keeping pace with inflation. Aged individuals need assistance in obtaining all the benefits they are entitled to and in learning how to manage their income wisely. Nurses should be aware of the impact economic welfare has on health status and should actively involve themselves in political issues that promote adequate income for all individuals.

LONELINESS

Loneliness and desolation emphasize all the misfortunes of people who are growing old. Children are grown and gone, friends and spouse may be deceased, and others who could allay the loneliness may avoid the aged individual because they find it difficult to accept the changes they see or to face the fact that they too will be old some day. Location in a sparsely populated rural area can geographically isolate older persons, and when they live in an urban area, they may be fearful of going

TABLE 3-2: RETIREMENT BUDGET: EXPENSES

Living Requirements	Current Monthly Expenses	Expenses After Retirement
Living accommodations		
Mortgage or rent		
Utilities (gas, electricity, water)		
Taxes		
Maintenance		
Telephone		
Food and other necessities		
Clothing		
Medical (doctor, dentist, medicine)		
Insurance		
Life		
Health		
Auto		
Other		
Loans and other credit		
Automobile expenses (gas, oil, repairs)		
Entertainment		
Subtotal		
Other expenses (10% of subtotal)		
Total		

outdoors. Hearing and speech deficits and language differences, which present communication barriers, can also foster loneliness. Insecurity resulting from multiple losses can cause suspiciousness of others and lead to a self-imposed isolation. At a time of many losses and adjustments, personal contact, love, extra support, and attention are needed—not isolation. These are essential human needs. Isn't it likely that a failure to thrive will occur in adults who feel unwanted and unloved just as it does in infants, who display anxiety, depression, anorexia, and behavioral and other difficulties when they perceive love and attention to be inadequate?

Nurses should attempt to intervene when isolation and loneliness are detected in an aged person. There are programs that provide telephone reassurance or home visits as a source of daily human contact, and the person's church may also provide assistance. Nurses can help the person identify and join social groups and sometimes even accompany him or her to the first meeting. A change in housing may be called for to provide a safe environment that is conducive to social interaction. If the aged person speaks a foreign language, relocation to an area in which members of the same ethnic group live can often remedy loneliness. Even pets are frequently very significant and effective companions to the aged.

It should be emphasized that being alone is not synonymous with being lonely. Periods of solitude are essential at all ages, providing us with the opportunity to reflect, analyze, and better understand the dynamics of our lives. Older individuals may want periods of solitude to reminisce and review their lives. Some individuals, young and old, prefer and choose to be alone and do not feel isolated or lonely in any way. Of course, attention should also be paid to the correction of hearing, vision, and other health problems which may be the cause of social isolation.

SOCIETAL PREJUDICE

It is not difficult to detect overt ageism in our society. Rather than showing appreciation for the vast contributions of the aged and their wealth of resources, society is beset with prejudices and lacks adequate provisions for them, thus derogating their dignity. The same members of society that oppose providing sufficient income and health care benefits for the aged enjoy an affluence and standard of living that was provided through the efforts of the aged.

Although the aged constitute the most diverse and individualized group, they continue to be stereotyped by misconceptions such as the following:

Old people are sick and disabled.

Most old people are in nursing homes.

Senility comes with old age.

Old people are unhappy.

People either get very tranquil or very cranky as they age.

Old people have lower intelligence and are resistant to change.

Old people aren't able to have sexual intercourse and aren't interested in sex anyhow.

There are few satisfactions in old age.

Since for a majority of older persons the above statements are not true, increased efforts are necessary to make the members of society aware of the realities of aging. Groups such as the Gray Panthers have done an outstanding job of informing the public about the facts regarding aging and the problems and rights of older adults. More advocates for the aged are needed.

Erik Erikson says that the last stage of the life cycle is concerned with integrity versus despair. Integrity results when the older individual derives satisfaction from an evaluation of his or her life. Disappointment with one's life and the lack of opportunities to redo one's past bring despair. The experiences of our entire lifetime determine whether our old age will be an opportunity for freedom, growth, and contentment, or a miserable imprisonment of our human potential.

REFERENCES

Atchley, Robert C. *The Sociology of Retirement.* Schenkman, Cambridge, Mass., 1975.

Brody, S. J. "Evolving Health Delivery Systems and Older People." *American Journal of Public Health,* 64:245, 1974.

Butler, Robert. "The Life Review: An Interpretation of Reminiscence in the Aged." *Psychiatry,* 26:65–76, 1963.

——— "The Life Review." *Psychology Today,* 5:49–51, December 1971.

Riley, Matilda W., and Foner, Ann. *Aging and Society, Vol. I: An Inventory of Research Findings.* Russell Sage Foundation, New York, 1968, p. 214.

4

CHANGES ASSOCIATED WITH THE AGING PROCESS

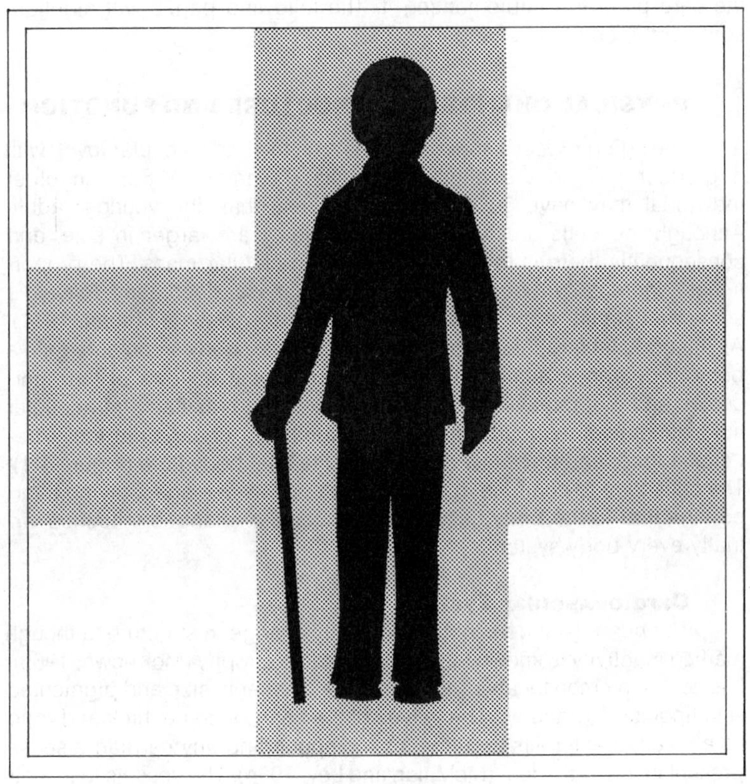

Living is a process of continual changes. Infants become toddlers, pubescent children blossom into young men and women, and dependent adolescents develop into responsible adult members of society. The type, rate, and degree of physical, emotional, psychological, and social changes experienced during this life process are highly individualized, being influenced by genetic factors, environment, diet, health, stress, and a variety of other factors.

That the process of change continues into old age is natural and to be expected. The multitude of changes that have occurred, during the life span of those who achieve old age, make old people appear physically, psychologically, and socially different in certain ways. However, they continue to share characteristics with younger individuals, and thus remain linked with all human beings. Understanding the changes experienced during the aging process will assist the nurse in caring for older individuals. Such an understanding will provide a foundation for the nurse's assessment and guidance and for adjusting the care plan and implementing it. The following pages will highlight some of the common changes.

PHYSICAL CHANGES IN STRUCTURE AND FUNCTION

The aging process shows its effects on the basic cellular level, with a gradual loss in the number of cells (Freeman, 1965). An older individual may have 30 percent fewer cells than the younger adult. Although the cells are fewer in number, they are larger in size, and consequently there is less of a reduction in cellular mass. The proportionate increase in body fat as the cell mass decreases leaves a somewhat similar appearance of the total body mass (Goldman, 1971). As the body fat atrophies with advanced age, the body's contours gain a bony appearance along with a deepening of the hollows of the intercostal and supraclavicular spaces, orbits, and axillae. Intracellular fluid decreases, although there is no significant changes in the extracellular fluid, and there is a decrease in the total body fluid (Figure 4-1). The cells tend to combine in irregular patterns as one ages, giving altered structure to the body tissues. These cellular changes influence virtually every body system.

Cardiovascular System

The heart itself does not significantly change in structure, although marked inactivity is known to promote cardiac atrophy (McKeown, 1965). It is not uncommon for an aged heart to be smaller in size and pigmented with lipofuscin granules. The valves of the heart become thick and rigid as a result of sclerosis and fibrosis, compounding any cardiac disease present in the individual (McMillan and Lev, 1964). The vessels lose their

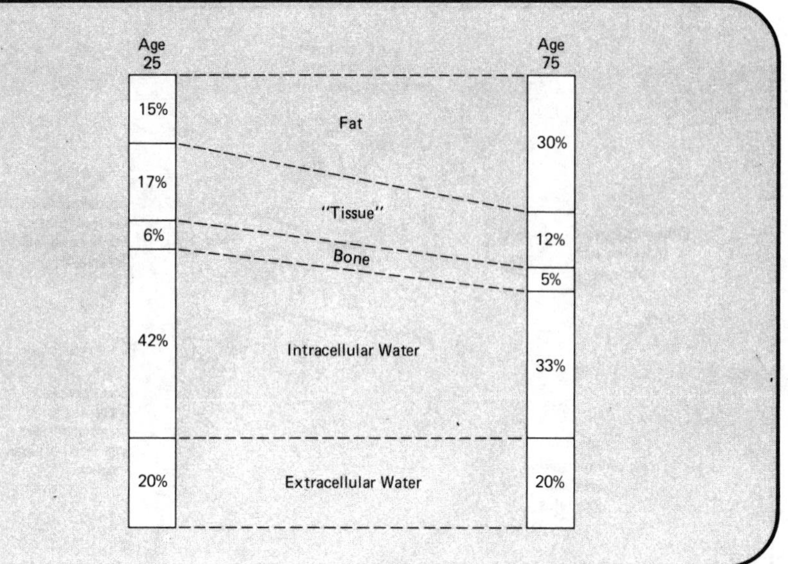

Figure 4-1. Distribution of major body components with age. (Source: R Goldman. *Journal of the American Geriatric Society, 18* (765). 1970.

elasticity, and muscular arteries in the head, neck, and extremities become more prominent.

There are various physiologic changes in the cardiovascular system that occur. A slower heart rate and decreased stroke volume cause decreases in cardiac output as high as 40 percent between the ages of 25 and 65 years (Brandfonbrener, Landowne, and Shock, 1955). Sudden stress is not managed well by the aged heart, as demonstrated by a lesser increase in pulse rate and a prolonged time for return to the previous rate (Goldman, 1971). The stroke volume may increase to compensate for this situation, which results in an elevation in blood pressure—although it is possible for the blood pressure to remain stable as a tachycardia progress to heart failure in the elderly (Harris, 1974). Oxygen utilization is less efficient, which may contribute to prolonged tachycardia in older individuals (Harris, 1974). There is a wide range into which the pulse rate may fall—from 44 to 108 beats per minute (Harris, 1974). Increased peripheral resistance contributes to a rising blood pressure, affecting both the systolic and diastolic pressures (Master and Lasser, 1961). Although Harris has considered hypertensive levels in the aged as being persistent elevations over 170 mmHg systolic and 95

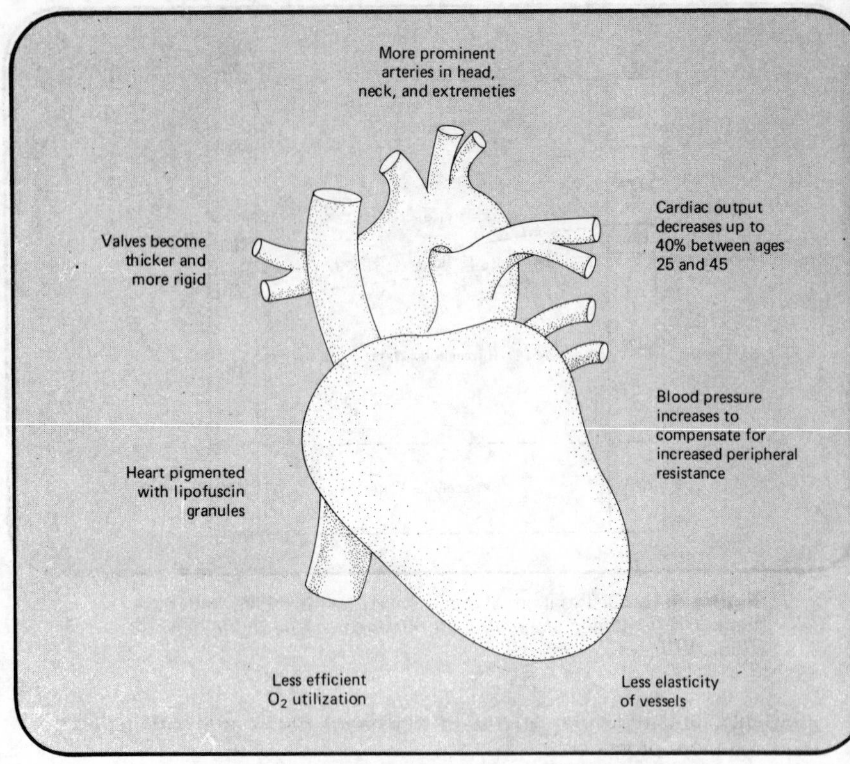

Figure 4-2. Cardiovascular changes with aging.

mmHg diastolic, Harris, Caird and Judge (1974) offer slightly higher upper limits of blood pressure (Table 4-1) and discourage treating blood pressures lower than these levels as hypertensive.

Respiratory System

The aged lung tends to be larger on inspection due to a loss of elasticity. This results in an increase in residual capacity of approximately 50 percent by age 90 (Mithoefer and Karetzky, 1968). The number of alveoli are reduced and are of increased size, as are the bronchioles and alveolar ducts. As the residual volume increases, the vital capacity is lowered (Norris, et al., 1956). The maximum breathing capacity is reduced. Total lung capacity is not significantly different in older individuals, however.

Age does not influence the blood carbon dioxide level (pCO_2)

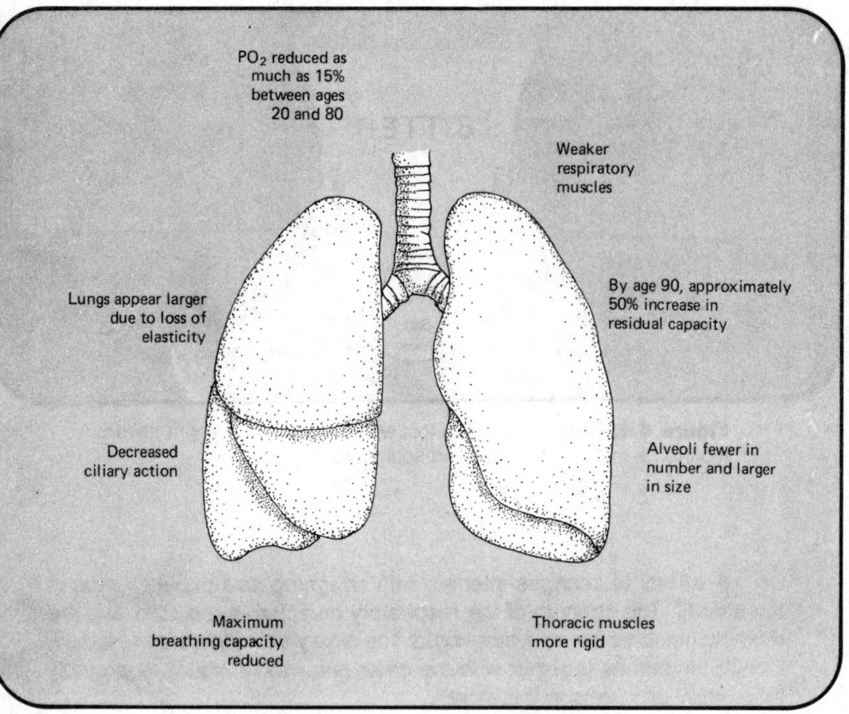

Figure 4-3. Respiratory changes with aging.

which remains at approximately 40 mmHg, but it does decrease the arterial blood oxygen level (pO_2) by 10 to 15 percent between the ages of 20 and 80 (Mithoefer and Karetzky, 1968). Thus an older individual may have a blood oxygen level of 75 mmHg.

TABLE 4-1: SUGGESTED UPPER LIMITS OF BLOOD PRESSURE IN OLD AGE

	mmHg for Men		mmHg for Women	
Age	Systolic	Diastolic	Systolic	Diastolic
60–69	195	100	200	110
70–79	195	105	210	110
80+	195	105	210	115

Source: F. I. Caird and T. G. Judge, *Assessment of the Elderly Patient*, Pitman Medical Publishing Co., New York, 1974, p. 34.

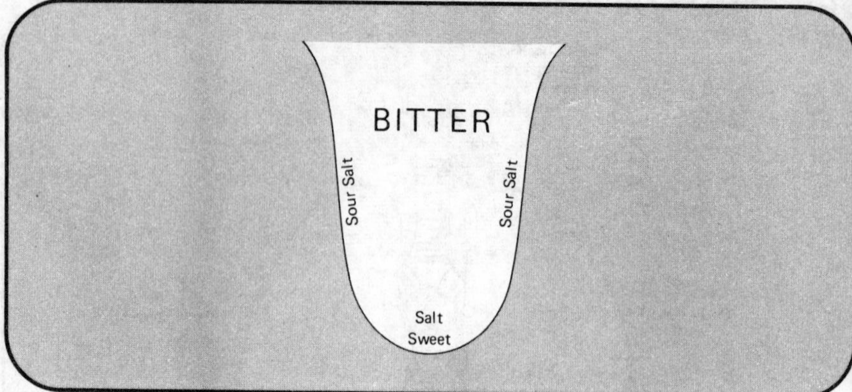

Figure 4-4. Taste sensations lost with age. Sweet and salt flavors tend to be lost before bitter and sour flavors.

A variety of changes interfere with coughing and expectoration in the elderly. The strength of the respiratory muscles is reduced and the thoracic muscles become more rigid. The ciliary activity is also reduced. Cough limitations together with the other respiratory changes promote respiratory problems in the elderly.

Gastrointestinal System

Although not as fatal as cardiovascular or respiratory problems, gastrointestinal problems are more discomforting and bothersome to older individuals. A contributing factor is the common loss of teeth due to poor dental care, environmental influences, or changes in gingival tissues. After age 30, peridontal disease is the major cause of tooth loss, and it is rare to find an individual who has not suffered severe tooth loss by age 70. The teeth in older adults may have a flatter surface and appear to be longer due to resorption of the gum tissue around the tooth's base. Taste sensation decreases with age, due to chronic irritation (as with pipe smoking) or to a wearing out or atrophy of taste buds. There is a tendency for the sweet sensations on the tip of the tongue to be lost earlier than the sour, salt, and bitter taste sensations (Figure 4–4).

Esophageal motility is decreased and the esophagus tends to become dilated. The lower esophageal sphincter relaxes and esophageal emptying is slower (Soergel et al., 1964). The stomach is

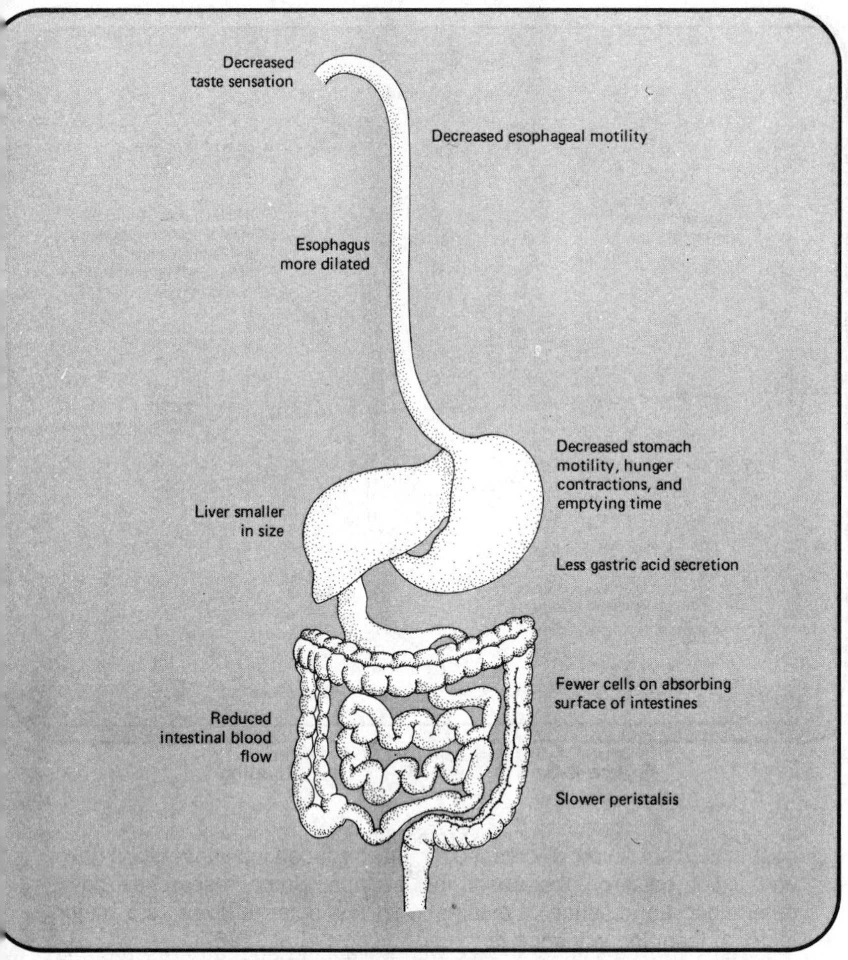

Figure 4-5. Gastrointestinal changes with aging.

believed to have decreased motility, along with decreases in hunger contractions, gastric acid secretion, and emptying time (Sklar, 1974). Some atrophy occurs throughout the small and large intestine, although research regarding the changes in the intestine is limited; constipation, common in the older population, is thought to be a result of slower colonic peristalsis. Absorption may be decreased due to change in

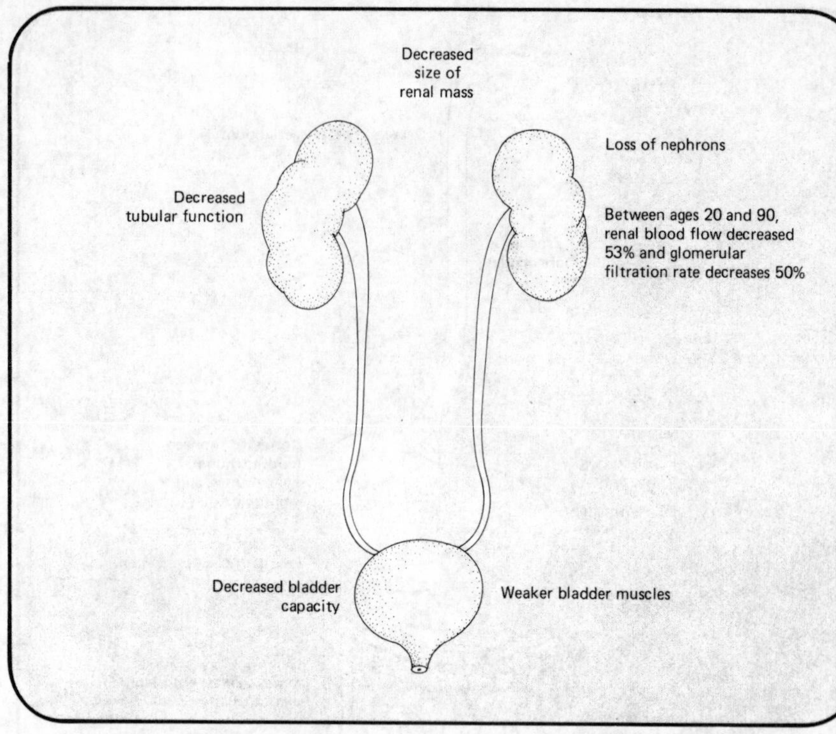

Figure 4-6. Urinary tract changes with aging.

gastric acid secretion, decreased motility, reduced intestinal blood flow, and fewer cells on the absorbing surface. Some researches have determined an absence of external anal sphincter reflexes as a major factor in fecal incontinence in the aged (Alva et al., 1967).

The liver is smaller in size with advancing age, and research has shown a reduction in splanchnic blood flow (Sherlock et al., 1971) and a decreased storage capacity (Calloway and Merrill, 1965). Total serum bilirubin, SGOT (serum glutamic oxalectic transaminase) SGPT (serum glutamic pyruvic transaminase), and alkaline phosphate values are not significantly altered with age.

Genitourinary System

The renal mass decreases in size with age, attributable to the loss of nephron units (Goldman, 1971). Renal tissue growth declines with age (Oliver, 1952), and atherosclerosis may promote atrophy of the kidney.

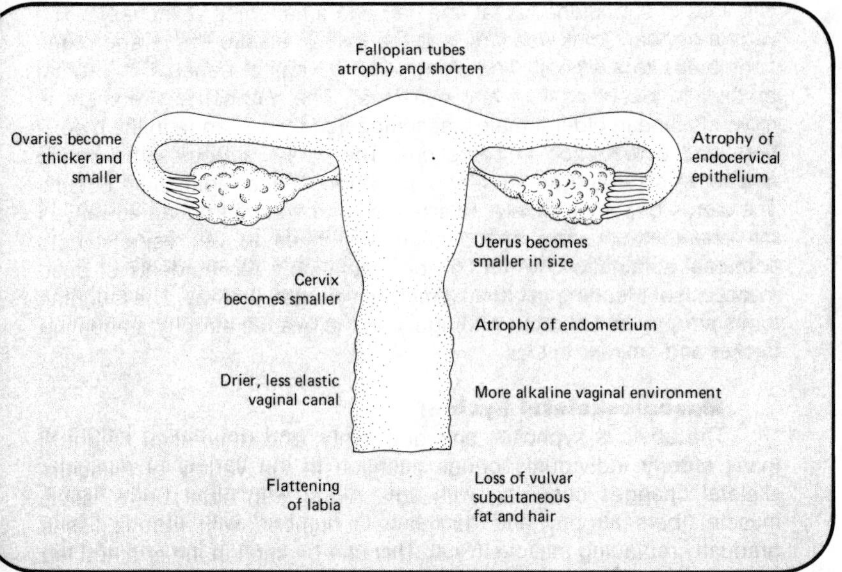

Figure 4-7. Changes in the female genitalia with aging.

These changes will alter renal function in a variety of ways. Renal blood flow decreases 53 percent and the glomerular filtration rate at age 90 is almost 50 percent less than it was at age 20 (Davies and Shock, 1950). Tubular function also decreases, demonstrated by increased problems in concentration of urine. The maximum specific gravity at age 80 has been shown to be 1.024, whereas at younger ages the maximum was 1.032 (Goldman, 1971). Decreased tubular function also affects reabsorption from the filtrate, making a 1^+ proteinuria in the aged, which is of no diagnostic significance (Kahn and Snapper, 1974). Decreased renal functioning is further displayed by an average blood urea nitrogen (BUN) of 21.2 mg% at age 70, whereas from ages 30 to 40 the average is 12.9 mg% (Kahn and Snapper, 1974).

The bladder undergoes changes during the aging process, including weakening of the bladder muscles and a decreased bladder capacity. Emptying of the bladder is more difficult and retention of a large volume of urine may result.

Prostatic enlargement is present in most elderly men, although rate and type varies with individuals. Three-fourths of the men over age 65 have some degree of prostatism (Jaffee, 1974). The female genitalia demonstrate many changes with age (Agate, 1963; Jeffcoate, 1967). The vulva, affected by hormonal changes, gains an atrophic appearance, with loss of subcutaneous fat and hair and a flattening of the labia. The vagina appears pink and dry, and the loss of elastic tissue and rugae contributes to a smooth and shiny looking vaginal canal. The vaginal epithelium becomes thin and avascular. The vaginal environment is more alkaline in older females, accompanied by a change in the type of flora and a reduction in secretions. The cervix atrophies, becoming smaller in size, and an atrophy of the endocervical epithelium occurs. The uterus becomes smaller in size also and suffers from an atrophy of the endometrium. The endometrium continues to be responsive to hormonal stimulation, which can be responsible for incidents of postmenopausal bleeding in older women on estrogen therapy. The fallopian tubes atrophy and shorten with age, and the ovaries atrophy, becoming thicker and smaller in size.

Musculoskeletal System

The obvious kyphosis, enlarged joints, and decreased height of many elderly individuals brings attention to the variety of musculoskeletal changes occurring with age. Along with other body tissue, muscle fibers atrophy and decrease in number, with fibrous tissue gradually replacing muscle tissue. This can be seen in the arm and leg muscles which become flabby and weak. Bone mass decreases, and the amount of bone mineral is reduced, contributing to the brittleness of older bones. While long bones do not significantly shorten with age, thinning disks and shortening vertebrae reduce the length of the spinal column. Height is reduced approximately two inches between ages 20 and 70 (Rossman, 1971). Varying degrees of kyphosis may occur, accompanied by a backward tilting of the head, and there are varying degrees of flexion at the wrists, hips, and knees.

In addition to structural change, slower movement is observed in older individuals. Muscle tremors may be present during resting states, believed to be associated with extrapyramidal system degeneration. The tendons undergo shrinkage and sclerosis, which causes a decrease in tendon jerks (Grob, 1974). Reflexes are lessened in the arms and nearly completely lost in the abdomen, but maintained in the knee. For a variety of reasons, muscle cramping may frequently occur.

Nervous System

It is difficult to describe with accuracy and exactness the nervous system's changes with age due to the dependence of this system's function on other body systems. For instance, cardiovascular difficulties may reduce cerebral circulation and be responsible for cerebral dysfunction. Declining nervous system function may be unnoticed, as changes are often nonspecific and slowly progressing. There is a delay in response and reaction time—especially reaction associated with

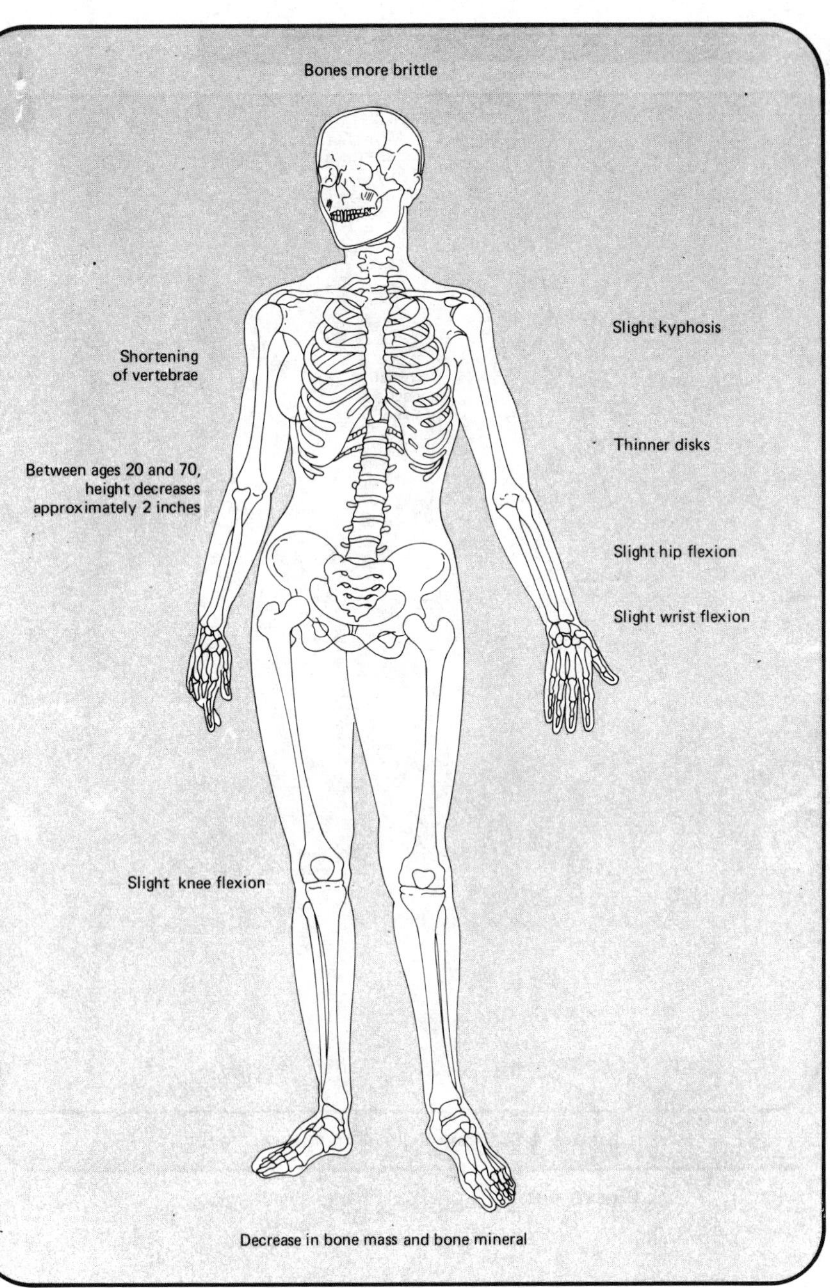

Figure 4-8. Skeletal changes with aging.

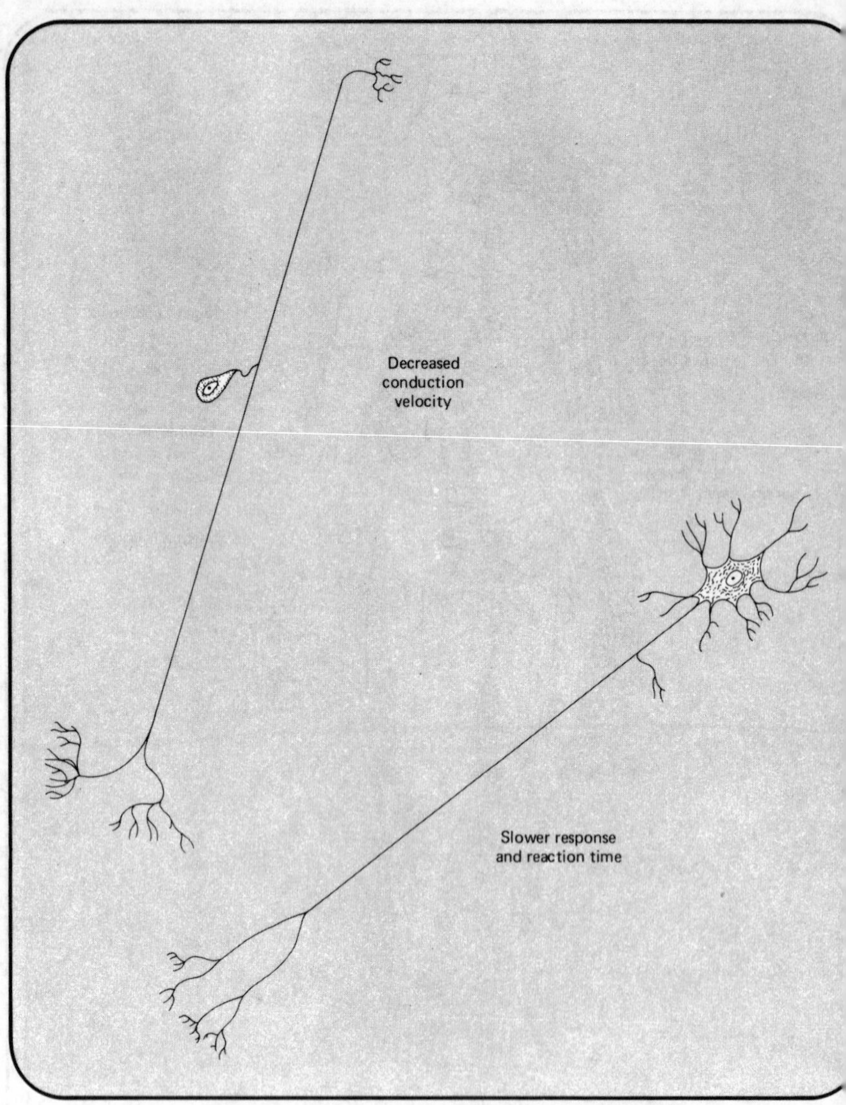

Figure 4-9. Neurological changes with aging.

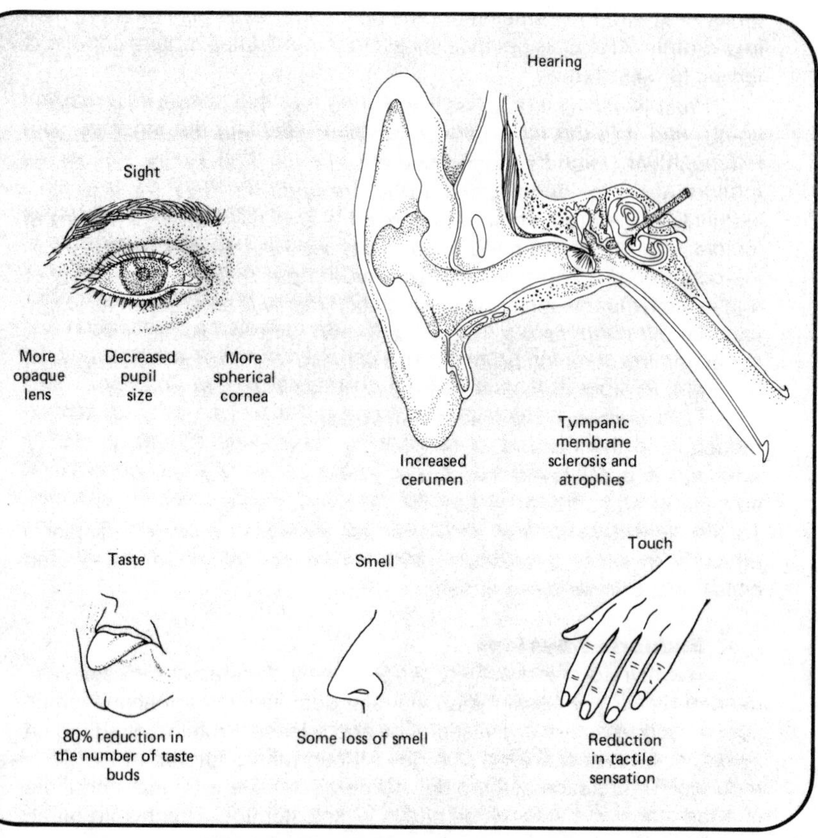

Figure 4-10. Sensory changes with aging.

stress. The conduction velocity has also been shown to decrease with age (Goldman, 1971).

Sensory Organs

The five senses becomes less efficient with increasing age, interfering in varying degrees with safety, normal daily functioning, and general well-being. Perhaps the greatest of such interferences results from changes in vision. Sclerosis of the pupil sphincter and a decrease in pupil size occur, making the pupil less responsive to light. The cornea becomes more spherical, and the lens opaque. Visual acuity decreases, as does the extent of the visual field, making peripheral vision more difficult. The light perception threshold increases and vision in dim areas or at night becomes more difficult. Older eyes also adapt to dark less rapidly. Also as is obvious, most older individuals require corrective lenses for assistance.

Presbycusis is a progressive hearing loss that occurs as a result of aging, and it is the most serious problem affecting the inner ear and retrocochlear. High-frequency sounds are the first to be lost as an individual ages; middle and lower frequencies may be lost subsequently. This problem causes speech to sound distorted. A variety of factors, including continued exposure to loud noise, may contribute to the occurrence of presbycusis. The middle ear displays the effects of age in the tympanic membrane, which commonly is sclerotic or atrophic. External ear changes are insignificant, with cerumen accumulation and impaction the common problem. The cerumen contains a higher amount of keratin in older individuals which contributes to that problem.

Taste sensation decreases with age and there can be an 80 percent reduction in the number of functioning taste buds (Goldman, 1971). Although it is observed that a loss in the sense of smell occurs with advancing age, this area has not received much research attention. Tactile sensation is also reduced, as observed in an old person's difficulty in sensing pressure, and discriminating temperatures, and occasional unawareness of pain.

Endocrine System

The thyroid gland activity progressively decreases with age, evidenced by a lower basal metabolic rate, decrease in radioactive iodine uptake, and less thyrotropin secretion and release. Protein-bound iodine levels in the blood do not change, although the total serum iodide is reduced. The release of thyroidal iodide decreases with age, and there is a reduction in the excretion of the 17-ketosteroids. The thyroid gland progressively atrophies, and loss of adrenal function can further decrease thyroid activity (McGavack, 1974a).

Much of the secretory activity of the adrenal cortex is regulated by ACTH, (adrenocorticotropic) a pituitary hormone. As ACTH secretion decreases with age, secretory activity of the adrenal gland also decreases (McGavick, 1974a). Although the secretion of ACTH does not affect aldosterone secretion, it has been shown that less aldosterone is produced and excreted in the urine of older persons (Flood et al., 1967). The secretion of glucocorticoids 17-ketosteroids, progesterone, androgen, and estrogen, also influenced by the adrenal gland, are reduced as well.

Pituitary activity is altered by age in a variety of ways. The growth hormone (STH-somatotrophic or growth hormone) is present in older and younger individuals in similar amounts, although the blood level may be reduced. Decreases are seen in adrenocorticotropic (ACTH), thyroid-stimulating (TSH), follicle-stimulating (FSH), luteinizing (LH), and luteotropic (LTH) hormones to varying degrees (McGavick, 1974b). Gonadal secretion declines with age, including gradual decreases in testosterone, estrogen, and progesterones (Pincus, 1956). With the exception of alterations associated with changes in plasma calcium level or dysfunction of other glands, the parathyroid glands maintain their function throughout life.

Integumentary System

In addition to the regular effects of the aging process, heredity, environment, diet, general health, activity, and exposure influence the condition of the skin. The changes in the integumentary system are easily recognized and include lines and wrinkles from the loss of subcutaneous fat; thinning, graying scalp hair; thicker hair in the nose and ears; skin pigmentation due to clustering of melanocytes; and less elastic and more delicate skin, due to decreased hydration and vascularity of the dermis (Burgeon and Burgeon, 1958). The fingernails become hard and brittle. The decrease in the number and function of the sweat glands results in a slight reduction in perspiration (Wells, 1954).

PSYCHOLOGICAL CHANGES

Psychological changes during the aging process cannot be isolated from concurrent physical and social changes. Sensory organ impairment can impede the interaction of older individuals both with their environment and with other persons, thus influencing their psychological status. Likewise, feeling useless and socially isolated may obstruct optimum psychological function. General health status, genetic factors, educational achievement, and activity are among the factors which influence psychological changes during the aging process. In light of the involvement of other factors in the psychological functioning of older adults, and the awareness that psychological changes differ among aged individuals, some general findings can be discussed.

Drastic changes in basic personality do not commonly occur as one ages. The kind and gentle old person was most likely that way when younger. Likewise, the cantankerous old person was probably not mild and meek in earlier years. Excluding pathological processes, the personality will be consistent to that of earlier years, possibly with more open and honest expression. The alleged "rigidity" of older persons is more a result of physical and mental limitations, rather than a personality change. For example, an older person's insistence that furniture not be rearranged may be interpreted as rigidity, but to someone coping with poor memory and visual deficits, this may be a wise safety measure. Changes in personality traits may occur in response to events which alter one's attitude toward oneself, such as retirement, death of a spouse, loss of independence, income reduction, and disability (Birren, 1964; Neugarten, 1968).

Memory may be altered with age, and usually memory for past events is superior to the retention and recall of more current information—even that presented seconds to minutes earlier. This explains why the older person who can't remember the name of the nurse who has cared for him all week can accurately recall the name of every member of his World War I outfit. Memory problems are more common in the presence of a poor health status. Evidence indicates changes in intelligence test scores with increasing age. Older individuals tend to generally do less well on intelligence tests involving spatial perception, decoding tasks, arrangement of geometric forms, and psychomotor performance in general. On the other hand, performance involving information, verbal comprehension, and arithmetic operations improves with age through the sixth decade (Botwinick, 1967). There is a correlation between the health status of the older individual and intelligence test scores.

In general, it is wise to interpret the findings related to intelligence and the aged with much caution, as results may indicate a problem with the measurement tool and method rather than with the person whose intelligence is being measured. Cross-sectional studies may be attempting to test similar information for different age groups; different environmental and educational advantages, as well as unique life experiences due to living in different periods of history, may cause the old and young to respond differently to similar questions and situations. Longitudinal studies are able to measure changes that occur in a specific generation as it ages; however, the costs and time involved with longitudinal studies have made this type of research scarce. In interpreting research associated with intelligence and the aged one must consider the aged population sampled. Were they representative of the aged population, or a sample from a nursing home? One must also consider the number sampled. Were the findings from 100 people generalized as representative of 20 million? The tool used for intelligence measurement is also a factor. Was it a written test with print too small for aged eyes to read? Did the test require the older person with a hearing deficit to listen for questions and directions? The relevancy of the test must also be determined. Was there a cultural or age bias in the items being tested?

Although learning ability is not seriously altered with age, other factors do interfere with learning in older individuals. These include motivation, attention span, problems in transfering information into the nervous system, perception deficits, and disease. Older individuals may display less readiness to learn and may depend on previous experience for solutions to problems rather than experiment with new problem-solving techniques. Differences in the intensity and duration of the older person's physiological arousal may make it more difficult to extinguish previous responses and acquire new material. The early phases of the learning process tend to be more difficult for older individuals than younger ones; however after a longer early phase, they are then able to keep equal pace. While there is little difference between old and young in verbal or abstract ability, older persons show some difficulty with perceptual motor tasks. There is some evidence indicating a tendency toward simple association rather than analysis.

Since it is generally more difficult to learn new habits when old habits exist which must be unlearned, relearned, or modified, this is a particular problem for individuals with a lifetime accumulation of habits. Habit reversal, such as performing a task in reverse order, is more difficult (Botwinick, 1967). There is little decline in the psychomotor performance of simple tasks with age, although there is some problem with a series of tasks that is complicated, coordinated, and continuous in sequence. As motor performance is slower, due to decreased neuromuscular activity, poor judgment may be displayed by older persons. The alterations in an old person's psychological ability are an individual matter determined by the challenges he or she faces, the stresses imposed, and the education, activity, experiences, and health of the particular person.

REFERENCES

Agate, J. *The Practice of Geriatrics.* Thomas, Springfield, Ill., 1963.

Alva, J., Mendeloff, A. I., and **Schuster, M. M.** "Reflex and Electromyographic Abnormalities Associated with Fecal Incontinence." *Gastroenterology,* 53:101, 1967.

Birren, J. E. *The Psychology of Aging.* Prentice-Hall, Englewood Cliffs, N.J., 1964.

Botwinick, J. *Cognitive Processes in Maturity and Old Age.* Springer, New York, 1967.

Brandfonbrener, M., Landowne, M., and **Shock, N. W.** "Changes in Cardiac Output with Age." *Circulation,* 12:577, 1955.

Burgeon, C. F. Jr., and **Burgeon, J. S.** "Aging and the Cutaneous System." Geriatrics, 13:391, 1958.

Caird, F. I., and **Judge, T. G.** "Assessment of the Elderly Patient." Pitman Medical Publishing Co., New York, Eng., 1974, p. 34.

Calloway, N. O., and **Merrill, R. S.** "The Aging Adult Liver, I: Bromsulphalein and Bilirubin Clearances." *Journal of the American Geriatrics Society,* 13:594, 1965.

Davies, D. F., and **Shock, N. W.** "Age Changes in Glomerular Filtration Rate, Effective Renal Plasma Flow and Tubular Excretory Capacity in Adult Males." *Journal of Clinical Investigation,* 29:496, 1950.

Flood, C., Gherondache, C., Pincus, G., Tait, J. F., Tait, S. A. S., and **Willoughby, S.** "The Metabolism and Secretion of Aldosterone in Elderly Subjects." *Journal of Clinical Investigation,* 46:960, 1967.

Freeman, J. T. "Body Composition in Aging." In Freeman, J. T. (ed.), *Clinical Features of the Older Patient.* Thomas, Springfield, Ill., 1965.

Goldman, Ralph. "Decline in Organ Function with Aging." In Rossman, I. (ed), *Clinical Geriatrics.* Lippincott, Philadelphia, 1971, pp. 19–21, 24, 30, 41.

Grob, David. "Common Disorders of Muscles in the Aged." In Chinn, A. B. (ed.), *Working with Older People: A Guide to Practice, Vol. IV: Clinical Aspects of Aging,* USPHS Pub. No. 1459, Rockville, Md., U.S. Health Services and Mental Health Administration, 1974, pp. 156–162.

Harris, R. "Special Features of Heart Disease in the Elderly Patients." In Chinn, A.B. (ed.), *Working with Older People: A guide to Practice, Volume IV: Clinical Aspects of Aging,* USPHS Pub. No. 1459, Rockville, Md., U.S. Health Services and Mental Health Administration, 1974, pp. 83, 89.

Jaffe, J. W. "Common Lower Urinary Tract Problems in Older Adults." In Chinn, A. B. (ed.), *Working with Older People: A Guide to Practice, Vol. IV: Clinical Aspects of Aging,* USPHS Pub. No. 1459, Rockville, Md., U.S. Health Services and Mental Health Administration, 1974, p. 142.

Jeffocoate, T. N. A. *Principles of Gynecology,* 3rd ed. Prentice-Hall (Appleton), Englewood Cliffs, N.J., 1967.

Kahn, A. I., and **Snapper, I.** "Medical Renal Diseases in the Aged." In Chinn, A. B. (ed.), *Working with Older People: A Guide to Practice, Vol. IV: Clinical Aspects of Aging,* USPHS Pub. No. 1459, Rockville, Md. U.S. Health Services and Mental Health Administration, 1974, p. 132.

McGavick, T. H. "Endocrine Changes with Aging Significant to Clinical Practice." In Chinn, A. B. (ed.), *Working with Older People: A Guide to Practice, Vol. IV: Clinical Aspects of Aging.* USPHS Pub. No. 1459, Rockville, Md. U.S. Health Services and Mental Health Administration, 1974, (a) p. 198, (b) p. 195.

Master, A. M., and **Lasser, R. P.** "Blood Pressure Elevation in the Elderly." In Breast, A. M., and Moyer, J. H. (eds.), *Hypertension: Recent Advances.* Lea & Febiger, Philadelphia, 1961.

McKeown, F. *Pathology of the Aged.* Butterworth, London, 1965.

McMillan, J., and Lev, M. "The Cardiopulmonary System in the Aged." In Powers, J. D. (ed.), *Surgery of the Aged and Debilitated Patient.* Saunders, Philadelphia, 1968, chap. 5.

Mithoefer, G. C. and **Karetzky, M. S.** In Powers, J. D. (ed.): *Surgery of the Aged and Debilitated Patient.* Saunders, Philadelphia, 1968 Chap. 5.

Neugarten, B. L. (ed.). *Middle Age and Aging.* Univ. of Chicago Press, 1968.

Norris, A. H., Shock, N. W., Lansdowne, M., and Falzone, J. S. "Pulmonary Function Studies: Age Differences in Lung Volume and Bellows Function." *Journal of Gerontology,* 11:379, 1956.

Oliver, J. "The Growth and Decline of the Renal Tissues." In Lansing, A. I. (ed.), *Cowdry's Problems of Aging,* 3rd ed. Williams & Wilkens, Baltimore, 1952.

Pincus. G. "Aging and Urinary Steroid Excretion." In Engle, E. T., and Pincus, G. (eds.), *Hormones and the Aging Process.* Academic Press, New York, 1956, pp. 1–18.

Rossman, I. *Clinical Geriatrics.* Lippincott, Philadelphia, 1971, p. 6.

Schonfield, David, and **Robertson, Elizabeth A.** "Memory Storage and Aging." *Canadian Journal of Psychology,* 20:228–236, 1966.

Sherlock, S., Beorn, A. G., Billing, B. H., and **Patterson, J. C. S.** "Splanchnic Blood Flow in Man by the Bromsulphalein Method: The Relation of Peripheral Plasma Bromsulphalein Level to the Calculated Flow" (J. Lab. Clin. Med., 35:923, 1950). In Rossman, I. (ed.), *Clinical Geriatrics.* Lippincott, Philadelphia, 1971, p. 34.

Sklar, M. "Gastrointestinal Diseases in the Aged." In Chinn, A. B. (ed.), *Working with Older People: A Guide to Practice, Volume IV: Clinical Aspects of Aging,* USPHS Pub. No. 1459, Rockville, Md., U.S. Health Services and Mental Health Administration, 1974, p. 124.

Soergel, K. H., Zboralske, F. F., and **Amberg, J. R.** "Presbyesophagus: Esophageal Mobility in Nonagenarians." *Journal of Clinical Investigation,* 43:1472, 1964.

Wells, G. C. "Senile Changes of the Skin in Man." *Journal of the American Geriatrics Society,* 2:535, 1954.

5

PRINCIPLES GUIDING GERONTOLOGICAL NURSING PRACTICE

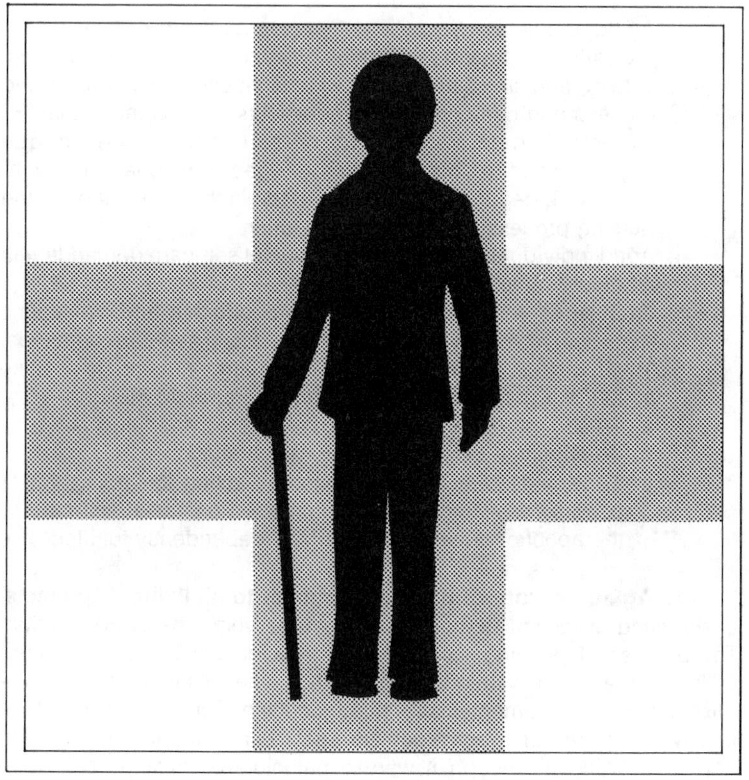

Scientific data regarding theories, life adjustments, and general changes associated with the aging process combined with selected information from psychology, sociology, biology, and other physical and social sciences are utilized in accurately, intelligently, and effectively applying the nursing process to the older population. It is the responsibility of the professional nurse to use these scientific data as the foundation for nursing practice and to make sure through educational and supervisory means that others to whom responsibility for care is delegated also utilize them.

Data from the variety of disciplines is incorporated also in the development of nursing principles—proven facts or theories that are accepted by society and that direct nursing actions. In addition to the general principles utilized in the delivery of care to all individuals, there are specific principles for the care of individuals in certain age groups or with particular health problems. The principles guiding gerontological and geriatric nursing practice, discussed in this chapter, are the following:

1. Aging is a natural process common to all living organisms.
2. Heredity, nutrition, health status, life experiences, environment, activity, and stress are factors which influence the normal aging process and demonstrate unique effects in each individual.
3. Scientific data related to normal aging and unique psychobiosocial characteristics of aged individuals are combined with general nursing knowledge in the application of the nursing process to the aged population.
4. Aged individuals share similar universal self-care demands with all other human beings.
5. Each aged individual has unique capacities and limitations regarding his or her ability to fulfill universal self-care demands.
6. The focus of gerontological and geriatric nursing is to take action in a planned, organized, and therapeutic manner:
   a. To strengthen the individual's self-care capacities
   b. To eliminate or minimize self-care limitations
   c. To provide direct care services by acting for, doing for, or partially assisting the individual when universal self-care or therapeutic demands cannot be independently fulfilled

***1.* Aging—a natural process common to all living organisms.** Every living organism begins aging from the very time of conception. The process of growing old helps the individual achieve the mature cellular, organ, and system functioning that is necessary for the accomplishment of developmental tasks throughout life. Constantly and continuously, every cell of every organism ages. Many people discuss and approach aging as though it were a pathological experience. When

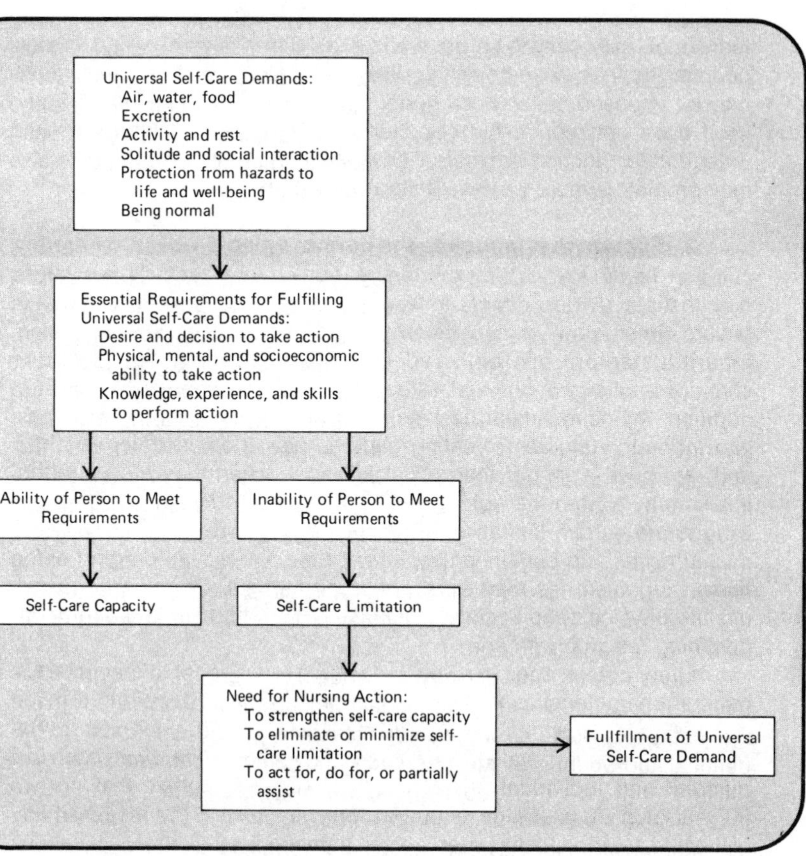

Figure 5-1. Relationship between nursing and the total self-care system.

asked what aging means to them, they usually respond with typical statements:

> *"Getting senile"*
> *"Looking gray and wrinkled"*
> *"Losing health and independence"*
> *"Becoming inflexible, demanding, and disinterested"*
> *"Having less satisfaction and happiness"*
> *"Returning to childlike behavior"*
> *"Suffering losses"*

Although each of the above responses may be true for a given older individual, they cannot be generalized as descriptive of aging in most people. Aging is not a crippling disease and although some limitations may be imposed as the body systems lose efficiency in function, aging itself does not reduce the opportunity for happiness, fulfillment, and independent function. An increased understanding of the aging process may promote a more positive attitude toward old age.

2. Factors that influence the normal aging process. Heredity, nutrition, health status, life experiences, environment, activity, and stress demonstrate unique effects in each individual. Among the variety of factors either known or hypothesized to alter the usual pattern of aging, inherited factors are believed by some researchers to produce chromosomal alterations that cause cells to age at a particular rate. In addition, malnourishment hastens the ill effects of the aging process, and laboratory studies of eating patterns have demonstrated that fish and rats have a longer than usual life span when they are underfed. Illness may hasten the aging process, reduce the human life span, or exaggerate certain limitations of advancing age. Exposure to environmental toxins and certain viruses may cause a more rapid aging of the human organism, as may overexertion and stress. On the other hand, mental, physical, and social activity may reduce the rate and degree of declining function with age.

Every person ages in a very individualized manner, although some general characteristics may be evident among most people in a given age category. Just as we wouldn't assume all 30-year-olds to be identical and would evaluate, approach, and communicate with each in a different and individualized manner, we must recognize that no two 60-year-olds, 70-year-olds, or 80-year-olds are alike. It is a responsibility of the nurse caring for the aged person to recognize the effects of various factors on a particular individual's aging process and how these effects are consequently displayed in the individual. An awareness of the unique aging patterns among people and a more individualized approach will enhance nursing practice with the older person.

***3.* Data and knowledge used in applying the nursing process to the aged population.** In nursing the aged, the scientific data related to normal aging and the unique psychobiosocial characteristics of aged individuals are combined with a general knowledge of nursing. The nursing process provides a systematic approach to the delivery of nursing service. It affirms that nursing actions are deliberate and purposeful, involving a combination of intellectual, interpersonal, and technical skills (Yura and Walsh, 1973). The scope of nursing includes more than following a medical order or performing an isolated task; the nursing process involves a wholistic approach to individuals and the care they require. Four activities are components of the nursing process: assessment, planning, implementation, and evaluation.

As discussed in previous chapters, the unique characteristics and changes associated with the aging process require that certain adjustments be made in the application of the nursing process to the aged. In addition to handling differences in laboratory values, data analysis, priorities, nursing techniques, etc., the nurse caring for the older individual must thoroughly understand the physiological and psychological differences and the unique socioeconomic problems and must utilize this knowledge when assessing, planning, implementing, and evaluating care. Chapter 6 provides a more thorough examination of the application of the nursing process to aged individuals.

4. Self-care demands. Aged individuals share similar universal self-care demands with all other human beings. Every human being has certain basic requirements for the optimum and integrated functioning of the total individual. These needs, or life's demands, categorized in a variety of ways, have been described by Dorothea Orem (*Nursing: Concepts of Practice*) as air, water, food; excretion; activity and rest; solitude and social interaction; avoidance of hazards to life and well-being; and being normal.

Through self-care practices, the individual performs activities independently and voluntarily to meet these universal life demands. Age, illness, and disability may interfere with an individual's ability to do so, and assistance may be required perhaps in the form of nursing services. Some explanation of the effects of aging on an individual's universal self-care demands, and related nursing considerations are discussed in Chapter 7.

5. Capacities and limitations regarding self-care. Each aged individual has unique capacities and limitations regarding his or her ability to fulfill universal self-care demands. Not all individuals can, do, or will meet their universal self-care demands similarly or equally. A variety of factors will determine the success with which these needs are met. Individuals are said to have *self-care* capacity when they are able to be independent and take responsibility for meeting these needs. When the individual's ability to fulfill a demand is partially or totally restricted, he or she is said to have a self-care limitation. Whether the aged person can handle the universal demands of daily living and the actions required to meet specific therapeutic demands, such as the self-administration of medications and complying with a low-sodium diet, depends on several factors, including (a) the desire and decision for action; (b) the required physical, mental, and socioeconomic means for taking action; (c) the knowledge, experience, and skills needed to perform the action.

a. ***Desire and decision for action.*** The value a person sees in performing the action, as well as the person's knowledge, attitudes, and beliefs, and degree of motivation influence the desire and decision for action. Limitations result if a person lacks desire or decides against action. If an individual isn't interested in preparing and eating meals because of social isolation and loneliness, a dietary deficiency may develop. A hypertensive individual's lack of desire and decision to forfeit potato chips and pork products in his or her diet because he or she does not think it is worth the benefit may pose a real threat to his or her health. The person who is not informed of the importance of physical activity may not realize the need to arise from bed during an illness, and consequently may develop complications. A dying individual, viewing dying as a natural process, may decide against medical intervention to sustain his or her life and may not comply with prescribed therapies.

   Values, attitudes, and beliefs are deeply established and not easily altered. While the nurse should respect the right of individuals to make decisions affecting their life, if limitations restrict their ability to meet self-care demands, the nurse can help by explaining the benefit of a particular action, providing information, and developing motivation. In some circumstances, as with an emotionally ill or mentally incompetent person, desires and decisions may have to be superceded by professional judgments.

b. ***Physical, mental, and socioeconomic means.*** Aged individuals may be able to remain active and involved in life if they have adequate financial resources. A person will be able to prevent contractures if he or she is physically able to have unrestricted motion. On the other hand, if individuals lack the finances to obtain necessary health care services or the energy to ambulate and feed themselves or the mental faculties to cross a street safely, self-care will be limited.

   It is the responsibility of nursing to minimize or reduce limitations imposed by physical, mental, and socioeconomic restrictions. Nursing services that assist in the reduction of limitations will be more fully discussed in Chapter 7.

c. ***Knowledge, experience, and skills.*** Limitations exist when the knowledge, experience, or skills required for a given self-care action are inadequate or nonexistent. An individual with a wealth of social skills is capable of a normal, active life that

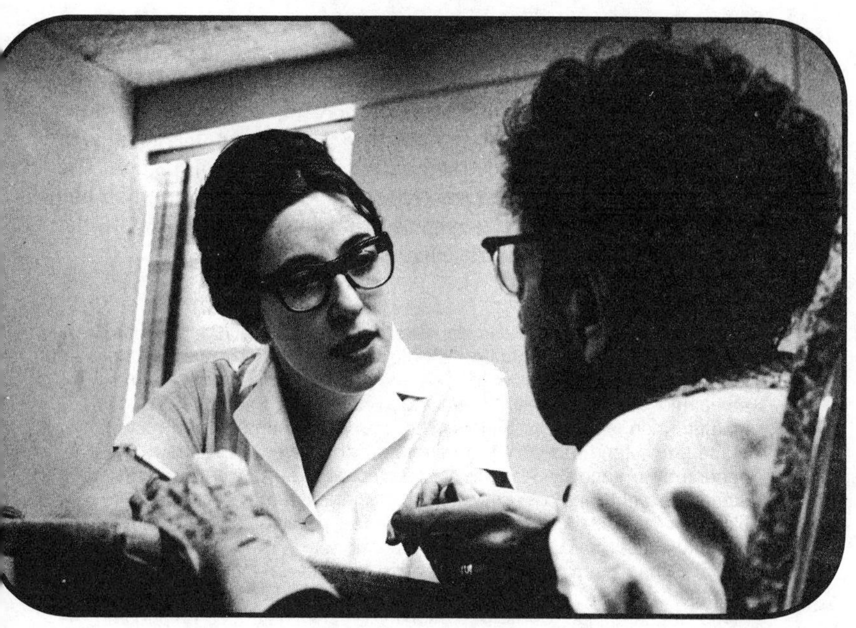

includes friendships and other social interaction. People who have knowledge of the hazards of cigarette smoking will be more capable of protecting themselves from health problems associated with this habit. On the other hand, an older man who is widowed may not be able to cook and provide an adequate diet for himself if he depended on his wife for meal preparation. The diabetic person who lacks skill in self-injection of insulin may not be able to meet his or her therapeutic demand for insulin administration. Specific nursing considerations for enhancing self-care capacities will be offered in other chapters.

***6.* Planned, organized, and therapeutic nursing action.** The nurses actions are directed toward (a) strengthening the individual's self-care capacities; (b) eliminating or minimizing self-care limitations; and (c) providing direct care services by acting for, doing for, or assisting the individual when universal self-care or therapeutic demands cannot be independently fulfilled.

An individual unaffected by illness, disability, advanced age, or limited resources may be fully able to perform the necessary actions related to universal self-care demands. These individuals may have no need for nursing services. Even when self-care actions cannot be performed and a limitation is present, nursing services can sometimes increase the individual's self-care capacity and reduce the limitation. At times, the self-care capacity cannot be temporarily or permanently improved and the self-care limitation cannot be eliminated. In these situations the nurse may have to perform the action, partially or totally, or assist other personnel or family members in performing the action. The following case will exemplify some types of needs an aged person has regarding universal self-care demands. It should be remembered that this sort of example is not all inclusive.

The Case of Mrs. D

Mrs. D, 78 years old, was admitted to a hospital service for acute conditions with the identified problems of a fractured neck of the femur, malnutrition, and a "disposition problem." Initial observation revealed a small-framed, frail-looking lady, with obvious signs of malnutrition and dehydration. She was well oriented to person, place, and time, and able to converse and answer questions quite coherently. Although her memory for recent events was poor, she selcom forgot to inform anyone who was interested that she neither liked nor wanted to be in the hospital. Her previous and only other hospitalization had been 55 years earlier!

Mrs. D had been living with her husband and an unmarried sister for more than 50 years when her husband died. For the five years following she had depended heavily on her sister for emotional support and guidance. Then, her sister died, which promoted feelings of anxiety, insecurity, loneliness, and depression. Living alone, she cared for her six-room home in the county with no assistance other than that from a neighbor who did the marketing for Mrs. D and occasionally provided her with transportation. A year later, on the day of her admission to the hospital, Mrs. D fell on her kitchen floor, weak from her malnourished state. Discovering her hours later, her neighbor called an ambulance which transported Mrs. D to the hospital. Once the diagnosis of fractured femur was established, plans were made to perform a nailing procedure and to correct her malnourishment and find a new living arrangement since her home seemed to demand more energy and attention then she was capable of providing.

Based on an assessment of Mrs. D's self-care capacities and limitations, a variety of nursing actions were planned to assist her in fulfilling the general universal self-care demands and specific therapeutic self-care demands imposed by her problems.

Nursing Actions Related to Universal Requirements

The chart that follows describes the nursing actions that are necessary in fulfilling the universal requirements for (1) air, food, and water; (2) excretion; (3) activity and rest; (4) solitude and social interaction; (5) avoiding hazards to life and well-being; and (6) being normal. These procedures can be related to caring for Mrs. D in the case described above.

UNIVERSAL REQUIREMENT	RELATED NURSING ACTION	TYPE OF ACTION
AIR		
	1. Maintain normal respirations	
	Preventing blockage of airway, or any other interference with normal breathing	Partially assisting
	Observing for and detecting respiratory problems early	Partially assisting
	2. Promoting active and passive exercises	
	Teaching and encouraging turning, coughing, and deep-breathing exercises	Strengthening self-care capacity
	Encouraging active exercises, such as using blow bottles and deep-breathing	Strengthening self-care capacity
	Performing passive range of motion exercise	Doing for
	3. Avoiding external interferences with respiration	
	Providing good room ventilation	Doing for
	Avoiding restrictive clothing, linens, or equipment	Doing for
	Positioning in manner conducive to best respiration	Partially assisting
	Preventing anxiety-producing situations, such as delays in answering call bell	Doing for
FOOD AND WATER		
	1. Stimulating appetite	
	Planning diet according to person's preferences, consisting with therapeutic requirements	Partially assisting
	Providing quiet, pleasant environment that allows for socialization with others	Doing for
	Stimulating appetite through appearance and seasoning of foods	Minimizing self-care limitation
	2. Planning meals	
	Reading menu selection to patient	Partially assisting
	Guiding choice of high-protein, carbohydrate, and vitamin- and mineral-rich foods	Minimizing self-care limitation
	Assessing food preferences and including them in menu selections	Acting for

UNIVERSAL REQUIREMENT	RELATED NURSING ACTION	TYPE OF ACTION
	3. Assisting with feeding	
	Conserving energy and promoting adequate intake by preparing food tray, encouraging rest periods, and feeding when necessary	Strengthening self-care capacity, doing for, and partially assisting
	4. Preventing complications	
	Not leaving solutions, medications, or harmful agents in location where they may be mistakenly ingested (especially when assessment indicates visual limitations)	Acting for
	Checking temperature of foods and drinks to prevent burns (especially when assessment indicates decreased cutaneous sensation)	Acting for
	Assisting in the selection of foods conducive to bone healing and correction of malnutrition	Partially assisting
	Observing fluid intake and output for early detection of imbalances	Minimizing self-care limitation
	Assessing general health status frequently to detect new problems or improvements that have resulted from changes in nutritional status (weight changes, skin turgor, mental status, strength, etc.)	Acting for and minimizing self-care limitation
EXCRETION		
	1. Promoting regular elimination of bladder and bowels	
	Guiding the selection of a diet high in roughage and fluids	Partially assisting
	Observing and recording elimination pattern	Acting for and minimizing self-care limitation
	Assisting with exercises to promote peristolsis and urination	Partially assisting
	Arranging schedule to provide regular time periods for elimination	Acting for
	Assisting with hygienic care of body surfaces	Partially assisting
	Providing privacy when bedpan is used	Acting for
	2. Developing good hygienic practices	
	Teaching importance and method of cleansing perineal region after elimination	Strengthening self-care

UNIVERSAL REQUIREMENT	RELATED NURSING ACTION	TYPE OF ACTION
	3. Preventing social isolation	
	Preventing, detecting and correcting body odors resulting from poor hygienic practices	Acting for, minimizing self-care capacity
ACTIVITY AND REST		
	1. Adjusting hospital routines to individual's pace	Strengthening self-care capacity
	Spacing procedures and other activities	Acting for
	Allowing longer periods of time for self-care activities	Minimizing self-care limitation
	2. Providing for energy conservation	
	Promoting security and relaxation through the avoidance of frequent changes of personnel	Acting for
	Allowing for short rest periods several times a day	Strengthening self-care capacity
	Controlling environmental noise, light, and temperature	Acting for
	3. Preventing complications associated with immobility (such as decubiti, constipation, renal calculi, contractures, hypostatic pneumonia, thrombi, edema, and lethargy)	
	Encouraging frequent change of position	Minimizing self-care limitation
	Motivating and rewarding activity	Strengthening self-care capacity
	Teaching simple exercises to prevent complications and improve motor dexterity	Strengthening self-care capacity
	Planning activities to increase independence progressively	Acting for and strengthening self-care capacity
SOLITUDE AND SOCIAL INTERACTION		
	1. Controlling environmental stimuli	
	Scheduling the same personnel to care for person	Acting for
	Maintaining a regular daily schedule	Strengthening self-care capacity
	Arranging for a roommate with similar interests and background	Acting for and strengthening self-care capacity
	Regulating the amount of visitors	Acting for
	Spacing activities and procedures	Acting for and minimizing self-care limitation

UNIVERSAL REQUIREMENT	RELATED NURSING ACTION	TYPE OF ACTION
	2. Promoting meaningful social interactions	
	Instructing others to speak clearly and sufficiently loud while facing the person	Strengthening self-care capacity
	Planning activities in which person can be involved	Strengthening self-care capacity
	Promoting and maintaining an oriented state	Strengthening self-care capacity and minimizing self-care limitation
	Displaying interest in person's social interactions and encouraging their continuation	Strengthening self-care capacity
	Initiating contacts with community agencies to develop relationships that can continue after discharge	Acting for and minimizing self-care limitation
	Assisting with grooming and dressing	Partially assisting and minimizing self-care limitation
	3. Providing opportunities for solitude	
	Providing several preplanned time periods during the day in which person can be alone	Acting for
	Providing privacy by pulling curtains around bed and making use of facilities such as chapel	Minimizing self-care limitation and partially assisting
AVOIDING HAZARDS TO LIFE AND WELL-BEING		
	1. Compensating for poor vision	
	Reading to person	Doing for and minimizing self-care limitation
	Writing information and labeling with large letters and color coding when possible	Minimizing self-care limitation
	Removing obstacles that could cause accidents, such as foreign objects in bed, clutter on floor, and solutions which could be mistaken as water	Minimizing self-care limitation and acting for
	Communicating this problem to other personnel	Acting for
	Initiating an ophthalmology referral	Acting for
	2. Compensating for decreased ability to smell:	
	Preventing and correcting odors resulting from poor hygienic practices	Partially assisting and minimizing self-care limitations

UNIVERSAL REQUIREMENT	RELATED NURSING ACTION	TYPE OF ACTION
	Detecting unusual odors early (may be symptomatic of infection)	Acting for
	3. Compensating for hearing loss	
	Speaking clearly and loudly while facing person	Minimizing self-care limitation
	Utilizing feedback techniques to make sure person has heard and understood	Minimizing self-care limitation
	Initiating referral to ear, nose, and throat clinic	Acting for
	4. Maintaining good skin condition	
	Inspecting for rashes, reddened areas, and sores	Doing for
	Assisting with hygienic practices	Partially assisting
	Giving back rubs, changing person's position frequently, and keeping person's skin soft and dry	Doing for Partially assisting and minimizing self-care limitation
	5. Preventing falls	
	Supporting person who is ambulating or being transported	Partially assisting
	Maintaining muscle tone	Strengthening self-care capacity
	Keeping bed rails up and supporting person in wheelchair	Doing for
	Providing rest periods between activities	Strengthening self-care capacity and minimizing self-care limitation
	Placing frequently used objects within easy reach	Partially assisting
	6. Maintaining proper body alignment	
	Utilizing sandbags, trochanter rolls and pillows	Minimizing self-care limitation and partially assisting
	Supportive person's affected limb when it is lifted or moved	Partially assisting and minimizing self-care limitation
	7. Seeking safe living arrangements in preparation for person's discharge	
	Evaluating patient's preferences, capacities, and limitations, in order to suggest appropriate arrangements	Acting for and partially assisting
	Initiating referral to social worker	Acting for
BEING NORMAL		
	1. Improving physical limitations where possible	

UNIVERSAL REQUIREMENT	RELATED NURSING ACTION	TYPE OF ACTION
	Assisting with reeducation for ambulation	Partially assisting and strengthening self-care capacity
	Exercising body parts to maintain function	Partially assisting and minimizing self-care limitation
	Encouraging patient to consume an adequate diet	Strengthening self-care capacity
	Initiating referral for audiometric examination to explore utility of hearing aid	Acting for Minimizing self-care limitation
	Initiating ophthalmology referral to explore utility of corrective lenses	Acting for and minimizing self-care limitation
	2. Maintaining familiar components of life-style	
	Adjusting hospital routine to person's home routine as much as possible	Acting for and minimizing self-care limitation
	Encouraging person to wear own clothing	Minimizing self-care limitation
	Providing person with personal items from home, pillow, blanket, photographs, and tea cup	Minimizing self-care limitation
	Providing leisure activities person is accustomed to	Minimizing self-care limitation and strengthening self-care capacity
	3. Promoting active participation	
	Providing person with opportunities to make own decisions whenever possible	Strengthening self-care capacity
	Involving person in care	Strengthening self-care capacity
	Stimulating and encouraging communication	Strengthening self-care capacity

The above principles of gerontological nursing practice are basic to the nursing care of older persons. These principles lay a solid foundation upon which specialized nursing actions for the aged can be developed. A truly professional gerontological nurse demonstrates a distinct and effective blend of cognitive and technical skills to achieve excellence in gerontological care. Only by utilizing sound valid data can nurses surpass the technical level of caring for the aged, and attain the realm of intelligent care of the aged.

REFERENCES

Orem, Dorothea E. *Nursing: Concepts of Practice.* McGraw-Hill, New York, 1971.

Yura, Helen, and **Walsh, Mary B.** *The Nursing Process: Assessing, Planning, Implementing and Evaluating,* 2nd ed. Prentice-Hall (Appleton), Englewood Cliffs, N.J., 1973.

6

THE NURSING PROCESS AND THE AGED

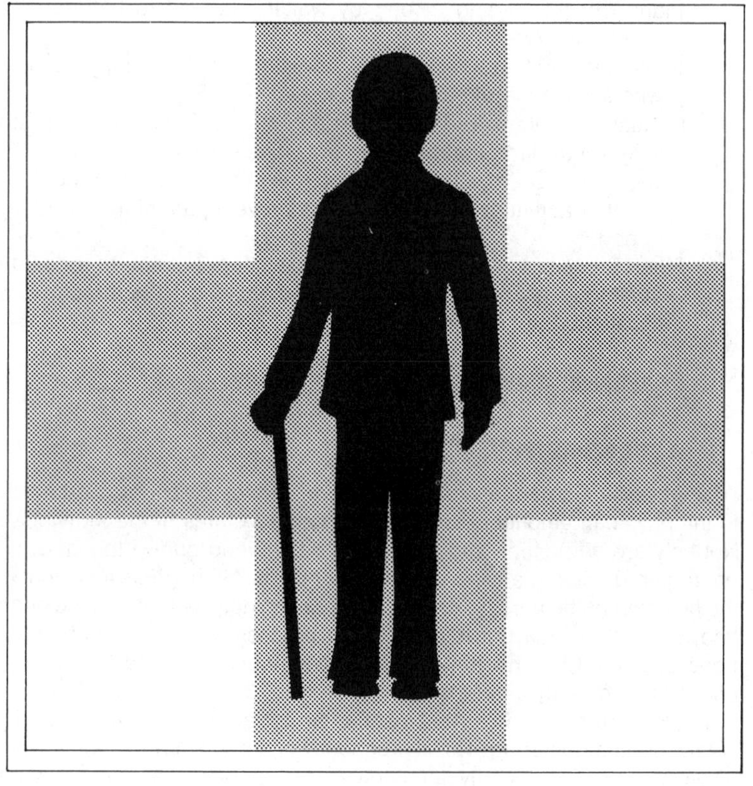

As mentioned in the previous chapter, the nursing process requires an orderly, organized, and intentional approach to the delivery of nursing services. When knowledge regarding both normal aging and the specific differences of aged persons is added, the result is a complete system of nursing care for aged individuals. There are four phases of the nursing process: (1) an initial assessment, (2) specific planning to compensate for limitations and to maintain and strengthen the capacities of the individual, (3) implementation of these plans through a variety of selected nursing actions, and (4) evaluation of the effectiveness of these actions in achieving the desired outcomes. This evaluation, in turn, provides feedback that may stimulate a reassessment and establishment of new plans, and so on. This sequence would apply to one isolated problem as follows:

Assessment: Patient frequently urinates in bed due to short time interval between feeling the sensation to void and actual voiding.
Plan: Prevent voiding in bed by walking patient to bathroom at regular intervals.
Implementation: Patient is walked to bathroom q 2h during daytime with assistance of nurse.
Evaluation: Patient did not void in bed entire day but was too fatigued to participate in other activities.
Assessment: Q 2h walks to bathroom expend the energy required for other activities, although it does prevent patient from voiding in bed.
Plan: Prevent voiding in bed by assisting patient to bedside commode q 2h during daytime and walking to bathroom with assistance of nurse once per shift.

Each phase is described in the sections that follow.

ASSESSMENT

Assessment pertains to the collection and review of data pertaining to the physical, emotional, and socioeconomic status of the individual. Not only are capacities and limitations determined during this activity, but required nursing actions are also identified. Although assessment is the first step of the nursing process, it is not an activity that is done once and forgotten. Instead, it is an ongoing process, whereby all observations and interactions are utilized to collect new data, recognize changes, and analyze needs.

Many nurses view assessment as an isolated nurse-client activity solely for data gathering. This is frequently observed during a clinic visit when a patient is initially interviewed or completes a questionnaire pertaining to health status. In institutional settings, the nurse may plan the first encounter with the patient and his or her family to include an interview and examination for baseline data collection. It is perfectly appropriate for this activity to be a separate one in some situations. However, it is also possible to integrate data collection into other activities, such as during an informal conversation at mealtime or during a back rub. Nurses who have an understanding of the type of essential information necessary for comprehensive and individualized care planning and delivery may know how to integrate the physical, emotional, and socioeconomic assessment with other contacts with individuals and their families, documenting their assessment later. Some nurses, due to individual preference or inexperience, may be inclined to use a nursing-history tool to guide them in their information gathering. Regardless of the approach, it is essential that standard, comprehensive, baseline data be collected and documented for all aged individuals, and that assessment be viewed as a dynamic process, rather than limited to an initial activity of the nurse-client relationship.

Of the various skills required in assessment, good communication is especially important if honest and thorough information is to result. The nurse must communicate the reason the information is being sought, how it will be used, and an assurance it will be managed discreetly and respectfully. Many persons have had limited experience in being interviewed by service agencies, and many may be reluctant to share their personal problems of financial status with "strangers." Time must be provided for the establishment of trust in the nurse in order for the individual to be willing to share information. In addition, language may have to be adjusted to meet the needs of the particular individual. For instance, a person may respond negatively when asked Do you ever expectorate in the morning? But when asked Do you ever bring up phlegm in the morning? or Do you ever have to cough or spit up in the morning? the person may better understand the question and respond accurately. Using common jargon can help the nurse obtain more accurate information. Many patients who do not understand the term *diuretics* know what is meant by *fluid pills*.

Patients may think of medications as being only those drugs prescribed by a physician and not contribute the information that they regularly take aspirin, antacids, or laxatives when asked if they're taking any medications. Identifying such lack of understanding or misconceptions during the assessment has important implications for care planning and delivery, especially in terms of the educational needs of the patient. The manner in which a question is presented can influence the accuracy of the response. Asking Do you ever have to use a laxative ? may elicit a negative response because the person may believe it is wrong to do so and be unwilling to make the admission. Rephrasing the question to How often do you have to use a laxative? may convey understanding that the person may have to occasionally use a laxative and make him or her more willing to give an honest response.

When asked for their age, elderly persons may forget whether they are 77 or 79 years old; but if asked for their birthdate, they may rapidly recall the exact day, month, and year. Instead of inaccurately labeling the person as confused, the nurse might make an assessment that memory for recent events is poor, and seek more information related to that characteristic. Emotional and neurological status, attention span, language barriers, and hearing, vision, and speech deficits can also be detected through the keen use of communication skills during the assessment process. The interview with the aged individual is complemented by, or sometimes, by necessity, substituted for, an interview with the individual's family. This not only creates a potential for further collection of information, but also actively involves the family in the person's care.

Physical examination of the aged person is part of the assessment process and, like the interview, is either separately defined or integrated into other care activities. The physical assessment by a nurse serves a different purpose from the physical examination by a physician. The physician may diagnose a specific degree of hearing loss. The nurse *recognizes* this loss and attempts to *assess* how this loss is managed by the patient and the way the care may have to be altered to compensate for this limitation. Likewise, the physician may be concerned with identifying the extent of disability caused by arthritic fingers. The nurse would be more concerned with identifying relief and supportive measures. The focus of the nurse's physical examination is to recognize capacities, limitations, and pathology, and also to establish how these factors will be managed, to analyze the effects of these factors on the individual's ability to fulfill universal self-care demands, and to identify nursing actions which may be required.

A nursing-history tool may be used as a guide to standardized and comprehensive data collection, and as a source for documenting the assessment in a consistent, organized, and easy manner. The tool utilized will vary to meet the needs of the individual agency and should be flexible enough to meet the unique needs of the client and the nurse in a particular situation. Some baseline data, beneficial to incorporate in the assessment may include the items discussed below.

***1.* Profile of patient.** Identifying information includes full name, sex, race, religion (including name and location of church, synagogue, etc.), date of birth, address, telephone number, languages spoken, and name of spouse or nearest contact person.

2. Profile of family. If the spouse is living, information should be obtained pertaining to his or her full name, date of birth, address, telephone number, occupation, and length of marriage. An assessment of the spouse's health status is also beneficial, not only in order to identify problems, but to evaluate the ability of this person to assist the patient should the need arise. If the spouse is deceased, it is useful to know the date and cause of death. Sometimes through exploring this information with the patient, unresolved grief, guilt, or other feelings are surfaced.

Names and addresses of children add helpful information to the record as do their ages and health status, which provide a realistic estimate of their ability to assist the patient. It is becoming increasingly common to find such situations as an ill 85-year-old whose only source of assistance with daily home care is an ill 68-year-old. (One in five aged individuals has a child over the age of 65!) Deceased children and the date and cause of death should also be explored, and profiles of any other members of the household should be obtained. Just because the aged person may have no living family does not mean that friends or boarders in the household aren't providing a strong support system.

The relationship with family members is useful to know. There are situations in which an elderly person would prefer living in a shabby room alone rather than in the new home of a daughter with whom he or she never got along. Likewise, if an elderly couple have had a satisfying marriage and have never been apart, the health team could make sure that when they are admitted to a nursing home, it is one in which they can share the same room and have their relationship respected.

3. Occupational profile. If the individual is employed, information pertaining to the type of work, length of time at the present job, and working hours should be collected. The type of work can give clues to occupationally caused illnesses and indicate the type of diversionary activities the patient may prefer. It may be useful to explore the individual's reason for working if he or she is of retirement age. Continuing employment due to the satisfactions obtained from the job and a sincere desire in wanting to remain employed will have different implications from disliking one's job but having to work due to financial necessity. If the person is unemployed or retired, it is useful to evaluate the reason. Being unemployed because one desires to retire and travel has different implications from unwanted mandatory retirement or being unemployed due to poor health. The length of unemployed time and the means of income are valuable to know and may help the nurse assess factors such as interests and financial concerns. Here again, the nurse should question the patient as to his or her occupational history.

***4.* Home profile.** The patient's home environment is essential to know, although this information is often overlooked by those who provide care for the aged in institutional settings. The home profile should include the type of dwelling, number of levels, location of bathroom and patient's bedroom, stairs climbed in an average day, location of nearest neighbor, availability of a telephone, type of community, safety hazards, and whether the person owns or rents the home. The capacity of the individual to fulfill responsibilities in the home should also be explored.

The nursing history should reflect the presence of pets in the household. This may appear to be an insignificant consideration, but to the aged individual a pet may provide an important source of satisfaction and companionship. Some aged individuals may resist an emergency hospitalization or new housing due to their concern about the welfare of their pet. Knowledge pertaining to the cause of certain health problems, allergies for instance, may also be revealed by collecting information regarding pets.

5. Economic profile. Various sources and amounts of income and whether the person is receiving all the benefits to which he or she is entitled should be ascertained. Sometimes the elderly aren't aware that they may qualify for certain benefits, or they may have been unable to understand the application process for these benefits. The monthly income should be balanced with the monthly expenses to evaluate the capacity of the individual to meet financial obligations. While obtaining this data, the nurse may learn that the aged person is eating a poor quality diet due to budget constraints or that he or she is fearful of losing a home through inability to pay the annual property tax. Clues to specific financial concerns should be sought while questioning the person about his or her financial status.

6. Health insurance. The type of health insurance and policy number is basic information. If there is no insurance, measures can be taken to enroll the person in a program suited for his or her needs. The lack of health insurance sometimes discourages people from seeking health care; it can be a source of stress should hospitalization be required.

***7.* Currently used health and social resources.** The names and locations of other physicians, social workers, visiting nurses, public health nurses, clinics, and hospitals involved with the individual should be recorded. They can provide additional insight into the patient and should be kept informed to promote continuity of care. It is important to obtain information and avoid duplication regarding community resources utilized by the patient, such as home health aides or delivered meals.

***8.* Social and leisure activities.** Knowing what organizations the person belongs to and his or her hobbies and interests helps guide the nurse in planning the care and also indicates the person's health status, energy level, and opportunities for socialization. Sometimes organizations to which the individual has belonged will provide visits and continued communication, should the individual be hospitalized or enter a nursing home.

***9.* Health history.** The health history of an aged person need not explore every childhood disease or minor health problem that has ever existed, unless this information is significant to the current health status. Information pertaining to a family tendency toward stroke, diabetes, heart disease, cancer, or hypertension may be more relevant. Health problems of current concern, or for which treatment is being obtained, should be recorded. A history of diabetes, hypertension, tuberculosis, and cancer should be indicated, even if the patient states that he or she is free of the disease at present. Major hospitalizations, surgeries, and fractures in the past may give insight into current problems and should be explored. Women should be questioned as to the number and course of pregnancies. Allergies to foods and other items and drug sensitivities should be recorded.

***10.* Current health status.** Current health problems should be recorded, and the patient's and family's knowledge and understanding of these problems should be ascertained. Perceptions regarding these problems should be indicated if significant—for example, the belief by an individual that his cancer was "caught" from his wife who recently died of the disease. Any limitations in functions or inability to perform the activities of daily living should be assessed, as well as the methods in which these problems are managed and coped with. Any particular appliance or prosthesis used in the management of health problems should be listed. The main concerns and goals of the patient and family in relation to the health status should be discussed and reflected in the assessment.

***11.* Medications.** The name and dosage of all medications which the older person is taking is vital information. The nurse should explore how and why the medication was obtained. The aged are as guilty as the young of self-prescription of medication! The time and method in which the medication is taken and the patient's understanding of the medication, its action, and its adverse effects should be indicated. Exploring this information with the individual will often give clues to errors in drug administration and drug related symptoms which he or she may be displaying. The nurse may also detect discrepancies. For example, a physician at one clinic may have prescribed a medication that combats the effect of a drug another physician has concurrently prescribed. The patient should be instructed to take all medications along when visiting a health facility or physician.

***12.* Physical status.** Assessment of physical status requires an examination of the person as well as an interview. Baseline values for vital signs should be established when the person is well in order to have comparative data available should the person's health status change. Although one of the vital signs may be severely altered in the aged, it may still fall within normal limits for the general adult population. For instance, normal body temperature in the aged may be as low as 95° F and a temperature of 98° F would be a severe elevation for that person, but it could be missed because it is a low normal for younger adults. Such a missed diagnosis can delay correction of the problem. The normal body temperature should be established, and the individual should be informed of his or her norm. Sometimes ancillary personnel who obtain a thermometer reading of 96° F in aged persons, believe there was an error in the way they performed the procedure, and record the temperature as 98.6° F to avoid "criticism" of their procedure. All nursing staff should understand that a lower body temperature in aged individuals can be the normal value for that person.

Unless the patient is unable to satisfactorily hold a thermometer in place sublingually, this should be the means of obtaining body temperature. Recent research indicates that for general assessment purposes, the most accurate recording of the body temperature is obtained by using the sublingual site. This site reflects temperature changes faster than the rectal site. Reduced blood flow to the lower bowel and the possible presence of feces may cause inaccurate rectal temperature readings. If the sublingual site cannot be used, the nurse can then use the axilla, if there is a stable and controlled environmental temperature. When no other site is possible or practical, a rectal temperature should then be obtained. Research indicates that an accurate oral reading is obtained by leaving the thermometer in place at least seven minutes. Rectal thermometers need only two minutes for an accurate reading in rooms of at least 72° F or greater, and three minutes in rooms under 72° F (Nichols and Kucha, 1972).

The rate, rhythm, and volume of the pulse should be noted during assessment of the older adult. The acceptable range for pulse rate is 50 to 100 beats per minute, although the elderly may occasionally have rates which fall beyond those boundaries. Irregularity of pulse rhythm is not uncommon in the aged, but it should be evaluated if the irregularity is due to digitalis toxicity, an electrolyte imbalance, or a disease process. A full, bounding pulse may occur in the presence of volume excess while a volume deficiency or electrolyte imbalance is demonstrated by a weak, thready pulse. The arteries of the aged may feel tortuous due to the loss of elasticity and smoothness with advancing age.

The rate, rhythm, and depth of the aged's respirations should be noted. The number of respirations may range within 14 to 18 per minute, although slower rates are not unusual in the aged. Irregularities of rhythm are not unusual either, and respirations similar to Cheyne-Stokes respirations may be evidenced during sleep. Depth of respirations is lessened as a result of reduced strength of the respiratory muscles and rigidity of the thoracic cage. An increase in respiratory rate and depth may indicate metabolic acidosis, while the opposite, accompanied by an irregular rhythm, occurs with metabolic alkalosis.

Increased peripheral resistance results in higher systolic and diastolic blood pressures in older individuals. Hypertensive levels in the aged are considered persistent elevations of 170 mmHg systolic and 95 mmHg diastolic, or greater. A shortening of the vertebral column also occurs with age and accompanies slight hip and knee flexion to produce a decreasing height. There is a tendency for weight gain in the fifth and sixth decades, which plateaus in the late sixth and seventh decades, and is followed by a gradual loss thereafter. Although the total body weight decreases in old age, there is an increase in the amount of body fat with age.

A urine sample should be evaluated as part of the individual's assessment. The color and clarity of the specimen should be noted, as well as the presence of any unusual characteristics. Due to the declining efficiency of the kidneys, several differences may be noted in the urine of the aged. A proteinuria of 1+ may result from decreased reabsorption from the filtrate and is usually of no diagnostic significance in the aged. An increased renal threshold for glucose may result in high blood glucose levels without evidence of glycosuria, decreasing the accuracy of urine testing for glucose. Older adults also have a lower specific gravity due to decreased ability to concentrate urine.

The entire surface of the body should be examined to assess the condition of the skin. Any skin breakage or wound should be described as to location and size. Specific measurements should be used; instead of describing a decubitus ulcer on the heel as being "small," give the exact measurement whenever possible in inches or centimeters. Rashes should also be distinctly described, and the location and characteristics of any discolored areas noted.

Hair should be described as to condition and amount. Whether the

TABLE 6-1: NORMAL RANGE OF JOINT MOTION FOR THE AGED

Joint	Range of Motion
Neck	Flexion, 45° Extension, 45° Rotation, 60° Laterat bend, 45°
Shoulder	Flexion, 150° Hyperextension, 30° Abduction (hand supine), 160° Abduction (hand prone), 110°
Elbow	Flexion, 160°
Wrist	Palmar flexion, 80° Dorsal flexion, 70° Ulnar flexion, 60° Radial flexion, 10° Rotation (internal and external), 90°
Thumb	Proximal phalange flexion, 70° Distal phalange flexion, 90°
Finger	Proximal phalange flexion, 90° Proximal phalange hyperextension 30° Middle phalange flexion, 120° Distal phalange flexion, 80°
Hip	Extension (lying prone), 5° Extension (standing), 30° Flexion (knee bent), 120° Flexion (knee straight), 90° Abduction, 35° Adduction, 30°
Knee	Flexion, 100° Hyperextension, 5°
Ankle	Dorsiflexion, 10° Plantar flexion, 40° Eversion, 25° Inversion, 35°
Great toe	Proximal phalange flexion, 35° Proximal phalange hyperextension, 75° Distal phalange flexion, 50°
Other toes	Proximal phalange flexion, 30° Proximal phalange hyperextension, 75° Middle phalange flexion, 80° Distal phalange flexion, 45°

hair is matted or well groomed may give clues to other problems, such as the inability to comb hair due to an immobile joint or a negative self-concept. Nails should be examined for breakage, discoloration, curving, and the presence of a fungal infection.

Assessment of mobility should consider not only individuals' ability to ambulate, but also the characteristics of their gait, the type of assistance required for ambulation, the length of time a person is able to ambulate without discomfort and fatigue, the ability to rise from a chair and toilet, and the ability to climb stairs. The capacity and limitation in regard to each factor should be described. The function of all limbs should be evaluated, with attention to the location and degree of any contracture, arthritis, paralysis, painful movement, and spasm. The nurse should attempt to identify the measures the older person employs to assist with or relieve any limitations in extremity function. It is also helpful to note which is the dominant hand of the individual. Table 6-1 shows the degrees of joint motion that are normal in aged individuals.

In regard to respiratory function, the older person should be questioned as to a history of orthopnea, dyspnea, shortness of breath, wheezing, asthma, coughing, and any other respiratory disturbance. The frequency of occurrence, precipitating factors, and the extent to which they limit the individual should be ascertained, as well as the measures used to assist with or relieve the problem. The present and past smoking history of the individual should be reviewed. A sputum specimen should be obtained and its characteristics noted. Circulatory function should be reviewed, and a history recorded of chest pain, tachycardia, edema, extremity cramps, palpitations, or any other symptom of poor cardiac function. The extent to which any problem limits the individual should be explored, as well as measures used to assist with or relieve the problem. The extremities should be examined for color, temperature, and equality of pulse. The presence of a pacemaker should be noted.

The nutritional status of the older person should be assessed by reviewing the quality and quantity of food and fluid intake. Food preferences, restrictions, and intolerances should be indicated, in addition to the usual meal pattern for the individual. Factors which cause and relieve indigestion, constipation, and diarrhea should be explored. Since poor dental status can restrict food intake and threaten nutritional status, part of the nutritional assessment should include an examination of teeth and/or dentures. Any adjustments that must be made for eating, such as nasogastric feedings or pureeing foods, should be made known.

Bladder function should be assessed with attention to the presence of nocturia, frequency, burning, urgency, incontinence, stress incontinence, and retention. The voiding pattern should be reviewed in regard to frequency and amount. The length of time any indwelling catheter or ostomy has been present should be recorded, and the technique of care should be described.

The frequency and characteristics of bowel movements should be ascertained, with consideration to any recent change in either. The frequency of occurrence and management of diarrhea and constipation should be explored. The presence of hemorrhoids, fecal incontinence, or an ostomy should be described in terms of length of time present and management.

Assessment of the older person's sensory status is vital and extremely beneficial to care delivery. The ability of the individual to hear regular sounds should be evaluated first. Can he or she hear a telephone ring or a door close? Does he or she understand all conversation? The ability to hear high-frequency sounds should then be evaluated; these sounds, which are most problematic for the aged, include the consonant sounds *f,z,s* and *sh*. To make sure lipreading isn't taking place, questions should be asked from the side of the person or from behind. The use of a hearing aid should be noted. Ears should be examined for cerumen impactions, not uncommon in the aged.

Visual capacities and limitations should be carefully reviewed, and the type, age, and source of corrective lenses should be noted as well as an assessment of night vision, peripheral vision, color discrimination, depth perception, and reading ability. The status of other senses is also important. Taste sensation can be evaluated by testing the individual's ability to differentiate among sweet, sour, salty, and bitter substances. Likewise, a variety of substances can be used in determining the individual's ability to detect different odors and temperatures. With the individual's eyes closed, the nurse can determine if the person can sense differences between hot and cold temperatures, sharp and dull sensations. Assessment of speech includes whether a speech is laryngeal or esophageal, or if aphasia exists. The location, degree, and type of any pain should be described with explanations of effective relief measures.

It is helpful to know rest and sleep patterns and the factors that interfere with or promote each. A thorough review of medications and other measures used to induce sleep may reveal other problems of which the nurse should be aware, such as alcohol or drug abuse or misuse. It should be remembered that more rest and less sleep is required by older people.

In assessing the reproductive systems of a woman, the date of her last gynecological examination should be obtained and she should be examined for the presence of any vaginal discharge, itching, lesions, breast masses, nipple discharge, and breast pain. (Older females have a more alkaline vaginal environment, predisposing them to more vaginal infections.) History of a mastectomy should be indicated, including the

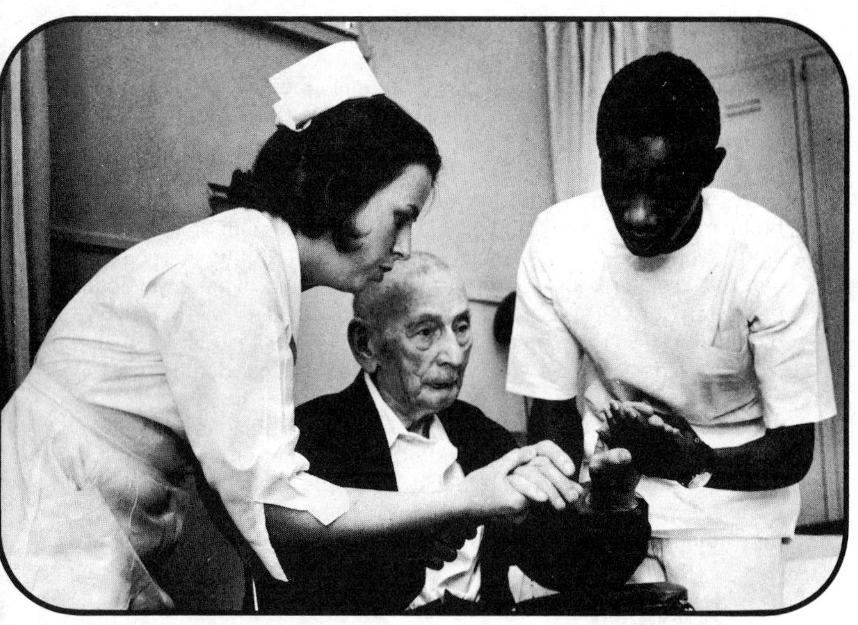

use of a prosthesis. Men should be evaluated for scrotal swelling, lesions, discharge, and impotency. A sexual history is useful to include. Attempts should be made to determine sexual interest, frequency of sexual activity, factors limiting sexual expression (psychosocial as well as physiological), attitude, and presence of dyspareunia.

***13.* Mental status.** Mental status can be evaluated throughout the assessment process by observing how alert the individual is, how well and how rapidly he or she responds to stimuli, and how lucidly he or she behaves. Orientation to person, place, and time can be determined indirectly throughout the interview or by questions such as Where do you live? What is the day and date? Why did you visit the hospital today? Who is your primary nurse? and Who is now president of the United States? Memory should also be assessed. *Old memory,* recall of events that have taken place in the past, can be assessed by asking questions such as What year did World War II end? This type of memory is usually good in the aged. *Short-term memory,* recall of events occurring up to 10 minutes after the information is introduced, can be assessed by techniques such as introducing yourself or giving a simple direction and immediately asking the individual to repeat what you said. The aged have more of a problem than the young have with this type of memory.

Long-term memory, events recalled at least 10 to 20 minutes after they have taken place, would be the ability to describe the medication schedule taught the previous day or to remember the day one visited a friend last week. This type of memory declines with age as well.

***14.* Emotional status.** Nursing observations and information from older persons and their family may indicate specific emotional problems. Attention should be paid to the presence of anxiety, depression, suspiciousness, fearfulness, emotional lability, nervous mannerisms, disinterest in self or life in general, and hyper or hypoactive behavior. Current stress factors in the individual's life should be explored along with coping mechanisms employed. It is also revealing to learn the older person's attitude and concerns about death.

Compilation of data. If the information obtained is compiled on a nursing history form, it will provide guidance and organization in data collection and ease in data retrieval. A sample of such a form is provided in the following pages (Table 6-2). The type of format will vary, depending on the type of information and the use to which it is put.

PLANNING

After the assessment phase, during which the nurse collects and analyzes quantitative and qualitative data pertaining to the individual, plans can be made for using nursing measures to alleviate the specific problems and needs that have become apparent. Since aged individuals may be experiencing a variety of physiological, psychological, and socioeconomic losses, some of their problems may require more immediate attention or be of greater concern than others. It is therefore necessary to establish *priorities* when planning for care, and if possible, to enlist the active participation of the individual for whom care is being planned. This approach respects the right of the individual to make decisions affecting his or her life. It also avoids conflicts that can arise from the differing opinions of individuals and nurses regarding priorities and avoids wasting human and material resources. The following case illustrates

> A visiting nurse was concerned about the housing situation of the 72-year-old woman she was caring for. The house this woman lived in was too large for the woman to clean adequately and consequently was unclean and cluttered. Leaking faucets, peeling wallpaper, and roaches added to the nurse's impression that it was necessary to seek new housing for the woman.
>
> The nurse worked diligently with the local housing authorities and social services department to locate an affordable apartment in a

TABLE 6-2: NURSING HISTORY FOR OLDER ADULTS

1. PROFILE OF PATIENT
Name ______ Sex ____ Race ____ Religion ____ Date of birth ______
Address ______ Telephone ______
Language spoken ______ Nearest contact person ______

2. PROFILE OF FAMILY

Spouse
____ Living
Health status:
Age:
Occupation:
____ Deceased
Year deceased:
Cause of death:
Others in household:

Children
____ Living
Names and addresses:
____ Deceased
Year deceased:
Cause of death:

3. OCCUPATIONAL PROFILE

____ Employed
Type of Work:
Length of employment
Working hours:
Sources of income:

____ Unemployed
Reason:
Length of unemployment:
Feelings about unemployment:
Previous occupations:

4. HOME PROFILE

____ Single dwelling
____ Multiple dwelling
____ Own
____ Rent
____ Telephone
____ Pets

Number of levels:
Location of bathroom:
Location of bedroom
Nearest neighbor:
Household responsibilities

5. ECONOMIC PROFILE
Sources of income:
Monthly income:
Monthly expenses:
Financial concerns:

6. HEALTH INSURANCE
____ Medicaid
____ Medicare
____ Blue Cross/Blue Shield
____ Other:
Policy number:

7. HEALTH AND SOCIAL RESOURCES CURRENTLY UTILIZED

____ Private M.D.
____ Hospital
____ Clinic

____ H.M.O.
____ Visiting Nurse
____ Public health nurse

____ Social worker
____ Meals on wheels
Other:

8. SOCIAL/LEISURE ACTIVITIES
Organization Membership:
Hobbies/Interests:

9. HEALTH HISTORY

____ Allergies
Food:
Drug:
Other:
____ Diabetes
____ Hypertension
____ Cancer

____ Hospitalizations:
____ Surgery:
____ Fractures:
____ Major health problems:

TABLE 6-2: NURSING HISTORY FOR OLDER ADULTS (Cont'd)

10. CURRENT HEALTH STATUS

Knowledge and Understanding of Health Problems:

Limitations of function or performance of ADL:

Management of Limitations:

Health goals:

11. MEDICATIONS

Name	Dosage	How and When Taken	How Obtained	Knowledge and Understanding of Medication
____	____	____	____	____
____	____	____	____	____
____	____	____	____	____
____	____	____	____	____
____	____	____	____	____
____	____	____	____	____

12. PHYSICAL STATUS

T ____ (A,O,R)
P ____
R ____

Height ____
Weight ____ (recent changes:)
BP ________ (sitting, standing, lying)

Urine:
S/A: ____
Specific gravity:
How obtained:
Characteristics:

Skin condition
____ Intact
____ Dry
____ Rash (describe)
____ Discoloration (describe)
____ Wounds (describe)

Hair condition:

Nail condition:

Mobility
____ Ambulatory
____ Nonambulatory
____ Ambulatory with assistance: (specify)
____ Able to rise from chair or toilet
____ Able to climb stairs

TABLE 6-2: NURSING HISTORY FOR OLDER ADULTS (Cont'd)

Extremity function

	Location	Degree of Limitation	Assistive/Relief Measures
Contracture			
Arthritis			
Painful movement			
Paralysis			
Spasm			
Amputation			
Dominant hand			

Respiration

	Precipitating Factors	Degree of Limitation	Assistive/Relief Measures
Orthopnea			
Dyspnea			
Shortness of breath			
Wheezing			
Asthma			
Coughing			

Sputum characteristics:
Smoking history: ____ Tracheostomy

Circulation

	Precipitating Factors	Degree of Limitation	Assistive/Relief Measures
Chest Pain			
Tachycardia			
Edema			
Cramping in extremities			

Equality of pulse, temperature, and color in extremities:

TABLE 6-2: NURSING HISTORY FOR OLDER ADULTS (Cont'd)

Nutrition

Teeth:	Dentures:	Chewing problems:
Number:	___ Partial—Complete	Swallowing problems:
Status:	Fit:	Feeding tube:

Date last dental exam:

	Precipitating Factors	Assistive/Relief Measures
Indigestion Constipation		
Diarrhea		

Usual meal pattern:	Fluid intake: Alcohol use:
Food preferences:	Food restrictions:

Bladder

___ Nocturia	___ Burning	___ Incontinence	___ Catheter
___ Frequency	___ Urgency	___ Stress incontinence	___ Ostomy

Voiding pattern:
Urine characteristics:

Bowel

___ Hemorrhoids	___ Pain during movement	___ Chronic constipation	___ Incontinence
___ Straining	___ Recent change in pattern	___ Chronic diarrhea	___ Ostomy

Stool

Bowel movement pattern:
Characteristics:

	Frequency of Use and Results Obtained	
Laxatives		
Suppositories		
Enemas		

Sensory status

	Degree of Limitation	Assistive/Relief Measures

TABLE 6-2: NURSING HISTORY FOR OLDER ADULTS (Cont'd)

Hearing
All sounds
High frequency

Vision
Full vision
Night vision
Peripheral vision
Reading
Color discrimination
Depth perception

Taste

Smell

Touch
Feels pressure and pain
Differentiates temperature
Speech
Pain

___ Hearing aid
Other sensory data:
___ Eyeglasses
___ Contact lenses
Date last vision exam:
Date last hearing exam:

Rest and sleep
___ Insomnia (describe)
___ Night restlessness
___ Night confusion
Medicines and alcohol used to induce sleep:
Factors interfering with rest:
Usual sleep and rest pattern:

Female reproductive factors:
___ Vaginal discharge
___ Itching
___ Lesions
___ Breast mass
___
Date last exam:
___ Nipple discharge
___ Breast pain
___ Mastectomy
(indicate right or left)
___ Prosthesis

Male reproductive factors
___ Scrotal swelling
___ Lesions
___ Discharge
___ Impotency

Sexual profile
___ Interest
___ Sexually active
___ Dyspareunia
___ Limitations:
Attitude:
Frequency:

---

13. MENTAL STATUS

___ Alert
___ Rapid response to verbal stimuli
___ Slow response to verbal stimuli
___ Confused
___ Stuporous
___ Comatose
Memory of recent events:

Orientation
___ Person
___ Place
___ Time
Attention span:
Memory of past events:

TABLE 6-2: NURSING HISTORY FOR OLDER ADULTS (Cont'd)

14. EMOTIONAL STATUS

____ Anxious	____ Hyperactive	____ Disinterest in life
____ Fearful	____ Hypoactive	____ Emotionally labile
____ Depressed	____ Suspicious	____ Suicidal

Self concept:	Current stress factors:

Attitude and concerns about death:

Other data:

Informant

____ Patient
____ Other (specify)

Signature of Nurse ______ Date

modern facility. She felt positive about her efforts to arrange for a housing improvement that would maintain the independence of the elderly woman in a community setting.

With excitement, the nurse shared her accomplishment with the old woman, anticipating that the woman would express delight at the improvement the new housing would bring to her life. Needless to say, the nurse was shocked to hear the woman refuse the new apartment. Didn't this woman understand? Was she confused? How could she deny an opportunity to leave her shabby house and move to a modern apartment?

If the participation of the elderly woman had been elicited initially in establishing plans for her housing problem, the nurse may have saved herself and others much time and energy and delivered more efficient and effective care. To this 72-year-old, maintaining the same house in which she had spent most of her lifetime was of utmost importance. The familiar furnishings, the memories, the yard in which her dog could romp, her friendly neighbor of long standing were all part of that old house. Of course, she didn't like the dirt and roaches either; but even though her limited efforts couldn't control the situation, maintaining her own home was worth the price. If the nurse had explored these factors with the elderly lady, and if they had jointly established priorities, perhaps the nurse's efforts could have focused on arranging a homemaker's service or exploring church groups or other local resources to obtain a handyman to make the necessary repairs at a nominal cost.

When developing plans, nurses should also enlist the cooperation of other professionals who will be involved in the care of the individual, such as the physician, social worker, physical therapist, nutritionist and paraprofessionals. Since older persons often have several interwoven problems, a multidisciplinary approach is essential. It is confusing to the older individual if each discipline exerts efforts toward different and sometimes conflicting goals. This reduces the therapeutic value of the care and is an ineffective and inefficient use of the time, energy, and human and financial resources of the various disciplines. Multidisciplinary interdependence, cooperation and respect are requirements for intelligent care of the aged.

The nurse should not only focus the care on management of existing problems, but also on the prevention of problems. Consideration is given to each of the universal self-care demands with this preventive planning, utilizing the data obtained from the nursing history. For example, from the assessment the nurse may have learned that the individual has occasional periods of depression which can lead to eating problems. Although there may be no current nutritional problem, planning can include arranging for the person to attend a senior citizen lunch program to provide an opportunity for socialization and enjoyment, in order to prevent poor eating habits from developing. Likewise, an older person's skin may be in fine intact condition when he or she is admitted to a hospital and placed on complete bedrest. To maintain this skin condition, the nurse would plan to turn the individual frequently, offering massages and using a bath oil when bathing the person.

In some agencies, plans are translated into nursing orders, which give specific direction to nursing actions by specifying exactly what is to be done, by whom, when, how, and where. Nursing orders provide for consistency and continuity in care through the selective identification and explicit description of particular nursing actions required for a given individual. In some agencies, nursing orders are sanctioned the way physician's orders have traditionally been sanctioned. Examples of nursing orders are:

Ambulate the patient from bedroom to dayroom q4h during daytime, with a staff member providing support on each side.
Reduce fluid intake to 300 ml between 6 P.M. and 6 A.M.
Instruct patient's daughter on wound-dressing technique and have her change dressings with nurse's assistance when she visits on Wednesdays.
Provide warm basin of water at bedside qAM in which patient can soak hands.
Wheel patient to room of Patient X at mealtime for a two-hour visit.
Arrange for staff member to assist patient's wife in taking patient outside in wheelchair this Sunday for two to three hours.

Call Social Service Department to arrange round-trip transportation and an escort for patient's clinic visit Friday at 10 A.M.

Obviously, the above nursing orders provide a greater understanding of what actions are required for the individual than vague directions, such as instruct family in care, encourage activity, provide socialization, prevent unnecessary incontinence.

Any staff member reading the nursing order knows exactly what the care planner had intended and also has a means of evaluating the effectiveness of the action. For example, if the nursing care plan stated "reduce fluid intake at bedtime," one care giver could interpret this as meaning only 100 ml after 9 P.M., another could interpret it as 500 ml after dinner, while to another it could mean no fluids after midnight. It would be difficult to evaluate the effectiveness of reducing fluid intake at bedtime to prevent nocturnal incontinence as there is no daily consistency or continuity of approaches. On the other hand, from the nursing order to "reduce fluid intake to 300 ml between 6 P.M. and 6 A.M.," the nurse can judge the effectiveness of the particular plan and identify exactly any change needed to result in the desired outcome.

Whether nursing orders or a nursing care plan form is used in a given agency, it is important to have plans in a written form and in a manner that is clearly understood and provides specific directions to anyone caring for the individual.

IMPLEMENTATION

Implementation involves action; it is the phase in which care planning is made operational. Whereas the assessment and planning phases of the nursing process require the use of more intellectual and interpersonal skills than technical ones, the implementation phase necessitates a proficient blend of all these skills. During the discussion of the focus of gerontological and geriatric nursing in the previous chapter, it was indicated that nursing actions are taken to (1) strengthen the individual's self-care capacities; (2) eliminate or minimize self-care limitations; and (3) provide direct care services by acting for, doing for, or partially assisting the individual when universal self-care or therapeutic demands cannot be independently fulfilled. When nurses are not directly responsible for all these actions, they can encourage and supervise any other individuals who perform them. The family or a neighbor or other personnel may be performing certain actions on behalf of the individual, and the nurse can provide guidance and coordinate actions. In such situations it is essential for the nurse to communicate to those responsible, providing significant data and relating the care plan with thoroughness.

Part of the nurse's responsibility will be to recognize when changes in the individual's capacities and limitations require a different provider of care for a given activity. Perhaps the patient has recovered from an illness and has restored energy and no longer requires an aide to assist with bathing; in this situation, the patient is the new care provider. On the other hand, if an aged individual becomes more limited in the ability for self-injection of insulin due to arthritic fingers, a visiting nurse may have to administer the insulin as the new care provider for this requirement. The nurse must be aware not only of the changing requirements for actions, but also of the changing requirements for persons to perform the actions.

EVALUATION

The fourth step in the nursing process is that of evaluation, whereby the degree to which plans and actions were effective in achieving desired outcomes is judged. If plans and actions continue to be effective and result in the desired outcomes, no change is necessitated. Some actions may have proven ineffective in achieving desired results, and specific alterations may be required in the care plan. Oversights or omissions may be detected, and additions may have to be made to the care plan. Thus, the evaluation process can result in no change, an alteration of the original plan, or an addition of new plans.

The individual for whom care is being provided, his family, and other care providers should be included in the evaluation process. It may be learned that although the action is bringing about the desired outcome, the action itself is not satisfactory to the individual or his care providers; perhaps a different action achieving the same result is necessary. For example, let us say the goal was to provide increased opportunities for socialization to an elderly widow living alone, and the actions planned included daily attendance at a senior citizen center. If the women has attended daily and developed friendships, the nurse can evaluate this action as effective in reaching the desired outcome. However, if the widow feels that visitng the center daily fatigues her to the extent that she is unable to perform her household responsibilities and is too expensive in terms of transportation costs, different plans to achieve a similar goal may be warranted. The nurse can alter the plan to provide a different means of transportation, to arrange for visits to the center on alternate days and for visitors to her home in between, and to obtain assistance for household chores. The nurse must not assume that a desired outcome has been necessarily achieved in the most preferable and beneficial manner to the individual.

Through evaluation, it is learned whether accurate, effective, and efficient planning and actions have taken place. Nursing audits are becoming an increasingly common means to evaluate nursing care. Several audit tools, such as the Slater Nursing Competencies Rating Scale and Phaneuf Audit are available to assist in this process. Increased research in the area of effective geriatric nursing practice is necessary to develop specific standards by which the application of the nursing process to aged individuals can be evaluated. Time, energy, and money can be saved by the aged person and the provider when useless plans and actions are recognized and replaced by those which will achieve the desired results.

7

ASSISTING THE AGED WITH UNIVERSAL SELF-CARE DEMANDS

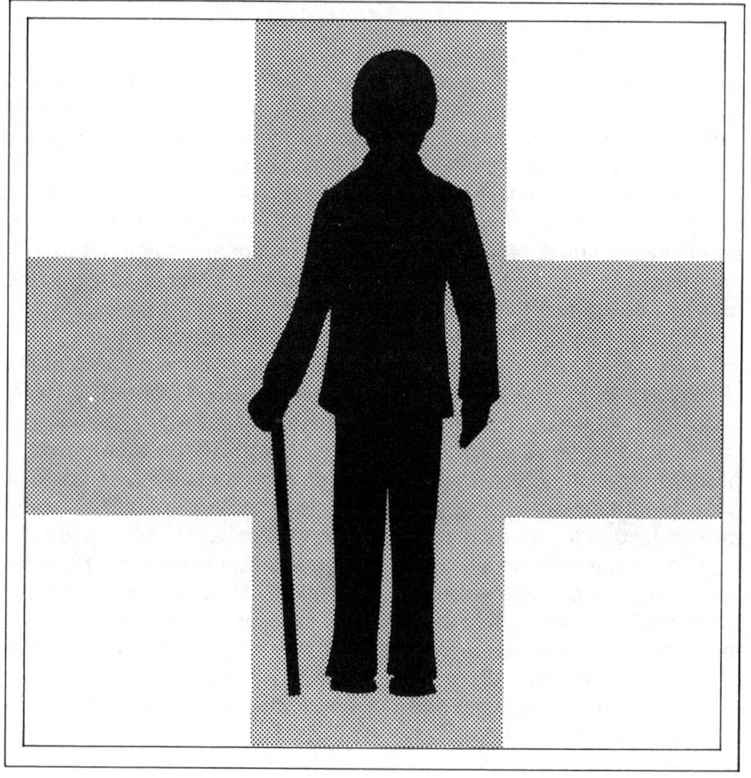

The nurse providing quality care for the older individual thinks and acts in a manner which demonstrates knowledge of (1) the unique psychobiosocial characteristics of aging; (2) the principles guiding gerontological and geriatric nursing practice; (3) the nursing process; and (4) expert clinical skills.

In this chapter, these areas of knowledge are combined to provide guidance in caring for aged persons. Each universal self-care demand is reviewed. The norms for fulfilling each demand and the limitations and potential capacities of aged individuals to do so are discussed. Measures which can assist the aged individual or the person providing care are presented.

AIR

The lungs lose elasticity with age, which results in an increased residual capacity. The alveoli are fewer in number and those which are present are of increased size. Bronchioles and alveolar ducts are of increased size as well. There is a loss of strength in the respiratory muscles and a rigidity of the thoracic muscles. Ciliary action is lessened with age also. These changes produce less respiratory activity, which gives an older person greater risk of developing upper respiratory infections. To prevent upper respiratory infections, respiratory activity should be promoted. Exercises, individually planned in view of the unique capacities and limitations of the individual, should be encouraged; these may benefit the total well-being of the individual, in addition to his respiratory function. Deep breathing exercises should be encouraged several times throughout the day with emphasis to forced expiration (Figure 7-1). The older person should attempt to cough and expectorate sputum following deep breathing exercises. Providing balloons or an inflatable toy to blow will assist in these exercises.

The aged should be advised to seek medical attention promptly, should any sign of a respiratory infection develop. Frequently, older people do not experience the chest pain associated with pneumonia to the same degree as younger adults, and they can be afebrile while possessing an infection. Thus, by the time symptoms become obvious, pneumonia can be in an advanced stage. The susceptibility of older people to drafts necessitates that indirect ventilation be utilized. Fibrositis, common in the aged, can be aggravated by chilling and drafts. Changes in the character of the sputum should also be reported, as it will be altered in the presence of certain disease processes. For example, the sputum will be tenacious, translucent, and grayish white with chronic obstructive pulmonary disease; purulent and foul smelling with a lung abscess or bronchiectasis; and red and frothy with pulmonary edema and left-sided heart failure.

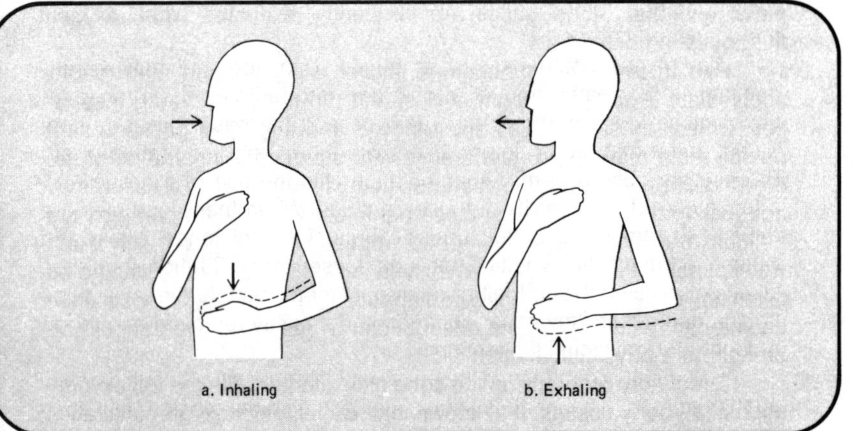

Figure 7-1. Breathing exercises for the aged should emphasize forced expiration: (a) With one hand below the ribs on the stomach and the other over the middle anterior chest, the individual should inhale to the count of one. The hand over the stomach should fall as the stomach moves downward; the hand over the chest should not move. (b) Exhale to the count of three. The hand over the stomach should rise as the stomach moves upward; the hand over the chest should not move.

The aged should be cautioned against periods of inactivity and bed rest due to the higher risk of upper respiratory infections. Some aged persons have been raised with the belief that when one is sick, one should go to bed. Family members with good intentions may encourage bed rest and inactivity for the aged person who is sick. Education by the nurse is required to teach the public the multitude of problems associated with immobility.

Approximately 80 percent of the aged have some degree of chronic obstructive pulmonary disease; thus, a higher amount of carbon dioxide retention can occur. The nurse should teach deep breathing exercises with forced expiration and encourage the person to do these exercises regularly. Carbon dioxide retention can cause adverse reactions to oxygen therapy, and the nurse should understand this and keenly observe for symptoms of carbon dioxide narcosis. These include confusion, muscle twitching, visual defects, profuse perspiration, hypotension, progressive degrees of circulatory failure, and cerebral depression, which may be displayed by increased sleeping to a deep comatose state. The nurse should be sure that oxygen is used prudently with the aged, that symptoms of carbon dioxide narcosis are recognized early, and that blood gases are frequently evaluated when oxygen therapy is indicated.

Hair in the nostrils becomes thicker with age and may readily accumulate a greater amount of dust and dirt particles during inspiration. Unless these particles are removed and the nasal passage kept patent, there may be an interference with the normal inspiration of air. Blowing the nose and mild manipulation with the use of a tissue may adequately rid the nostrils of these particles. When these particles are difficult to remove, a cotton tipped applicator, moistened with warm water or normal saline solution may help loosen them. Caution should be taken not to insert the cotton tipped applicator too far into the nose since trauma can result. Any nasal obstruction not easily removed should be brought to a physician's attention.

Circulatory problems in the aged may interfere with the full oxygenation of all body tissues. It is known that less efficient oxygen utilization is a factor in prolonged tachycardia in many aged persons. Efforts to promote good circulation should be encouraged. Activity, range of motion exercises, frequent change of position, warmth, skin massage, gentle friction during bathing, and the avoidance of circulation interferences (such as garters or tight fitting shoes), will assist in improving circulation. Hypotension should be prevented, as this reduces cerebral circulation and subsequently decreases the amount of oxygenation to that tissue; this is an important consideration for the older person on antihypertensive therapy. Aged persons and those who care for them should be aware that blood pressure normally rises with age, and what may be a hypertensive level for a 40-year-old may fall within a normal boundary for the older adult.

FOOD AND WATER

Painless, intact gums and teeth will promote the ingestion of a wider variety of food. The ability to meet nutritional requirements in old age is influenced by basic dental care throughout one's lifetime. Poor dental care, environmental influences, poor nutrition, and changes in the gingival tissue commonly contribute to severe tooth loss in older persons. After the third decade of life, periodontal disease becomes the first cause of tooth loss, and by age seventy, a majority of people have lost all their teeth. Obviously, a lifetime of poor dental care cannot be reversed. Geriatric dental problems should be prevented early in the individual's life. Geriatric dentistry is a young specialty, but unfortunately those who have access to this service do not always have the financial means to avail themselves of it.

Through education, the nurse should make the public aware of the importance of good, regular dental care and oral hygiene at all ages and that aging alone doesn't necessitate the loss of teeth. The use of a toothbrush is more effective in improving gingival tissues and removing soft debris from the teeth than are swabs or other soft devices. However, care should be taken not to traumatize the tissues, as they are more sensitive in the aged and easily prone to irritation. Dental problems should be readily corrected as they can affect virtually every system of the body. Loose teeth should be extracted as they can possibly be aspirated and cause a lung abscess.

Many aged persons believe that having dentures eliminates the necessity for dental care. The nurse should correct this misconception and encourage continued dental care for the individual with dentures. Lesions, infections and other diseases can be detected by the dentist and can lead to the prevention of serious complications. Also, changes in tissue structure may have affected the fit of the dentures and necessitate a readjustment. Poor fitting dentures need not always be replaced; sometimes they can be lined to ensure a proper fit. This should be made known to the older person who may resist correction out of concern for the expense involved. Most importantly, dentures should be used and not kept in a pocket or dresser drawer! Wearing dentures will allow proper chewing and may encourage including a wider variety of foods in the diet.

A poor appetite resulting from decreased taste sensation can also have adverse effects on the aged's nutritional status. Taste receptors are lost with age due to atrophy of the taste buds, chronic irritation, or general wearing out. The receptors on the tip of the tongue lose the most sensation, and these include the taste receptors for sweet and salt. The taste buds for bitter and sour tastes remain which make old people think most foods taste bitter. Those involved with the aged should recognize this factor and understand the reason why an older person may add seemingly excessive amounts of salt and sugar to their food. These taste deficiencies compound the difficulties in adjusting to a limited sodium or sugar diet, which is so frequently prescribed for the aged. The use of salt and sugar substitutes and other flavoring, such as lemon, should be considered to compensate for this taste limitation. Special efforts should be made to serve food attractively, and the use of wine to stimulate the appetite may prove beneficial.

Indigestion and food intolerance are common in the aged due to decreased stomach motility, less gastric secretion, and a slower emptying time. The older person frequently attempts to manage these problems by using antacids or limiting food intake—both potentially predisposing the person to other risks. Other means to manage these problems should first be explored. Several smaller meals may help reduce indigestion and promote a regular blood glucose level throughout the day, from which various benefits may also be realized. Fried foods may be replaced by broiled, boiled, or baked ones. If an intolerance to a particular food exists, substitution with a tolerable food of equal nutritional value should be made. Sitting in a high Fowler's position will increase the size of the abdominal and thoracic cavities, provide more room for the stomach, and facilitate swallowing and digestion. Adequate fluid intake and activity will also promote digestion.

Constipation is a common problem among the aged due to slower peristalsis, inactivity, and less bulk and fluid in the diet. If food intake is reduced to relieve discomfort, this can threaten nutritional status. Laxatives, another relief measure, can result in diarrhea, which is also threatening to the aged's nutritional status. Constipation should be recognized as a frequent problem of the aged and preventive measures should be emphasized. Plenty of fluids, fruits, vegetables, and activity should be encouraged, as should providing regular and adequate time allowances for a bowel movement. Laxatives should be considered after other measures have proven ineffective, and then should be used with discretion. Mineral oil should not be used by the aged, as the fat soluble vitamins A, D, and E can dissolve in and be excreted with this substance, producing deficiencies of these vitamins.

Since malnourishment is a potential threat to the aged, it should be carefully observed for. The variety of factors contributing to this problem include decreased taste and smell sensations for food; reduced mastication capability; slower peristalsis; decreased hunger contractions; reduced gastric acid secretion, causing poor absorption of nutrients and minerals; and less absorption of nutrients due to reduced intestinal blood flow and fewer cells on the absorbing surface of the intestines. Socioeconomic factors are commonly responsible for malnourishment in the aged as well. The appearance of the aged may be misleading and cause a malnourished state to be undetected. An aged person who appears obese due to the presence of increased amounts of adipose tissue can actually be malnourished.

Malnourishment in the aged may be first demonstrated through symptoms of mental confusion, easily judged as senility and mistakenly treated as a separate problem. The nurse should carefully explore the quality as well as the quantity of food intake and engage in diet instruction as needed. The ability of the person to market and to purchase and prepare foods should be examined to assess the need for food stamps, delivered meals, or the service of a home health aide. Participation in a senior citizen lunch program or the arrangement of a mealtime visitor can eliminate poor eating habits resulting from social isolation. A review of the individual's budget may reflect the need for financial assistance to provide adequate money for food expenses.

The diet of the aged should reflect a *lower quantity* and *higher quality* of food (Figure 7-2). Less carbohydrates and fats are required in

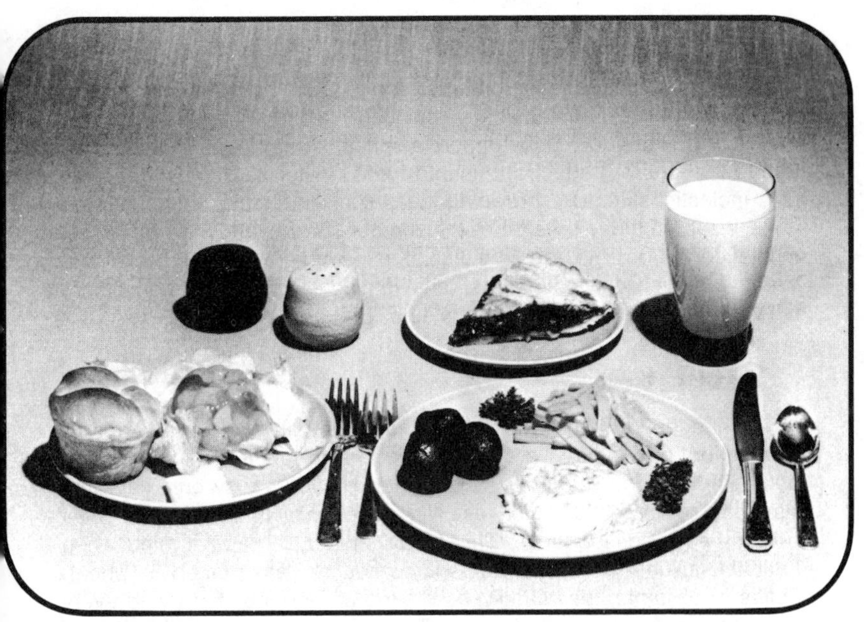

Figure 7-2. The diet of the aged should reflect a lower quantity and higher quality of food. (U.S. Dept. of Agriculture)

the diets of older adults. The decreased ability of the older person to maintain a regular blood glucose level emphasizes the need for a reduced carbohydrate intake. Sometimes, a high carbohydrate diet stimulates an abnormally high release of insulin which in turn causes hypoglycemia. (Here again, mental confusion may be the symptom presented.) At least a gram of protein per kilogram of body weight is necessary for the renewal of body protein and protoplasm, and for the maintenance of enzyme systems. Several protein supplements are available commercially and may be useful additives to the elderly's diet. Although the ability to absorb calcium decreases with age, calcium is still required in the diet to maintain a healthy musculoskeletal system as well as to promote the proper functioning of the body's blood clotting mechanisms. Unless other problems dictate differently, older women should have approximately 1600 calories, and older men, 2200 calories in a well-balanced daily diet.

The fluid consumption of older adults should range between 2500 and 3000 ml daily. The aged's daily fluid intake should be carefully evaluated to ascertain if this requirement is being met. Lack of motivation, avoidance of nocturia and frequency of urination, fear of incontinence, and inability to independently obtain or drink fluids are among the factors which could restrict fluid consumption. This fluid restriction can not only predispose the older person to infection, constipation, and decreased bladder distensibility, but can lead to a serious fluid and electrolyte imbalance. Dehydration, a serious threat to the older person due to the already reduced amount of body water, is demonstrated by dry, inelastic skin, dry brown tongue, sunken cheeks, concentrated urine, elevated blood urea (above 60 mg per 100 ml), and in some cases, mental confusion. The aged are also affected more by overhydration due to decreased cardiovascular and renal function—a consideration if there is ever a therapeutic need for intravenous fluids.

EXCRETION

Changes in the urinary tract with age may give rise to a variety of elimination problems. One of the great annoyances results from a decreased bladder capacity. Some aged bladders may only have the capacity to hold 200 ml or less, and frequency is common in older persons as a consequence. This factor should be kept in mind when individuals, unable to independently ambulate, are placed in wheelchairs. If possible, they should be offered an opportunity to void every two hours to prevent incontinence. Trips and activities should also be planned to allow for bathroom breaks at frequent intervals. Not only do older people find more frequent voiding necessary throughout the day, but night frequency may pose a bothersome problem as well. Often, kidney circulation may be decreased when the aged individual is in an upright position. When the recumbent position is assumed, circulation improves, promoting kidney function. Thus, voiding may be required a few hours after the individual lies down, promoting nocturia.

With the increased light-perception threshold making night vision difficult, nocturia could predispose the aged individual to accidents and threaten safety. Night-lights should be present to improve visibility during trips to the bathroom, and any clutter or environmental hazards which could promote a fall should be removed. Reduced fluids several hours prior to bedtime may lessen episodes of nocturia; if several episodes of nocturia continue to occur nightly, the person may need medical evaluation to ensure that no urinary tract problem exists. The aged and those caring for them should be aware that the longer-acting diuretics, such as the thiazides, even when administered in the morning, can cause nocturia.

Bladder muscles weaken with age which may promote retention of large volumes of urine. Women may experience retention from a fecal impaction, and men from prostatic hypertrophy, which is present to some degree in most older males. Symptoms of retention include urinary frequency, straining, dribbling, a palpable bladder, and a feeling by the individual that the bladder has not been emptied. This retention may predispose the older person to the risk of developing a urinary tract infection. Good fluid intake and efforts to enhance voiding should be emphasized. Attempts to tighten the muscles through contraction exercises, and mild massage over the bladder area may assist in preventing urinary retention. Sphincter control may be improved by exercises such as tightening the perineum muscles and stopping the urine flow midstream when voiding.

The efficiency of the kidneys in filtration functions decreases with age, an important factor in the elimination of drugs. The nurse should look for signs of adverse drug reactions resulting from an accumulation of toxic levels of the medication. Higher blood urea nitrogen levels may result from reduced renal function, causing lethargy, mental confusion, headache, drowsiness, and several other symptoms. Decreased tubular function may cause problems in the concentration of urine; the maximum specific gravity at 80 years of age has been shown to be 1.024 while the maximum for younger ages is 1.032. Decreased reabsorption from the filtrate makes a proteinuria of 1.0 usually of no diagnostic significance. The renal threshold for glucose is increased, a serious concern since an older person may then be hyperglycemic without evidence of glycosuria. False negatives in diabetic urine testing can occur for this reason. Urine screening for the presence of a urinary tract infection may also produce false negatives, as it may exist without evidence of proteinuria.

Bowel function is often a major concern of the aged, many of whom were raised with the belief that anything but a daily bowel movement is abnormal. Slower peristalsis, inactivity, reduced food and fluid intake, and the ingestion of less bulk foods are frequently responsible for constipation in the aged. Decreased sensory perception may cause the signal for bowel elimination to go unnoticed and promote constipation.

Laxative abuse as a reaction to constipation is common in the aged, and the habitual use of laxatives should be discouraged. Magnesia based preparations can reduce the already reduced amount of gastric acids, and the problem of vitamin depletion from the use of mineral oil has already been mentioned. There is the serious risk that the use of laxatives and enemas can predispose the older person to dehydration. Education is necessary to help the aged, and those providing care for them, understand that daily bowel elimination is not necessary.

A good fluid intake, a diet rich in fruits and vegetables, activity, and the establishment of a regular time for bowel elimination can be beneficial in maintaining a regular elimination pattern. As there is a tendency in the aged for incomplete emptying of the bowel at one time, time should be provided for full emptying, and for repeated attempts at subsequent times. Those caring for the older person should understand that there may be a need for the aged to have a bowel movement one-half to one hour after the initial movement. Sometimes, an older person's request to be taken to the bathroom or to have a bedpan for a bowel movement just after he has had one is viewed as an unnecessary demand and ignored; it is then wondered why fecal incontinence has occurred. It is useful for the aged to attempt to have a bowel movement following breakfast, as the morning activity following a period of rest and the ingestion of food and fluid stimulate peristalsis. Suppositories may occasionally be necessary to stimulate elimination, and they should be administered one-half hour before bowel elimination is desired. Fecal softeners are commonly prescribed to promote elimination in the aged.

Fecal impaction may occur as a result of constipation. Preventive measures to avoid constipation are the best approach to this problem. Observation of the frequency and character of bowel movements may indicate the development of fecal impaction; a defecation record is a must for the older person in a hospital or nursing home. Symptoms to note include distended rectum, abdominal and rectal discomfort, oozing of fecal material around the impaction (often mistaken as diarrhea), and palpation of a hard fecal mass during digital examination of the rectum. This problem should receive the attention of a health professional and be immediately corrected. Removal of fecal impactions should be attempted with care. Sometimes an oil retention enema will soften the impaction and facilitate its passage through the rectum. If this initial procedure is not effective, it may be essential to break up the impaction with a lubricated gloved finger. Inserting 60 ml of hydrogen peroxide prior to the digital attempt at removal will sometimes assist in breaking the impaction.

Itching and discomfort around the rectum may occur as a result of poor hygienic practices or dryness resulting from reduced secretions of the mucus membrane. Scratching and dryness can irritate the tissue and possibly lead to skin breaks and infection. Regular thorough cleansing with soap and water, followed by the application of a lubricant in small quantities, may prevent this problem. Coarse toilet tissue should always be avoided.

Flatulence, not uncommon in the aged, is caused by constipation, irregular bowel movements, certain foods, and poor neuromuscular control of the anal sphincter. Achieving a regular bowel pattern and avoiding flatus-producing foods may relieve this problem, as may the administration of certain medications intended for this purpose. Discomfort associated with the inability to expel flatus may occasionally occur in the aged. Increased activity may provide relief, as may a knee-chest position, if possible. A flatus bag consisting of a rectal tube with an attached plastic bag that prevents the entrance of air into the rectum can also be used (Figure 7-3).

Elimination of wastes through the skin must also be considered.

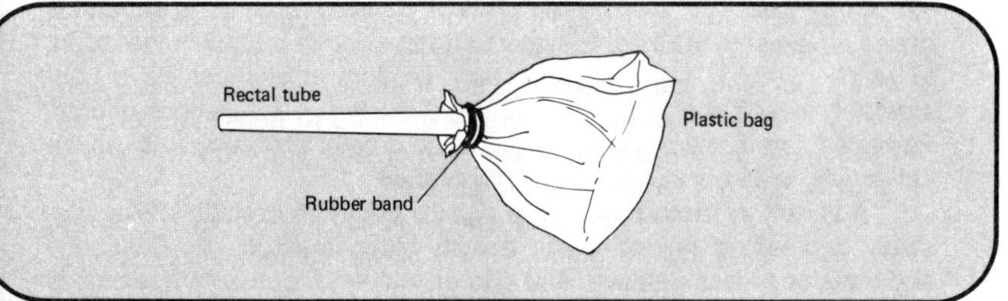

Figure 7-3. A flatus bag can be made by attaching a plastic bag to a rectal tube.

Perspiration and oil production is decreased with age, making less frequent bathing necessary for older adults. Reduced hydration and vascularity of the dermis make the skin less elastic and more delicate. Consequently, dryness, itching, and breakage of the skin can result from bathing too frequently. Unless another problem warrants a different pattern, complete bathing is not required more than every third or fourth day. Partial sponge baths to the face, axillae, and perineum on a daily basis should prevent odor and irritation. Neutral or superfatted soaps and bath oils should be used for bathing, followed by the application of skin softeners and moisterizers. Tub baths are not only effective for good cleansing, but enhance circulation and provide an opportunity to exercise stiff joints. (Safety considerations during tub baths will be discussed later in this chapter.) Showers may also be enjoyed by the aged and the use of shower chairs and other appliances may assist with this activity. The individual's unique bathing habits, schedule, and preferences should be appreciated and respected, as should the right to privacy and protection from exposure during bathing activities.

ACTIVITY

Through activity, many physical, psychological, and social benefits are gained. Physical activity aids respiratory, circulatory, digestive, excretory, and musculoskeletal functions. Mental activity maintains mental functioning and promotes a sense of normality. Multiple health problems, such as atherosclerosis, joint immobility, pneumonia, constipation, decubiti, and insomnia, can be avoided when an active state is maintained.

Maintaining a physically active state is a challenge not only for the aged, but for most of the adult population. Fewer and fewer occupations require hard physical labor, and those which still do usually utilize technological inventions to perform the more strenuous tasks. Television viewing and spectator sports are popular forms of recreation. Automobiles, taxicabs, and buses provide transportation to destinations once conveniently walked. Elevators and escalators minimize the extent to which climbing stairs is necessary. Modern appliances have considerably eased the physical energy expended in household chores. Perhaps future generations will have even greater problems with physical activity than our current aged population.

A variety of factors affect the aged's ability to be active. Progressively decreasing thyroid gland activity slows metabolism. Response and reaction time is delayed, and approximately 10 percent more time is required for impulses to travel along the pathways of the nervous system. Muscle fibers atrophy and decrease in number; fibrous tissue gradually replaces muscle tissue, evidenced in flabby and weak arm and leg muscles. Immobility, weakness, and pain of the joints often results from arthritis problems in aged persons. Hormonal changes contribute to thinning and weakening of the bones, and muscle cramping occurs more easily. Less blood is pumped by the heart due to decreases in cardiac function, causing the physical stress associated with activity to be poorly managed. Rising from a lying or sitting position may cause a 60 mm drop in blood pressure and lead to uncomfortable dizziness or fainting. Activity may be further reduced by urinary frequency or incontinence, sensory losses, social isolation, limited financial resources to participate in recreational activities, and inability to maintain pace with a hurried society.

Considering such interferences with activity, special efforts are demanded by the aged and those caring for them to maintain and promote an active state. Education should be provided to teach the public and care providers the importance of physical activity for the aged. Sometimes, families believe they are assisting their older family members by allowing them to be sedentary. Often, assisting with household responsibilities not only enhances good functioning of the body's systems, but promotes a sense of worth by providing an opportunity for productivity. Older people should be taught that although physical activity may be more uncomfortable or demanding than inactivity, additional health problems and disability may be spared in the future. Motivation is necessary at times to stimulate interest in physical activity. For instance, encouraging membership in a senior citizen's club can often motivate many other types of activity, such as providing the incentive to get out of bed, prepare a good breakfast, eat, bathe, dress, and travel to the club destination. Those involved with the aged can provide motivation by demonstrating a sincere interest in the individual's activities. Recognizing the person's housekeeping efforts, using his or her handmade gifts, commenting on a well-groomed appearance, and asking about the latest club activity are small but meaningful ways to reinforce the aged's positive efforts toward maintaining an active state.

Exercises are valuable at any age and are of much benefit to the elderly. Capitalizing on the regular activities of daily living is one means to provide exercise. During a shower or bath the older person can perform flexion and extention exercises under the guise of cleansing and drying various body parts. Dishwashing can be a means of exercising stiff finger joints with the assistance of warm water. Deep breathing and limb exercises can be incorporated into the period between awakening and rising from bed. Foot, leg, shoulder, and arm circling can be done while watching a regular television program. Often, a regular exercise schedule can be established and maintained with greater success when it is integrated into other routine activities since there is more tendency to forget or omit exercises when they are an isolated activity. Figure 7-4 depicts several exercises which may be beneficial to the aged.

Exercises should be paced throughout the day, and fatigue from exercising should be avoided because of chance of muscle pain and cramping. Morning exercises loosen stiff joints and muscles and encourage activity, while bedtime exercises promote relaxation and encourage sleep. If an older person is not accustomed to a great deal of physical activity, exercises should be introduced gradually and increased according to readiness. Some tachycardia may normally occur during the exercises and continue for several hours thereafter. Longer periods of time must be allowed for the older person to perform exercises, and rest periods should follow. Warm water and warm washcloths or towels wrapped around the joints may ease joint motion and facilitate exercising.

As the weaker, thinner, and more brittle bones of the elderly are more easily fractured, these persons should avoid forceful exercise of an immobilized joint, jumping and running exercises, and strenuous sports. Elderly persons with cardiac or respiratory problems should seek advice from their physician as to the amount and type of exercise best suited for their unique capacities and limitations. At times, the older person may need partial or complete assistance with exercises. The nurse or other care providers may find it helpful to remember these points:

1. All body joints should be exercised through their normal range of motion at least three times daily (see Table 6-1 in the previous chapter).
2. The joint and the distal limb should be supported during the exercise.
3. A joint should not be forced past the point of resistance or pain.

Figure 7-5 shows some equipment that can assist the nurse in moving and exercising the elderly.

Psychological activity is as vital to the total well-being of the elderly

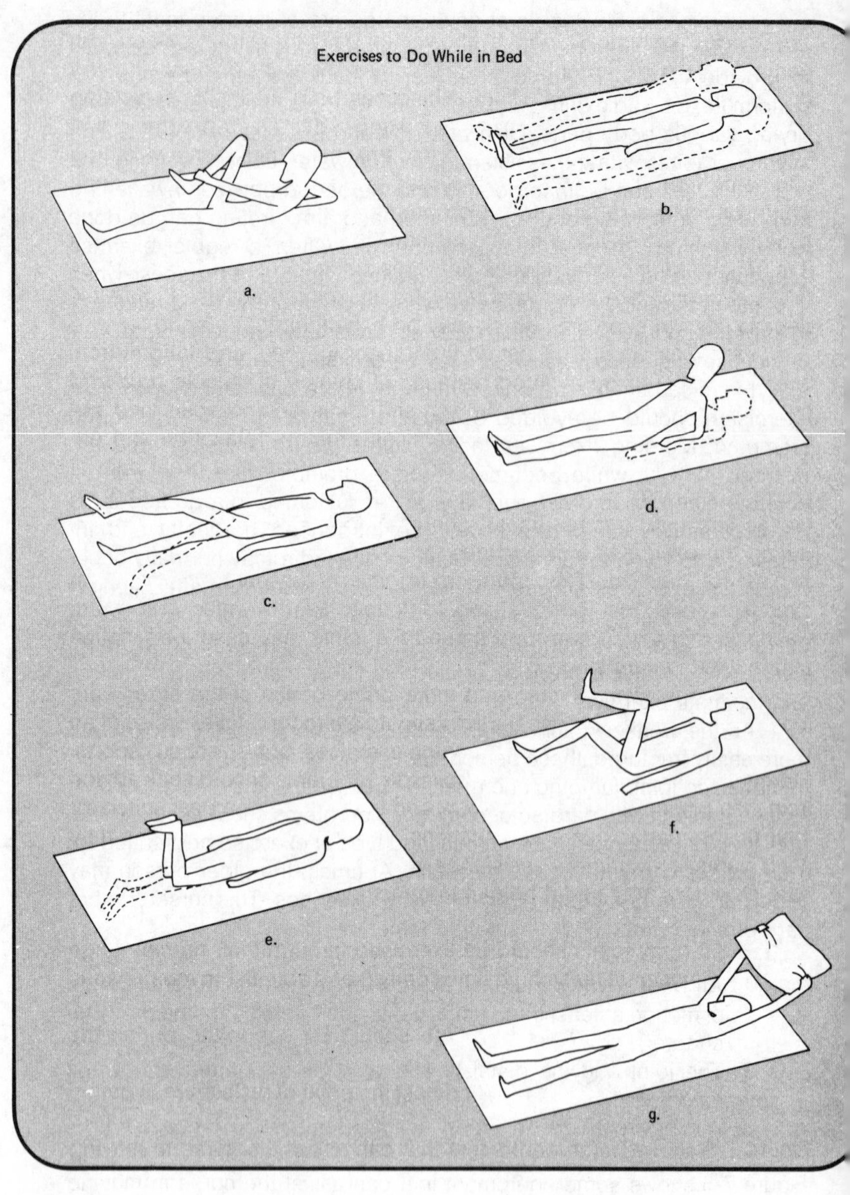
Exercises to Do While in Bed
a.
b.
c.
d.
e.
f.
g.

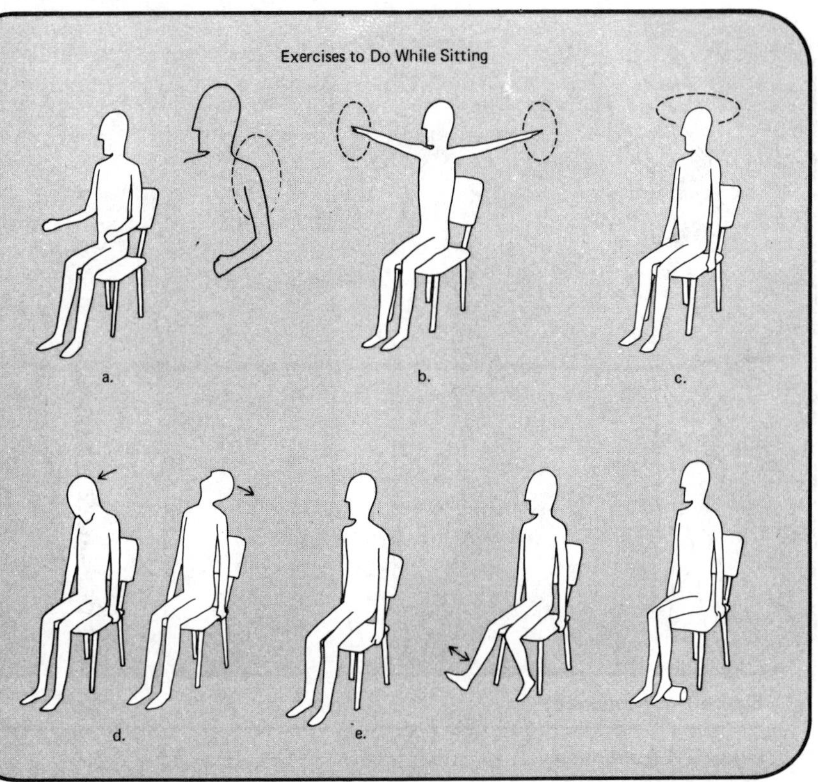

Figure 7-4. Exercises to do while in bed: (a) Flexing knee with opposite hand holding foot for assistance. (b) Rolling from side to side. (c) Scissorlike crossing of legs. (d) Raising chest. (e) Flexing knees while lying on abdomen. (f) Bicycling. (g) Lifting pillow over head with arms straight. Exercises to do while sitting: (a) Circling motion of shoulder joint with arm at side. (b) Circling arms. (c) Rotating head. (d) Flexing and extending neck. (e) Pushing up in chair with use of arms. (f) Kicking legs while sitting. (g) Rolling foot on tin can. All exercises can be built into regular activities. Exercises to do anytime: (a) Rolling pencil on hard surface. (b) Flexing fingers around pencil. (c) Exaggerating chewing motions. (d) Rubbing back with towel. (e) Tightening rectoperitoneal muscles. (f) Holding stomach in to tighten abdominal muscles.

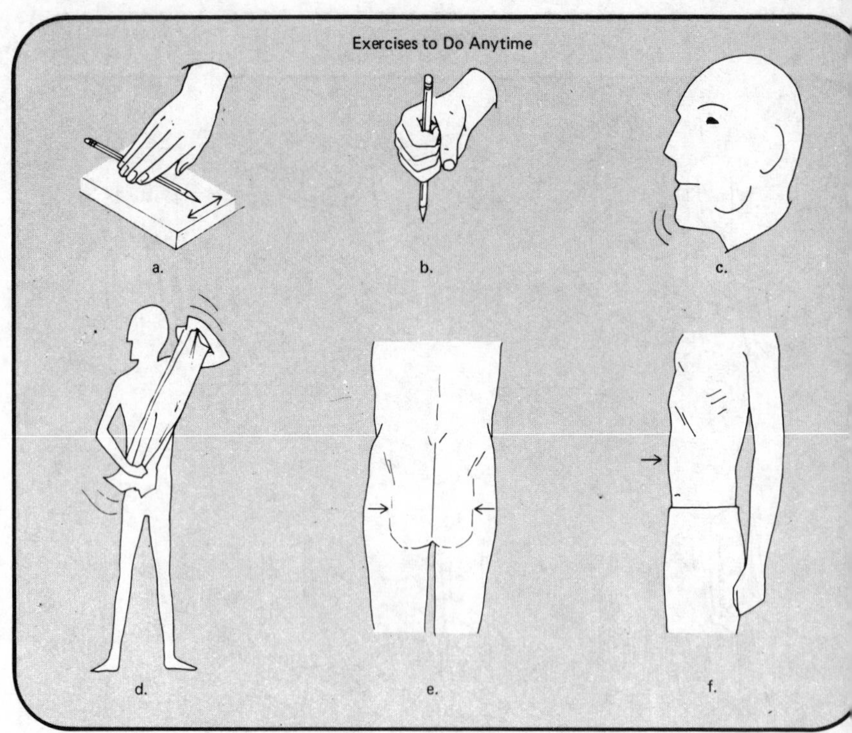

Figure 7-4 (*continued*)

as physical activity. Stimulation and challenges help the older mind maintain lucid functioning. Barring the existence of health problems, the personality and interests will remain consistent throughout an individual's lifetime. The assertive, independent young woman will most likely resent not having a role in decisions involving her and being addressed in a patronizing manner when she grows old. The couple who enjoyed nightclub entertainment throughout the years will not suddenly cease this activity when they begin to be considered old. Likewise, the individual who preferred privacy and solitude when young will most likely not live gregariously when aged. Activities for the aged should be planned according to the unique interests of the given individual. Old age may also be a time for the development of new hobbies and interests; *old people can learn and enjoy new activities.* As mentioned earlier, pets are frequently a source of interest, activity, and companionship for the elderly.

If it is expected that an aged person will be forgetful and confused, and if the person is treated as though this were true, he or she will most likely become forgetful and confused. On the other hand, if the person is expected to keep oriented to current events and relate on an equal basis with others, he or she will most likely remain alert, aware, and mentally active. Thus a self-fulfilling prophecy often dictates the activities in which old people will engage.

Two basic rules should guide those involved with psychological activity of the aged. First, the individual's psychological status should be assessed and psychological stimulation should be provided based on the person's unique capacities and limitations. In other words, *avoid stereotyping the aged.* Some aged individuals may derive psychological satisfaction from discussing a football game with friends at the local tavern, while others may seek satisfaction from completing a foreign language course at the local college. Individual differences, preferences, and abilities must be considered and appreciated. Second, adequate time and patience must be afforded the aged. Slower passage of impulses through the nervous system, sensory deficits, and the vast storehouse of information that is triggered off and has to be sorted through in response to psychological stimuli are just a few of the factors that interfere with rapid reactions in older people.

REST

Satisfying, regular activity promotes rest and relaxation. Greater amounts of rest are required by older people and should be interspersed with periods of activity throughout the day. Upon awakening, the older persons should spend several minutes resting in bed and stretching their muscles, followed by several more minutes of sitting on the side of the bed before rising to a standing position. This will reduce the morning stiffness of the muscles and prevent dizziness and falls resulting from postural hypotension. Some aged individuals may focus all of their activity in the early part of the day so that they will then have their evening free. For instance, the early morning hours may be invested in household cleaning, marketing, club meetings, gardening, cooking, and laundering so that these activities will be completed before evening. The evening hours may then be spent watching television, reading, or sewing. This pattern may be an outgrowth of many years of employment, whereby the individual worked eight hours during the early day and relaxed in the evening. Older people need insight into the advantages of pacing activities throughout the entire day and providing ample periods for rest and naps between activities. The nurse may need to review the daily activities and assist the person in developing a schedule that more equally distributes activity and rest throughout the day.

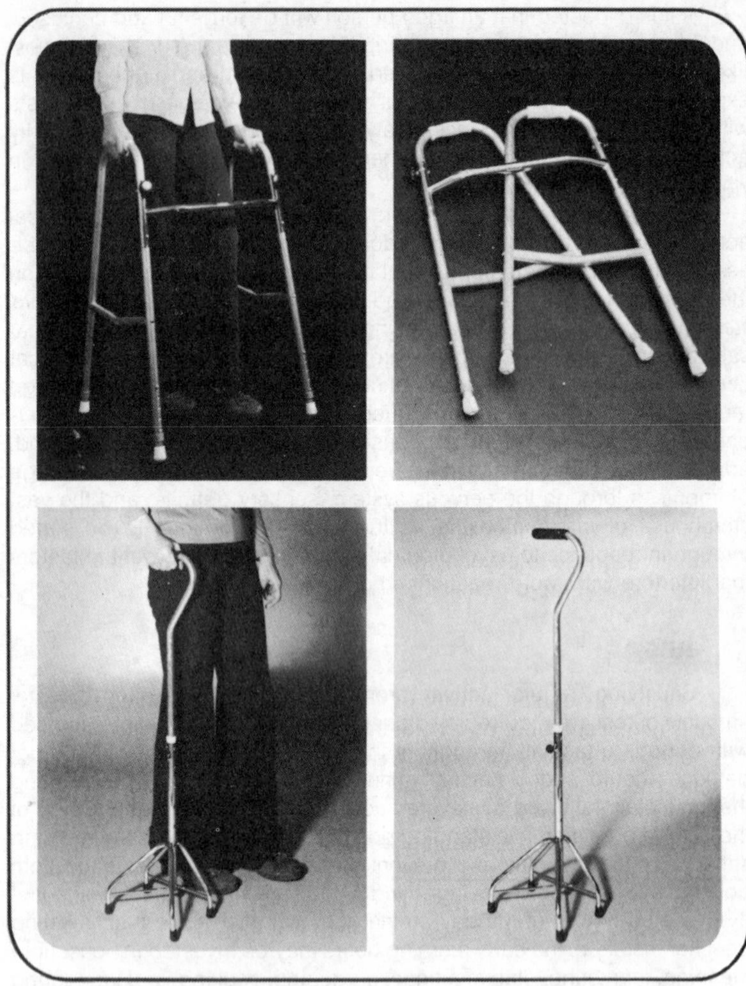

Figure 7-5. Various equipment can be used to assist patients with ambulation and transfer activities. (Courtesy of Maddak, Inc. Subsidiary of Bel-Art Products, Pequannock, N.J.)

Although more rest is required by the aged individual, the length of time required for sleep is reduced. Five to seven hours of night sleep is sufficient for the aged and longer periods may be harmful to their physical and mental functioning. The aged sleep less soundly and may frequently have their sleep interrupted by muscle cramps and tremors, environmental interferences, and nocturia. Older persons may be initially disoriented and confused when wakening in a dark room, and this possibility, combined with visual deficiencies and postural hypotension, may predispose them to accidents. A night-light should be provided in the person's bedroom, and if possible, bathroom lighting should remain on throughout the night. Clutter and furniture should not obstruct the pathway from the bedroom to the bathroom. It may be beneficial to provide a urinal, bedpan, or bedside commode in the older person's room if the bathroom is on a different floor of the house.

The attachment of side rails to the bed may be a beneficial protective measure for the older person at home. This not only prevents falls from bed, but it assists the individual with movement and provides a means of orientation to place. It is important for individuals to feel confident that they can remove these rails to get out of bed or that someone will be readily available to help them do so when necessary. Occasionally, hospital or nursing home patients will resist having side rails due to fear of staff delays in helping them out of bed. These patients need verbal and also behavioral reassurance that they are not trapped and unable to get up. Falls resulting from attempts to climb over the side rails may be prevented by prompt staff response to calls for assistance.

Vision and hearing limitations produce difficulties for care providers who need to communicate necessary questions, warnings, or directions during the night. Whispering to avoid awakening other sleeping individuals will not wake an aged person who has a reduced ability to hear or whose hearing aid is removed, and lipreading is difficult in dimly lit bedrooms. Focusing a flashlight on the lips of the speaker can help the individual read lips, and cupping the hands over the ear and speaking directly into it can aid hearing. A stethoscope can also be used to amplify conversation by placing the earpieces into the individual's ear and speaking into the bell portion.

It is not uncommon for the aged to have difficulty falling asleep. Much too often, the first means employed to encourage sleep is the administration of a sedative. Although the use of medications for the aged population is discussed in detail in Chapter 22, it is worthwhile to mention here that sedatives must be used with utmost care. Barbiturates should be used with extreme caution. They are general depressants, especially to the central nervous system, and they can significantly depress some vital body functions, lowering basal metabolic rate even more than it already is and decreasing blood pressure, mental activity, and peristalis to the extent that other problems may develop. The aged may be more susceptible to many of the adverse reactions to barbiturates. Nonbarbiturate sedatives are not without their problems either, and they should be used only when absolutely necessary. Due to the prolonged half-life of medications in the elderly, the effects of sedatives may exist into the daytime and result in confusion and sluggishness. (To compound the problem, these symptoms are sometimes treated with other medications!) Occasionally, sleeping medications will also reverse the individual's normal sleep rhythm. Sedatives may decrease body movements during sleep and predispose the older person to the many complications of reduced mobility.

Alternatives to sedatives should be used to induce sleep whenever possible. The activity schedule of the individual should first be evaluated. If he has been inactive in a bed or wheelchair all day, most likely he will not be sleepy at bedtime. Including more stimulation and activity during the day may be a solution. The amount of time alotted for sleep should also be evaluated. With a reduced demand for sleep, it should not be expected that the older person who goes to bed at 8 P.M. should be able to sleep until 8 A.M. the following day. A warm bath at bedtime can promote muscle relaxation and encourage sleep, as can a back rub, alleviating pain or discomfort, and finding a comfortable position. A quiet environment, at a temperature preferred by the individual, should be provided. Electric blankets can also promote comfort and relaxation.

Changes in sleep patterns may indicate signs of other problems in the elderly. Although early morning rising is not unusual for the aged, a sudden change to earlier awakening or insomnia may be symptomatic of emotional disturbance. Sleep disturbances may also arise from cardiac or respiratory problems which produce such difficulties as orthopnea and pain from poor peripheral circulation. Restlessness and confusion during the night may be a display of an adverse reaction to a sedative. Nocturnal frequency may be a clue to the presence of diabetes. It is important to assess the quality and quantity of sleep in the aged.

SOLITUDE AND SOCIAL INTERACTION

The axiom that people are social beings holds true for the aged as well. Through social interaction, we share our joys and burdens, derive feelings of normality, validate our perceptions, and maintain a link with reality. The aged, however, may face unique obstacles in their attempts to interact with others due to a variety of intrinsic and extrinsic factors.

The ability to communicate is an essential ingredient for social interaction, and sensory deficits in the aged may interfere with this process. Presbycusis may cause speech to be inaudible or distorted, as can impacted cerumen, a common problem in the aged. Older people may be quite self-conscious of this limitation and avoid situations in which they must interact. In turn, others may avoid them due to this difficulty. Telephone conversation can be affected by this problem, limiting social contact even further for the individual who may be socially isolated for other reasons. (Approximately one-tenth of the aged have some difficulty hearing on the telephone.) Corrective measures for hearing problems should be explored. An audiometric examination can determine whether the particular hearing problem can be improved by the use of a hearing aid, which should not be purchased without such an examination. It is not uncommon to find an older person attempting to correct a hearing problem independently by purchasing a hearing aid from a private party. Not only can this produce disappointing results, but it can waste hundreds of dollars from an already limited budget.

Inability to adjust to the presence of the aid and the distortion of sound caused by the amplification of environmental noise in addition to speech may cause rejection of its use. The nurse should encourage its use, offering support to the individual during this adjustment phase, suggesting that the aid be worn for progressively longer periods each day until the person feels comfortable with it and that it not be used in noisy environments such as airports, train stations, stadiums, etc. The aid should be checked to make sure that the earpiece is not blocked with cerumen and that the battery is working. This appliance may easily correct a hearing problem and reintroduce the older person to a socially active world. If a hearing aid will not solve the problem, efforts should be made to speak clearly and distinctly, in a low frequency but at an audible level while facing the individual. Shouting should be avoided, as it raises the high-frequency sounds, which the older person already has difficulty hearing, causing even greater hearing difficulties. Cupping the hands over the less deficient ear and talking directly into the ear may be helpful. Using gestures and pictures and pointing to items while talking about them can assist.

The nurse should examine the elderly's ears frequently for cerumen accumulation and gently irrigate the ear with a warm saline or hydrogen peroxide and water solution. The aged should understand that irrigation is superior to the use of cotton tipped applicators, which may push the cerumen back into the ear canal and cause an impaction. It is beneficial for the nurse to educate the public as to the effects of environmental noise on their health and their risk of developing presbycusis. Nurses should be actively involved themselves and encourage the involvement of others in legislation controlling noise pollution, as well as the enforcement of such legislation.

The ability to see is equally important to communication. Most elderly persons require some form of corrective lens and approximately half of the individuals identified as legally blind each year are 65 years of age or older. Visual limitations can make communication quite problematic since facial expressions and gestures, which are just as important as the words, may be missed or misinterpreted. Lipreading to compensate for hearing deficits may be difficult and written correspondence may be limited because independent reading and writing become almost impossible tasks. Remaining aware of current events through newspapers and socialization through card playing and other games may thus be hampered. For visual deficit, one of the first assistive measures is a thorough eye examination, including tonometry, by an ophthalmologist. The importance of an annual eye examination, not only to detect vision changes and needs for alterations in corrective lenses, but also for early discovery of problems such as cataracts and glaucoma and other disease processes, must be stressed to the older person. Limited financial means and satisfaction with one's old pair of eyeglasses may cause the aged to neglect regular vision examinations.

To compensate for visual limitations, one should face the individual when speaking and exaggerate gestures and facial expressions. To compensate for the poor peripheral vision old people commonly have, one should approach the individual from the front and seat the person facing those with whom he is interacting. Ample lighting should be provided; several soft indirect lights are superior to a single bright glaring light. Interaction can be promoted by using games and playing cards with enlarged figures (see Figure 7-6), telephone dials with enlarged numbers that glow in the dark, and cassette recorders. Books and magazines with large print and recordings of current events and popular literature can provide a source of recreation and a means of keeping informed.

Because of declining physical function, the older person may have less energy to invest in social interaction. Urinary frequency and incontinence make the individual reluctant to engage in social activities, as do stiff, painful joints and other discomforts. Changes in appearance may alter the individual's self-concept and interfere with the motivation for and quality of social interaction. Although many of these problems cannot be eliminated, nursing intervention can help reduce the limitations they cause. Education of younger adults regarding the normal aging process can enhance their sensitivity and patience, and help them understand the socialization problems an aged person faces, perhaps thereby helping them learn how to minimize and manage these limitations when they grow old. Assuring the aged that their problems are shared by many others and that some of their limitations are a natural part of aging may help them feel "normal," and thus promote social interaction. The nurse can help review and perhaps readjust the person's activity schedule to conserve energy and maximize opportunities for social interactions. Medication schedules should be planned so that during periods of social activity analgesics will provide relief, tranquilizers won't sedate, diuretics won't reach their peak, and laxatives won't become most effective. This is common sense, but often overlooked. Likewise, fluid intake and bathroom visits prior to engagement in activities should be planned to reduce the fear or actual occurrence of "accidents," and activities planned for the aged should provide for frequent break periods for visits to the bathroom. Very often, the control of these minor obstacles can facilitate social interaction.

Given the capacity to interact socially and manage their own problems, the aged must then deal with social factors over which they have no control. Their circle of friends and relatives may become smaller through deaths, and a limited budget may necessitate giving food and shelter priority over social activities. A youth-oriented, fast-paced society may not provide an atmosphere conducive to active social involvement. If the disengagement theory is valid (see Chapter 2), how can the human need for social interaction be satisfactorily fulfilled by the aged? Nurses may discover the importance of influencing society in order to gain acceptance for the aged and obtain opportunities for them to remain socially active. Fortunately, most older people have close relationships with siblings, and most have at least one child less than an hour away whom they see at least weekly.

Solitude is also important for most human beings. It offers a rest from the many stimuli and interactions to which we are regularly exposed and provides for introspection, whereby insights into ourselves, others, and our environment are gained. Reflecting on and analyzing life's events help us to develop and to understand life. Periods of solitude are therapeutic to the aged. Unresolved feelings from earlier years may be worked through and resolved, resulting in personal satisfaction. In reminiscing, evaluating, and understanding the dynamics of life's earlier events and achievements, older people can find a satisfaction with the quality of their life that helps compensate for their multiple losses. They can also gain a new perspective on themselves and others. The death of friends, spouse, and others and the realization of one's own mortality necessitate thought regarding the reality of death and dying.

Time should be provided daily in which no interruptions interfere with solitude. How often are meaningful thoughts and resolutions to unfinished business interrupted by a care provider who wants to distribute a medication or take the individual to the dayroom or change bed linens? Often, busy care providers with a multitude of tasks to complete are not sensitive to the fact that elderly persons who appear to be doing nothing are performing a psychological task as important as any other task that might be performed for them at that time. Designated areas, such as a corner of the dayroom, or a bedroom, should be provided for privacy and respected as such. It must be remembered that solitude and loneliness

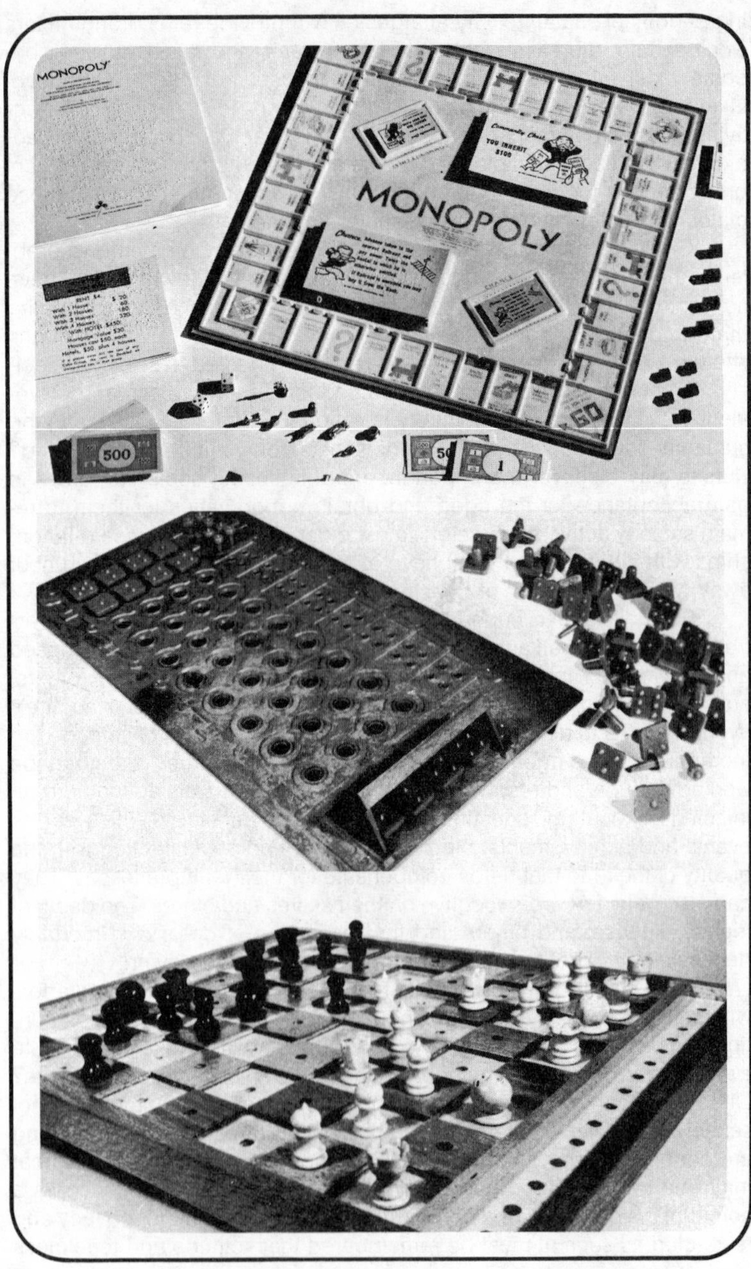
MONOPOLY
Community Chest
YOU INHERIT
$100
MONOPOLY
500
1

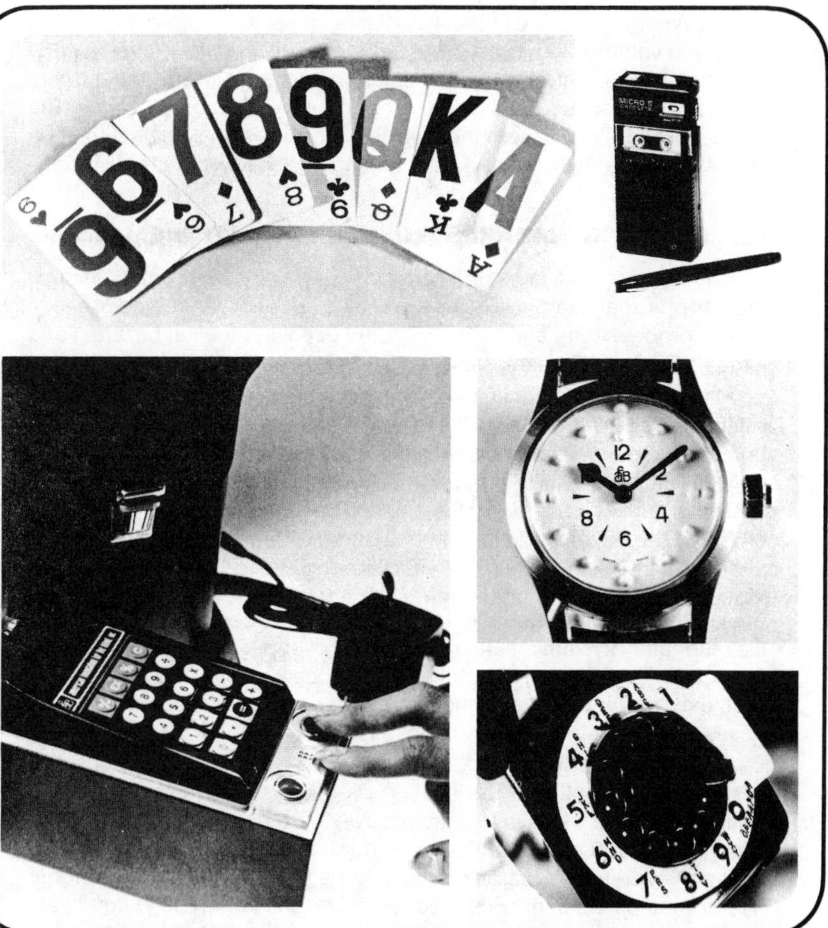

Figure 7-6. Special equipment can help the visually impaired engage in recreational activities: (a) Backgammon, Monopoly, dominoes, checkers, and dice sets with raised and depressed markings. (DiMartini, American Foundation for the Blind.) (MONOPOLY is Parker Brothers' registered trademark for its real estate trading game equipment (c) 1935, 1946, 1961. Photograph courtesy of Parker Brothers.) (b) Jumbo cards with oversized symbols and numbers, and portable radios and cassette recorders. (General Electric) (More information on aids and appliances for the visually impaired can be obtained from the American Foundation for the Blind, 16 West 16th St., New York, N.Y. 10011.)

are not synonymous. The nurse may discover that some aged individuals enjoy and value sitting alone in the park for hours and may forfeit a party invitation for a quiet evening at home. To *choose* solitude differs from being socially isolated and not have opportunities for social activity. The nurse must carefully assess the degree of solitude and social interaction and assist in achieving and maintaining a healthy balance of both.

AVOIDING HAZARDS TO HEALTH AND WELL-BEING

Protective measures to maintain health and well-being include regular physical examination; avoidance of alcohol, drug, and tobacco abuse; proper eating and activity; control of environmental hazards; and early correction of health problems. Due to lack of knowledge, ability, or good judgment, people occasionally expose themselves to, or neglect to protect themselves from, hazards to health and well-being. It is clear that neglecting regular Pap smears for the early detection and treatment of cervical cancer is a threat to a woman's life; that being unaware of the pollutants released from a local industry prevents the community from correcting the hazard; and that not having the benefit of regular dental care risks a child's health. While encountering similar problems to those of other age groups the aged face additional challenges that may pose unique threats and require special nursing considerations. Changes in the respiratory system create a greater risk of upper respiratory infection; changes in the urinary tract create a predisposition for a variety of urinary problems and infections; a more alkaline vaginal environment predisposes older females to some infections.

The lower body temperature of the aged can cause infectious processes to go unnoticed. The healing process is generally slower, and wounds that take 31 days to heal in a 20-year-old, take 55 days in a 40-year-old and 100 days in a 60-year-old (Manney). Normal absorption of food and excretion of waste products are altered, and there is a higher risk of malnourishment. Reduced pressure and ability to differentiate temperature create the danger of injury and breakage to the aged's more delicate and fragile skin. Brittle bones, resulting from reduced bone minerals, can fracture under the amount of stress that would not affect younger bones. Unrestricted activity is harder to achieve, and yet a multitude of problems associated with immobilization are quick to occur. Adverse reactions to drugs often occur and these problems remain untreated because mental confusion, the early sign of disease or drug problems, is often misjudged as senility. Those caring for the aged can help protect them from hazards to health and well-being by recognizing the potential threats discussed above and by understanding the following facts regarding normal values for this age group.

Body temperature is lower in the aged and may normally be as low as 95° F (35°C). The individual whose normal temperature is 96° F may be febrile at 99° F, but he or she may not be identified as such because this temperature is within a normal range for the general adult population. For every 1° F (0.6°C) temperature increase, the pulse increases from 7 to 10 beats per minute. If there is a delay in detecting the increase in metabolic, respiratory, and pulse rates which occur with an elevation in body temperature, serious complications can develop. Pulse rates can fall within a wide range, from 50 to 100 beats per minute, and frequently, the rhythm is irregular. Although an irregular rhythm may be of no diagnostic significance, there is a possibility that it is indicative of a problem, for example, digitalis toxicity.

Although the elderly may have a slow and irregular respiratory rate, the average number of respirations per minute ranges between 14 and 18. Systolic and diastolic blood pressures are higher in the aged as a result of increased peripheral resistance. Persistent elevations above 170 mmHg systolic and 95 mmHg diastolic are considered hypertensive levels in the elderly. (Caird and Judge suggest that normal upper limits can be 195/105 for a male over 80 years of age and 210/115 for a female, and that if these individuals are asytomatic, they need not receive antihypertensive therapy.). Attempting to reduce blood pressure to a level that is normal for younger adults can cause a reduction in cerebral blood flow and, consequently, a reduction in cerebral function. Health professionals should understand this phenomenon and not refer every older person with a blood pressure of 160/90 for treatment; this is costly to the older person and an inefficient use of a health professional's time. The nurse should inform the public of the higher blood pressure levels with advanced age during hypertension screening programs.

As can be seen, regular assessment is important in order to establish baseline norms for the aged individual and recognize changes in these norms. The aged person should be informed of the normal values of his or her vital signs, and these values should be documented on a permanent record. If an older person suddenly begins to display symptoms of senility, the cause may be hidden unless the previous norm for blood pressure has been established and is known by the health care provider. If examination reveals a blood pressure of 140/70, this could be interpreted as normal. However, if the previous blood pressure had consistently been 190/90, the person may now be hypotensive.

The older person's safety may also be threatened by certain visual changes with aging. Older eyes adapt less quickly to light and dark, see less well in dim areas, have greater difficulty with depth perception and peripheral vision, discriminate low-tone colors (such as blues and greens) less well, and may have more opaque lenses. These factors predispose the aged to many accidents. A small light should be left on throughout the night, and night driving should be discouraged. Bright lights and glare should be avoided by using several small lights instead of one large one, by filtering bright sunlight through sheer drapes or stained-glass windows, and by placing the older person's bed or chair so that it does not face a bright window.

To compensate for reduced peripheral vision, the individual should be approached from the front rather than from the back or side, and furniture and frequently used items should be arranged in full view. Altered depth perception may hamper the ability to detect changes in levels, and this may be helped by providing good lighting, eliminating clutter on stairways, painting the stairs a contrasting color, and using signals to indicate when a change in level is being approached. The filtering of low-tone colors should be considered when decorating areas for the aged; bright oranges and yellows and contrasting colors on doors and windows may be appealing and assistive. The problem with seeing low-tone colors should be considered when teaching urine testing to older diabetics since they must differentiate these colors to detect glycosuria. Cleansing solutions, medications, and other materials should be labeled in large letters to prevent accidents or errors.

Directions and warnings may also be missed due to poor hearing. Explanations and directions for diagnostic tests, medication administration, or other therapeutic measures should be explained in written as well as verbal form. The individual should live close to someone with adequate hearing who can tell him or her of fire alarms or other warnings. Decreased sense of smell may also cause the older person to miss life-saving warnings, such as the different scents of mouthwash and juice. Electric stoves may be helpful in preventing gas intoxication from the inability to detect a gas odor. The loss of taste receptors may cause the aged to use excessive amounts of sugar and salt in the diet, a possible health hazard. Reduced tactile sensation to pressure from shoes, dentures, or an unchanged position can cause skin breakdown, and inability to discriminate temperatures can cause burns.

Slower response and reaction times may prove to be safety hazards. Older pedestrians may misjudge their ability to cross streets as traffic lights change, and older drivers may not be able to react quickly enough to avoid accidents. Stove burns while cooking are also a danger, one compounded by visual problems. Slower movement and poor coordination subject the older person to falls and other accidents. Loose rugs, slippery floors, clutter, and poor-fitting shoes and slippers should be eliminated. Railings should be present on stairways and bathtubs. Rubber mats or nonslip strips are a must in the bathtub, where fainting and falls often occur as a result of reduced blood pressure—first from the warm bath water which dilates the peripheral vessels and then again from rising to a standing position. Using a stool in the tub and resting before rising are useful measures. Since poor judgment, denial, or lack of awareness of their limitations may prevent them from protecting their health and well-being, older people should be advised not to take risks such as window washing or climbing on a ladder.

With the vast number of medications used by older population, it is important to avoid inappropriate or unwise use of them. Feedback should be obtained to evaluate the understanding the individual has of his or her medications and their administration. All adverse reactions and special precautions should be written down and explained to the individual and the family. The necessity of the medication should be periodically reevaluated and it should be discontinued if there is no real therapeutic need for the drug any longer. Side effects may be demonstrated differently in the aged, and they should be anticipated and detected early. As many drugs are required in lower dosages for older persons, the lowest possible effective dose should be used. Additional problems and precautions with drug use in the elderly are discussed in Chapter 22. Since the aged are more susceptible to hazards, require a longer recovery period, and are prone to more complications when an illness develops, the most effective means of managing threats to health and well-being is to prevent them from occurring. The environmental checklist below suggests some preventive devices.

Environmental Checklist

Smoke detector
Telephone
Fire extinguisher
Vented heating system
Minimal clutter
Proper food storage
Adequately lighted hallways and stairways
Handrails on stairways
Even floor surface, easy to clean and requiring no waxing and free of loose scatter rugs and deep pile carpets
Unobstructed doorways, painted a different color from wall for easy visibility
Bathtub or shower with nonslip surface, safety rails, and no electrical outlets nearby
Windows easy to reach and open
Ample number of safe electrical outlets, preferably 3 feet higher than level of floor for easy reach
Safe stove with burner control on front
Shelves within easy reach to avoid need for climbing
Faucet handles that are easy to operate
For wheelchair use, doorways and hallways that are clear and wide enough for passage; ramps and/or elevators; bathroom layout to provide for wheelchair maneuvering; and sinks, stoves, tables, and cabinets low enough for reach from wheelchair

BEING NORMAL

The desire to be normal is important at any age. The aged, however, may find many unique challenges in achieving feelings of normality for two general reasons. First, our society's definition of normal is based upon a young model. Just observing advertisements and walking through a department store reflects our country's bias for the young. Those who can't keep pace or conform to the styles and activities of the young are in a sense viewed as abnormal. Second, knowledge of what is normal for the aged is rather recent and still developing. Not only lay people, but many health professionals don't know or understand norms for the aged. Consequently, wasted time, energy, and money is invested in achieving norms for the aged that are inappropriate or hazardous. Daily baths, shouting to compensate for hearing loss, inappropriate reduction of blood pressure, and determining fever by values used for the young are just several of the practices which may indicate poor utilization of existing knowledge. The nurse can be a more effective practitioner and a significant consumer advocate by educating others regarding normality in the aged.

Certain physiological changes may cause the aged to feel abnormal in reference to their appearance. A reduction in height occurs as thinning disks shorten the vertebral column. This is compounded by postural changes, such as slight hip and knee flexion, and in many individuals, kyphosis with a backward tilting of the head. Height reductions may even be more obvious because span and length of the upper extremities remain the same. With the exception of the face, body hair is lost and scalp hair commonly becomes thin and gray. The clustering of melanocytes causes some skin pigmentation to accompany the lines and wrinkles resulting from a loss of subcutaneous fat. Women may be disturbed at the facial hair and breast tissue atrophy what occurs with age, and men may find prostatic hypertrophy and baldness common problems. Tooth loss, dry skin, swollen joints, hard and brittle fingernails, and many other factors cannot be altered; but measures can be employed to promote a good appearance in the elderly.

Attractive clothing and jewelry may offset bodily changes. Cream-based cosmetics offer protection from sun and wind exposure and are also of psychological value. Shampooing the hair once or twice monthly can improve hair condition, and with regular brushing and scalp massage in between, this is all that is really necessary for the aged. Wigs can be worn and hair dyes may be used. (Rinses and vegetable dyes are less harmful than heavy metal and aniline-based dyes.) Facial hair can be removed by the use of tweezers, pumice stones, chemical agents or electric needles; mole hair should not be pulled but carefully cut with scissors to avoid trauma. Soaking will ease the task of cutting nails, and podiatry services may prove beneficial. Gauze or cotton placed gently under a curved nail may facilitate its straight growth. (These should be changed daily and removed for baths.) Creams and lotions may be used to soften skin. The aged should be motivated to practice good grooming habits and maintain an attractive appearance.

The effects of declines and alterations in body function on one's ability to feel and act normal should be considered by the nurse, and attempts should be made to provide the most normal life-style attainable in light of these limitations. Certain factors may make it difficult for the aged to adjust to the rapid rate of societal change and technological advancement. Performing a series of complicated, coordinated tasks may be problematic for the aged and reliance on previous experience may supersede creative problem-solving techniques. In addition, memory for past events may be far superior to memory of recent facts. Imagine how difficult it must be for an older person who has cooked with a gas stove for over 50 years to comprehend and learn the use of a microwave oven! Some of the normal daily demands of today's world may be difficult for the aged to fulfill.

Although a fuller discussion of sexuality and the aged is provided in Chapter 20, it may be useful to mention a few points here. It is normal for the aged to desire sexual satisfaction and be able to engage in sexual activity. Masters and Johnson have found through their research that sexual expression is more inhibited by social and psychological forces than by physical ability. The nurse should encourage older people to express their sexuality and should convey the importance of understanding and appreciating this to family members and others providing care for the aged. Ridicule, lack of privacy, and demeaning reactions to sexual behavior can prevent the aged from experiencing the psychological and physiological benefits of sexuality. Older males, whose responsiveness and intensity of pleasure may be reduced, should be encouraged to worry less about the actual performance of the sex act and to focus more on the importance of sharing love, warmth, and intimacy. This advice is applicable to older females as well. Hormonal imbalances may cause dyspareunia for the aged female, but hormonal replacement can often improve this problem. Health professionals and the public in general may have to change old attitudes and encourage sexual activity—if only for its therapeutic value alone.

In our society one's worth is often determined by one's productivity. Changing requirements for skills, the abundance of young workers, and rigid retirement policies often force the older worker out of the labor force, and the retired person may have feelings of worthlessness having no productive role to fill. Nuclear families and day-care centers often eliminate the traditional roles for grandparents. As a nonproductive member of society the aged individual often cannot help feeling abnormal. Some solutions to this problem are to discontinue discriminatory hiring practices and provide a capable older person with equal opportunity for employment; to abandon mandatory retirement practices; and to utilize the rich pool of wisdom and skills accumulated throughout the older person's lifetime by establishing employment or volunteer programs. Obviously, one can remain a valuable member of society when retired, and if society's attitude reflected this, the negative feelings associated with unemployment might be reduced. The financial security to live a full and satisfying life should also be something everyone can expect when retirement occurs.

Long-term goals should include programs to educate the public for aging. Youth should be helped to gain insight into the assets and problems of old age, and an appreciation and respect for the older members of society. Gaining an understanding of aging as a normal and natural process may encourage the development of a healthy attitude toward growing old. Learning how to prepare for old age through preventive health practices, the development of leisure activities, the accumulation of financial assets, periods of trial retirement prior to actual retirement, intelligent life planning, and increased legislation to promote health, security, and safety for the aged should be promoted.

REFERENCES

Caird, F. I. and Judge, T. G. *Assessment of The Elderly Patient.* Pitman, New York, 1974, p. 34.

Manney, James R. *Aging in American Society.* University of Michigan, Wayne State University, Ann Arbor, Mich., 1975, p. 27.

8

CARDIOVASCULAR PROBLEMS

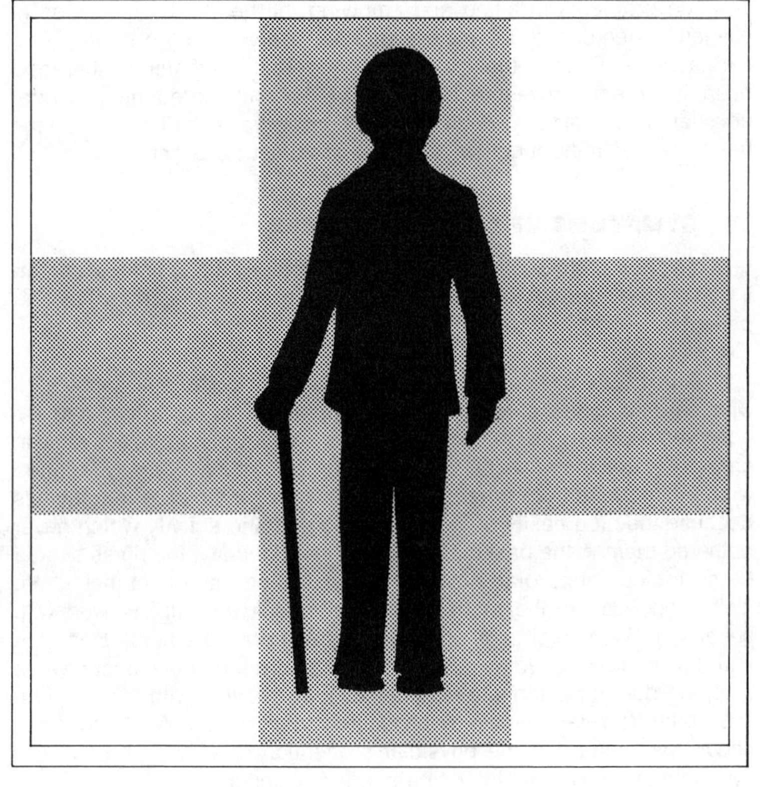

The geriatric nurse frequently encounters persons with some form of cardiovascular disease. Heart disease increases with age and most deaths due to cardiovascular disease are in the aged population. The number one cause of death in individuals 65 years of age or older is cardiovascular disease. A review of some of the heart changes associated with the aging process promotes understanding of the reasons for cardiac problems in old age. The heart either remains the same or becomes smaller in old age than it was during middle adulthood, and the older heart has a deeper brown color. Subpericardial fat is present in greater amounts, and there is evidence of endocardial thickening and sclerosis. The aorta and arteries are less elastic, and the carotid artery may become kinked to the extent that it is mistaken for an aneurysm. The heart valves thicken and become more rigid.

The reduced efficiency of the heart is manifested in a variety of ways. Heart contractions may be weaker and cardiac output reduced. The lessened elasticity of the aorta and the presence of atrial atrophy produce problems in filling and emptying the heart. The utilization of oxygen is decreased, as are the cardiac reserve and the capacity for cardiac work. Despite these changes and reduced efficiency, the aged heart is able to meet the demands of daily life adequately. Under unusual circumstances, when stress places increased demands on the heart, the declining function of the heart is most apparent.

SYMPTOMS OF CARDIAC DISEASE

The gerontological nurse must be particularly alert to clues indicatint possible cardiac disease, either visible or as described by the patient.

Shortness of breath. The most common complaint associated with cardiac disease is shortness of breath. This symptom can be observed by the nurse when patients have to interrupt normal activities in order to "catch their breath" and when they become noticeably fatigued with minimal exertion. When patients refuse to participate in activities because they tire easily or indicate that a specific activity which never bothered them in the past, now causes them difficulty, the nurse should be suspicious of cardiac disease. An unjustified complaint that "there isn't enough air in the room to breathe" should also be viewed with suspicion. Sleep problems should be explored by the nurse since the inability to breathe fully, and the fear that death may occur while sleeping due to inadequate respirations may interfere with the individual's ability to relax and enjoy an entire night's sleep. Acute dyspnea should be brought to the physician's attention quickly as it can be a symptom of myocardial infarction in aged patients.

Chest pain. Acute or recurrent chest pain, a common complaint associated with cardiac disease, is difficult to assess. The pain described by the aged person may be atypical for cardiac disease as a result of altered pain sensation in old age. With the high prevalence of respiratory, gastric, and musculoskeletal problems in aged individuals, this symptom can also be attributed to some other existing disorder. The nurse should note the time of onset and the characteristics, location, duration, and other factors associated with incidents of chest pain.

Cheyne-Stokes respiration. This symptom is common in the aged and may be an indication of cardiac disease. The nurse should be alert in making observations and in noting patient's comments about having insomnia, which is frequently caused by Cheyne-Stokes respiration.

Changes in cerebral function. Occasionally, such changes are thought to be a result of the aging process, but this may actually be a symptom of cardiac disease and consequent poor cerebral circulation. The nurse should detect early the development of vertigo, mental confusion, change in mental status, or behavioral changes.

Edema. Edema is frequently a symptom of cardiac disease, especially with right-sided heart failure. Subtle clues which may be indicative of edema should be recognized, such as the inability to remove a previously removable wedding band, the complaint that shoes suddenly feel tight and an increase in weight.

Other Symptoms. Coughing and wheezing are symptoms which may reflect left-sided heart failure, and hemoptysis is frequently associated with congestive heart failure and pulmonary edema. As mentioned with chest pain, this group of symptoms may be attributed to respiratory disorders that are present in the aged individual. Some symptoms that occur with cardiac disease in younger adults, such as pain, anorexia, vomiting, frequency, and nocturia, occur less commonly in an old person with cardiac disease.

Since the early detection and diagnosis of cardiac disease can be difficult because of (1) a slow, gradual rate in the progress of symptoms,(2) an easy confusion of cardiac symptoms with those of other systems, and (3) an atypical manifestation of symptoms, keen, accurate nursing observations are especially important.

Electrocardiogram

A basic diagnostic aid in cardiovascular disease in the aged is the electrocardiogram. Even in the absence of disease, there are some

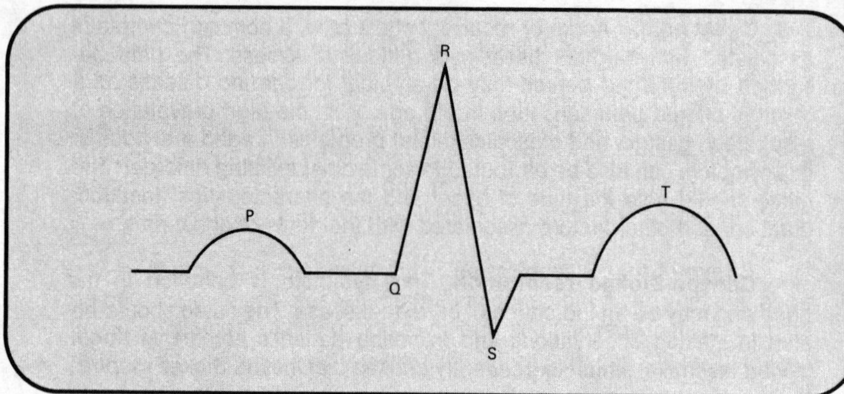

Figure 8-1. Normal adult EKG.

changes in the electrocardiogram of older persons with which the nurse should be familiar. For a basis of comparison, a normal adult EKG reading is shown in Figure 8-1, with parts labeled. In the aged, there is a reduced voltage of the waves and a slight prolongation of all intervals due to the slower conduction of impulses through the pacemaker, conduction system, and myocardium. Figure 8-2 shows a hypothetical EKG of an aged person superimposed on the normal adult EKG from Figure 8-1. The P wave may normally be smaller in the aged. The P-R interval shows no significant change while the QRS interval is slightly longer. The QT interval may show an increase, but it remains within the normal limit, and the T wave will appear lower. As can be seen, these changes do not produce a significant difference in the appearance of the EKG.

COMMON CARDIOVASCULAR DISEASES OF THE AGED

Although other cardiovascular diseases may occur in older persons, those most encountered by the gerontological nurse have been selected for this chapter. Only factors particularly relevant to the aged patient are discussed, and the nurse is encouraged to refer to medical-surgical textbooks for a complete review of the diseases presented.

Congestive Heart Failure

The incidence of congestive heart failure increases with age and is an especially potential complication in older patients with arteriosclerotic heart disease. The variety of conditions that can precipitate congestive heart failure in the aged include coronary artery disease, hyperten-

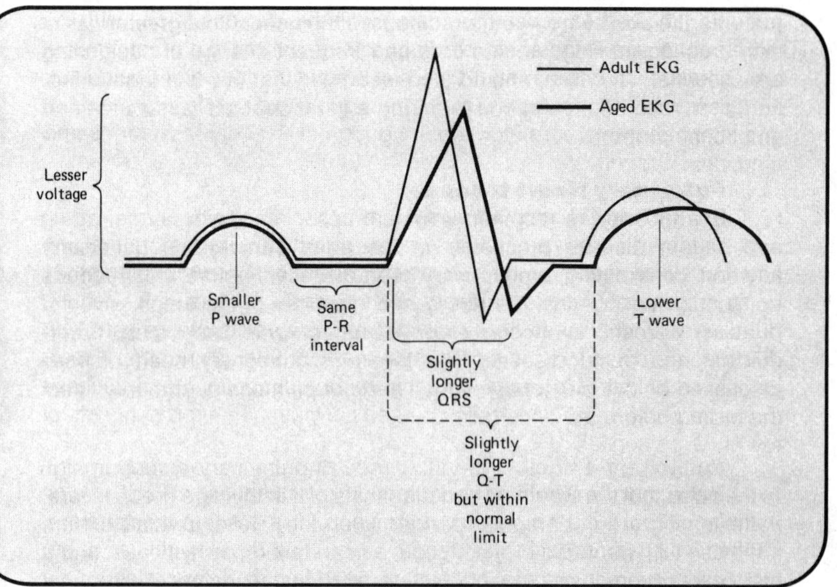

Figure 8-2. Age-related EKG changes superimposed on normal adult EKG.

sive heart disease, cor pulmonale, mitral stenosis, subacute bacterial endocarditis, bronchitis, pneumonia, congenital heart disease, and myxedema. Nurses should closely monitor patients with any of these conditions and detect indications of congestive heart failure. Symptoms of this problem which may develop in aged patients include mental confusion, insomnia, wandering during the night, agitation, depression, anorexia, nausea, weakness, shortness of breath, orthopnea, and bilateral ankle edema. The detection of any of these symptoms should be promptly communicated to the physician.

The management of congestive heart failure in the aged is basically the same as in middle-aged adults, commonly consisting of bedrest, digitalis, diuretics, and a reduction in sodium intake. The patient may be allowed to sit in a chair next to the bed; complete bedrest is usually discouraged to avoid the potential development of thrombosis and pulmonary congestion. The patient should be assisted into the chair and adequately supported. While sitting, the patient should be observed for signs of fatigue, dyspnea, changes in skin color, and changes in the pulse.

The nurse should be aware that the presence of edema and the poor nutrition of the tissues associated with this disease, along with the more fragile skin of the aged, predisposes the patient to a greater risk of skin breakdown. Regular skin care and frequent change of positioning are essential. The nurse should also recognize that this is a frightening, and often recurring, condition requiring a great deal of reassurance and emotional support.

Pulmonary Heart Disease

Changes in the respiratory system associated with normal aging and certain disease processes in the aged can reduce pulmonary function, contributing to pulmonary heart disease. Factors which reduce pulmonary function include decreased elasticity of the lungs, alveolar dilation, fibrosis, kyphosis, emphysema, chronic bronchitis, tuberculosis, and mitral disease. The forms of pulmonary heart disease discussed below, pulmonary emboli and cor pulmonale, primarily affect the older person.

Pulmonary emboli. The incidence of pulmonary emboli is high in the aged, but the detection and diagnosis of it in this age group is rare. Patients who are in particular danger when they develop this problem are those with fractured hip, congestive heart failure, arrhythmias, and a history of thrombosis. Immobilization and malnourishment, frequent problems in the aged population, can contribute to pulmonary emboli. Symptoms which should be observed include mental confusion, apprehension, increasing dyspnea, slight temperature elevation, pneumonitis, and an elevated sedimentation rate. Older patients may not experience chest pain due to altered pain sensations, or their pain may be attributed to other existing problems. A lung scan or angiography may be done to confirm the diagnosis and establish the location, size, and extent of the problem. Treatment of pulmonary emboli in the aged does not significantly differ from that employed for the young.

Cor pulmonale. *Acute* cor pulmonale is usually a result of a massive pulmonary embolus, respiratory infection, atrial fibrillation, or chronic failure. This is often a problem experienced by older hemiplegics. With the exception of the use of morphine or barbiturates, treatment is the same as for younger adults. *Chronic* cor pulmonale is primarily a result of emphysema. This disease can develop into acute cor pulmonale, and nursing measures should focus on preventing this from happening. Treatment does not differ from that for the young, including antismoking education.

Coronary Artery Disease

Coronary artery disease is the popularly used phrase for ischemic heart disease. There is an increased prevalence of coronary artery disease with advanced age, so that some form of this disease exists in most persons 70 years of age or older.

Anginal syndrome. A symptom of myocardial ischemia, the angina syndrome presents itself in an atypical pattern, creating difficulty in detection. Pain may be diffuse and of a less severe nature than described by younger adults. The first indication of this problem may be a vague discomfort under the sternum, frequently following a large meal. The type of pain described and the relationship of the onset of pain to a meal may cause the patient, and the health professional, to attribute this discomfort to indigestion. As this condition progresses, the patient may experience precardial pain radiating down the left arm. The recurrence of anginal syndromes over many years can result in the formation of small areas of myocardial necrosis and fibrosis. Eventually diffuse myocardial fibrosis occurs leading to myocardial weakness and the potential risk of congestive heart failure.

Nitroglycerine has proved beneficial in the prevention and treatment of anginal attacks. As this drug may cause a drop in blood pressure, the patient should be cautioned to sit or lie down after taking this tablet to prevent fainting episodes and falls. To prevent swallowing the tablet and thus blocking its absorption, patients should be reminded not to swallow their saliva for several minutes following sublingual administration. Specific information on nitroglycerine is offered in Chapter 22. Long-acting nitrates are usually not prescribed for the aged. To prevent anginal syndromes, the patient should be taught and helped to avoid these factors which may aggravate this problem, such as cold wind, emotional stress, strenuous activity, anemia, tachycardia, arrhythmias, and hyperthyroidism.

Myocardial infarction. A cardiac problem frequently seen in older persons, especially in men with a history of hypertension and arteriosclerosis, myocardial infarction can have a delayed or missed diagnosis in the aged due to an atypical set of symptoms and the frequent absence of pain. Symptoms include pain radiating to the left arm, the entire chest, the neck, and abdomen; moist, pale skin; decreased blood pressure; low-grade fever; and an elevated sedimentation rate. Output should be observed since partial or complete anuria may develop as this problem continues. Arrhythmias may occur, progressing to fibrillation and death if untreated. Cardiac rupture may also occur, especially in older women.

The trend in treating myocardial infarction has been to reduce the amount of time in which the patient is on bedrest and to replace complete bedrest with allowing the patient to sit in an armchair next to the bed. The patient should be assisted into the chair with minimal exertion on his part. Arms should be supported to avoid strain on the heart. Not only does this armchair treatment help to prevent many of the complications associated with immobility, but it also prevents pooling of the blood in the pulmonary vessels, thereby decreasing the work of the heart.

Since aged persons are more susceptible to cerebral and intestinal bleeding, close nursing observation for signs of bleeding is essential if anticoagulants are used in the patient's treatment. Nurses should be alert to signs of developing pulmonary edema and congestive heart failure, potential complications for the geriatric patient with a myocardial infarction. These and other observations, such as persistent dyspnea, cyanosis, decreasing blood pressure, rising temperature, and arrhythmias, reflect a problem in the patient's recovery and should be promptly brought to the physician's attention.

Acute coronary insufficiency. Arterial narrowing and myocardial damage and increased cardiac stress can result in acute coronary insufficiency. Symptoms of this problem which the nurse can recognize include a low-grade fever and prolonged chest pain. Treatment includes the use of oxygen and analgesics, as well as rest. Areas of necrosis can develop after repeated episodes of this problem, leading to diffuse fibrosis.

Hypertension

The incidence of hypertension increases with advancing age and is a problem which the gerontological nurse commonly encounters in practice. Many aged people have a high blood pressure due to the vasoconstriction associated with aging, which produces peripheral resistance. Hyperthyroidism, parkinsonism, Paget's disease, anemia, and a thiamine deficiency can also be responsible for hypertension. Usually, if the older person's blood pressure is equal to or greater than 200 mmHg systolic and 100 mmHg diastolic, and if the person is symptomatic, treatment is initiated. The nurse should carefully assess the patient's blood pressure by checking it several times with the person in standing, sitting, and lying positions. Anxiety, stress, or activity prior to the blood pressure check should be noted, as these factors may be responsible for a temporary elevation. The anxiety of being examined by a physician or of preparing for and experiencing a visit to a clinic frequently cause an elevated blood pressure in a usually normotensive individual.

Awakening with a dull headache, impaired memory, disorientation, confusion, epistaxis, and a slow tremor may be symptoms of hypertension. The presence of these symptoms with an elevated blood pressure reading usually warrants treatment. Hypertensive older patients are advised to rest, reduce their sodium intake, and if necessary, reduce their weight. Aggressive antihypertensive therapy is discouraged for older persons due to the risk of a sudden dangerous decrease in blood pressure. Nurses should observe for signs indicating a blood pressure which is too low to meet the patient's demands, such as dizziness, confusion, syncope, restlessness, and drowsiness. An elevated blood urea nitrogen level may also be present. These signs should be observed for and communicated to the physician if they appear. In the management of the older person who is hypertensive, it is a challenge to achieve a blood pressure level which is high enough to provide optimum circulation while being low enough to prevent serious related complications.

Arrhythmias

Digitalis toxicity, hypokalemia, acute infections, hemorrhage, anginal syndrome, and coronary insufficiency are some of the many factors which cause an increasing incidence of arrhythmias with age. Of the causes mentioned, digitalis toxicity is the most common.

The basic principles of treatment of arrhythmias do not vary much for older adults. Tranquilizers, digitalis, and potassium supplements are part of the therapy prescribed. Patient education may be warranted to help the individual modify diet, smoking, drinking, and activity patterns. The nurse should be aware that digitalis toxicity can progress in the absence of clinical signs and that the effects can be evident even two weeks after the drug has been discontinued. The aged have a higher mortality rate from cardiac arrest than other segments of the population, emphasizing the necessity for close nursing observation and early problem detection, to prevent this serious complication.

Tachycardia. Tachycardia is one form of conduction disturbance seen in older persons. The most common types are *paroxysmal atrial tachycardia* and *ventricular tachycardia*. With the exception of acute myocardial infarction, ventricular tachycardia—a serious problem for young and old—does not frequently occur. However, ventricular tachycardia has been noted at the time of a person's death and for minutes following clinical death. Decreased blood pressure, impaired cerebral circulation, and congestive heart failure may develop if tachycardia is not corrected.

Premature contractions. Atrial and ventricular premature contractions are cardiac arrhythmias experienced by the aged. Premature contractions can be caused by gastrointestinal disturbances, stress, and agents such as coffee, tea, alcohol, and tobacco. If not corrected, this problem can lead to a serious ventricular arrhythmia.

Atrial fibrillation. As a result of severe cardiovascular disease, hyperthyroidism, high fevers, digitalis intoxication, and pulmonary emboli, atrial fibrillation can occur. If it is prolonged, it encourages the development of an atrial thrombus and thus prompt treatment is important. Signs of a possible embolus should be observed for. Dyspnea and chest pain may indicate a pulmonary emboli, while an emboli lodged in the mesenteric arteries will cause abdominal pain. Discolored urine may result from a renal emboli, and changes in cerebral function may indicate an emboli there.

Heart block. Arteriosclerosis, digitalis overdose, quinidine, certain poisons, and changes in the heart structure can cause heart block. Older persons experiencing heart block have a greater risk of suffering cardiac standstill and Stokes-Adams attack—whereby unconsciousness and possible seizures occur as a result of hypoxia from interrupted cerebral circulation.

Bacterial Endocarditis

Subacute bacterial endocarditis. This may be a potential complication experienced by aged patients with staphylococcal, fungal, and other infections and with collagen disorders, diabetes, and a history of recent surgery; also by patients who have been receiving steroids, cancer chemotherapy, and antibiotics for a long period of time. Diagnosis can be complicated in aged persons because of such nonspecific symptoms as anorexia, fatigue, weight loss, anemia, mental confusion, weakness, pallor, tachycardia, and an elevated sedimentation rate. The difficulty in relating these symptoms to subacute bacterial endocarditis in the aged contributes to the high mortality associated with this problem. As this disease progresses, atrial fibrillation and heart failure may occur. The treatment for this problem in the aged is similar to that employed for younger persons.

Acute bacterial endocarditis. This occurs in the aged to a significantly lesser degree than the subacute form, but with similar difficulty in diagnosis because its symptoms are like those of many other geriatric problems.

Rheumatic Heart Disease

Rheumatic heart disease may occur in aged people who either have had rheumatic fever earlier in life or have had acute episodes during old age. Older individuals who have rheumatic fever suffer moderate joint discomfort, sudden soreness and diffuse redness of the throat, enlarged lymph nodes, and a temperature elevation. Any joint lesions are more disabling to the elderly. It is not unusual for repeated episodes to occur, and the nurse should be alert to symptoms in patients with a history of this disease. With proper therapy, the prognosis for an older person with acute rheumatic fever is favorable, and rheumatic heart disease, which occurs more often in elderly women, can be prevented. Residual valvular deformities from acute rheumatic fever progress differently in each individual. Usually, the mitral and aortic valves are most affected. Some persons have minimal limitations because of adequate compensation by the myocardium; some develop murmurs, hypertension, atrial fibrillation, and congestive heart failure. Aggressive therapy for the disease itself is usually not warranted, and the emphasis is on managing the symptoms and any complications that develop.

Syphilitic Heart Disease

Ten percent of the heart disease in persons 50 years of age or older is a result of syphilis. Aged persons with syphilitic heart disease may have contracted the disease at a time when a definite stigma was attached to venereal diseases, and open discussion and education regarding these diseases was nonexistent or minimal. The individual may have been fearful or felt guilty or may not have noticed or been aware of the significance of the associated symptoms, and therefore may not have sought treatment. Treatment before the 1940s, when penicillin was developed, may have been inadequate and ineffective in eliminating the disease. Older persons who have had recent exposure to syphilis may be reluctant to seek treatment because they are concerned about what others might think of sexual activity in old age.

The first sign of syphilitic heart disease may occur years after the initial infection. The valvular defect most frequently associated with this disease is aortic insufficiency, whereby a leak in the aortic valve during diastole causes blood to be forced back into the left ventricle. The systolic blood pressure is increased, the diastolic blood pressure is reduced, and the pulse pressure is significantly greater. When the heart is no longer able to compensate for these changes, cardiac failure can occur. The most effective treatment may be the replacement of the damaged valve with a ball-valve prosthesis, a procedure viewed with increasing optimism for the aged.

Congenital Heart Disease

Due to the limited medical and surgical correctives for congenital defects that were available when today's aged population was young, people born with serious heart problems most likely did not survive to adulthood. Thus, congenital heart disease is not very common among the aged and is sometimes unrecognized as such. It is believed that some of the arrhythmias, murmurs, and other cardiac diseases found in the geriatric patient are caused by congenital lesions.

Atrial and ventricular septal defects. These are the most common congenital heart defects discovered in the aged. Symptoms of atrial septal defect are similar for all ages, except that older people may have a higher pulse rate, increased blood pressure, dyspnea, recurrent bronchopneunomia, and a greater incidence of coronary artery disease. Most patients with ventricular septal defects are asymptomatic, although they may experience fatigue and episodes of heart failure. Surgery is sometimes effective in improving both these defects in older persons.

NURSING CONSIDERATIONS

The prevention of cardiovascular problems in all age groups should be a primary concern of the nurse. By teaching people of all ages to identify and lower the risk factors related to cardiovascular disease, the nurse will also be contributing to people's optimum health and functioning. The nurse should emphasize the importance of proper nutrition, the relationship of cholesterol and obesity to heart disease, and the benefits of regular exercise. Many Americans today exert minimal physical activity during the workweek and fill the weekend with gardening, swimming, tennis, housecleaning etc., when they should be distributing exercise throughout the entire week. In the absence of a special exercise regimen, one can take advantage of simple daily opportunities, such as using stairs instead of an elevator, walking short distances instead of driving, and making a list of exercises to perform while watching a favorite television show.

Moderation should be recommended in alcohol consumption, and cigarette smoking should be discouraged. The nurse should realize that a smoking habit is difficult to break and should employ methods to educate people regarding the multiple health problems associated with it. Smokers should also be assisted in finding antismoking programs that meet their unique needs. Regarding the association of stress and heart disease, the nurse should review a person's stresses, coping mechanisms, and outlets for stress, promoting insight into factors that can increase the risk and measures that can reduce the risk of heart disease. The nurse should remember that it is much easier to establish good habits early in life than to change long-established practices.

As mentioned throughout this chapter, diagnosis of cardiovascular disease in the aged is often complicated and difficult. Emphysema, hiatus hernia, gall bladder disease and other disorders may mistakenly be assigned responsibility for or mask symptoms of cardiovascular disorders. As the person that probably has the most direct contact with the patient, the nurse should observe closely for even the most subtle clue indicating a possible cardiovascular problem, including those learned in conversations with the patient. Comments such as "My chest felt like it had a butterfly in it while I was mowing the lawn, but it went away" or "Sometimes I wake up from my sleep feeling like someone has a pillow over my face" should be explored further. The same patients who made these comments may have responded negatively when asked by the physician if they had ever experienced chest pain or shortness of breath. It will facilitate diagnosis if such findings are communicated to the physician.

The type of diagnostic measures utilized for older patients with possible cardiovascular disease will not differ greatly from those used with younger patients, and the same nursing measures should be applied. Due to sensory deficits, anxiety, mental confusion or limitations in memory, the older patient may not fully understand or remember the explanations given for the diagnostic measures employed. The nurse should prepare the patient for tests, offer full explanations on a meaningful level, reinforce the teaching provided, and allow the patient to discuss questions and concerns openly. Families should also be part of this process. Commonly, procedures which seem relatively minor to the nurse, such as frequent checks of vital signs, may be alarming to the unprepared patient and family.

Although the basic care of the cardiovascular patient is similar for young and old, there are some specific considerations for the geriatric patient. The edema associated with many cardiovascular diseases may promote skin breakdown, especially in older people who have more fragile skin. Frequent change of position is vital. The body should be supported in proper alignment, and arms and legs should not be allowed to hang off the side of a bed or chair. Clothing and restraints should be checked frequently to make certain that they haven't become constricting due to increased edema. Areas of the body that receive pressure should be protected and should be massaged frequently. If the patient is to be on a stretcher, an examining table, or an operating-room table for a long period of time, the nurse should place protective padding on pressure areas beforehand to provide comfort and prevent skin breakdown. When much edema is present, excessive activity should be avoided. Activity increases the circulation of fluid and also of toxic wastes in the fluid, which can subject the patient to profound intoxication. The nurse should note changes in the patient's edematous state; a tape measure will provide quantitative data.

Accurate observation and documentation of fluid balance is especially important. Within any limitations prescribed by the physician fluid intake should be encouraged, in order to prevent dehydration, to which the aged are more susceptible, and facilitate diuresis (water is effective for this). Fluid loss through any means should be measured; volume, color, odor, and specific gravity of urine should be noted. The patient's weight should be obtained daily. If intravenous fluids are being administered, careful monitoring is essential. Excessive fluid infusion results in hypervolemia, subjecting the aged to the risk of congestive heart failure. It should be remembered that an intravenous glucose solution could stimulate the increased production of insulin, resulting in a hypoglycemic reaction if this solution is abruptly discontinued without an adequate substitute for the intravenous glucose.

Vital signs must be checked frequently, with careful attention to any changes. A temperature elevation can reflect an infection or a myocardial infarction. Remember that the body temperature for the aged may be normally lower and that it is important to have collected data on normal conditions as a basis for comparison. It is advisable to detect and correct temperature changes promptly. A temperature elevation increases metabolism, which in turn increases the body's requirements for oxygen and causes the heart to work harder. A decrease in temperature slows metabolism, which causes less oxygen consumption and thereby less carbon dioxide production and fewer respirations. A rise in blood pressure indicates increased demands on the heart. Headache, dizziness and nosebleed may indicate elevated blood pressure. Chronic hypoxia may be the cause of increased blood pressure, and the nurse should evaluate the patient for this factor. A decreased blood pressure is associated with a reduced cardiac output, vasodilation, and a lower blood volume. Hypotension can result in insufficient circulation to meet the body's needs. Symptoms of mental confusion and dizziness could indicate insufficient cerebral circulation resulting from a reduced blood pressure. Pulse changes are also significant. In addition to cardiac problems, tachycardia could indicate hypoxia due to an obstructed airway. Bradycardia could be associated with digitalis toxicity.

Oxygen is frequently administered in the treatment of cardiovascular diseases, and in aged patients it requires most careful use. Hypoxia should be closely observed for. Patients using a nasal catheter may breathe primarily by mouth and reduce oxygen intake. Although a face mask may remedy this problem, it does not guarantee a sufficient oxygen inspiration. The aged patient may not demonstrate cyanosis as the initial sign of hypoxia; instead he or she might be restless, irritable, and have dyspnea. These signs can also indicate high oxygen concentrations and consequent carbon dioxide narcosis, which is a particular risk to aged patients receiving oxygen therapy. Although blood gas levels will provide data revealing these problems, early correction is facilitated by keen nursing observation.

The nurse may have to help patients fulfill their nutritional needs and encourage older patients to eat if they have cardiovascular disease and suffer from anorexia. Favorite foods attractively served may overcome this, and several smaller meals throughout the entire day rather than a few large ones will compensate for poor appetite and reduce the work of the heart. The cardiovascular patient should be encouraged to maintain a regular intake of glucose, the primary source of cardiac energy. Patient education is frequently necessary regarding low-sodium, low-cholesterol, and/or low-calorie diets. It is not uncommon for the aged to have difficulty accepting a new diet. Ethnic dishes, often an important component of older people's culture, may not be allowed because of prescribed dietary restrictions. This can be a significant sacrifice for the older person, and many choose not to comply at all rather than to forfeit these dietary pleasures. The nurse can offer support to the aged person as these difficult dietary adjustments are made.

Involving patients in setting their own priorities and negotiating compromises in their diet may be worthwhile. A realistic although imperfect diet with which the patient is satisfied is more likely to be complied with than an ideal one that is meaningless to the patient. Older patients may need assistance in developing menus that observe their dietary restrictions. Lists of preferred foods along with notations regarding their sodium, cholesterol, and caloric content should be developed and assessed. It is more meaningful and efficient to focus only on foods commonly eaten by the patient and provide a description of the sodium, cholesterol, or caloric intake, depending on the type of restriction (see Table 8-1). Aged patients should also understand that carbonated drinks, certain analgesic preparations, commercial alkalizers and homemade baking soda mixtures, which they commonly employed for relief of indigestion, also contain sodium.

Reduced activity increases risks of constipation, and to avoid this problem and fecal impaction, ample fluid intake and dietary items that promote bowel elimination should be provided to maintain regular bowel function. Straining due to constipation, enemas, and removal of fecal impactions can cause vagal stimulation and be dangerous to the cardiovascular patient. If the patient is on bed rest, range-of-motion exercises can promote circulation and prevent complications resulting from immobilization; with complete bed rest, passive range-of-motion exercises will cause muscle contractions that compress peripheral veins and thereby facilitate the return of venous blood.

Patients who are weak or who fall asleep while sitting should have their head and neck supported to prevent hyperextension or hyperflexion of the neck. All aged persons, not only cardiovascular patients, can suffer a reduction in cerebral blood flow due to the compression of vessels during this hyperextension and hyperflexion. Those with congestive heart failure need good positioning and support. A semirecumbent position with pillows supporting the entire back maintains good body

TABLE 8-1: PARTIAL LIST SHOWING SODIUM CONTENT OF PREFERRED FOODS

	Sodium Content	Restriction Required
Meat, Poultry, and Fish		
Ham hock	High	√
Lean beef	Low	
Oysters	Low	
Corned beef	High	√
Dairy Group		
Skimmed milk	Low	
Cheddar cheese	High	√
Fruits and Vegetables		
White turnips	High	√
Glazed fruits	High	√
Kale	High	√
Pickled onions	High	√
Canned peas	High	√
Peanut butter	High	√
Apple	Low	
Breads and Cereals		
Puffed wheat	Low	
Baking powder biscuits	High	√

alignment, promotes comfort, and also assists in reducing pulmonary congestion. Cardiac strain is reduced by supporting the arms with pillows or armrests. Footboards help prevent foot-drop contracture, and patients should be instructed in how to use them for exercising also.

If hepatic congestion develops, drugs may detoxify more slowly. As the aged may already have a slower rate of drug detoxification, the nurse must be acutely aware of signs indicating an adverse drug reaction. Digitalis toxicity should be especially observed for in older persons. Nausea, vomiting, arrhythmias, and a slow pulse are among the signs which may indicate this problem. Since hypokalemia sensitizes the heart to the effects of digitalis, it should be prevented through proper diet and possibly the use of potassium supplements.

The patient who must manage anginal attacks should be helped to identify factors that precipitate attacks and to review the proper use of nitroglycerin—including its use when an attack is anticipated, such as during a stressful event, rather than after the attack occurs. Since the pain associated with a myocardial infarction may be similar to that of angina, the patient should be instructed to notify the physician or nurse if pain is not relieved by nitroglycerin. The patient's chart should include the factors that precipitate attacks, as well as the nature of the pain and how the patient describes it, the method of management, and the usual number of nitroglycerin tablets used to alleviate the attack.

Relaxation and rest are both important in the treatment of cardiovascular disease, and it is wise to remember that a patient who is at rest is not necessarily relaxed. The stresses from hospitalization, pain, ignorance and fear regarding disability, alteration in life-style, and thoughts about death can cause the aged to become anxious, confused, and irrational. Reassurance and support are needed, including full explanations of diagnostic tests, institutional routines, and other activities. Opportunities should be provided for the patients and their families to discuss questions, concerns, and fears openly. An often unasked question of aged patients relates to the restrictions cardiac disease imposes on sexual activity. Health professionals should not neglect to review any necessary limitations in sexual activity thinking aged patients aren't interested. This may be a serious concern to the geriatric patient, and it requires open discussion. Explanations of any necessary restrictions and changes in life-style should emphasize that the patient need not become a "cardiac cripple" for the remainder of his or her life. Most patients can still live a normal life and should be assured of this.

9

PERIPHERAL VASCULAR DISEASE

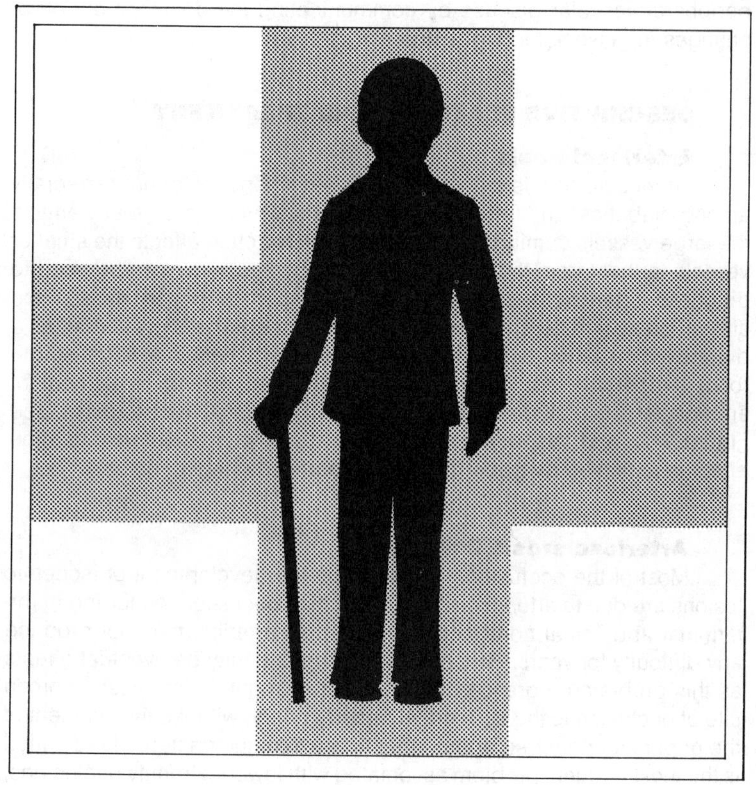

Blood vessels throughout the body undergo changes with age which contribute to a variety of peripheral vascular diseases. A loss of elasticity causes the vessels to dilate and elongate, and the tortuous nature of the vessels can be detected by the naked eye. Greater amounts of calcium, cholesterol, and other lipids are found in arteries, and increased amounts of connective tissue and mucopolysaccharides in the intima. There is also a reduced efficiency in the valves.

Many signs and symptoms of peripheral vascular disease can be noted during the initial assessment of the patient or while assisting with basic care; generalized edema, chills, and pallor, for example, might be suspect. Thick, dry nails and thin, scaling skin are subtle indications of poor circulation, and drowsiness, dizziness, and memory disturbances can be caused by insufficient cerebral circulation. Possible signs revealed by examination of the patient include pain, skin discoloration, altered skin temperature, and changes in the size of a limb or a portion of the body. Nurses can assist in the detection and management of peripheral vascular disease by communicating the development of, or changes in, associated signs and symptoms.

DESCRIPTIVE FEATURES AND TREATMENT

Arteriosclerosis

Arteriosclerosis is a common problem among the aged, especially among diabetics, and unlike atherosclerosis, which more greatly affects the large vessels coming from the heart, it most often affects the smaller vessels farthest from the heart. Arteriography and X-ray can be used to diagnose arteriosclerosis; and oscillometric testing can assess the arterial pulse at different levels. If surface temperature is evaluated, as a diagnostic measure, the nurse should keep the patient in a warm, stable room temperature for at least one hour before testing. Treatment of arteriosclerosis includes bed rest, warmth, Buerger-Allen exercises (see Figure 9-1), and vasodilators. Occasionally, a permanent vasodilation effect is achieved by performing a sympathetic ganglionectomy.

Arteriosclerosis Obliterans

Most of the occlusions that result in the development of ischemic lesions are due to arteriosclerosis. Aortoiliac occlusion, occurring in the terminal abdominal aorta and common iliac arteries, may not produce any difficulty for years. Rest pain and gangrene may be eventual effects as this problem progresses. In the lower extremities the most common site of occlusion is the superficial femoral artery, with the involvement of the popliteal artery tree or the tibial artery tree. Intermittent claudication is the most frequent problem associated with lower-extremity occlusions,

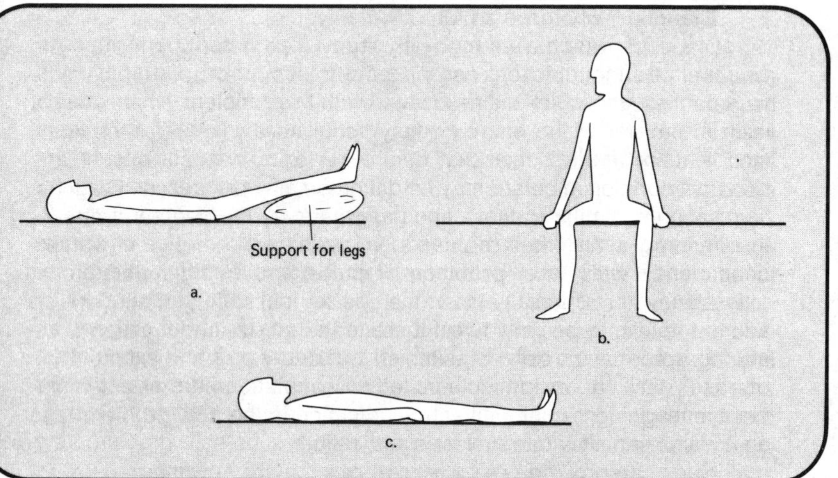

Figure 9-1. Buerger-Allen exercises: (a) Patient lies flat with legs elevated above the level of the heart until blanching occurs (approximately two minutes). (b) Patient lowers legs to fill the vessels and exercises feet until the legs are pink (approximately five minutes). Patient lies flat for approximately 5 minutes before repeating the exercises. Entire procedure is done five times, or as tolerated by the patient, at three different times of the day. The nurse should assist the patient with position changes since postural hypotension can occur. Tolerance and effectiveness of the procedure should be noted.

although some patients do develop ischemic rest pain, neuropathy and, less frequently, ulcers and gangrene. Treatment of arteriosclerosis obliterans depends on the location.

Arterial Embolism

Aneurysms, atrial fibrillation, myocardial infarction, atherosclerosis, and arteriosclerosis are among the problems which give rise to arterial emboli, which lodge primarily in the lower-extremity and brachial arteries. The aged are seriously threatened by gangrene and death from an undetected or untreated embolism, and the nurse should therefore be alert to indicative symptoms and signs. Coldness and numbness below the location of the embolism may prevent the aged from feeling pain until the condition progresses. Any pressure or constriction to the affected part should be avoided. Anticoagulation therapy, which, as discussed in Chapter 22, requires close nursing supervision, and embolectomies have proven beneficial.

Special Problems of the Diabetic

Diabetics, who have a high risk of developing peripheral vascular disease and associated complications, commonly display the neuropathies and infections associated with this problem, which affects vessels throughout the entire body. Arterial insufficiency can present itself in several ways: rest pain may occur as a result of intermittent claudication; arterial pulses may be difficult to find or totally absent; and skin discoloration, ulcerations, and gangrene may be present. Diagnostic measures, similar to those used to determine the degree of arterial insufficiency with other problems, include oscillometry, elevation-dependency tests, and palpation of pulse and skin temperature at different levels. Especially when there is the possibility of surgery, an arteriography may be done to establish the exact size and location of the arterial lesion. The treatment selected will depend on the extent of the disease. Walking can promote collateral circulation and may be sufficient management if intermittent claudication is the sole problem, and analgesics can provide relief from rest pain.

Since many of today's older diabetics may have witnessed severe disability and death among other diabetics they have known throughout their lives, they need to be assured that improved methods of medical and surgical management—perhaps not even developed at the time their parents and grandparents had diabetes—increase their chances for a full, independent life. Specific nursing measures used in the care of the older diabetic with peripheral artery disease are provided later in this chapter.

Aneurysms

Advanced arteriosclerosis is usually responsible for the development of aneurysms in aged persons, although they may also result from infection, trauma, syphilis, and other factors. Sometimes they can be seen by the naked eye and are able to be palpated as a pulsating mass; sometimes they can only be detected by X-ray. A thrombosis can develop in the aneurysm, leading to an arterial occlusion or rupture of the aneurysm—the most serious complications associated with this problem.

Aneurysms of the abdominal aorta most frequently occur in older people. Patients with a history of arteriosclerotic lesions, angina pectoris, myocardial infarction, and congestive heart failure more commonly develop aneurysms in this area. A pulsating mass, sometimes painful, in the umbilical region is an indication of an abdominal aorta aneurysm. Prompt correction is essential since if not corrected, rupture can occur. Fewer complications and deaths result from surgical intervention prior to rupture. Among the complications which the aged can develop after surgery for this problem are hemorrhage, myocardial infarction, cerebral vascular accident, and acute renal insufficiency. The nurse should closely observe for signs of postoperative complications.

Aneurysms can also develop in peripheral arteries, the most common sites being the femoral and popliteal arteries. Peripheral aneurysms can usually be palpated, and a diagnosis can be established in this manner. The most serious complication associated with peripheral aneurysms is the formation of a thrombus, which can occlude the vessel and cause loss of the limb. As with abdominal aorta aneurysms, early treatment reduces the risk of complications and death. The lesion may be resected with replacement of the portion of the vessel removed—commonly with a prosthetic material. For certain patients, a lumbar sympathectomy can be performed. The nurse should be aware that these patients can develop a thrombus postoperatively and assist the patient in preventing this complication.

Varicose Veins

Varicosities, a common problem in the aged, can be caused by lack of exercise, jobs entailing a great deal of standing, and losses of elasticity and strength associated with the aging process. Varicosities in all ages can be detected by the dilated, tortuous nature of the vein, especially the veins of the lower extremities. The person may experience dull pain and cramping of the legs, sometimes severe enough to interfere with sleep. Occasionally dizziness may occur as the patient rises from a lying position due to the localization of blood in the lower extremities and reduced cerebral circulation. The effects of the varicosities make the skin more susceptible to trauma and infection, promoting the development of ulcerative lesions, especially if the patient is obese or diabetic.

Treatment of varicose veins is aimed toward reducing venous stasis. The affected limb is elevated and rested to promote venous return. Exercise, particularly walking, will also enhance circulation. The nurse should make sure that elastic stockings and bandages are properly used and not constricting and that the patient is informed of the causes of venous status (e.g., prolonged standing, crossing the legs, wearing constricting clothing), in order to prevent the development of complications and additional varicosities. Ligation and stripping of the veins require the same principles of nursing care which would be used for other age groups undergoing this surgery.

Venous Thromboembolism

An increasing incidence of venous thromboembolism is found among the aged. Patients who have been on bed rest or have had recent surgery or fractures of a lower extremity are high risk candidates. Although the veins in the calf muscles are the most frequently seen sites of this problem, it also occurs in the inferior vena cava, iliofemoral segment, and various superficial veins. The symptoms and signs of venous thromboembolism depend on the vessel involved. Clues which the nurse should be alert for include edema, warmth over the affected area, and pain in the sole of the foot. Edema may be the primary indication of thromboembolism in the veins of the calf muscle since it is not unusual for discoloration and pain to be absent in aged persons with this problem. If the inferior vena cava is involved, there will be bilateral swelling, aching and cyanosis of the lower extremities, engorgement of the superficial veins, and tenderness along the femoral veins. Similar signs will appear with involvement of the iliofemoral segment, but only on the affected extremity.

The location of the thromboembolism will dictate the treatment employed. Elastic stockings or bandages, rest, and elevation of the affected limb may be used to promote venous return. Analgesics may be given to relieve any associated pain. Anticoagulants may be administered and surgery may be performed as well. The nurse should help the patient to avoid situations that cause straining and to remain comfortable and well hydrated.

NURSING CONSIDERATIONS

Preventing problems such as peripheral vascular disease from developing is an important part of nursing. Health education should emphasize the importance of exercise, such as walking to promote circulation, and of not sitting with legs crossed or standing for prolonged periods of time. Obesity, which can interfere with venous return, should be avoided. Clothing that might interfere with circulation should be pointed out, for example, garters, tight-fitting shoes, girdles, and tight slacks. Instruction in such measures can prevent complications from, and avoid the development of, vascular problems. The use of tobacco should be discouraged as it may cause arteriospasms. To prevent thrombus formation, immobility and hypotension should be prevented. The physician may prescribe Buerger-Allen exercises (see Figure 9-1), and the nurse should instruct the patient, and perhaps a family member, in the proper method of doing them, including how to provide comfort for the patient while they are done and how to use any support hose or special elastic stockings correctly.

Persons with peripheral vascular disease must pay special attention to the care of their feet, which should be bathed and inspected daily. To avoid injury, the patient should not walk in bare feet. Any foot lesion or discoloration should promptly be brought to the attention of the nurse or physician. These patients may easily develop fungal infections from the moisture produced by normal foot perspiration. The aged frequently

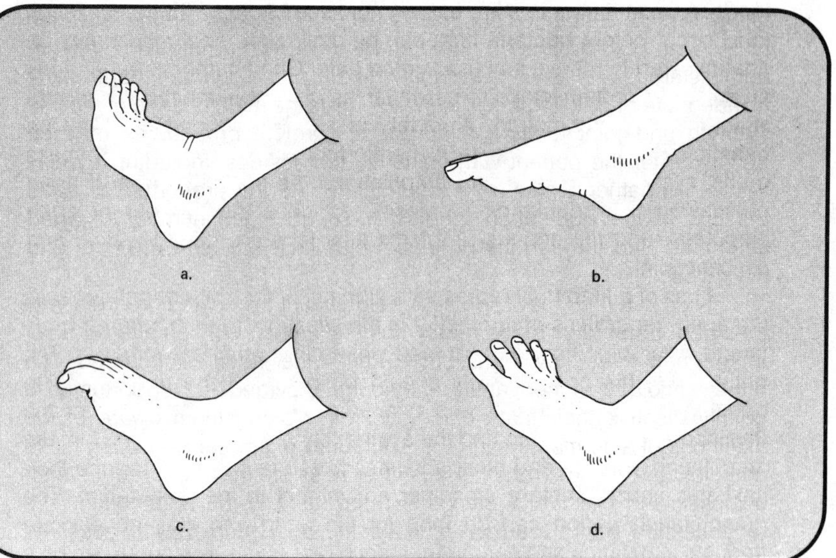

Figure 9-2. Foot and toe exercises: (a) Foot flexion. (b) Foot extension. (c) Curling toes. (d) Moving toes apart.

develop fungal infections under their nails, emphasizing the importance of regular, careful nail inspection. If untreated, a simple fungal infection can lead to gangrene and other serious complications. Placing cotton between the toes and removing shoes several times throughout the day will help keep the feet dry. Shoes should be large enough to avoid any pressure and safe enough to prevent any injuries to the feet, and they should be aired after wearing: patients should be encouraged to have several pairs of shoes, if possible, and rotate their use. Laces should not be tied tightly because they can exert pressure on the feet. Socks should be changed regularly, and to prevent possible irritation from dyes, colored socks should be discouraged. Although the feet should be kept warm, the direct application of heat to the feet, as with heating pads, hot water bottles, and soaks, can increase the metabolism and circulatory demand, thereby compounding the existing problem. Figure 9-2 shows some exercises which may benefit the patient with peripheral vascular disease.

Ischemic foot lesions may be present in patients with peripheral vascular disease. If eschars are present, they should be loosened to allow drainage. Debridement should be performed with care to avoid bleeding and trauma. Chemical debriding agents are sometimes utilized. Systemic antibiotic agents can be helpful in controlling cellulitis. Topical antibiotics are usually not used because epithelialization must occur before bacteria flora can be destroyed. Analgesics may be administered to relieve any associated pain. Good nutrition, particularly an adequate protein intake, is essential, as is the maintenance of muscle strength and joint motion. A variety of surgical procedures may be beneficial for the patient with ischemic foot lesions, including bypass grafts, sympathectomies, and amputations. As the proportion of aged persons in the population increases, so does the number of aged amputees, and the serious problems they face are both physical and psychosocial.

Loss of a limb may represent a significant loss of independence to the aged, regardless of the reality of the situation. With an altered body image, new roles may be assumed while other roles are forfeited. The patient and his or her family should be provided the opportunity to openly discuss their fears and concerns. Making them aware of the likelihood of a normal life and the availability of appliances which make ambulation, driving, and other activities possible may help reduce their anxieties and promote a smoother adjustment to the amputation. The rehabilitation period can be long for the aged and may necessitate frequent motivation and encouragement by the nurse. The nurse can be a valuable support person to the patient and the family during this difficult process.

It is hoped that the nurse will explore medical-surgical nursing literature for a complete discussion of general care of the patient with peripheral vascular disease.

10

CANCER

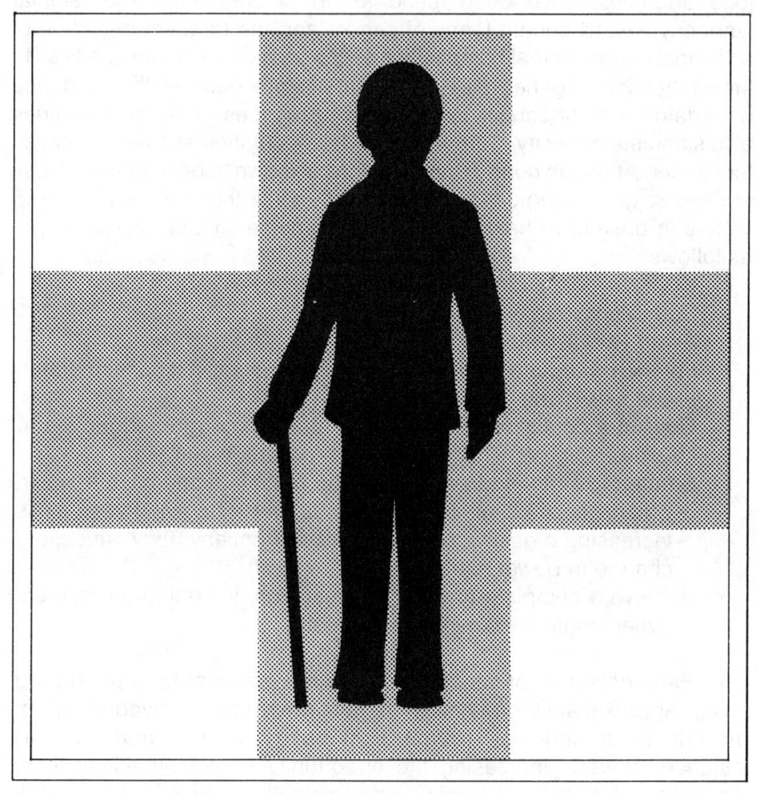

Cancer, a serious problem at any age, is the second leading cause of death among the older population. The incidence of cancer increases with age until the ninth decade, when a tendency for fewer new cases in proportion to that age group is noted. Although the prevalence of most carcinomas is higher among the aged, some forms, such as cervical cancer and sarcomas, are diagnosed less frequently in older persons. Cancer tends to progress more slowly and run a less aggressive course in the aged.

ETIOLOGY AND DETECTION

The exact etiology of cancer is presently unknown, but several factors have been associated with it. Chronic irritation, from pipe smoking for instance, has been known to promote lesions which can become cancerous. Radiation can alter cellular activity and cause abnormal cell growth. Certain agents, such as air pollutants and some food additives, have been found to be carcinogenic. The familial tendency toward certain forms of cancer and the frequent detection of abnormal chromosomal composition of cancer cells raise questions as to the relationship of genes to cancer. Relationships between the incidence of certain forms of cancer in the dietary practices of certain countries also stimulate curiosity. Currently there is speculation as to a viral cause for cancer. Although none of these factors is known to be a definite cause of cancer, gerontological nurses can recognize them as predisposing factors in preventive health practices. The nurse should advise people as follows:

Do not smoke.
Avoid excessive alcohol intake.
Follow a well-balanced diet, avoiding extremes in food temperature and seasoning.
Consult a dentist for poor-fitting dentures or jagged-edged teeth.
Use protection against excessive exposure to sun.
Be alert to signs and symptoms that might indicate cancer: a sore which doesn't heal, unexplained weight loss, a painless mass, increasing digestive problems, blood from any body orifice, or a change in bowel habits.
Receive a complete physical examination, including a rectal and gynecological examination, regularly.

Early detection of cancer improves the potential for a good prognosis. Approximately one-half of the sites that cancer invades can be directly examined—the breast, oral cavity, rectum and skin, for instance—thereby increasing the opportunity for abnormalities to be discovered during a routine physical examination. Unfortunately, people do not always seek regular checkups, waiting, instead, until they feel ill. By the time the disease has progressed to the extent that it causes symptoms, valuable treatment time may be lost and the chances of a good prognosis reduced. Also, symptoms produced by cancer in a particular site may be confused with other problems; for example, constipation associated with cancer of the colon may mistakenly be attributed to poor peristalsis in the aged. If baseline information has been obtained through the nursing assessment, it can provide comparative data for the nurse to use when changes indicating cancer are suspected. An extensive review of cancer facts will not be provided here. Since the general principles of diagnosis and management are similar for old and young, the nurse should consult medical-surgical texts for more information.

FACTORS RELEVANT TO THE GERONTOLOGICAL NURSE

The gastrointestinal system is frequently the location of cancerous growths. A squamous cell form of cancer may develop on the lip, primarily involving the lower lip. Exposure to sun and irritation from a pipe, teeth, or dentures are among the contributing factors. Cancer of the lip can metastasize to the cervical lympth nodes. Vitamin-B deficiencies, syphilis, excessive smoking, and pressure from jagged edged teeth or dentures can promote cancer of the mouth. Cancer of the tongue can metastasize to local lymph nodes, although it does not usually metastasize to other body organs, and the tonsils can also develop cancer that affects the surrounding lymph nodes. Since bleeding is a symptom that may indicate cancer in this site, and since this symptom can initially be misjudged as hemoptysis, the nurse should carefully examine the mouth and throat when bleeding occurs to more accurately differentiate the cause of the problem. Cancer of the tonsils may be secondary to breast cancer.

There is an increasing incidence of lung cancer, especially among males. A great deal of evidence links a history of smoking to the development of lung cancer. Symptoms of this problem include dyspnea, fever, weakness, cyanosis, and hemoptysis—all of which may be confused with symptoms of other respiratory diseases, thus delaying diagnosis. Without early detection and treatment, metastasis throughout the entire body can occur.

Cancer of the pharynx also requires keen observation and assessment for early detection. Associated symptoms are soreness of and bleeding from the throat and a slight deafness. Cancer of the pharynx may be a result of metastasis from cancer of the esophagus, heart, bronchi, or palate. Tobacco, alcohol, tuberculosis, and irritation from highly seasoned foods may contribute to cancer of the stomach and the esophagus (which is of higher incidence in men). Cancer of the stomach tends to have a poor prognosis due to the difficulty in early diagnosis. Symptoms of stomach cancer—cachexia, weight loss, anemia, hypoalbuminemia, and dyspepsia—are often attributed to other causes, which interferes with early detection. A change in bowel habits, a sign which nurses are often able to detect, should give suspicion as to cancer of the intestines. General symptoms, such as anemia, diarrhea, and weight loss, which can be attributed to other causes, may be indications of cancer of the cecum.

Most persons who develop cancer of the colon and rectum are aged; cancer of the colon occurs more often in females, and cancer of the rectum in males. Cancer of the ascending colon can produce cryptic anemia and a dull pain, which may be easily confused with gallbladder pain. Cancer of the ascending colon can metastasize to the sacral plexus, producing sciatic or back pain. Cancer of the descending colon and rectum can produce anorexia, weight loss, fatigue, weakness, constipation, diarrhea, and bloody, mucus stools. Many masses in this area can be detected through a digital examination; the nurse should make sure the patient is not impacted prior to a digital examination so that a fecal impaction is not confused for a mass. Since cancer in the lower bowel does remain localized for a long time, early surgery is beneficial.

Breast cancer is a serious problem among older women. Any lump in the breast after menopause should give rise to suspicion of breast cancer. Older women should receive instruction regarding the proper method of breast examinations and become familiar with the normal contour of their breasts (Figure 10-1). They should be encouraged to examine their breasts regularly on a specific day of the month, such as their birthday or the day a pension check arrives. Often, a woman will be able to note a change in her breasts more quickly than the physician who examines her several times a year. Any dimpling of the skin or discharge from the nipples should be evaluated. Although cervical cancer does not occur as frequently among older females, they should still be encouraged to receive regular Pap smears and thorough gynecological examinations. Some older women believe that after menopause they needn't be concerned about seeing a gynecologist unless definite symptoms appear; the nurse should be certain to clarify this misconception and encourage regular examinations.

Cancer of the prostate gland is not an uncommon problem for older men, and regular examination of the prostate gland is essential for early detection. A small percentage of benign hypertrophies develop into malignancies, thereby emphasizing the importance of periodic reevaluation of benign prostatic hypertrophy. Cancer at this site is known to metastasize to the pelvis, vertebrae, and brain. Hematuria may be an

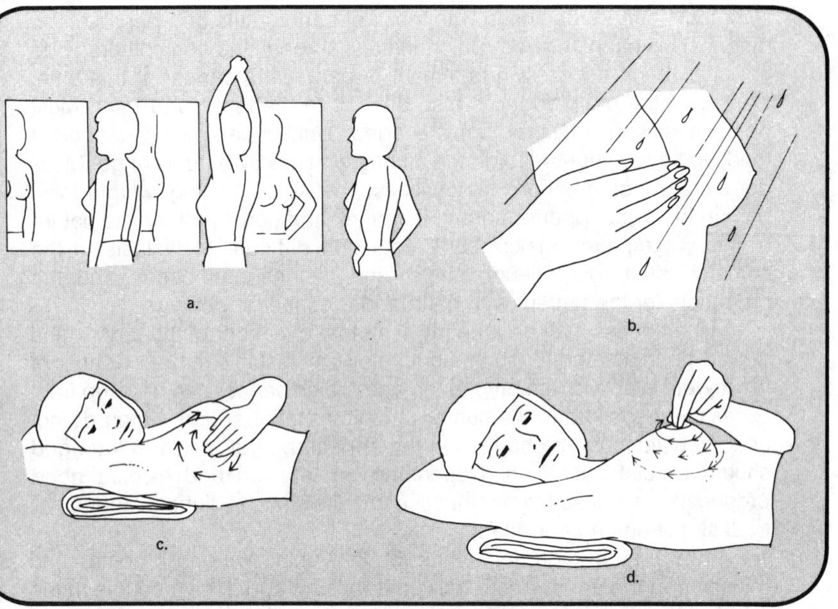

Figure 10-1. Self-examination of breasts: (a) With arms straight at side, arms over head, and hands on hips while flexing chest muscles, inspect breasts before a mirror to detect swelling, changes in contour, dimpling, nipple change, or any other differences. (b) While in tub or shower, run hand over breast with fingers flat to detect thickening or lumps. (c) Inspect breasts while lying down, with folded towel under shoulder of side being examined and arm of that side behind head. (d) With fingers flat, examine outer portion of each breast, progressing in a circular motion around circumference of breast. Move fingers one inch toward center and repeat until entire breast is examined. Then gently squeeze nipple to detect any discharge. (Additional information is available from the American Cancer Society.)

indication of cancer within the genitourinary system and should receive prompt evaluation. Older males tend to have a higher incidence of bladder cancer. Cancer within this system can metastasize to the lungs, liver, lymph nodes, and other organs if not corrected.

Cancer of the pancreas, more prevalent among males, is a difficult problem to diagnose and treat in the aged. Symptoms may include anorexia, weakness, weight loss, dyspepsia, epigastric pain radiating to the back, diarrhea, constipation, obstructive jaundice, and depression and other emotional changes. Sometimes venous thrombosis occurs, believed to be caused by an elevation in serum trypsin. Since these symptoms can be confused with those of pancreatitis and peptic ulcer, diagnosis is often delayed. Unfortunately, surgery and chemotherapy do not offer much success in treatment of pancreatic cancer at this time. Cancer of the gallbladder is also difficult to diagnose and treat. Most persons having this problem are aged. Unlike pancreatic cancer, it tends to have a higher incidence among women. Symptoms of gallbladder cancer include anorexia, weakness, nausea, vomiting, weight loss, pain in the right upper quadrant, jaundice, and constipation. The nature of these symptoms makes early detection difficult. Metastasis to the common duct, peritoneum, lungs, and ovaries can occur, and the prognosis for the patient with gallbladder cancer is poor.

Hoarseness may be an early symptom of cancer of the larynx, and should be evaluated for such. Fortunately, metastasis is rare. Cancer of the thyroid gland is rare among the aged. Skin cancer can develop from excessive exposure to the sun or chronic irritation. Sores which do not heal, new lesions, or changes in the appearance of moles in the aged should arouse suspicion. Depending on location and size, a good prognosis can result from the use of excision, radiation, and electrodesiccation and currettage.

There is a high incidence of leukemia, lymphosarcoma, and myeloma in the aged. Acute leukemia runs an aggressive course in the aged, although chemotherapy is often successful in producing remissions. Chronic lymphocytic leukemia or myeloma, on the other hand, is not an aggressive disease in the aged. Multiple myeloma can be extremely painful and disabling to the aged, but fortunately, the incidence of this disease is lower in older age groups. Hodgkin's disease tends to run a more aggressive course in the aged. Anemia, leukopenia, and thrombocytopenia occur with both multiple myeloma and Hodgkin's disease in the aged.

As mentioned earlier, treatment of cancer in the aged will be basically similar to treatment methods selected for younger adults, striving toward cure with minimal limitation. Surgery may prove beneficial but it should be remembered that the aged are a higher surgical risk. The benefits of chemotherapy must be weighed against the side effects it may cause in the aged. A therapeutic ratio is usually sought whereby the optimum effect is achieved with the least toxicity. Individualized decisions for cancer management are based on the general health status of the person, the form of cancer, the expected outcome, and the preferance of the patient. At no time should treatment be discouraged or withheld due to age alone.

The nurse is a key figure in cancer management. It may be the nurse who first detects a symptom of cancer and who can facilitate a prompt diagnosis. The nurse can offer support and explanations during the diagnostic process. Once a positive diagnosis is made, the nurse can help the patient work through the denial, anger, depression, and other reactions frequently associated with a new diagnosis of cancer. While providing hope, the nurse can also guide the patient toward a realistic understanding of the outcomes of his or her disease. If disability and death are to be expected, the patient and his family may need strong nursing support as they learn to accept and plan for these consequences. On the other hand, patients with a good prognosis should be encouraged not to self-impose limitations or become "emotional cripples" as a result of having had a diagnosis of cancer. Within a realistic framework, all patients with cancer should be inspired to maintain a normal life-style and maximize their existing capacities.

When the terminal stage of cancer is reached, additional nursing intervention may be required to compensate for the patient's increasing limitations. The relief of pain is a priority for terminally ill patients. Concern as to the reality of the pain or the risk of narcotic addiction should not prevent the administration of analgesics. A low dosage should be administered initially, with periodic reevaluations as to the need for dosage change. To reduce stress and preserve energy of the terminal patient, analgesics should be given to *prevent* pain and not only *correct* it once it has already occurred. The nurse should observe the nature of the pain as the disease progresses; as death approaches, less pain may be sensed, and consequently less analgesics required to provide relief. Small, frequent feedings of foods enjoyed by the patient may compensate for poor appetite and promote a better food intake. Vitamin and protein supplements may be beneficial. An ample fluid intake should be maintained.

The skin should be kept clean, dry and unbroken. Due to the general debilitated state of the patient, skin breakdown may be a greater risk. Frequent skin care can provide cleanliness, comfort, and prevention of breakdown. Comfort is important, physically and psychologically. Certain forms of cancer produce an unpleasant odor, and the nurse should maintain an attractive appearance of the patient, especially in light of any disfigurement, weight loss, jaundice, or other changes which may be taking place. Positioning should provide optimum comfort. Environmental considerations—such as adequate ventilation, soft lights, and a clean area—mean a great deal to the bedridden patient and the family. Opportunities for conversations should be provided. The terminally ill patient and the family may need to discuss their relationships, feelings, and the impending death. Involvement of the clergy may provide valuable support to them. The skills of the nurse may determine if the patient's death will be an unnecessarily traumatic experience, or one of beauty and dignity.

11

RESPIRATORY PROBLEMS

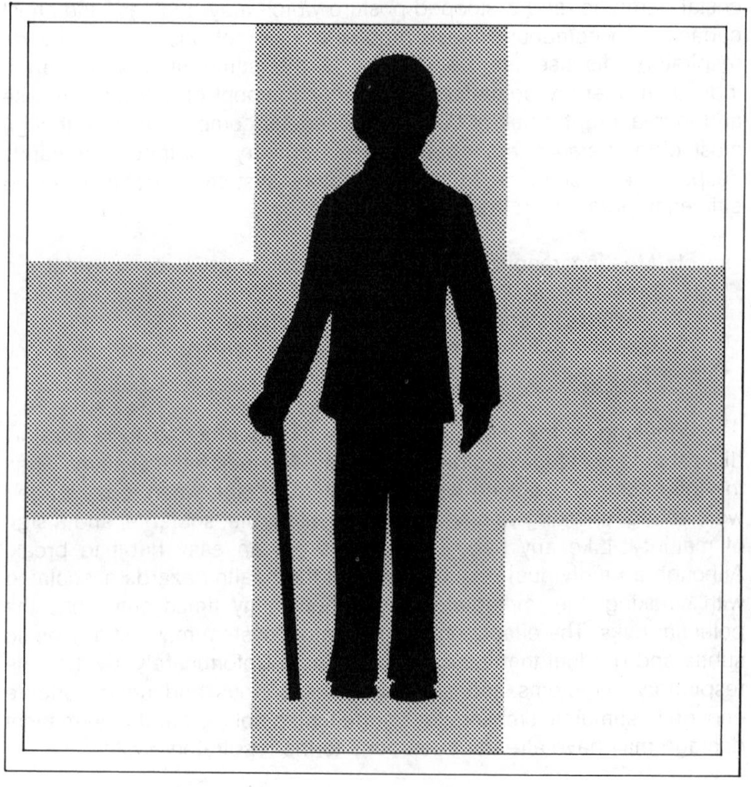

Respiratory problems are among the more common and life-threatening disorders the aged experience. Influenza and pneumonia are the fourth leading causes of death, and bronchitis, emphysema, and asthma rank eighth. In addition to the high mortality that results, respiratory diseases impose many limitations that prevent aged people from enjoying an active, full life. Various aging changes, which increase the susceptibility and decrease the capacity of a person to manage these disorders, may explain their high prevalence among the aged. In general, the respiratory system functions less efficiently with advancing age. The lungs lose their elasticity and increase in size, contributing to a higher residual volume and lower vital capacity. The lung capillaries are fewer in number. Bronchioles and alveoli lose elasticity as well. The blood oxygen level (PO_2) may be 75 mmHg instead of 90–95 mmHg, as it is in younger adults; however, the blood carbon dioxide level (PCO_2) tends to remain the same.

Respiratory limitations may also be imposed by other changes associated with aging, such as a more rigid rib cage, ossification of costal cartilage, and a stooped posture which may decrease the chest capacity. To compound these problems, it is not unusual for several respiratory diseases to be present at the same time in an aged individual, thereby complicating the management of any one disease and increasing the risk of developing serious complications. Although most older persons are able to meet ordinary respiratory demands despite these changes to the respiratory system, there is reduced efficiency primarily in the following areas:

1. Meeting respiratory demands under unusual or stressful circumstances
2. Lower resistance to respiratory infections
3. Greater difficulty managing a respiratory problem once one develops

Smoking is the most important factor contributing to respiratory disease. Many of today's older smokers started their habit at a time when the full effects of smoking weren't realized. In fact, when today's aged were young, smoking was considered fashionable, sociable, and a sign of maturity. Like any habit, smoking is not an easy habit to break. Although an individual may be aware of the health hazards associated with smoking, the immediate gratification many times outweighs the potential risks. The effects on the respiratory system may initially be so subtle and gradual that they are not noticed. Unfortunately, by the time respiratory symptoms and signs become serious and uncomfortable enough to stimulate smokers to change their smoking habits, permanent damage may have already been done to the respiratory system.

TABLE 11-1: DEATH RATES FOR RESPIRATORY DISEASES BY SEX AND AGE

	Influenza and Pneumonia	Emphysema
Male		
15–24	2.4	0
25–44	5.7	0.6
45–64	30.0	22.0
65 and over	266.1	151.4
Female		
15–24	1.6	0
25–44	4.0	0.3
45–64	15.0	6.0
65 and over	171.1	22.3

Source: U.S. Bureau of the Census, *Statistical Abstract of the United States: 1975.* 96th Ed., Washington, D.C., 1975, p. 61, No. 86. Death rates per 100,000 for 1973.

Smoking is the major cause of chronic bronchitis. Smokers have a higher incidence of respiratory disease and a higher incidence of complications with respiratory disease than nonsmokers. Commonly, smokers have a productive cough, episodes of shortness of breath, and a reduced breathing capacity. Also, smokers have twice the incidence of lung cancer. Gerontological nurses should be actively involved with preventing young persons from developing a smoking habit. Education as to the health problems associated with smoking and positive reinforcement to nonsmokers may promote the health of future aged persons. Local health departments and respiratory disease associations provide specific information on various antismoking programs and strategies to help smokers forfeit their habit, and the nurse can help make smokers aware of these programs.

COMMON DISORDERS IN THE AGED

Pneumonia

Pneumonia is common in the aged, especially bronchopneumonia, and as mentioned, it is one of the leading causes of death in this age group. There was a time when pneumonia in an aged person meant death, but fortunately the discovery of antibiotics has significantly reduced the mortality and morbidity associated with this disease. There are several factors contributing to the high incidence. Changes to the respiratory system with age may cause poor chest expansion and more shallow breathing. The aged may have other respiratory diseases which promote mucus formation and bronchial obstruction. Upper respiratory infection is more frequent in the aged, especially since they already have a lowered resistance to infection. The reduced sensitivity of pharyngeal reflexes in many aged persons may promote aspiration of foreign material. Also, the aged are more likely to be debilitated and immobile.

The signs and symptoms of pneumonia may be altered in older persons. A serious pneumonia may exist without symptoms being evident. Pleuritic pain, for instance, may not be as severe as that described by younger patients. Differences in body temperature may cause little or no fever to be present. Symptoms may include a slight cough, fatigue, and rapid respiration. Confusion, restlessness, and behavioral changes may occur as a result of cerebral hypoxia. Nursing care for the geriatric patient with pneumonia is similar to that employed for the younger patient. Close observation for subtle changes is especially important. A complication which the aged patient may develop is paralytic ileus, prevented by mobility.

Asthma

Some aged have been affected with asthma throughout their lives, some develop it during old age. The symptoms and management do not differ much from those of other age groups. Epinephrine, antibiotics, and occasionally adrenocorticosteroids are used in treating older asthmatics. Because of the added stress asthma places on the heart, older asthmatics have a high risk of developing complications such as bronchiectasis and cardiac problems. The nurse should assist in detecting causative factors and should educate the patient regarding early recognition and prompt attention to an asthma attack when it does occur. Careful assessment of the aged asthmatic's use of aerosal nebulizers is advisable. Cardiac arrhythmias leading to sudden death may be risked by the overuse of sympathomimetic bronchodilating nebulizers (Stolley, 1972).

Chronic Bronchitis

Many aged persons demonstrate the persistent, productive cough and wheezing and the recurrent respiratory infections and shortness of breath caused by chronic bronchitis. As with many other chronic respiratory diseases, these symptoms may develop gradually, sometimes taking years for the full impact of the disease to be realized, at which time the patients notice increased difficulty breathing in cold and damp weather due to bronchospasm. They experience more frequent respiratory infections and greater difficulty in managing them. Episodes of hypoxia begin to occur as mucus obstructs the bronchial tree and causes carbon dioxide retention. As the disease progresses, emphysema may develop and death may occur from obstruction. The management of this problem, aimed at removing bronchial secretions and preventing obstruction of the airway, is similar for all age groups. Older patients may need special encouragement to maintain a good fluid intake and expectorate secretions. The nurse can be most effective in preventing the development of chronic bronchitis by discouraging chronic respiratory irritation, such as from smoking, and by helping the aged to prevent respiratory infections.

Emphysema

Of increasing incidence in the aged population is the progressive, chronic, and obstructive lung disease emphysema. Factors causing this destructive disease include asthma, chronic bronchitis, and chronic irritation from dusts or certain air pollutants. Cigarette smoking also plays a major role in the development of emphysema. The symptoms are slow in onset and initially may resemble those of the changes in the respiratory system that come with age, causing many patients to have delayed identification and treatment of this disease. Gradually, increased dyspnea is experienced, which is not relieved by sitting upright as it may have been in the past. A chronic cough develops. As more effort is required for breathing and as hypoxia occurs, fatigue, anorexia, weight loss, and weakness are demonstrated. Recurrent respiratory infections, malnutrition, congestive heart failure, and cardiac arrhythmias are among the more life-threatening complications the aged can experience from emphysema.

Treatment usually includes postural drainage, intermittent positive pressure breathing, bronchodilators, the avoidance of stressful situations and breathing exercises, which are an important part of patient education (Figure 11-1). Cigarette smoking should definitely be stopped. The older patient especially may have a problem with adequate food and fluid intake, requiring special nursing attention. If oxygen is utilized, it must be done with extreme caution and close supervision. It must be remembered that for this patient, a low oxygen level rather than a high carbon dioxide level stimulates respiration. The older patient with emphysema is a high risk candidate for the development of carbon dioxide narcosis. Respiratory infections should be prevented, and any which do occur, regardless of how minor they may seem, should be promptly reported to the physician. Sedatives, hypnotics, and narcotics may be contraindicated because the patient will be more sensitive to these drugs. Patients with emphysema need a great deal of education and support to be able to manage this disease. It is very difficult to adjust to the fact that one has a serious chronic disease requiring special care or even a change in life-style. The patient must learn to pace activities, avoid extremely cold weather, administer medications correctly, and recognize symptoms of infection.

Tuberculosis

The incidence of tuberculosis is increasing among the aged, and a high incidence is found in institutional settings. Rather than a new infection, the aged usually experience a reactivation of an earlier infection which was either asymptomatic or improperly treated. Diagnosis may be delayed, either because the classic symptoms are not demonstrated or because symptoms resemble changes associated with the aging process. For instance, anorexia and weakness may be the primary symptoms. Night sweats may not occur due to reduced diaphoresis with advanced age. Likewise, fever may not be detected due to alterations in the aged's body temperature. These factors emphasize the importance of periodic evaluation for this disease. Screening for tuberculosis should be performed for all patients entering a hospital or facility for geriatric care, and, periodically, groups of aged persons, such as golden age clubs and senior citizen associations, should be checked.

Treatment follows the same principles as for any age group, basically consisting of rest, good nutrition, and medications. Some of the side effects of medications commonly prescribed for tuberculosis have special implications for aged persons. Streptomycin can cause damage to the peripheral and central nervous systems, demonstrated through hearing limitations and disequilibrium. The safety hazards created by these adverse reactions are significant to the aged. Para-aminosalcylic acid can cause irritation to the gastrointestinal tract, anorexia, nausea, vomiting, and diarrhea—predisposing the aged to the risk of malnutrition. In addition, changes in gastric secretions can cause these tablets to pass through the gastrointestinal system without being dissolved, thereby preventing a therapeutic benefit. Stools should be examined for undissolved tablets. Isoniazid, although not as toxic as the other drugs mentioned, can have toxic effects on the peripheral and central nervous systems. The nurse must continuously assess the patient for the appearance of adverse reactions from such medications.

A diagnosis of tuberculosis can be extremely difficult for older persons to accept. Having lived through a time when people with tuberculosis were sent away to sanitariums for long periods of time, they may be unaware of new approaches and fear institutionalization. Believing they might infect family and friends, they may avoid contact with others, promoting social isolation. It is also possible that other people will fear contracting the disease and be reluctant to maintain social contact. Education of patients, their family, and friends is essential in order to clarify these misconceptions, promote a normal life-style.

Two different types of breathing exercises include pursed lip breathing and diaphragm retraining exercises. Since their purpose is to effect a change in the patient's breathing pattern, both should be shown to the patient as a simultaneous effort.

Instruction should include the following:

1. Inhale a normal breath through the nose to the count of one to humidify and cleanse the air.
2. Relax and exhale to the count of three using pursed lips to facilitate CO_2 elimination.
3. Neither gasp for the next breath nor force air out past the count of three. The goal is to develop a slow respiratory rate with an inspiratory-expiratory ratio of 1:3 or 1:4.
4. Place one hand (hand A) below the ribs on the stomach. Place the other hand (hand B) over the middle anterior chest. During exhalation, firmly press hand A inward and upward on the stomach to assist the lungs in expelling air. Concentrate on increasing stomach movement (hand A will rise on expiration and fall on inspiration) and decreasing chest movement (hand B should not move).

By permission of Hilary D. Sigmon, R.N., M.S.N., Clinical Specialist, Johns Hopkins Hospital.

Figure 11-1. Breathing exercises.

Patients should be taught their responsibilities in managing this disease. Medication is essential for the treatment of tuberculosis, and since the aged person may have a problem remembering to take it, nurses should devise a system for helping the patient remember how to administer the medication. For example, medications and denture cream could be placed in the same box so that during daily denture care medications would be remembered; the patient, a family member, or a visiting nurse could fill seven envelopes with medications, labeling them for each day of the week, and devise a chart for recording when medication is taken; a family member or friend could call the patient daily to ask whether medication was taken. With prompt and proper therapy, the aged person can recover from tuberculosis with minimal residual effects.

Lung Cancer

It is uncertain whether the increased incidence of lung cancer in the aged population is due to more cases of lung cancer actually occurring or improved diagnostic tools and greater availability of medical care. Lung cancer occurs more frequently in men, and there is a higher mortality from lung cancer among Caucasions. Cigarette smokers have twice the incidence of nonsmokers. There is also a high incidence among individuals who are chronically exposed to agents such as asbestos, coal gas, radioactive dusts, and chromates. This emphasizes the significance of obtaining thorough information regarding a patient's occupational history as part of the nursing assessment. Although conclusive evidence is presently unavailable, there is some association between the presence of lung scars (such as those resulting from tuberculosis and pneumonitis) and lung cancer.

The individual may have lung cancer long before any symptoms develop. This suggests that individuals at high risk should be regularly screened and should obtain periodic roentgenograms to detect this disease in an early stage. Dyspnea, coughing, chest pain, fatigue, anorexia, wheezing, and recurrent upper respiratory infections are part of the symptomatology seen as the disease progresses. Diagnosis is confirmed through chest roentgenogram, sputum cytology, bronchoscopy, and biopsy. Treatment may consist of surgery, chemotherapy, or radiotherapy, requiring the same type of nursing care for patients of any age with this diagnosis.

Lung Abscess

A lung abscess may result from pneumonia, tuberculosis, a malignancy, or trauma to the lung. Aspiration of foreign material can also cause a lung abscess and this may be a particular risk to aged persons who have decreased pharyngeal reflexes. Symptoms, resembling those of many other respiratory problems, include anorexia, weight loss, fatigue, temperature elevation, and a chronic cough. Sputum production may occur, but this is not always demonstrated in aged persons. Diagnosis and management are the same as for other age groups. Modifications for postural drainage, an important component of the treatment, will be discussed later in this chapter. Since protein can be lost through the sputum, a high-protein, high-caloric diet should be encouraged to maintain and improve the nutritional status of the aged patient.

Bronchiectasis

Bronchiectasis does not occur as frequently in older age groups as it does in the young. Aged persons can develop this problem from chronic bronchitis, asthma, recurrent upper respiratory infections, or aspiration of foreign material. There is also some belief that the weakening of the bronchioles with increased age causes a breakdown of the alveolar and bronchiolar walls. The most outstanding symptoms that older persons demonstrate are a temperature elevation and a chronic cough that produces large amounts of foul-smelling sputum. Diagnostic measures and treatment are similar to those for other age groups. Postural drainage, modified for the aged, and a high-protein high-caloric diet are essential components of the treatment plan.

NURSING CONSIDERATIONS

Respiratory problems are serious for aged individuals. They are at greater risk of developing respiratory complications in association with other diseases and also as a result of changes in the respiratory system with age. Once respiratory diseases have developed, close monitoring of the patient's status is required to minimize disability and prevent mortality. Close nursing observation can prevent and detect respiratory complications. Changes in the rate and volume of respirations can indicate respiratory problems, as can distended neck veins. A sudden increase in pulse can occur with hypoxia. Chronic hypoxia can cause an elevated blood pressure. Changes in mental status may also be associated with hypoxia. The nurse should assist the patient in the removal of secretions and regularly check for the patency of the airway. Body temperature should be frequently checked for elevations, not only to detect an infectious process, but to prevent stress on the cardiovascular and respiratory systems as they attempt to meet the body's increased oxygen demands imposed by an elevated temperature.

Since the aged may have reduced cough efficiency, the nature of the cough and the quality and quantity of sputum production should be observed and documented. To avoid embarrassment, some individuals learn to suppress a chronic cough; the nurse can ascertain this during her assessment by asking the patient to take several deep breaths, which will usually trigger any chronic cough. On the other hand, excessive coughing must be controlled to conserve energy and prevent added stress to the aged heart. The cautious use of medications, especially of diuretics and digitalis, is necessary because drug metabolism can be altered by situations reducing the body's oxygen. For optimum respiratory function the nurse should encourage correct posture, a good diet, the avoidance of obesity, paced activity, prophylactic influenza vaccines, diaphragmatic exercises, protection against and early treatment of upper respiratory infection, regular respiratory examination, and the avoidance of immobility.

One special measure of significance for aged patients with respiratory disorders is the accurate administration of oxygen, which must be used with extreme caution (Figure 11-2). If oxygen is prescribed for home use, the patient and the family must be thoroughly instructed in its safe and correct use. Frequent evaluations of arterial blood gases are essential. The nurse should evaluate the value of one method of oxygen administration over another. Older patients who breathe by mouth or have poor control in keeping their lips sealed most of the time, may not receive the full benefit of a nasal cannula. An emaciated older person whose facial structure does not allow for a tight seal of a face mask may lose a significant portion of oxygen through leakage. A patient who is insecure and anxious inside an oxygen tent may spend oxygen for emotional stress and not gain full therapeutic benefit. When nurses identify problems with the route of oxygen administration, they should make the physician aware of what method would be most effective for the particular patient. The oxygen flow should be checked frequently for any interruption or blockage from an empty oxygen tank, kinked tubing, or any other cause. The patient should be evaluated for hypoxia and suctioned when necessary. The nasal passages should be regularly cleaned to maintain patency. It must be remembered that some aged patients will not become cyanotic when hypoxic, thus close nursing observation for insufficient oxygenation is essential.

Postural drainage is commonly prescribed for the removal of bronchial secretions in certain respiratory diseases. The general procedure is the same for the aged, with some modifications. If aerosal medications are prescribed, they should be administered preceding the postural drainage. The position for postural drainage depends on the individual patient and on the portion of the lung involved. The older patient should change positions slowly and have a few minutes rest between position changes to allow for accommodation to the new position. The usual last position for postural drainage—lying face down across the bed with the head at floor level—may be stressful for the aged and cause adverse effects. The nurse can consult with the physician as to the advisability of this particular position and possible alterations to meet the needs of the individual patient. Cupping and vibration facilitate drainage of secretions; it should be remembered that old tissues and bones are more fragile and may more easily become injured. The nurse should discontinue the procedure and inform the physician if dyspnea, palpitation, chest pain, diaphoresis, apprehension, or any other signs of distress occur. Thorough oral hygiene and a period of rest should follow postural drainage. Documentation of the tolerance of the procedure and the amount and characteristic of the mucus drained is essential.

Coughing to remove secretions is important in the management of respiratory problems; however nonproductive coughing may be a useless expenditure of energy and stressful to the older patient. A variety of measures can be employed to promote effective coughing. Hard candy and other sweets increase secretions, thereby loosening the cough. Breathing exercises, as shown in Figure 11-1 will promote a productive cough. The patient can be instructed to take slow, full respirations, forcefully exhaling with pursed lips. The focus should be on relaxing abdominal muscles during inspiration and contracting them during

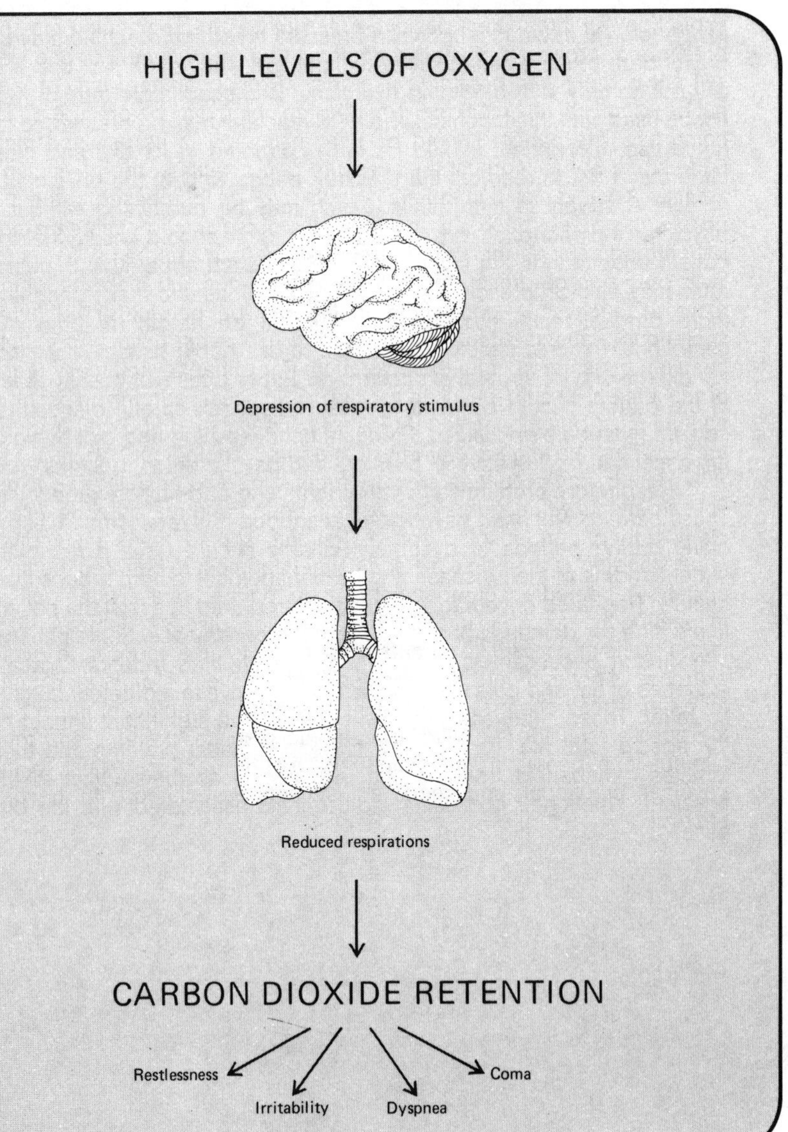

Figure 11-2. Oxygen must be administered to the aged with caution. High levels of oxygen can depress the respiratory stimulus in the brain, thereby reducing respiration and promoting carbon dioxide retention.

expiration. An intermittent positive-pressure breathing machine may be prescribed, proving especially beneficial to a weak patient or one who will not comply with breathing exercises. Bronchodilators may or may not be used with this machine. The IPPB machine may be prescribed for home use; the patient should be fully instructed in its use and must understand not to readjust the pressure gauge without the physician's advice. A variety of humidifiers, which may be purchased without a physician's prescription, are available; the nurse should ensure that the patient understands the safe, correct use of such apparatus. Expectorants may also be prescribed to loosen secretions and make coughing more productive. A good fluid intake will be helpful in liquifying secretions. Patients should be advised to use paper tissues, not cloth handkerchiefs, for sputum expectoration. Paper bags within easy reach of the patient should be used for tissue disposal; careful disposal of sputum must be emphasized. Frequent hand washing and oral hygiene are essential, having several physical and psychological benefits.

Respiratory problems are very frightening and anxiety producing. These patients will need psychological support and reassurance, especially during periods of dyspnea. Patients should have a complete understanding of their disease and its management to help reduce their anxiety. Repeated encouragement may be required to assist the patient in meeting the demands of a chronic respiratory disease. Some patients may find it necessary to spend most of their time indoors to avoid extremes of hot and cold weather; some may move to a different climate for relief. These changes in life-style may have a significant impact on the aged's total life. As with any chronic disease, patients and their families can benefit from nursing intervention as they adjust to the physical, emotional, and social adjustments associated with the disease.

12

DIABETES

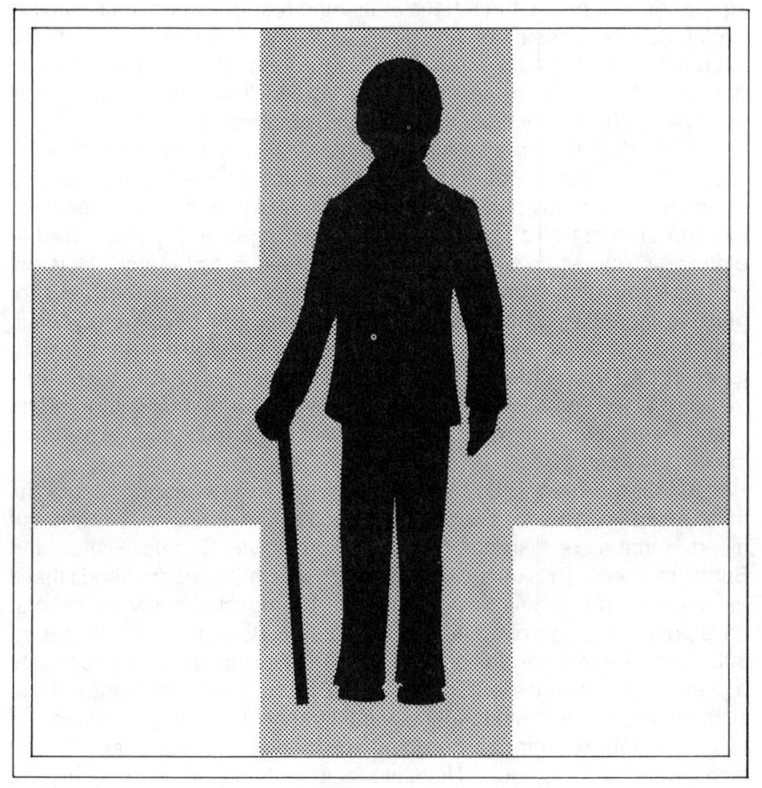

A proficient blend of various kinds of knowledge and skills is required in nursing diabetics, and older diabetics, with their unique set of problems, present an even greater challenge. Diabetes, the seventh leading cause of death among the aged, has a particularly high prevalence among blacks and among persons 65 to 74 years of age. Consequently, nurses have to be adequately informed of how the detection and management of diabetes in aged persons differs from that in others. The increasing number of individuals achieving old age, and the expanding health care services for the aged further emphasize the necessity for nurses to become prepared in meeting the needs of older diabetics.

DIAGNOSIS

Several explanations are offered for the high prevalence of hyperglycemia among the aged. Some researchers claim that a physiologic deterioration of glucose tolerance occurs with increasing age (Andres, 1967). Others believe that the high prevalence of glucose intolerance is a result of an increase in the incidence of diabetes throughout the general population. Regardless of the reason behind glucose intolerance in the aged, it is agreed that different standards must be applied in evaluating their glucose tolerance.

Early diagnosis of diabetes in older persons is often quite difficult. The classic symptoms of diabetes may be absent, leaving nonspecific symptoms as the only clues. Some indications of diabetes are orthostatic hypotension, stroke, gastric hypotony, impotence, neuropathy, glaucoma, dupuytren's contracture, and infection. Laboratory tests, as well as symptoms, may be misleading. Since the renal threshold for glucose increases with age, older individuals can be hyperglycemic without evidence of glycosuria, thus limiting the validity of urine testing for glucose. Fasting blood sugar testing is not a dependable diagnostic measure since some aged individuals may have a normal fasting blood sugar level while experiencing significant hyperglycemic levels after meals (Rifkin and Ross, 1971a).

Of all the diagnostic measures, the glucose tolerance test is the most effective, and to avoid a false positive diagnosis, it is recommended that more than one test be performed (McDonald, Fisher, and Burnham, 1965). The American Diabetes Association recommends that a minimum of 150 grams of carbohydrate be ingested daily for several days prior to the test; older malnourished individuals may be prescribed 300 grams. Recent periods of inactivity, stressful illness, and inadequate dietary intake should be communicated to the physician, since these situations can contribute to glucose intolerance. In such circumstances, more accurate results can be obtained if the test is postponed to one month after the episode. Nicotinic acid, ethacrynic acid, estrogen,

TABLE 12-1: AGE-RELATED GRADIENTS FOR GLUCOSE TOLERANCE TESTS

U.S.P.H.S. Standard Values*			Age-Related Gradients Based on U.S.P.H.S. Values		
Sample Time		Point Values (2 points = Diabetes)	55–64 Years	65–74 Years	75–85+ Years
Fasting	110	1	110	110	110
1 Hour	170	½	180	190	200
2 Hour	120	½	130	140	150
3 Hour	110	1	120	130	140

Source: Charles R. Shuman, *Special Problems of the Older Diabetic,* scientific exhibit at the AMA Clinical Convention, Cincinnati, Ohio, November 26–29, 1972.
Note: Increments of 10 mg/% added to one- two- and three-hour values in standard curve for each decade; fasting values remain unchanged.
* Values given for venous whole blood in mg/%-plasma values are 15% higher.

furosemide, and diuretics can decrease glucose tolerance and should not be administered prior to testing. Monoamine-oxidase inhibitors, propranolol, and high dosages of salicylates may lower blood sugar and also interfere with testing.

The usual nursing measures are applied during glucose tolerance testing of the aged. If unusual symptoms develop during the test, such as mental confusion, it is important to tell the physician. Those interpreting the glucose tolerance test may find it beneficial to utilize age-related gradients (Table 12-1). For each decade after age 55, 10 mg/% are added to the standard values at the first, second, and third hours. Thus, a glucose level which would be significantly elevated for a 35-year-old may be within normal limits for an 85-year-old.

MANAGEMENT

Although the basic principles of diabetic management are applicable to all age groups, special considerations and adjustments must be made for the older diabetic. It is impractical and unrealistic to expect that individuals who have established specific practices over the past six or seven decades will drastically alter their life-style when diagnosed as diabetics. Many compromises may be required by the diabetic individual *and* the professionals managing his or her care.

Educating the Older Diabetic

Once the diagnosis has been confirmed, a teaching plan should be established by the nurse. Diabetes is known as a serious and chronic problem to most lay individuals, and it is frightening to have it diagnosed in oneself. Fear and anxiety can interfere with the learning process for newly diagnosed older diabetics, who may have witnessed the crippling or fatal effects of diabetes in others and associate them with themselves. Having lived through a period in which diabetes was not able to be successfully managed and was always severely disabling or fatal, the older individual may not be aware of the advancements in diabetic management. Insulin was isolated in 1921, when many of today's elderly were children and young adults.

Elderly persons may be depressed or angry that this disease further threatens the short period of their remaining life; they may question the "trade-off" value in exchanging an unrestricted life-style for a potentially longer but restricted life. Concerns may arise as to how a special diet and medications will be afforded on an already limited budget. Social isolation may develop from fear of becoming ill in public or facing restrictions that make diabetics different from their peers. They may question their ability to manage their diabetes independently and worry that institutionalization will be necessary. These and a multitude of other concerns which the older diabetic may have must be recognized and dealt with by the nurse to reduce the risk of other limitations and to promote the individual's self-care capacities. Reassurance, support, and information can reduce barriers to learning about and managing diabetes. The following steps, helpful in any patient education situation, may offer guidance in teaching the older diabetic.

1. ***Assessment of Readiness to Learn.*** Discomfort, anxiety and depression may block learning and the retention of knowledge. Relieving these symptoms and allowing time for patients to develop to the point where they desire and can cope with information may be necessary.
2. ***Assessment of Learning Capacities and Limitations.*** This would include consideration of educational level, language problems, literacy, present knowledge, willingness to learn, cultural background, previous experience with the illness, memory, vision, hearing, speech, and mental status.
3. ***Outline of What to Teach.*** Your outline should not only be specific and clear, but should also consider learning priorities. Nurses sometimes feel obligated to teach every last detail about an illness, compacting a multitude of new facts and procedures into a short time frame. Most people need time to receive, absorb, sort, and translate new information into behavioral changes; the elderly are no different. Altered brain function or slower responses may further interfere with learning

in the aged. Patients and their families should have a role in setting teaching priorities; the most vital information should be given first, followed by other relevant material. Visiting nurses and other resources should be used after hospital discharge to continue the teaching plan if the proposed outline is not completed during the hospitalization.

4. ***Altering the Teaching Plan in View of Capacities and Limitations.*** The nurse may feel that an explanation of the physiological effects of diabetes is significant for new diabetics. However, the older person who tends to be confused or has a poor memory may not have long-range benefit from this type of information. It may be better to use that time to reinforce diet information or to make sure the most significant information required for self-care is retained.
5. ***Preparing the Patient for the Teaching-Learning Session.*** Patients should understand that education is an integral part of care and not just icing on the cake. Whenever possible, a specific time should be arranged in advance to avoid conflict with other activities and to allow the family to be present if desired.
6. ***Providing an Environment Conducive to Learning.*** An area that is quiet, clean, relaxing, and free from odors and interference will help to create a good atmosphere for learning. Distraction should be minimal, especially in view of the aged's reduced capacity to manage multiple stimuli.
7. ***Using the Most Effective Individualized Educational Method.*** The nurse must recognize the limitations of standard teaching aids and the importance of individualized methods. An aid that was successful for one person may not be effective for another. The variety of sophisticated audio-visual aids that are commercially prepared and available in many agencies as resources for nurses are impressive; but they may not necessarily be effective for the given patient. The quality of an audio cassette may be excellent, but it is of little benefit to the older person with a hearing problem. A slide presentation, even slowly paced, may present facts more rapidly than can be absorbed by an older person with delayed response time. The print on a commercial pamphlet may appear minute to older eyes. The language used in many commercial materials may not be one to which the person is accustomed. Original handmade aids suited for the individual's unique needs may have a value equal to or greater than commercially prepared ones. Selectivity in methodology is essential.

8. ***Using Several Approaches to the Same Body of Knowledge.*** The greater number of different exposures to new material, the higher the probability that the material will be learned. Combine verbal explanation with flipcharts, diagrams, pamphlets, demonstrations, discussions with other patients, and audio-visual resources.
9. ***Leaving Material with the Patient for Later Review.*** It is often helpful to summarize the teaching session in writing, using language familiar to the patient. This provides concrete material which the patient can independently review later and also share with the family.
10. ***Reinforcing Key Points.*** Reinforcement should be regular and consistent, with all staff members supporting the teaching plan. For example, if the objective of the nurse caring for the patient has been to increase competency in self-injection of insulin, then the person substituting on the nurse's day off should comply with the established objectives rather than administering the insulin for the individual. Informal reinforcement of information during other daily activities should also be planned.
11. ***Obtaining Feedback.*** Evaluate whether the patient and family have accurately received and understood the information communicated. This can be done by observing return demonstrations, asking questions, and listening to discussions among patients.
12. ***Periodic Reevaluating.*** To ascertain retention and effectiveness of the teaching sessions, informally reevaluate at a later time. Remember that retention of information may be especially difficult for the older individual.
13. ***Documentation.*** Describe specifically what was taught, when, who was involved, what methodology was used, the patient's reaction and understanding, and future plans for remaining learning needs. This assists the staff caring for patients during their hospitalization and also serves as a guide for those providing continued care after discharge.

Care and Health Supervision

One factor which must be considered in the management of the older diabetic is that the ability to handle a syringe and vial of insulin may be decreased due to arthritic fingers. Several return demonstrations of this skill should be performed during the hospitalization, especially on days in which arthritis discomfort is actively present. As most elderly persons have some degree of visual impairment, the ability to read the

TABLE 12-2: INSULINS USED IN THE MANAGEMENT OF DIABETES MELLITUS

Types of Insulin	Onset of Action	Peak	Duration
Fast-acting			
Injection: Regular, unmodified	20–30 min	1–2 hr	5–8 hr
Zinc suspension: prompt, crystalline (Semi-Lente)	50–60 min	2–3 hr	6–8 hr
Medium-acting			
Globin, with zinc	1–2 hr	8–16 hr	18–24 hr
Isophane suspension (NPH)	1–2 hr	10–20 hr	28–30 hr
Zinc suspension (Lente)	1–2 hr	10–20 hr	20–32 hr
Long-acting			
Zinc suspension, extended (Ultra-Lente)	4–6 hr	16–24 hr	24–36 hr
Protamine zinc suspension (Protamine Zinc)	4–6 hr	16–24 hr	24–36 hr

calibrations on an insulin syringe must be evaluated. The yellowing of the lens with age tends to filter out low-tone colors, such as blues and greens; since these colors are frequently used to identify various levels of glycosuria in urine testing kits, it is important to assess the older individual's ability to discriminate these shades. Older individuals may also be limited in their ability to purchase and prepare adequate meals due to financial, energy, or social limitations. Since this can interfere with management of the illness, Meals on Wheels, food stamps, the assistance of a neighbor, and other appropriate resources should be utilized to assist the individual.

Altered tubule reabsorption of glucose may lead to inaccurate results from urine testing. As mentioned, the older individual can be hyperglycemic without being glycosuric. On the other hand, higher blood glucose levels are common in the aged, and minimal or mild glycosuria is not usually treated with insulin (Rifkin and Ross, 1971b). Although nurses aren't responsible for prescribing the insulin coverage, they need to be aware that the insulin requirements of the older diabetic are individualized. Responses to various insulin levels are to be carefully observed and communicated to the physician. Table 12-2 reviews the various insulins that may be prescribed. As insulins are selected not only for their timing but for their specific tolerance by the patient, the nurse must be careful to administer the correct type of insulin prescribed. The patients must understand that they cannot borrow a vial of insulin from a friend if their supply should become exhausted.

Attempts should be made to maintain a consistent daily food

intake, as the insulin dosage is prescribed to cover a specific amount of food. This may be a problem if the elderly person has a minimal food intake during the week when alone but an increased intake when visiting with family on weekends or if he or she skimps on meals when the budget is thinning. Sociological and psychological factors can influence consistent food intake as much as physical factors. The nurse and physician must carefully assess, plan, and manage insulin needs in view of the individual's unique problems and life-style. Special attention must also be paid to the aged in a hosptial or nursing home setting to ensure that food intake is regular and adequate.

At times, oral agents are prescribed for the elderly diabetic. Chlorpropamide (Diabinese) is an oral hypoglycemic agent with approximately six times the potency of tolbutamide. It is readily absorbed in the gastrointestinal tract, reaching its maximum level in 2 to 4 hours, and is slowly excreted in the urine. The biological half-life of chlorpropamide is normally 36 hours, with most of the dose excreted within 96 hours. Chlorpropamide is contraindicated in individuals having severe impairment of hepatic, renal, or thyroid function. This drug can prolong the action of barbiturates, a consideration for gerontological nurses since elderly patients may be receiving both medications. Close nursing observation is essential when patients receiving oral hypoglycemic agents are prescribed antibacterial sulfonamides, phenylbutazone, salicylates, probenecid, dicoumarol or MAO (monoamine oxidase) inhibitors, since these drugs can potentiate a hypoglycemic reaction. Chlorpropamide may cause an exaggerated hypoglycemic effect in individuals with Addison's disease.

If hypoglycemia occurs in the patient receiving chlorpropamide it could be prolonged. A slightly higher blood glucose level is considered acceptable for adequate functioning in the aged, and therefore the nurse should note and communicate to the physician observations indicating dysfunction from a reduced blood sugar level; perhaps a higher than "normal" glucose level will promote optimum function in a given individual. Adverse reactions to chlorpropamide include pruritus, rash, jaundice, dark urine, light-colored stools, diarrhea, low-grade fever, and sore throat. Tolbutamide, acetohexamide, tolazamide and phenformin are among the other oral hypoglycemic agents which may be prescribed. Suggestions, special precautions, and adverse reactions for these drugs resemble those mentioned with chlorpropamide.

Some individuals only need oral hypoglycemic agents to control their diabetes. Those on insulin therapy who have lost weight or have not been ketoacidotic may have their insulin substituted by oral hypoglycemic agents. Still others will need periodic changes in their insulin dosages to meet changing demands. These factors, combined with other management difficulties in the older diabetic, necessitate frequent reevaluation of the patient's status. The continuation of health supervision is an essential part of diabetic management.

Complications

The elderly are subject to a long list of complications from diabetes and have a greater risk of developing these complications than younger adults. Hypoglycemia seems to be a greater threat to older diabetics than ketoacidosis, and this is especially problematic due to the possible presentation of a different set of symptoms. The classic tachycardia, restlessness, perspiration, and anxiety may be totally absent in the older individual with hypoglycemia. Instead, any of the following may be the first indication of the problem: behavior disorders, convulsions, somnolence, confusion, disorientation, poor sleep patterns, nocturnal headache, slurred speech, and unconsciousness. The nurse must be careful not to mistake signs of hypoglycemia with "senility" as this may delay detection and correction of this serious problem. Uncorrected hypoglycemia can cause tachycardia, arrhythmias, myocardial infarctions, cerebrovascular accident, and death.

Peripheral vascular disease is a common complication in the older diabetic, influenced by the poorer circulation and atherosclerosis often associated with increased age. Symptoms may range from numbness and weak pulses to infection and gangrene. The nurse should identify and promptly communicate symptoms of peripheral vascular disease. Education of the patient in proper foot care can help reduce the risk of this problem. Another significant vascular problem of older diabetics is retinopathy with consequent blindness. Individuals who are hypertensive or who have had diabetes for a long period of time have a greater risk of developing this complication. Hemorrhage, pigmentory disturbances, edema, and visual problems are manifested with this problem.

A variety of additional complications face older diabetics. They may develop neuropathies, demonstrated through tingling sensations, pain, paresthesias, nocturnal diarrhea, tachycardia, and postural hypotension. They have twice the mortality rate from coronary artery disease, twice the mortality rate from cerebral arteriosclerosis, and a higher incidence of urinary tract infections. There is a higher risk of problems developing with virtually every body system. Early detection of complications is essential and can be facilitated by nursing intervention and patient education. Competent management of the older diabetic is an extremely skillful and vital activity, posing a great challenge and responsibility to the practice of nursing. The recognition of differences in symptomatology, diagnosis, management, and complications is crucial.

REFERENCES

Andres, R. "Diabetes and Aging." *Hospital Practice,* 2:63, 1967.

McDonald, G. W., Fisher, G. F., and Burnham, C. "Reproducibility of the Oral Glucose Tolerance Test." *Diabetes,* 14:473, 1965.

Rifkin, H., and Ross, H. "Diabetes in the Elderly." In Rossman, I. (ed.), *Clinical Geriatrics.* Lippincott, Philadelphia, 1971. (a) p. 391; (b) p. 400.

13

MUSCULOSKELETAL PROBLEMS

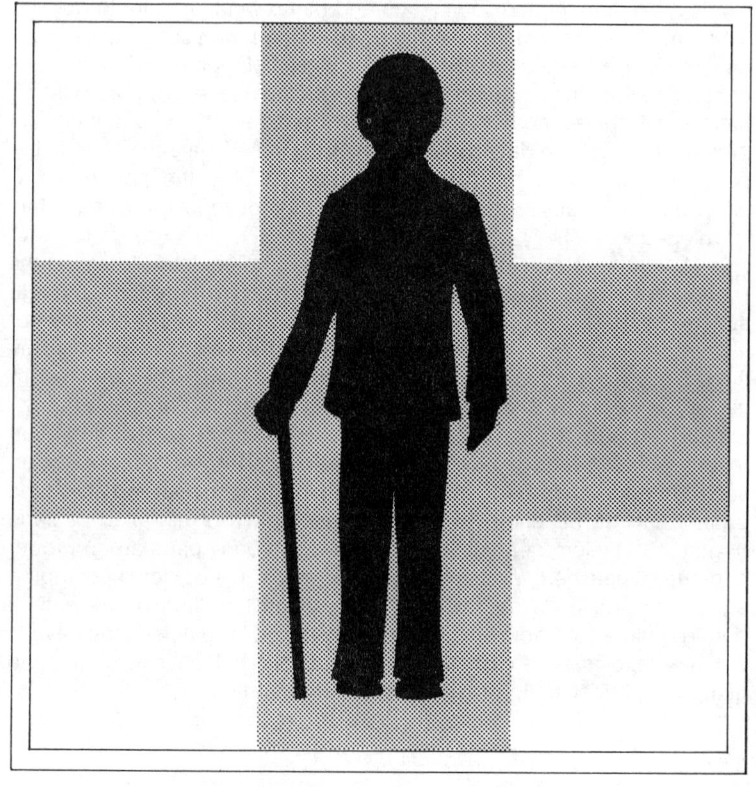

It is the rare older individual who does not experience some degree of discomfort, disability, or deformity from musculoskeletal disorders. In addition to the influence of diet, heredity, stress, and hormonal balances on the status of the musculoskeletal system, changes associated with the aging process also contribute to these problems. With age, there is a reduction in the number of muscle fibers and in muscle strength and endurance. Some wasting of the skeletal muscle occurs, and a loss of bone minerals causes the bones to become more brittle. Muscle movements and tendon jerks are decreased. Some joints become more mobile due to stretching of the ligaments; others stiffen and lose some range of motion. Hip and knee flexion, kyphosis of the dorsal spine, and shortening of the vertebral column can be evidenced by a reduction in height as an individual ages.

Pain frequently accompanies musculoskeletal problems. Degenerative changes in the tendons and arthritis are often responsible for painful shoulders, elbows, hands, hips, knees, and spine, and cramps, especially during the night, are commonly experienced in calves, feet, hands, hips, and thighs. Joint strain and damp weather more frequently cause musculoskeletal pain in the aged than in the young. The gerontological nurse should assess the musculoskeletal pain and note in the documentation the location, nature, duration, severity, precipitating factors, and relief measures used by the patient. This information can provide the baseline data by which changes in the characteristics of the pain can be measured. Also, the nurse can help the patient avoid situations that cause pain and to seek prompt relief once pain has developed.

A variety of nursing measures can be implemented to assist the patient with musculoskeletal pain. Heat often will relieve muscle spasms, and a warm bath at bedtime accompanied by blankets or clothing to keep the extremities warm can reduce spasms and cramps throughout the night and promote uninterrupted sleep. Passive stretching of the extremity also may be helpful in controlling muscle cramps. Excessive exercise and musculoskeletal stress should be avoided. Pain in the weight-bearing joints can be helped by resting those joints; supporting the parts under the painful joint when moving and lifting the patient can be beneficial, as can the assistance of a walker or cane (Figure 13-1). Correct positioning, whereby all body parts are in proper alignment, can help prevent and manage pain. Accidental bumping against the patient's bed or chair, and rough handling of the patient during routine care activities must be prevented. The nurse may have to emphasize to other care providers the need for gentleness in turning and lifting the patient while providing support to all limbs.

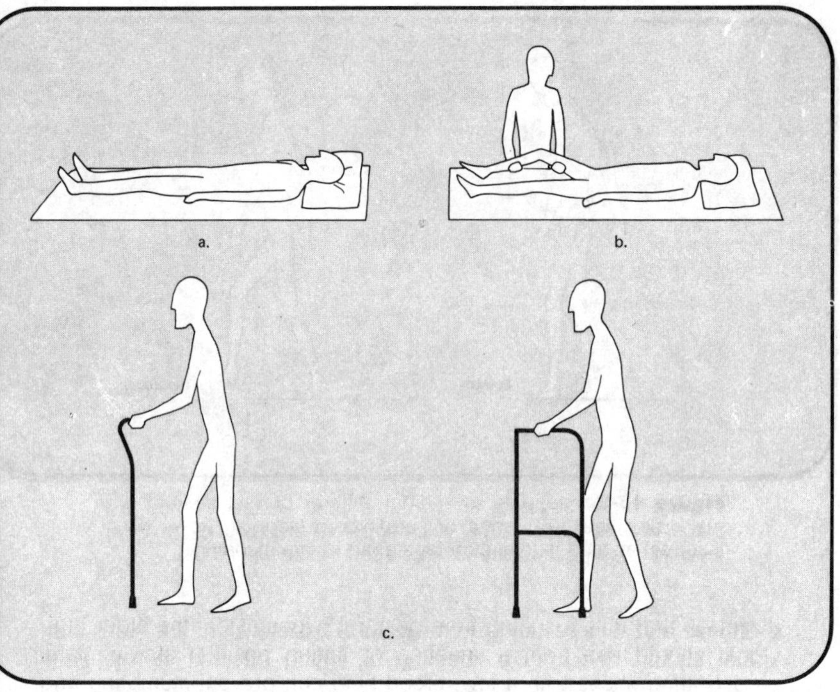

Figure 13-1. Methods for reducing musculoskeletal pain: (a) Good body alignment. (b) Support of parts of limb adjacent to painful joint when moving or lifting. (c) Use of walker or cane.

DISORDERS AND RELATED NURSING CARE

Fractures

Trauma, cancer metastasis to the bone, osteoporosis, and other skeletal diseases contribute to fractures in aged persons. The neck of the femur is a common site for fractures in the aged, especially in older females (Habermann, 1971). Not only do the more brittle bones of the aged fracture more easily, but their rate of healing is longer than in younger persons, potentially predisposing the aged to the many complications associated with immobility. Knowing that the risk of fracture and its multiple complications is high among the aged, the gerontological nurse must aim toward prevention, drawing on the effectiveness of basic commonsense measures. Since their coordination and equilibrium are poorer, the aged should be advised against climbing on ladders or chairs to reach high places and similarly risky activities. To prevent

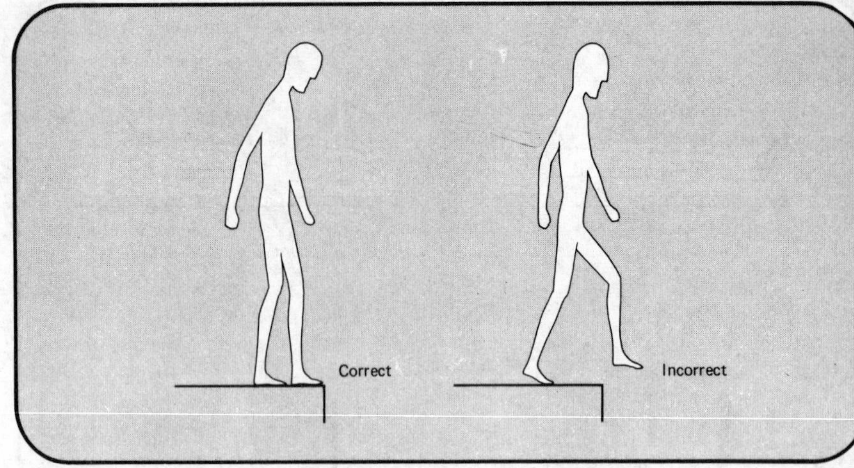

Figure 13-2. Stepping to or from a curb: Correct method is to place both feet near edge of curb before stepping up or down. Incorrect method is to stretch legs apart before stepping.

dizziness and falls resulting from postural hypotension, the older individual should rise from a kneeling or sitting position slowly. Safe, proper-fitting shoes with a low, broad heel can prevent stumbling and loss of balance, and handrails for climbing stairs or rising from the bathtub provide support and balance.

Placing both feet near the edge of a curb or bus before stepping up or down is safer than a poorly balanced stretch of the legs (Figures 13-2). The aged person should be reminded to carefully notice where he or she is walking to avoid tripping in holes and damaged sidewalks or slipping on pieces of ice. Since older eyes are more sensitive to glare, sunglasses may be helpful for improving vision outdoors. A nightlight is extremely valuable in preventing falls during night visits to the bathroom. Loose rugs and clutter on floors and stairs should be removed. Since even the most healthy aged person can experience some confusion when waking during the night, bedrails can be used to prevent falls from bed and attempts at sleepwalking, whether at home or away. Putting the bed against a wall with a straight chair at the other side is an effective substitute.

As mentioned, fractures heal more slowly in the aged, and the risk of complications is great. Pneumonia, thrombus formation, decubiti, renal calculi, fecal impaction, and contractures are among the complications that special nursing attention can help prevent. Activity, within the limits determined by the physician, should be promoted, including deep-breathing and coughing exercises, isometric and range-of-motion exercises, and frequent turning and position changes. Fluids should be encouraged, and the characteristics of the urine output noted. Good nutrition will facilitate healing and increase the resistance to infection and other complications. Joint exercises and proper positioning can prevent contractures. Correct body alignment can be maintained with the use of footboards, trochanter rolls, and sandbags. Keeping the skin dry and clean, preventing pressure, stimulating circulation through massage, and frequent turning may reduce the risk of decubiti. Sheepskin, water beds, and alternating-pressure mattresses are beneficial, but they do not substitute for good skin care and frequent position changes.

As early as possible, the patient should be mobilized. It is not unusual for the patient to fear using the fractured limb and avoid doing so. Explanations and reassurance are required to help the patient understand that the healed limb is safe to use. Since progress in small steps may be easier for the patient to tolerate physically and psychologically, the first attempt at ambulation may be to stand at the bedside, the next to walking to a nearby chair, and the next to walk to the bathroom. Initially, it may be helpful for two people to assist the patient with ambulation, especially since weakness and dizziness are not uncommon. The principles of nursing management for specific types of fractures are available in medical-surgical nursing textbooks and the reader is advised to explore that literature for more detailed information.

Osteoarthritis

Osteoarthritis is the deterioration and abrasion of joint cartilage, with the formation of new bone at the joint surfaces. This problem is increasingly seen with advanced age, affecting women more than men. Unlike rheumatoid arthritis, osteoarthritis arthritis does not cause inflammation, deformity, and crippling—a fact that is reassuring to the affected individual who fears the severe disability he has seen in persons with rheumatoid arthritis. The wear and tear of the joints as an individual ages is thought to have a major role in the development of osteoarthritis. Excessive use of the joint, trauma, obesity, and genetic factors may also predispose an individual to this problem. There is a high incidence of osteoarthritis in patients with acromegaly. Usually osteoarthritis affects several joints rather than a single one. Weight-bearing joints are those most affected, the common sites being the knees, hips, vertebrae, and fingers, and the classic symptoms associated with arthritis are present—aching, stiffness, and limited motion of the joint.

Systemic symptoms do not accompany osteoarthritis. Crepitation on joint motion may be noted, and the distal joints may develop bony nodules (Heberden's nodes). The patient may notice that the joints are more uncomfortable during damp weather and periods of extended use. Rest will help relieve the joint aching, as will heat and gentle massage. Although isometric and mild exercises are beneficial, excessive exercise will cause more pain and degeneration. Analgesics may be prescribed to control pain, and splints, braces, and canes offer support and rest to the joints. The importance of maintaining proper body alignment and using good body mechanics should be emphasized in educating the patient. Weight reduction may improve the obese patient's status and should be encouraged. It is beneficial if a homemaker's service or other household assistance relieves the patient of strenuous activities that cause the joints to bear weight. Occupational and physical therapists can be consulted for assistive devices to promote independence in self-care activities.

Rheumatoid Arthritis

Rheumatoid arthritis affects many persons, young and old; it is commonly seen among the aged. The deformities and disability associated with this disease primarily begin during early adulthood, peaking during middle age; in old age, greater systemic involvement occurs. This disease occurs more frequently in women and in persons with a family history of this problem (Habermann, 1971). The joints affected by rheumatoid arthritis are extremely painful, stiff, swollen, red, and warm to the touch. Joint pain is present during rest or activity. Subcutaneous nodules over bony prominences and bursae may be present, as may deforming flexion contractures. Systemic symptoms include fatigue, malaise, weakness, weight loss, wasting, fever, and anemia.

Encouraging patients to rest and thus providing support to the affected limbs is helpful. Limb support should be such that decubiti and contractures are prevented. Splints are commonly made for the patient in an effort to prevent deformities. Range-of-motion exercises are vital to maintain musculoskeletal function; the nurse may have to assist the patient with active exercises. Physical and occupational therapists can provide assistive devices to promote independence in self-care activities, and heat, gentle massage, and analgesics can help to control pain. In addition, patients with rheumatoid arthritis may be prescribed antiinflammatory agents, corticosteroids, antimalarial agents, gold salts, and immunosuppressive drugs. The nurse should be familiar with the many toxic effects of these drugs and detect them early.

The patient with rheumatoid arthritis and the family need considerable education to be able to manage this condition. Patient education should include a knowledge of the disease, treatments, administration of medications and identification of side effects, exercise regimen, use of

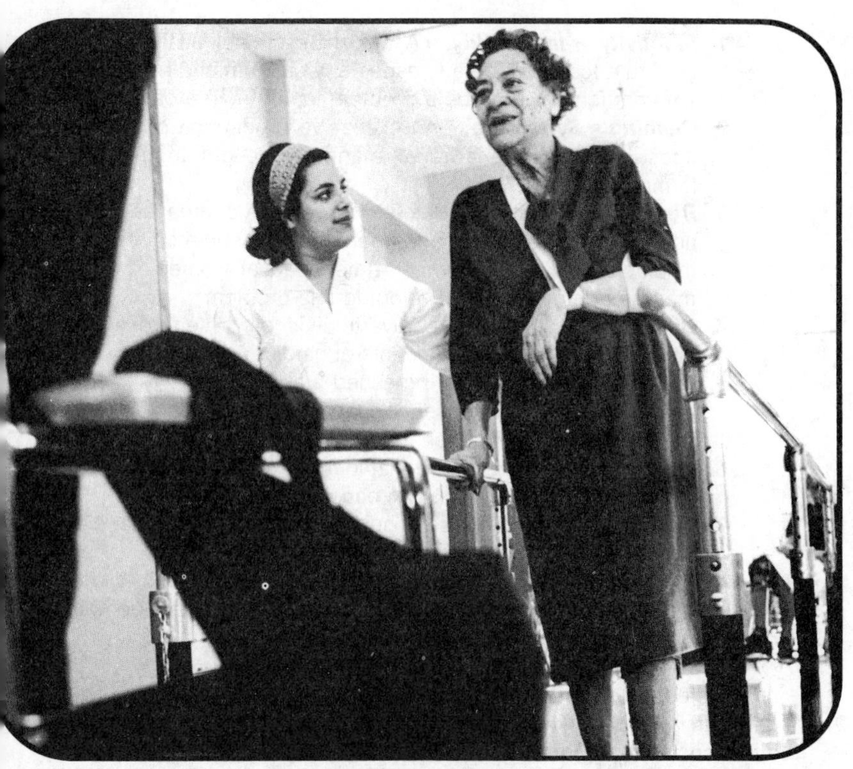

assistive devices, methods to avoid and reduce pain, and an understanding of the need for continued medical supervision. Accepting this chronic disease is not an easy task, either for the patient or the family. The patient may be a prime target for a salesperson offering a quick "cure" or "relief" for arthritis and should be advised to consult the nurse or physician before investing many dollars of an already limited budget on useless fads.

Osteoporosis

Osteoporosis is the most prevalent metabolic disease of the bone, primarily affecting adults in middle to late life. Demineralization of the bone occurs, evidenced by a decrease in the mass and density of the skeleton. Any problem in which there is inadequate calcium intake, excessive calcium loss, or poor calcium absorption can cause osteoporosis. Many of the potential causes listed below are problems commonly found among aged persons.

1. ***Inactivity or Immobility.*** A lack of muscle pull on the bone can lead to a loss of minerals, especially calcium and phosphorus. This particularly may be a problem for limbs in a cast.
2. ***Cushing's Syndrome.*** An excessive production of glucocorticosteroids by the adrenal gland is thought to inhibit the formation of bone matrix.
3. ***Reduction in Anabolic Sex Hormones.*** A decreased production or loss of estrogens and androgens may be responsible for insufficient bone calcium. Postmenopausal women, therefore, may be at high risk of developing this problem.
4. ***Diverticulitis.*** Excessive diverticulitis can interfere with the absorption of sufficient amounts of calcium.
5. ***Hyperthyroidism.*** This increased metabolic activity causes a more rapid bone turnover. Bone resorption occurs at a rate faster than bone formation, causing osteoporosis.
6. ***Poor Diet.*** An insufficient amount of calcium, protein, and other nutrients in the diet can cause osteoporosis.
7. ***Heparin.*** Prolonged use of heparin can increase bone resorption and inhibit bone formation.
8. ***Diabetes Mellitus.*** Although the direct relationship is uncertain at this time, diabetes can contribute to the development of osteoporosis.

Osteoporosis may cause kyphosis and a reduction in height. Spinal pain can be experienced, especially in the lumbar region. There may be a tendency for the bones to fracture more easily. Some patients may be asymptomatic, however, and not be aware of the problem until it is detected on X-ray. Treatment depends on the underlying cause and may include calcium supplements, vitamin D supplements, hormones, anabolic agents, fluoride, or phosphate. A diet rich in protein and calcium is encouraged. Braces may be used to provide support and reduce spasms. A bedboard is also beneficial and should be recommended. The patient must be advised to avoid heavy lifting, jumping or other activities that could result in a fracture. Persons providing care to the patient must remember to be gentle when moving, exercising, or lifting these patients since fractures can occur easily. (Compression fractures of the vertebrae are a potential complication of osteoporosis). Range-of-motion exercises and ambulation are important to maintain function and prevent greater damage.

Osteitis Deformans (Paget's Disease)

Osteitis deformans is a metabolic disease of the bone which produces excessive bone resorption and deposits. Although the exact cause is unknown, developmental defects, chronic inflammation of the bone, and wear and tear to the skeletal system throughout the years are thought to be contributing factors. This disease primarily involves middle-aged and aged males. The common sites affected are the skull, lumbar vertebrae, sacrum, pelvis, and long bones. The deformities most commonly displayed include enlargement and thickening of the skull, kyphosis, and bowing of the femur and tibia. Bone pain is usually present, as is the tendency for the bones to fracture easily. Complications to other organs may result, such as paraplegia due to pressure on the spinal cord and blindness due to pressure on the optic nerve. Symptomatic treatment is usually employed. Pain control and the prevention of complications are the major goals. Since osteitis deformans predisposes the individual to bone sarcoma, close observation and periodic evaluation are needed to identify this problem. In general, the prognosis associated with this disease is very poor.

NURSING CONSIDERATIONS

A good diet is important in preventing and managing musculoskeletal problems. A well-balanced diet, rich in proteins and minerals, will help maintain the structure and function of the bones and muscles. In addition to the quality of the diet, attention also must be paid to the quantity. Obesity places strain on the joints which aggravates conditions like arthritis. Weight reduction will frequently ease musculoskeletal discomforts and reduce limitations, and it should be stressed when gerontological nurses counsel individuals of all ages on intelligent aging.

Pain relief is essential in promoting optimum physical, mental, and social function. Aching joints may prevent aged persons from properly caring for their basic needs, managing their household, and maintaining social contact. To enrich the quality of an older person's life, every effort should be made to minimize or eliminate pain—whether by proper positioning, gentle massage, heat, analgesics, or passive stretching to relieve muscle cramps. Situations which are known to cause pain—such as heavy lifting and damp weather—should be avoided whenever possible. Diversional activities can prevent the patient's preoccupation with pain. The family may need support and education in learning to understand and assist the patient during episodes of pain. The patient should be helped to achieve a balance between the maximum level of activity and the least degree of pain.

Activity promotes optimum musculoskeletal function and reduces the many complications associated with immobility. Fear of reinjuring a healing bone or causing pain, however, may cause the patient to limit his or her activities unnecessarily. Realistic explanations describing the healing process or the benefit of exercise to aching joints are most

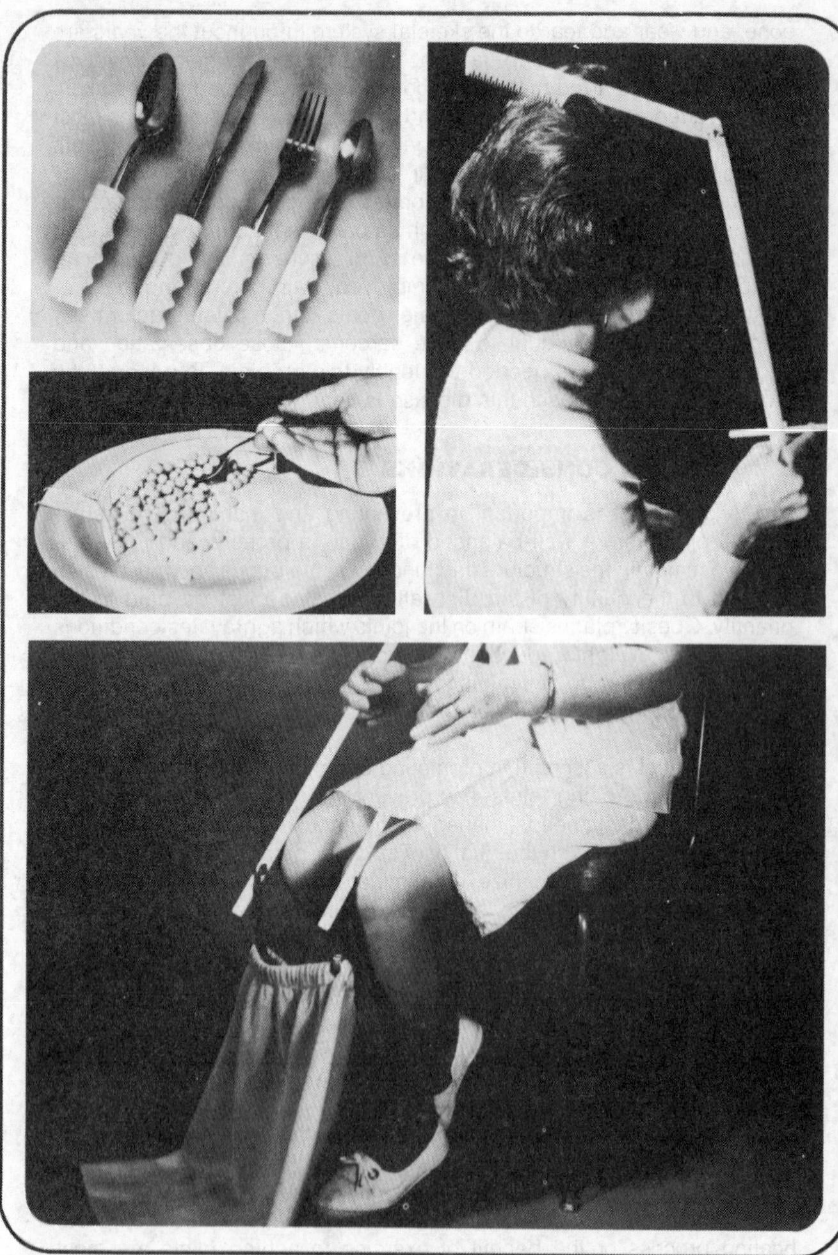

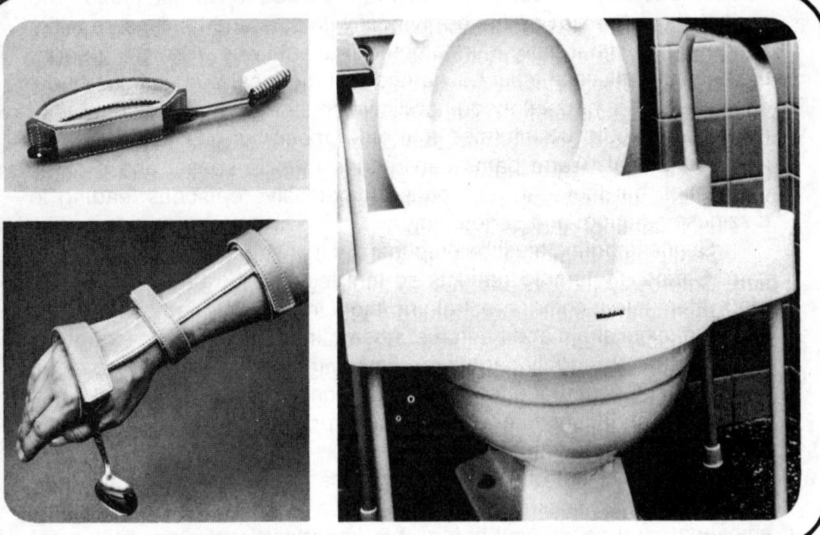

Figure 13-3. Self-care devices can help the patient achieve maximum independence: (a) Set of 4 built-up hand utensils. (b) Long-handled comb. (c) Food-bumper. (d) Dressing sticks with carter clips. (e) Universal ADL cuff. (f) Dorsal wrist splint. (g) Tall-Ette with safety bars. (Courtesy of Maddak Inc. Subsidiary of Bel-Air Products, Pequannock, N.J.)

important. Patients and families can benefit from an understanding of the hazards arising from immobility; sympathetic family members who believe they are helping the patient by allowing him or her to remain inactive may be more willing to encourage activity if they are aware of the harm immobility can cause. Continued support, encouragement, and positive reinforcement by the gerontological nurse can help the patient considerably.

Safety considerations are essential for all aged persons due to the high incidence of accidents and musculoskeletal injuries and the prolonged healing period. Prevention includes paying attention to the area where one is walking, climbing stairs and curbs slowly, using both feet for support as much as possible (Figure 13-2), using railings and canes for added balance, wearing properly fitting, safe shoes for good support, and avoiding trousers, nightgowns, or robes that are long enough to get caught by a shoe or slipper. Since heat is frequently used by aged persons to relieve joint pain or muscle spasm, attention must be paid to its safety hazards. Altered cutaneous sensations may allow burns from excessively hot soaks or hot water bottles to go unnoticed. The patient should be advised to apply heat with care and to measure water temperature (with a dairy thermometer). Patients who also have peripheral vascular disease must be warned that the local application of heat can cause extra circulatory demands which their body will be unable to meet; they should be informed that other means of pain relief may be more beneficial. Warm baths can reduce muscle spasm and provide pain relief, but they can also cause hypotensive episodes leading to dizziness, fainting, and serious injury.

Gentle handling must be emphasized in instructing those providing care. Carelessly turning patients so that legs hit the bedrail or "dropping" them into a chair or restraining them in an unaligned position can lead to muscle strain and fractures. Attempting to use force to straighten a contracture or roughly handling a limb without support can also result in fractures. Gentle handling will prevent unnecessary musculoskeletal discomfort and injury. Limbs should be supported below and above the joint for safety and comfort.

Since any loss of independence associated with the limitations imposed by musculoskeletal problems has a serious impact on physical, emotional, and social well-being, it is important for the gerontological nurse to explore all avenues to help patients minimize limitations and strengthen capacities, thus promoting the highest possible level of independence. Canes and walkers can enhance independence in ambulation, and self-care devices can often be obtained through physical and occupational therapists to help patients eat, bathe, and care for themselves (Figure 13-3).

REFERENCES

Habermann, E. T. "Orthopaedic Aspects of the Lower Extremities." In Rossman, I. (ed.), *Clinical Geriatrics*. Lippincott, Philadelphia, 1971, p. 311.

14

HEMATOLOGIC PROBLEMS

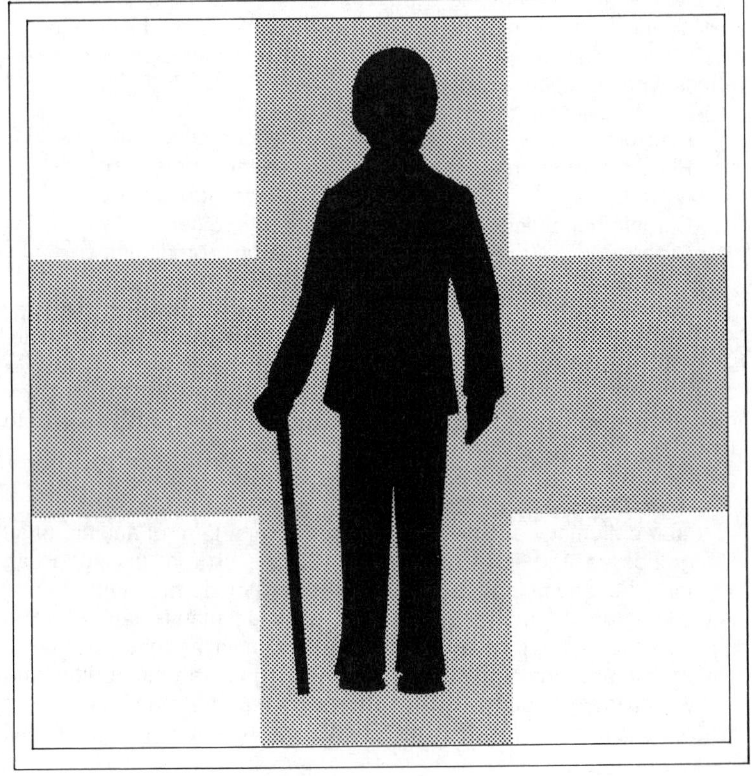

Hematologic problems are not uncommon in the aged, and lymphosarcoma, chronic lymphocytic leukemia, reticulum cell sarcoma, macroglobulinemia, and multiple myeloma are of high incidence. Anemia occurs with such frequency in aged persons that it is often mistakenly considered a normal consequence of growing old. These and other hematologic diseases which reduce the aged person's capacity to deal with stress are believed to be a result of several aging factors, including atrophy of the thymus and lymph nodes, impaired cutaneous hyper-reactivity, decreased immunoglobulin production in response to stress, increased lymphocytes in the bone marrow, and a reduction in the circulating red cell mass.

TYPES OF ANEMIA AND RELATED NURSING CONSIDERATIONS

As mentioned, while anemia is a common problem in the aged, it is not a normal condition. In addition to the fatigue and pallor which usually accompany this problem, the aged may demonstrate a greater susceptibility to infection, mental confusion, angina attacks, and episodes of congestive heart failure. Certain problems are associated with the various types of anemia in the aged.

Poor diet
Rheumatoid arthritis
Uremia
Chronic hepatitis
Cirrhosis
Prostatic hypertrophy
Diabetes
Cancer, especially of the hematopoietic organs and digestive tract
Peptic ulcers
Chronic bronchitis
Tuberculosis
Urinary-tract infections and other chronic or subacute infections

In addition to treatment, a thorough evaluation of the patient is needed to detect any underlying disease causing the anemia.

Iron Deficiency Anemia

Iron deficiency anemia is the most common form of anemia in all age groups. In addition to poor dietary intake of iron, the aged can develop this anemia as a result of hemorrhoidal bleeding, peptic ulcers, or impaired absorption of iron. The clinical manifestations of this imparied tissue nutrition are dry inelastic skin, headache, dizziness, fatigue, thin and brittle hair, atrophy of the tongue, and thin, brittle, and easily breakable fingernails. Blood tests confirm the diagnosis of iron deficiency anemia, and a misdiagnosis can result if problems that reduce iron-binding capacity and serum iron are also present—such as rheumatoid arthritis and chronic infection. Because anemia in the presence of an adequate iron intake can indicate poor absorption, bleeding, or other problems, a complete review of the older person's diet is essential. Theurapeutic measures, similar to those used with younger patients, include correcting any underlying cause, maintaining good nutrition, and using iron preparations. The patient should be instructed to administer the iron after meals and preferably not with dairy products.

It is important for the nurse to assist in the *prevention* of iron deficiency anemia through the encouragement of a well-balanced diet and a good nutritional status. Helping the aged patient obtain food stamps, introducing the patient to lunch programs, encouraging the correction of dental problems, teaching about diet, and providing guidance in the purchase of the best quality foods within limited budgets can be beneficial. The nurse can also discuss with the physician the value of iron supplements as a prophylactic measure.

Pernicious Anemia

Pernicious anemia is found mostly in aged patients (Maekawa, 1976), where it is usually accompanied by a reduced platelet and white blood cell count. A vitamin B-12 deficiency is the cause of pernicious anemia, which is frequently associated with cancer of the stomach. Accompanying the usual symptoms of anemia are premature graying or whitening of the hair; atrophy of the tongue, with a flattening of the papillae; and leg edema. Gastrointestinal changes contributing to this disease may cause anorexia, weight loss, diarrhea, constipation, and other related symptoms. The central nervous system may also be involved, depending on the extent of the problem. The treatment plan is the same at all ages. The patient needs to understand that monthly vitamin B-12 injections will be required for the remainder of his or her lifetime. Since gastric cancer is of greater incidence in patients with pernicious anemia, close follow-up and periodic stool examination are essential.

Folic Acid Deficiency

Folic acid deficiency is one of the major causes of nutritional anemia. Persons with limited fruit and vegetable intake are more likely to develop this form of anemia. Although folic acid deficiency is most commonly found in alcoholics, it is wise to realize that many aged persons risk developing this problem because a limited budget prevents them from including fruits and vegetables in their diet. Treatment consists of folic acid therapy, which, fortunately, can be replaced by good nutrition once the serum folic acid level has returned to normal.

OTHER HEMATOLOGIC DISEASES

Hodgkin's Disease and Multiple Myeloma

Hodgkin's disease in the aged and multiple myeloma are associated with anemia, leukopenia, or thrombocytopenia. Since symptomatology, diagnostic measures, and therapy for Hodgkin's disease are similar to those described for other age groups, the reader is advised to explore medical-surgical nursing literature for a complete review of this disease, which runs a more rapid and aggressive clinical course in the aged.

Multiple myeloma, more frequently diagnosed in middle-aged persons, has a decreasing incidence with age. Pathological fractures are a particular risk in aged people with multiple myeloma. Not only are these problems disabling in themselves, but they can pose serious threats to the aged as a result of emboli, pneumonia, and complications resulting from immobility. Mental confusion, behavioral changes, and coma are threats resulting from hypercalcemia associated with this disease. Many supportive measures to control pain and close observation for signs of complications are required of the nurse.

Leukemias

Leukemias have a higher incidence in aged people, where they (1) have an insidious onset; (2) manifest nonspecific symptoms which interfere with early diagnosis; (3) are difficult to manage; and (4) have a complicated course. A review of leukemias, readily available in medical-surgical literature, will not be presented here. However, there are some factors that are unique to the aged. *Acute leukemia* runs an aggressive course in the aged, is difficult to manage, and has a poor prognosis. *Chronic lymphoctic leukemia,* which is the most common leukemia in the aged, progresses slowly. With *chronic myeloid leukemia,* the associated spleen and liver enlargement may not develop in the aged.

Special nursing considerations. Although aged patients with leukemia require the same general care as younger patients, the gerontological nurse must be especially alert to complications. The aged are already at higher risk of infection than the young, and a disease like leukemia compounds that risk. Infections must be prevented and promptly treated if they occur. Since the aged do not manage the stress of hemorrhage well, this complication should be prevented; if it should occur, it should be readily detected and promptly treated. Radiation therapy and chemotherapy may cause nausea, vomiting, stomatitis, anorexia, and other problems which threaten the nutritional status of the patient. Careful attention to the prevention of mouth trauma, avoidance of extremes in the temperature and seasoning of food, and the encouragement of a good diet are beneficial. The patient's psychological state may be affected by changes in body image resulting from chemotherapy, radiation, or surgery. Maintaining the best possible appearance, through wigs and attractive clothing, for instance, and allowing patients to vent their reactions openly and discuss their disease may help them cope with these difficult adjustments.

REFERENCES

Maekawa, T. "Hematologic Diseases." In Steinberg, F. U. (ed.), *Cowdry's, The Care of the Geriatric Patient,* 5th ed. Mosby, St. Louis, 1976, p. 159.

15

GASTROINTESTINAL PROBLEMS

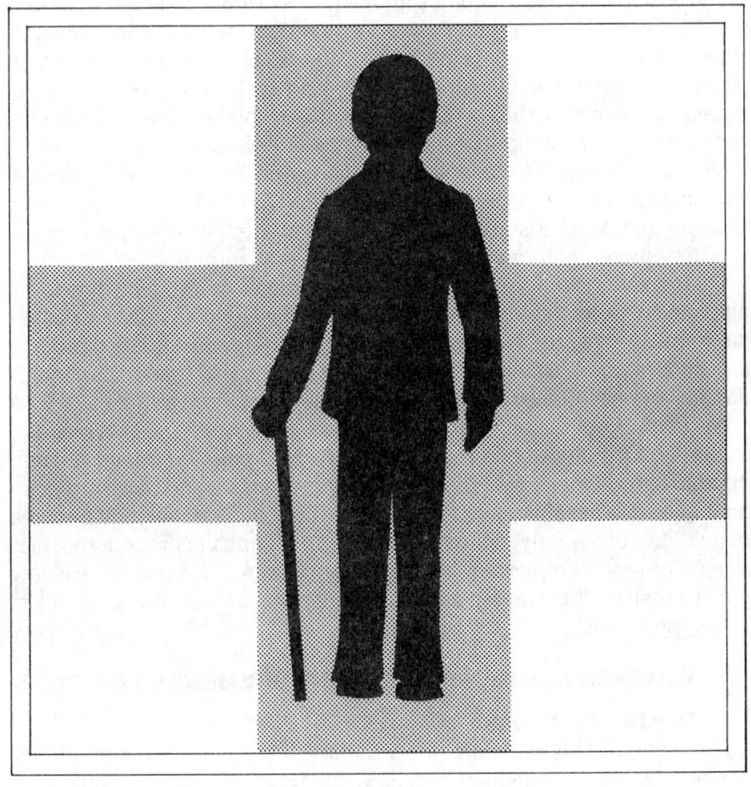

The gastrointestinal system becomes the most problematic body system with age and is the frequent cause of many complaints voiced by older persons. All gastrointestinal symptoms increase with advancing age. Problems that occur in the absence of any organic cause include indigestion, belching, diarrhea, constipation, nausea, vomiting, anorexia, weight loss, and flatulence. The aged have a higher incidence of cancer throughout the gastrointestinal tract, and also of high incidence are biliary tract disease, intestinal obstruction, and peptic ulcer. Gallbladder disease with cholelithiasis is a frequently diagnosed condition in older persons. In the absence of disease, there is no significant change in the functions of the liver, gallbladder, and pancreas.

A variety of factors related to the aging process contribute to the high incidence of gastrointestinal problems. A majority of the aged have lost most or all of their teeth, often needlessly. There is a reduction in taste sensation, particularly affecting the taste buds for sweet and salt, and poor appetite is not uncommon. Less gastric acid is secreted, and the stomach mucosa becomes thinner. The stomach takes a longer period of time to empty, and hunger contractions are reduced. Although supporting scientific data is inadequate, there is believed to be some atrophy throughout the intestines, colon, and rectum. Absorption is reduced by fewer absorbing cells on the walls of the intestines. Peristalsis becomes slower throughout the entire system. Secretory activity is altered, and salivary amylase secretion is lower. There is a decrease in pepsin secretion, and pancreatic enzymes. The changes in secretory function affect the absorption of all nutrients—protein absorption being affected more than fat and carbohydrate absorption.

The diagnosis of gastrointestinal problems is difficult due to an atypical symptomatology, which easily causes confusion with other problems. Among the tests frequently used to diagnosis these problems are barium swallow, esophagoscopy, gastroscopy, gastric analysis, barium enema, cholecystogram, sigmoidoscopy, and proctoscopy. A great deal of education, reassurance, and comfort should be provided for the aged during these procedures, many of which demand uncomfortable introductions of equipment into body orifices and awkward positioning on hard examination tables. Since the aged patient may become dehydrated or hypoglycemic if kept NPO for diagnostic procedures, prolonged or repeated periods of restricted nourishment intake necessitate close nursing observation and assessment to detect development of these problems.

COMMON DISORDERS AND REQUIREMENTS FOR CARE

Dental Problems

Continued dental care is important throughout an individual's lifetime. Dental examination can be instrumental in the early detection and prevention of many problems that affect other body systems. Poor teeth can restrict food intake, which can cause constipation and malnourishment; they also detract from appearance, which can affect socialization, and this in turn can result in a poor appetite, which can also lead to malnourishment. Periodontal disease can predispose the aged to systemic infection. Although dental care is important in preventing these problems, financial limitations prevent many aged persons from seeking dental attention. Some aged persons have the misconception that dentures eliminate the need for regular visits to the dentist. Others, like many younger persons, fear the dentist. The nurse should encourage regular dental examination and promote dental care, explaining that serious diseases can be detected by the dentist and helping patients find free or inexpensive dental clinics. Understanding how modern dental techniques minimize pain can alleviate fears. Although older persons may not have had the benefit of fluoridated water or fluoride treatments when younger, topical fluoride treatments are as beneficial to the teeth of the aged as they are to younger teeth. Patients should be instructed to inform their dentists about health problems and medications they are taking to help them determine how procedures need to be modified, what healing rate to expect, and which medications cannot be administered.

Dental problems can be caused by altered taste sensation, a poor diet, or a low-budget carbohydrate diet with excessive intake of sweets, which can cause tooth decay. Deficiencies of the vitamin B complex, hormonal imbalances, hyperparathyroidism, diabetes, osteomalacia, Cushing's disease, and syphilis can be underlying causes of dental problems in the aged, and certain drugs, such as aspirin and dilantin, can also play a part. The aging process itself takes its toll on teeth, surfaces are commonly worn down from many years of use, varying degrees of root absorption take place, and loss of tooth enamel increases the risk of irritation to deeper dental tissue (Goldman, 1971; Rowe, 1976). While benign neoplastic lesions occur more frequently than malignant ones, cancer of the oral cavity, especially in males, is of increasing incidence with age, as is moniliasis, which is often associated with more serious problems, such as diabetes or leukemia. It should not be assumed that all white lesions found in the mouth are moniliasis—biopsy is important to make sure they are not cancerous. Periodontal disease, damaging the soft tissue surrounding teeth and supporting bones, is of high incidence among the aged, and although they occur less frequently in older people, dental caries are a problem as well.

Good oral hygiene is especially important to the aged, who already may be having problems with anorexia or food distaste. Teeth, gums, and tongue can be helped by regular brushing using a soft toothbrush, which can also be used in gentle gum massage for people with dentures.

Daily flossing of natural teeth should be performed, and brushing may be better than using swabs, even for the teeth of unconscious patients. Since the buccal mucosa is thinner and less vascular with age, trauma to the oral cavity should be avoided. The nurse should notify the dentist and physician of an atonic or atrophic tongue, lesions, mucosa discoloration, loose teeth, soreness, bleeding, or any other problem identified during inspection and care of the oral cavity.

Esophageal Diverticulum

Dysphagia, gagging, and the regurgitation of undigested food are among the clues indicating esophageal diverticulum. The accumulation and decomposition of food in the diverticulum may cause the breath to have an extremely foul odor. A particularly dangerous complication of this disorder for older people is aspiration, which leads to many serious respiratory problems. A barium swallow confirms the diagnosis, and surgical intervention usually follows. Close nursing observation is important postoperatively to detect leakage from the esophagus, which could cause the formation of a fistula. Nasogastric feedings, discussed at the end of this chapter, are employed until the patient can progress to oral feedings.

Hiatus Hernia

The incidence of hiatus hernia increases with age and tends to affect females more than males (Straus, 1971a; Hodkinson, 1975a). It is estimated that over 50 percent of all aged persons are affected by this disease. Heartburn, dysphagia, belching, vomiting, and regurgitation are common symptoms associated with hiatus hernia. These symptoms are especially problematic when the patient is in a recumbent position. Pain, sometimes mistaken for a coronary, and bleeding may also occur. Diagnosis is confirmed by a barium swallow and esophagoscopy. A majority of patients are managed medically. If the patient is obese, weight reduction can minimize the problems. A bland diet may be recommended, as may the use of milk and antacids for symptomatic relief. Several small meals rather than three large ones are of extreme benefit in bringing about improvement, and may also be advantageous to the aged in coping with other age-related gastrointestinal problems. Eating before bedtime should be discouraged. Some patients may find it beneficial to sleep in a partly recumbent position.

Cancer of the Esophagus

Most persons affected by cancer of the esophagus are aged. This disease commonly strikes between the ages of 60 and 65 years and is of higher incidence in males, blacks, and alcoholics (Straus, 1971a; Berman and Kirsner, 1976b). Poor oral hygiene and chronic irritation from tobacco, alcohol, and other agents contribute to the development of this problem. Dysphagia, excessive salivation, thirst, hiccups, anemia, and chronic bleeding are symptoms of this disease. Barium swallow, esophagoscopy, and biopsy are performed as diagnostic measures. Treatment consists of an esophagectomy, and a poor prognosis is not uncommon among aged patients. Benign tumors of the esophagus are rare in the aged.

Peptic Ulcer

Although peptic ulcers occur most frequently at younger ages, the incidence of this problem is on the rise for the aged (Straus, 1971b). Older females develop ulcers more often than older males, and most frequently, these ulcers are gastric rather than duodenal (Berman and Kirsner, 1976b). In addition to stress, diet, and genetic predisposition as causes, particular factors are believed to account for the increased incidence of ulcers in the aged, including longevity, more precise diagnostic evaluation, and the fact that ulcers can be a complication of the increasingly prevalent disorder chronic obstructive pulmonary disease. Drugs commonly prescribed for the aged that can increase gastric secretions and reduce the resistance of the mucosa include aspirin, reserpine, tolbutamide, phenylbutazone, colchicine, and adrenal corticosteroids.

Early symptoms commonly associated with peptic ulcer may not occur in the aged patient, and pain, bleeding and perforation may be the only indication of this problem. Diagnostic and therapeutic measures resemble those employed for younger adults. The nurse should be alert to complications associated with peptic ulcer, which may be especially threatening to the geriatric patient. Constipation or diarrhea can be caused by antacid therapy, and pyloric obstruction can result in dehydration, peritonitis, hemorrhage, and shock.

Cancer of the Stomach

Although stomach cancer is of lower incidence in the aged, it is not uncommon. The incidence is greater among men, in patients with pernicious anemia or atrophy of the gastric mucosa, and in persons between the ages of 75 and 85 years (Straus, 1971c; Berman and Kirsner, 1976c). Anorexia, epigastric pain, weight loss, and anemia are symptoms of gastric cancer. Bleeding may occur, as can enlargement of the liver. Symptoms related to pelvic metastasis may also develop. Diagnosis is confirmed by barium swallow and gastroscopy with biopsy. Surgical treatment consisting of a partial or total gastrectomy is preferred. Unfortunately, the aged have a poor prognosis with gastric cancer.

Superior Mesenteric Vascular Occlusion

The aged, especially aged males, experience superior mesenteric vascular occlusion more frequently than younger adults do (Straus, 1971d). This occlusion usually involves the jejunum and ileum. Congestion, obstruction, peritonitis, and ischemic necrosis can result from this problem, seriously threatening the aged person's life. Pain, vomiting, abdominal distention, and bloody diarrhea are symptoms associated with superior mesenteric vascular occlusion. Surgical intervention, possibly a bowel resection, is employed, and the prognosis is not favorable for the aged.

Abdominal Angina

Arterial insufficiency may cause the aged patient to experience abdominal angina. Upper abdominal pain after meals and while walking (relieved by a recumbent position) are manifestations of this problem. Back pain also may be a symptom. Aortography is used to diagnose abdominal angina. Medical management is preferred and will include a feeding schedule of several small meals instead of three large ones. Sometimes surgical intervention is employed to replace the involved artery.

Diverticulosis and Diverticulitis

Multiple pouches of intestinal mucosa in the weakened muscular wall of the large bowel, known as *diverticulosis,* are common among the aged. Chronic constipation, obesity, hiatus hernia, and an atrophy of the intestinal wall muscles with aging contribute to this problem. Slight bleeding may occur with diverticulosis, and usually a barium enema identifies the problem. Surgery is not performed unless severe bleeding develops. Medical management is most common and includes a bland diet, weight reduction, and avoidance of constipation. Bowel contents can accumulate in the diverticuli and decompose, causing inflammation and infection. This is known as *diverticulitis.* Although less than half the patients with diverticulosis develop diverticulitis, most patients who do are aged. Older men tend to experience this problem more than any other group (Straus, 1971e).

Overeating, straining during a bowel movement, alcohol, and irritating foods may contribute to diverticulitis in the patient with diverticulosis. Pain in the left lower quadrant, similar to that of appendicitis but over the sigmoid area, is a symptom of this problem. Nausea, vomiting, constipation, diarrhea, low-grade fever, and blood or mucus in the stool may also occur. These attacks can be severely acute or slowly progressing; while the former can cause peritonitis, the latter can also be serious due to the possibility of lower-bowel obstruction resulting from scarring and abscess formation. In addition to the mentioned complica-

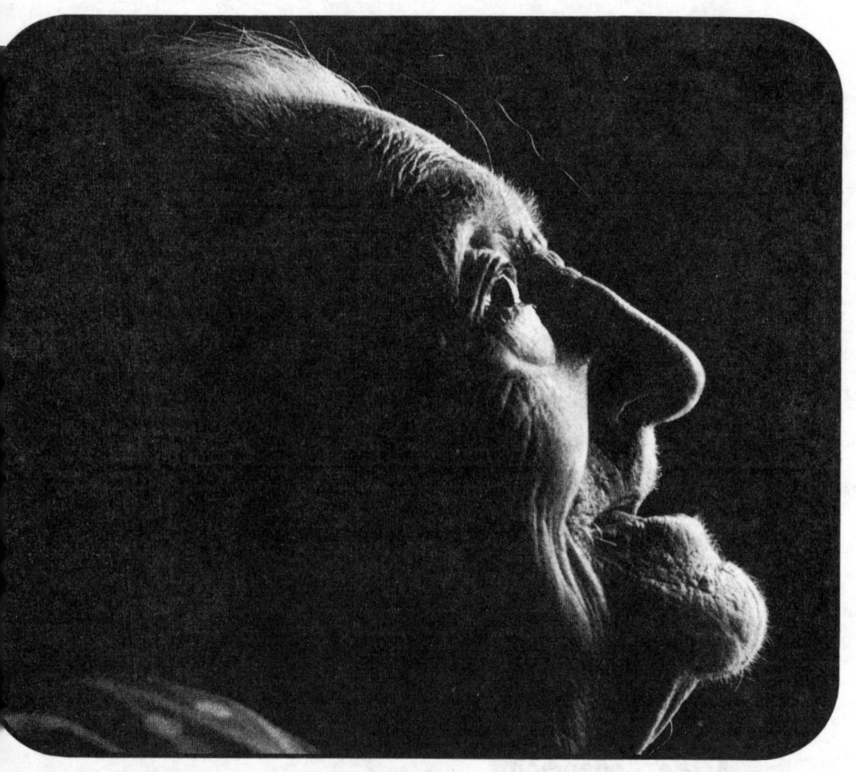

tions, fistulas to the bladder, vagina, colon, and intestines can develop. During the acute phase, efforts are focused on reducing infection, providing nutrition, relieving discomfort, and promoting rest. Usually nothing is ingested by mouth and intravenous therapy is employed. When the acute episode subsides, the patient is taught a low-residue diet. Surgery, performed if medical management is unsuccessful or if serious complications occur, may consist of a resection or temporary colostomy. Continued follow-up should be encouraged.

Cancer of the Colon

Cancer at any site along the large intestine is common in the aged and affects both sexes equally. The sigmoid colon and rectum tend to be frequent sites for carcinoma. Bloody stools, a change in bowel function, epigastric pain, jaundice, anorexia, and nausea may be symptoms of this problem, although the pattern of symptoms frequently varies for each person. Some older patients ignore bowel symptoms, believing them to be from constipation, poor diet, or hemorrhoids. The patient's description of his bowel problems is less reliable than a digital rectal examination, which detects half of all carcinomas of the large bowel and rectum (Straus, 1971f; Hodkinson, 1975b). The standard diagnostic tests, including barium enema and sigmoidoscopy with biopsy, are used to confirm the diagnosis. Surgical resection, with anastomosis or the formation of a colostomy, is usually performed. Medical-surgical nursing textbooks can provide information on this surgery, and nurses should consult them for specific guidance on caring for patients in this condition.

It is important to realize that a colostomy can present many problems for the aged. In addition to having to adjust to many bodily changes with age, a colostomy presents a major adjustment and a threat to a good self-concept. The aged may feel that a colostomy further separates them from society's view of normal. Socialization may be impaired by the patient's concern over the reactions of others, or by his fear of embarrassing episodes. Reduced energy reserves, arthritic fingers, slower movement, and poorer eyesight are among the problems which may hamper the aged's ability to care for a colostomy, thus causing dependency on others to assist with this procedure. This need for assistance may be perceived as a significant loss of independence for the aged. Tactful, skilled nursing intervention can promote a psychological as well as physical adjustment to a colostomy. Continued follow-up is beneficial to assess the aged patient's changing ability to engage in this self-care activity, identify problems, and provide ongoing support and reassurance.

Acute Appendicitis

Although acute appendicitis does not frequently occur in aged persons, it is important to note that it can occur and that it may present altered signs and symptoms in the aged. The severe pain which occurs in younger persons is absent in aged persons, whose pain may be minimal and referred. Fever may also be minimal, and leukocytosis may be absent. These differences often cause a delayed diagnosis. Prompt surgery will increase the patient's prognosis. Unfortunately, delayed or missed diagnosis and the inability to improve the general status of the patient before this emergency surgery can lead to greater complications and mortality in aged persons with appendicitis.

Chronic Constipation

It is not uncommon for the aged to be bothered by and concerned about constipation. An inactive life-style, less bulk and fluids in the diet, depression, and laxative abuse contribute to this problem. Certain medications will promote constipation, such as opiates, sedatives, and aluminum hydroxide gels. Dulled sensations may cause the signal for bowel elimination to be unnoticed, leading to constipation. Not allowing sufficient time for complete emptying of the bowel can also cause constipation. (It should be remembered that the aged may not fully empty the bowel at one sitting and it is not unusual for a second bowel movement to be required one-half hour after the initial one.) A diet high in bulk and fluid and regular activity can promote bowel elimination, and particular foods that patients find effective—prunes, chocolate pudding, etc.—can be incorporated into the regular diet. Providing a regular time for bowel elimination is often helpful; the mornings tend to be the best time for the aged to empty their bowels. Sometimes rocking the trunk from side to side, and back and forth while sitting on the toilet will stimulate a bowel movement. Only after these other measures have failed should medications be considered.

Older persons may need education concerning bowel elimination. The misconception that daily bowel movements are necessary must be corrected with realistic explanations. Safe use of laxatives should be emphasized to prevent laxative abuse. The patient should be aware that diarrhea resulting from laxative abuse may cause dehydration and be a serious threat to life. The aged in a hospital or nursing home setting may benefit from a stool chart which reflects the time, amount, and characteristics of bowel movements. This chart can help the nurse prevent constipation and impaction by providing easily accessible data regarding bowel function. Even aged persons in the community can benefit from the use of a stool chart which they can maintain.

Chronic constipation which does not improve with the usual measures may require medical evaluation, including anal, rectal, and sigmoid examinations to determine the presence of any underlying cause.

Fecal Impaction

Constipation frequently leads to fecal impaction in the aged. The absence or an insufficient amount of stool should create suspicion regarding an impaction. What may appear to be diarrhea may occur as a result of oozing of liquid feces around the impaction. While taking a rectal temperature the nurse may detect a resistance to the thermometer and find feces on the thermometer when it is withdrawn. A movable mass may be palpated by digital examination. The best approach to fecal impactions is to prevent them from developing; the preventive measures discussed with constipation should be exercised. Once the impaction has developed it must be softened, broken, and removed.

Since policies may vary, the nurse is advised to review the permissive procedures of her employing agency to ensure that removal of a fecal impaction is an acceptable nursing action. An enema, usually oil retention, may be prescribed to assist in the softening and elimination process. Manual breaking and removal of feces with a lubricated gloved finger will promote removal of the impaction. Sometimes, injecting 50 ml of hydrogen peroxide through a rectal tube will cause breakage of the impaction as the hydrogen peroxide foams. Care should be taken not to traumatize or exert the patient during these procedures.

Cancer of the Pancreas

Pancreatic cancer, which occurs most frequently in thin aged men, is a difficult disease to detect until it has reached an advanced stage (Straus, 1971g; Hodkinson, 1975c). Anorexia, weakness, weight loss, and wasting are generalized symptoms, which are easily attributed to other causes. Dyspepsia, belching, nausea, vomiting, diarrhea, constipation, and obstructive jaundice may occur as well. Fever may or may not be present. Epigastric pain radiating to the back may be experienced. This pain is relieved when the patient leans forward and is worsened when a recumbent position is assumed. Surgery is performed to treat this problem. Unfortunately, the disease is so advanced by the time diagnosis is made that the prognosis is usually poor.

Biliary Tract Disease

The incidence of gallstones increases with age and affects women more frequently than men (Hodkinson, 1975d; Straus, 1971h). Pain is the primary symptom associated with this problem. Diagnostic and treatment measures include the standard ones prescribed for adults of any age. Obstruction, inflammation, and infection are potential outcomes of gallstones and should be observed for. Cancer of the gallbladder primarily affects older persons, especially aged females (Straus, 1971i). Fortunately, this disease does not occur very frequently. Pain in the right upper quadrant, anorexia, nausea, vomiting, weight loss, jaundice, weakness, and constipation are the usual symptoms. Although surgery may be performed, the prognosis for the patient with cancer of the gallbladder is poor.

NURSING CONSIDERATIONS

Preventive measures that should be incorporated into the care of geriatric patients in an effort to avoid many of the gastrointestinal problems they commonly experience include the following:

Good dental hygiene
Regular physical and dental examinations
Weight control
A diet of the proper quantity and quality
Avoidance of constipation

Through teaching, supporting, and guiding, the nurse can help the aged comply with these measures and enhance gastrointestinal function.

Gavage feedings may be required to supply nutrition for some aged patients. When feeding the patient in this manner and instructing others how to gavage feed, certain points must be remembered. The patient should be placed in a sitting or high Fowler's position during the feeding to prevent aspiration. Prior to instilling the solution, the Levin tube must be checked to make sure it is in the stomach and has not slipped out of place. This is done as follows:

1. Using a 20-ml syringe and aspirating stomach contents
2. Injectioning 5 ml of air into the tube and listening with a stethoscope for a swishing sound as the air enters the stomach
3. Placing the end of the Levin tube in a glass of water so that the absence of regular air bubbles and coughing indicate that the tube is in the stomach

When it has been established that the Levine tube is in the stomach, the feeding can be given. The flow of the solution is not to be fast or forceful. For the geriatric patient, the solution reservoir may achieve a good flow if held at the level of the patient's nose. Rapid feeding can cause discomfort and regurgitation. The nurse or some other care provider should remain with the patient during the feeding; attaching the reservoir to a pole and allowing the feeding to flow in unattended could lead to serious complications and death. Dyspnea, coughing, cyanosis, or any other unusual sign necessitates that the feeding be discontinued and that a physician be notified. Because the time required for stomach emptying is greater in older persons, they should remain in an upright position for at least one-half hour after the feeding. To prevent the entry of air into the stomach, the tube is clamped, except during instillation of solution.

Figure 15-1 demonstrates the proper way to anchor the tube to the patient's face. The tube is not to be pulled and taped to the side of the nose; this causes the tube within the nasal passage to place pressure on the nasal mucosa, predisposing the aged's fragile skin to breakdown in that area. Sometimes, applying a small amount of lubricant in the nostril will prevent irritation. The nostrils are to be cleansed and kept patent. Gentle manipulation with a cotton-tipped applicator can be effective in removing dried crusts and preventing any interference with breathing. Frequent oral hygiene is also essential. It is the policy of some agencies to irrigate the Levine tube at intervals to maintain patency; the nurse is advised to review the standard gastric feeding procedure of her agency and learn the recommended practices.

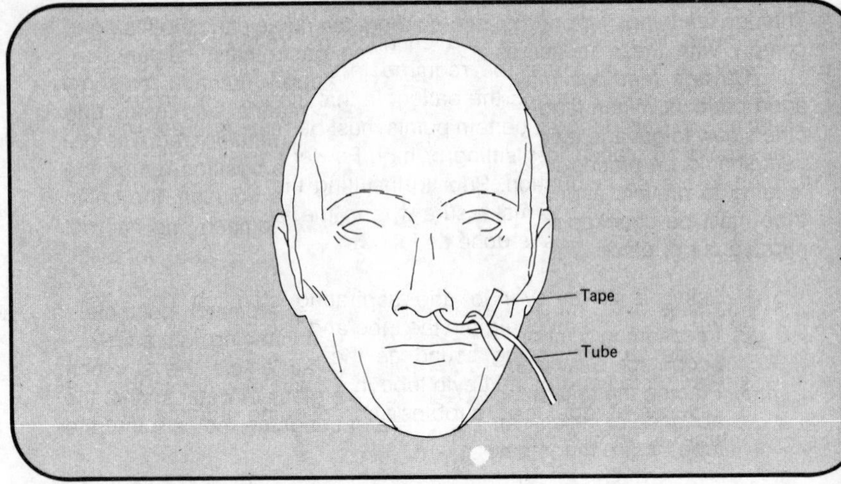

Figure 15-1. Proper anchoring of nasogastric tube to prevent irritation and breakdown of the nasal mucosa.

In some chronic care settings, the aged patient may be receiving gastric feedings over a long period of time. If this is the situation, special attention must be paid to the development of complications associated with prolonged use of a nasogastric tube, including respiratory infection, ulceration anywhere along the area in which the Levine tube is located (especially the nasal and gastric mucosa), sinusitis, and esophagitis. Regular assessment is required by the gerontological nurse to determine the continued need for gastric feeding. These feedings should be used only if the patient is unable to ingest food orally. At no time is tube feeding to be employed only because it is a faster and easier way to feed an older patient.

Since aged persons may have poor appetites, every effort should be made to promote an adequate food intake. A variety of foods that the older person can easily cut, manage, chew, and digest and that are attractively served will facilitate eating. A pleasant, colorful, odor-free environment, an opportunity for socialization, and ample time to allow for the slower movements of the older person should be provided. For many aged persons, a nutritional diet of the right quality and quantity will promote and maintain a high enough level of physiological and mental functioning to prevent the development of gastrointestinal disorders.

REFERENCES

Berman, P. M., and **Kirsner, J. B.** "Gastrointestinal Problems." In Steinberg, F. U. (ed.), *Cowdry's, The Care of the Geriatric Patient,* 5th ed. Mosby, St. Louis, 1976. (a) p. 95; (b) p. 96; (c) p. 97.

Goldman, R. "Decline in Organ Function with Aging." In Rossman, I. (ed.), *Clinical Geriatrics.* Lippincott, Philadelphia, 1971, p. 30.

Hodkinson, H. M. *An Outline of Geriatrics.* Academic Press, New York, 1975. (a) p. 108; (b) p. 113; (c) pp. 110–111; (d) p. 111.

Rowe, N. H. "Dental Surgery." In Steinberg, F. U. (ed.), *Cowdry's, The Care of the Geriatric Patient,* 5th ed. Mosby, St. Louis, 1976, p. 301.

Straus, B. "Disorders of the Digestive System." In Rossman, I. (ed.), *Clinical Geriatrics.* Lippincott, Philadelphia, 1971. (a) p. 186; (b) p. 187; (c) p. 188; (d) p. 190; (e) p. 194; (f) p. 196; (g) p. 198; (h) p. 199; (i) p. 200.

16

GENITOURINARY PROBLEMS

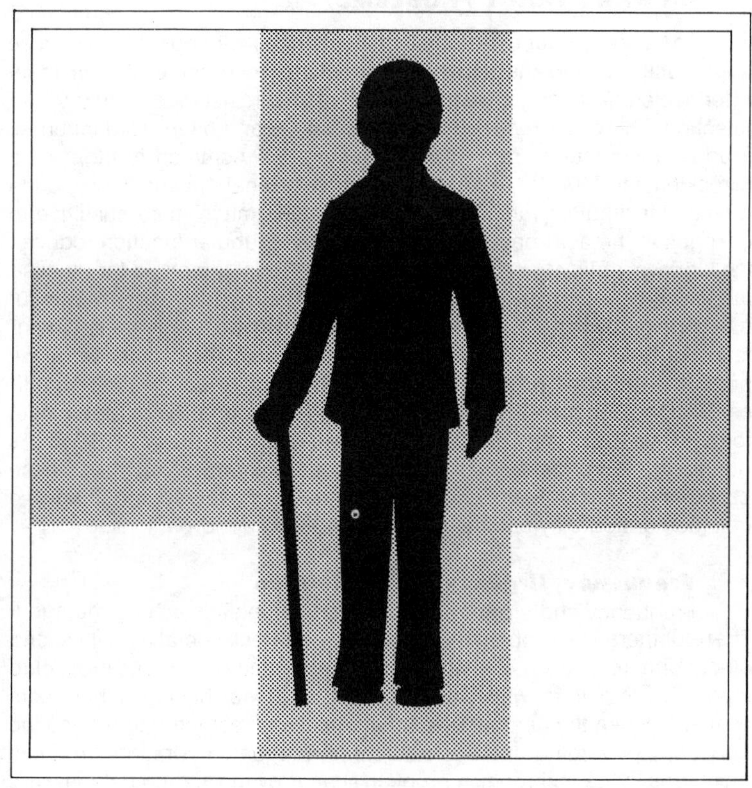

Genitourinary problems in older adults, while bothersome, potentially life threatening, and frequently occurring, are disorders which the aged are often reluctant to discuss. Some feel embarrassment or distaste at making others aware of these problems. Others fear societal reactions to an older person's concern about sexual function or believe symptoms of genitourinary disorders are merely a result of changes with age. Occasionally, the aged may associate genitourinary problems with sexual "wrongdoing" and feel guilty over the development of these disorders. These factors, along with reluctance to obtain gynecological and urologic examinations, often delay early detection and treatment. The nurse is in a position to develop a close relationship with the geriatric patient and can be a key person in identifying problems of the urinary tract and reproductive system. By demonstrating sensitivity, acceptance, and an understanding of the patient's problems, the nurse can facilitate medical attention.

URINARY TRACT PROBLEMS

The urinary tract undergoes many changes with age. Muscles lose their elasticity, and the supportive structures lose some of their tone. Arteriosclerotic changes reduce this system's resistance to injury and infection. There is a reduced bladder capacity and often residual urine. Bladder diverticulae, rare in older women, are common in older men (Brocklehurst, 1971a). There is a reduction in renal plasma flow and the glomerular filtration rate. The kidneys become much more sensitive to changes in the acid-base balance. Decreased tubular function reduces the kidneys' ability to concentrate urine. The renal threshold for glucose increases, so that an older person can be hyperglycemic without evidence of glycosuria. Although proteinuria with an abnormal sedimentation rate may be an early indication of chronic renal disease, a 1+ proteinuria may be present in older adults, usually being of no significance if the sedimentation rate is normal. The blood urea nitrogen level for a 70-year-old may be 21.2 mg% whereas it averages 12.9 mg% during the third decade of life (Kahn and Snapper, 1974a). These changes manifest themselves in a variety of ways, producing the common urologic symptoms observed in many aged persons.

Frequency, Urgency, and Retention

Frequency and urgency are common complaints among the aged. These bothersome problems can interfere with rest, social activities, and other normal functions. The affected individual may avoid bus trips, club meetings, and long walks due to the fear of not having a bathroom available when the need arises. If fluid intake is restricted to reduce the frequency of voiding, there is a threat to adequate hydration. Frequent night trips to the bathroom, a problem shared by most aged persons, are disruptive to sleep and can result in falls due to poor vision in dimly lit areas, blood pressure changes when rising from a lying position, disorientation, and reduced coordination. Limiting fluids at bedtime may be helpful, but this should be counterbalanced by adequate fluid intake during the entire day. Diuretics should be administered so that their peak is not reached during sleeping hours. Good lighting throughout the night and a bedside commode may also prove valuable. Since nocturia, urgency, and frequency can indicate infection or a variety of disease processes, thorough medical evaluation should be encouraged.

Urinary retention may be another problem, and the most common causes of this in the aged are fecal impactions in older women and prostatic hypertrophy in older men (Brocklehurst, 1971b). Urinary retention is also associated with a neurogenic bladder.

Urinary Incontinence

A common and bothersome problem of the aged that requires sensitive and skillful nursing attention is urinary incontinence. Changes that cause sphincter relaxation, altered bladder reflexes, and missed signals to void contribute to this problem. Urinary tract infections can cause temporary periods of incontinence. Tabes dorsalis, diabetic neuropathy, myasthenia gravis, and cerebral cortex lesions are responsible for incontinence as a result of neurogenic bladder. Certain medications used in the management of Parkinson's disease can exaggerate existing urinary tract lesions (Jaffe, 1974a). Incontinence also can be a result of mechanical causes, such as prostatic enlargement, calculi, and tumors. Incontinence can be quite problematic since irritation and breakdown of the aged patient's fragile skin is risked and the patient is subject to the development of urinary tract infection. In addition, odors, embarrassment, and fear of social inacceptance cause the aged to avoid active socialization.

The initial nursing action in caring for the incontinent patient is to arrange for a medical evaluation—to determine the cause of the problem, ensure treatment if possible, and provide a realistic assessment for use in rehabilitation. While specific nursing interventions are determined by the cause of the incontinence, there are some general measures that can prove beneficial. Observing and recording incidents of incontinence can reveal a pattern for scheduling bathroom trips and use of bedpans. Regularly asking patients whether they need to void and promptly answering calls for assistance can often prevent unnecessary episodes of bedwetting. Since concentrated urine can irritate the bladder and cause incontinence, fluids should be forced, unless another condition contraindicates this measure. Incontinence can be diminished by upright positioning during voiding (including while using the bedpan), which reduces the amount of urine retained, and by staying at the commode or urinal for several minutes after voiding to ensure complete emptying. Exercises to tighten the perineum while sitting, and interrupting the flow of urine midstream can improve sphincter control.

For dribbling or stress incontinence, women may find it helpful to wear sanitary pads, and men may benefit from the use of a condom catheter. Thorough, frequent cleansing of the perineal area and genitalia are essential. If an indwelling catheter is utilized, the patient should be observed closely for signs of infection. There are differences of opinion about how frequently an indwelling catheter should be changed and the nurse is encouraged to consult with the physician or review the policy of her agency. Intermittent catherterization is gaining popularity, and patients and their families may need to be instructed in this technique. In some geriatric settings it has been found that incontinence is reduced when patients wear their own clothing—a strategy with multiple benefits.

The nurse can assist patients in the development of a program for bladder training. The success of this program depends upon the patients' physical capacity to regain bladder control, their comprehension of the program, and their motivation. Therefore, a complete assessment of capacities and limitations and joint planning with the patient are prerequisites to the initiation of this regimen. When the patient is fully prepared to begin the program, a schedule is developed indicating the times for voiding. Usually, two hour intervals are planned first, with increased intervals as the patient's progress indicates and reduced intervals during the night. Approximately one-half hour prior to the time scheduled, the patient should drink a full glass of fluid and make a conscious effort to retain urine. At the scheduled time, the patient should attempt to void; if there is difficulty, massaging the bladder area or rocking forward and backward may facilitate voiding (Figure 16-1). It is important to keep an accurate record of intake and output and of the patient's responses to the training program and its effectiveness. The essential role for the nursing staff in this procedure is to make sure the schedule is strictly adhered to by all. Inconsistency on the part of the nursing staff will be destructive to the progress of patients and denigrating to their efforts. Conversely, positive reinforcement and encouragement are most beneficial to the patient during this difficult program.

Urinary Tract Infections

Infections of the urinary tract are not uncommon in the aged, especially in institutional settings. They are second to pulmonary disorders as the most frequent cause of fever in older persons (Jaffe, 1974b). Primarily responsible for urinary tract infections are escherichia coli in wcmen and B. proteus in men. The presence of any foreign body in the urinary tract or anything that slows or obstructs the flow of urine—such as immobilization, urethral strictures, neoplasms, or a clogged indwelling

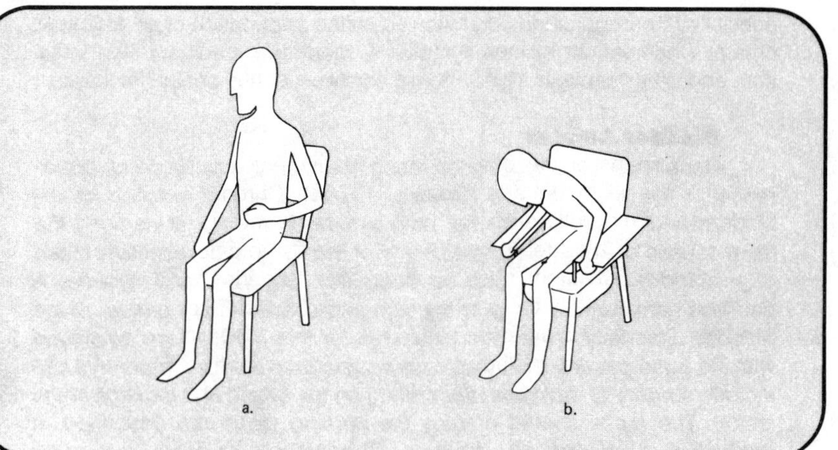

Figure 16-1. Measures to facilitate voiding: (a) Massaging bladder area. (b) Rocking back and forth.

catheter—predisposes the individual to these infections. They can result from poor hygienic practices or improper cleansing after bowel elimination, from a predisposition created by low fluid intake and excessive fluid loss, and from hormonal changes, which reduce the body's resistance. Persons in a debilitated state or who have neurogenic bladders, arteriosclerosis, or diabetes also have a high risk of developing infections.

The gerontological nurse should be alert to the signs and symptoms. Early indicators include burning, urgency, and fever. Awareness of the patient's *normal* body temperature helps the nurse recognize the presence of fever, for instance, 99° F in a patient whose normal temperature is 96.8° F. Some urologists believe that many urinary tract infections in the aged seem asymptomatic due to unawareness of elevations in normal temperature. The gerontological nurse can significantly facilitate diagnoses by informing the physician of temperature increases.

As a urinary tract infection progresses, retention, incontinence, and hematuria may occur. Treatment is aimed at establishing adequate urinary drainage and controlling the infection through antibiotic therapy. The nurse should carefully note the fluid intake and output. Forcing fluids is advisable, providing the patient's cardiac status doesn't contraindicate this action. If an indwelling catheter is utilized, attention should be paid to preventing infection and maintaining an unobstructed urinary flow. Regular meatus care for the patient with an indwelling catheter may consist of thorough cleansing followed by the application of an antibiotic cream. Observation for new symptoms, bladder distension, skin irritation, and other unusual signs should continue as the patient recovers.

Bladder Cancer

Neoplasms of the bladder reach their peak incidence of occurrence in the sixth decade (Bowles, 1976a). Chronic irritation of the bladder and cigarette smoking, both avoidable factors, are among the main causes of bladder tumors. Some of the symptoms resemble those of a bladder infection, such as frequency, urgency, and dysuria. A painless hematuria is the primary sign and characterizes cancer of the bladder. Standard diagnostic measures for this disease are employed with the aged patient, including cystoscopic examination. Treatment can include surgery or radiation, depending on the extent and location of the lesion. The nurse should employ the nursing measures described in medical-surgical nursing literature. Observation for signs indicating metastasis, such as pelvic or back pain, is part of the nursing care for these patients.

Bladder Diverticula

Bladder diverticula, usually occurring in numbers rather than singularly, may be present in aged individuals. Since they predispose the individual to infection, antibiotic therapy and surgical correction are typically major parts of the treatment plan.

Renal calculi

Renal calculi occur most frequently in middle-aged adults. In the aged, the formation of stones can be caused by immobilization, infection, changes in the pH or concentration of urine, chronic diarrhea, dehydration, excessive elimination of uric acid, and hypercalcemia. Pain, hematuria, and symptoms of urinary tract infection are commonly associated with this problem, and gastrointestinal upset may also occur. Standard diagnostic and treatment measures are used for the aged, and the nurse can assist by preventing urinary stasis, by providing ample fluids, and by facilitating prompt treatment of urinary tract infections.

Glomerulonephritis

Most frequently, chronic glomerulonephritis already exists in aged persons who develop an acute condition. It is possible for the symptoms of this disease to be so subtle and mild that they are initially unnoticed. Clinical manifestations include fever, fatigue, nausea, vomiting, anorexia, abdominal pain, anemia, edema, elevated blood pressure, and an increased sedimentation rate. Oliguria may occur, as can proteinuria and hematuria. Headache, convulsions, paralysis, aphasia, coma, and an altered mental status may be a consequence of cerebral edema associated with this disease. Diagnostic and treatment measures do not differ significantly from those used with the young. The use of antibiotics, a restricted sodium and protein diet, and close attention to fluid intake and output are basic parts of the treatment plan. If the aged person is receiving digitalis, diuretics, or antihypertensive drugs, close observation for cumulative toxic effects resulting from compromised kidney function must be observed for. The patient should be evaluated periodically after the acute illness is resolved for detection of exacerbations of chronic glomerulonephritis and signs of renal failure.

Pyelonephritis

Pyelonephritis is the most commonly diagnosed renal problem in the aged female. Although urinary obstruction is the primary cause of this disease in older persons, there is some thought that autoimmune reactions may have some relationship as well. Symptoms of this problem vary from mild to severe. Dull back pain, fever, gastrointestinal upset, frequency, dysuria, burning, bacteriuria, and pyuria are usually present with acute pyelonephritis. As the chronic form develops, progressive kidney damage leads to polyuria, anorexia, weight loss, fatigue and the classic symptoms associated with uremia. Aged patients have been found to have no fever and no voiding difficulty, however, even when high bacterial counts have been present (Kahn and Snapper, 1974b). The treatment depends on the causative factor and usually includes antibiotic therapy to eliminate the causative organism, correct the obstruction, and strengthen the patient's resistance. As with glomerulonephritis, periodic evaluation for the recurrence of infection and close follow-up are essential.

PROBLEMS IN THE FEMALE REPRODUCTIVE SYSTEM

Changes and disease processes common in old age contribute toward various problems in the female reproductive tract, many of which could be corrected or more easily managed through early detection. Unfortunately, older women do not always get regular gynecologic examinations, and by the time the symptoms produce enough discomfort to motivate them to do so, chances for a good prognosis can be significantly reduced. Some older women, having delivered their children at home, never had a gynecologic examination in their entire lifetime. Others mistakenly think that this procedure is not necessary for women over childbearing age. Some find it an embarrassing and uncomfortable procedure, and some have limited finances that must be spent attending to more disturbing medical problems.

Inquiry into the frequency of gynecologic examinations is an essential component of nursing assessment, and education should be provided regarding the continued importance of such examinations in old age. Health departments that offer examinations free or inexpensively to women attending family planning and prenatal clinics would provide a valuable service by extending their availability to the older woman, especially since she is more likely to be living on a lower income. Long-term care facilities should also recognize their importance and provide for them.

Infections and Tumors of the Vulva

The vulva loses hair and subcutaneous fat with age, and this is accompanied by a flattening and folding of the labia. A general atrophy occurs as well. These changes cause the vulva to be more fragile and more easily susceptible to irritation and infection. *Senile vulvitis* is the term used to describe vulvar infection associated with hypertrophy or atrophy. Vulvar problems in the aged may reflect serious disease processes such as diabetes, hepatitis, leukemia, and pernicious anemia. Incontinence and poor hygienic practices can also be underlying causes of vulvitis. Pruritis is the primary symptom associated with vulvitis. Patients who are confused and noncommunicative may display restlessness, and the nurse may discover that they are suffering from irritation and thickening of the vulvar tissue as a result of scratching. Initially, treatment is aimed at finding and managing any underlying cause. A good nutritional status assists in improving the condition, as does special attention to cleanliness. Sitz baths and local applications of saline compresses or steroid creams may be included in the treatment plan. Special attention is required to keep the incontinent patient clean and dry as much as possible. Sometimes alcohol is injected into the subcutaneous tissue of the perineum to provide relief.

Although pruritis is commonly associated with vulvitis, it may be a symptom of a *vulvar tumor*. Pain and irritation also may be associated with this problem. Any mass or lesion in this area should receive prompt attention and be biopsied. The clitoris is commonly the site of a vulvar malignancy. Cancer of the vulva may be manifested by large, painful, and foul-smelling fungating or ulcerating tumors. The adjacent tissues may also be affected. A radical vulvectomy is usually the treatment of choice and tends to be well tolerated by the aged female. Less commonly used is radiation therapy, which is not tolerated as well as surgery. Early treatment, prior to metastasis to inguinal lymph nodes, promotes a good prognosis.

Problems of the Vagina

Vaginitis. With advancing age, the vaginal epithelium thins, and this is accompanied by a loss of tissue elasticity. Secretions become alkaline and of lesser quantity. The flora changes, affecting the natural protection the vagina normally provides. These changes predispose the older female to the common infection, *senile vaginitis*. Soreness, pruritis, burning, and a reddened vagina are symptoms, and the accompanying vaginal discharge is clear, brown, or white. As it progresses, this vaginitis can cause bleeding and adhesions.

Local estrogens in suppository or cream form are usually effective in treating senile vaginitis. Nurses should make sure that patients understand the proper utilization of these topical medications and do not attempt to administer them orally. Acid douches may also be prescribed, and if the patient is to administer a douche at home, it is important to emphasize the need to measure the solution's temperature with a dairy thermometer. Altered receptors for hot and cold temperatures and reduced pain sensation in many aged persons predispose the patient to burns from solutions excessively hot for fragile vaginal tissue. Good hygienic practices are beneficial, not only in the treatment but also in the prevention of vaginitis.

Cancer of the vagina. Cancer of the vagina is rare in older females, resulting more frequently from metastasis than from the vaginal area as a primary site (Birnbaum, 1974). All vaginal ulcers and masses detected in aged females should be viewed with suspicion of malignancy and be biopsied. Since chronic irritation can predispose women to vaginal cancer, those who have chronic vaginitis and or who wear a pessary should obtain Pap smears frequently. Treatment is similar to that used for younger women and may consist of radiation or surgery, depending on the extent of the carcinoma.

Problems of the Cervix

With age, the cervix becomes smaller, and this is accompanied by an atrophy of the endocervical epithelium. Occasionally the endocervical glands can seal over, causing the formation of nabothian cysts. As secretions associated with these cysts accumulate, fever and a palpable tender mass may be evident. It is important, therefore, for the aged female to receive regular gynecologic examinations in which the patency of the cervix can be checked.

Cancer of the cervix. The incidence of cervical cancer decreases with age. Although most endocervical polyps are benign in older females, they should be viewed with suspicion until biopsy confirms a benign diagnosis. Vaginal bleeding and leukorrhea are signs of cervical cancer in aged females. Pain does not commonly occur. As the disease progresses, the patient can develop urinary retention or incontinence, fecal incontinence, and uremia. Treatment of cervical cancer can include radium or surgery.

Problems of the Uterus

The uterus decreases in size with age, becoming so small in some older women that it cannot be palpated on examination. It is important to note that the endometrium does continue to respond to hormonal stimulation.

Cancer of the endometrium. Cancer of the endometrium is not uncommon in the aged and is of higher incidence in obese, diabetic and hypertensive women. Any postmenopausal bleeding should give rise immediately to suspicion of this disease. Dilation and curettage usually are done to confirm the diagnosis since not all cases are detected through Pap smears alone. Treatment consists of surgery, radiation, or a combination of both. Early treatment can prevent metastasis to the vagina and cervix. Endometrial polyps can also cause bleeding and should receive serious attention since they could be indicative of early cancer.

Problems of the Fallopian Tubes and Ovaries

Although masses are occasionally detected in the fallopian tubes, they rarely present any significant problem to the aged female. The primary changes the fallopian tubes undergo with age are shortening, straightening, and atrophy. The ovaries also atrophy with age, becoming smaller and thicker. It is possible for them not to be palpable during the gynecologic examination, due to their decreased size. *Ovarian cancer* is occasionally diagnosed in the aged female. The clinical manifestations of this disease include bleeding, ascites, and the presence of multiple masses. Treatment may consist of surgery or radiation. Benign ovarian tumors commonly occur in the aged and surgery is usually required to differentiate them from malignant ones.

Perineal Herniation

As a result of the stretching and tearing of muscles during childbirth and of the muscle weakness associated with advanced age, perineal herniation is a common problem among older women. Cystocele, rectocele, and prolapse of the uterus are the types most likely to occur. Associated with this problem are lower back pain and pelvic heaviness and a pulling sensation, classic symptoms. Urinary and fecal incontinence, retention, and constipation may also occur. Sometimes the female is able to feel pressure or palpate a mass in her vagina. These herniations can make intercourse difficult and uncomfortable. Although rectoceles do not tend to worsen with age, the opposite is true for cystoceles, which will cause increased problems with time. Surgical repair is the treatment of choice and can be successful in relieving these problems. If surgery cannot be performed, the patient is usually fitted for a pessary, although this method is discouraged since the pessary can cause ulceration and infection.

Dyspareunia

Dyspareunia is a common problem among aged females but is not necessarily a normal consequence of aging. Nulliparous women experience this problem more frequently than women who have had children. Since vulvitis, vaginitis, and other gynecologic problems can contribute to dyspareunia, a thorough gynecologic examination is important, and any lesions or infections should be corrected to alleviate the problem. All effort should be made to help the aged female achieve a satisfactory sexual life. A more detailed discussion of sexual problems is offered in Chapter 23.

Breast Problems

The breasts atrophy with age, sagging more and hanging at a lower level. Some retraction of the nipples may occur as a result of shrinkage and fibrotic changes. Linear firm strands may develop on the breasts due to fibrosis and calcification of the terminal ducts.

Cancer of the breast. Due to the visual manifestations of decreased fat tissue and atrophy in aged women's breasts, it is not unusual for tumors, possibly present for many years, to become more evident. Since breast cancer is a leading cause of cancer deaths in aged as well as younger women, regular breast examinations should be encouraged. A more detailed explanation of breast examination is presented in Chapter 10. Diagnostic and treatment measures for women with breast cancer are the same at any age.

PROBLEMS OF THE MALE REPRODUCTIVE SYSTEM

Benign Prostatic Hypertrophy

A majority of aged men have some degree of benign prostatic hypertrophy (Howell, 1970; Jaffee, 1974c). Symptoms of this problem progress slowly but continuously; they include hesitancy, decreased force of urinary stream, frequency, and nocturia. As the condition progresses, dribbling, poor control, overflow incontinence, and bleeding may occur. Unfortunately, some men are reluctant or embarrassed to seek prompt medical attention and may develop kidney damage by the time symptoms are severe enough to motivate them to be evaluated.

Treatment can include prostatic massage and the use of urinary antiseptics. The most common prostatectomy approach used for aged men with prostatism is transurethral surgery. The patient should be reassured that this surgery will not cause impotence. On the other hand, realistic explanations are needed so that the patient understands that this surgery will not guarantee a sudden rejuvenation of sexual performance.

Cancer of the Prostate

Prostatic cancer is of increasing incidence with age. Although this disease can be asymptomatic, a majority of prostatic cancers can be detected by rectal examination—emphasizing the importance of regular physical examinations. Benign hypertrophy should be followed closely since it is thought to be associated with prostatic cancer, the symptoms of which can be similar (Hodkinson, 1975). In addition, symptoms such as back pain, anemia, weakness, and weight loss can develop as a result of metastasis. If metastasis has not occurred, treatment may consist of radiation or a radical prostatectomy; the latter procedure will result in impotency. Estrogens may be used to prevent tumor dissemination. Palliative treatment, employed if the cancer has metastasized, includes radiation, transurethral surgery, orchiectomy, and estrogens. General principles associated with these therapeutic measures are applicable to the aged patient. Many men are able to continue sexual performance after orchiectomy and during estrogen therapy; the physician should be consulted for specific advice concerning the expected outcomes for individual patients.

Tumors of the Penis, Testes, and Scrotum

Cancer of the penis is rare and tends to occur more frequently in men who have not been circumcised (Bowles, 1976b). It appears as a painless lesion or wartlike growth on the prepuce or glans. The resemblance of this growth to a chancre can cause a misdiagnosis or a reluctance on the part of the patient to seek treatment. A biopsy should be done of any penile lesion. Treatment may consist of radiation and local excision for small lesions and partial or total penile amputation for extensive lesions. Uncommon in the aged but usually malignant when they do occur are testicular tumors; testicular enlargement and pain and enlargement of the breasts are suspicious symptoms. Chemotherapy, radiation, and orchiectomy are among the treatment measures. Scrotal masses, usually benign, can be caused by conditions such as hydrocele, spermatocele, varicocele, and hernia. Symptoms and treatment depend on the underlying cause and are the same as for younger males.

NURSING CONSIDERATIONS

A basic nursing action for early detection of genitourinary problems is to encourage regular physical examinations for every aged person, including examination of the reproductive organs. Subtle clues of disturbances, such as nocturia and problems in sexual performance, should not be considered a result of aging without thorough medical evaluation. The nurse must understand that genitourinary problems may not be easy for geriatric patients to discuss; they require a great deal of sensitivity and respect from the nurse involved. Related to this is the need for respecting the dignity and privacy of the individual during urologic and gynecologic examinations. In overcoming patients' embarrassment at having others care for urinary drainage or perform treatments on their genitalia, a matter-of-fact but respectful approach and an understanding attitude on the part of the nurse are valuable assets. Exposure should be prevented, and this holds true for disoriented and unconscious patients as well. In addition, the nurse should be certain that ancillary staff and others working with aged patients demonstrate an understanding that few patients are intentionally incontinent, that few are not bothered or embarrassed by their incontinence, and that making an incident over it usually serves no therapeutic value and can be quite demeaning. A review of information regarding the genitourinary system is also useful for the aged patient. Some may believe that a particular sexual event caused their problem; others may believe that a urinary problem will alter their sexual performance. Realistic explanations help alleviate anxiety, fear, and guilt, and increased patient understanding can increase compliance. It is useful to include the spouse in such educational sessions.

REFERENCES

Birnbaum, S. J. "Geriatric Gynecology." In Chinn, A. B. (ed.), *Working with Older People*, Vol. IV. U.S. Dept. of Health, Education, and Welfare, 1974, p. 150.

Bowles, W. T. "Urologic Surgery." In Steinberg, F. U. (ed.), *Cowdry's, The Care of the Geriatric Patient*, 5th ed. Mosby, 1976. (a) p. 278; (b) p. 282.

Brocklehurst, J. C. "The Urinary Tract." In Rossman, I. (ed.), *Clinical Geriatrics*. Lippincott, Philadelphia, 1971. (a) p. 222; (b) p. 226.

Hodkinson, H. M. *An Outline of Geriatrics*. Academic Press, New York, 1975, p. 129.

Howell, T. H. *A Student's Guide to Geriatrics*. Staples, London, 1970, p. 173.

Jaffe, J. W. "Common Lower Urinary Tract Problems in Older Persons." In Chinn, A. B. (ed.), *Working with Older People*, Vol. IV. U.S. Dept. of Health, Education, and Welfare, 1974. (a) p. 144; (b) p. 141; (c) p. 142.

Kahn, A. I., and **Snapper, I.** "Medical Renal Diseases in the Aged." In Chinn, A. B. (ed.), *Working with Older People*, Vol. IV. U.S. Dept. of Health, Education, and Welfare, 1974. (a) p. 131; (b) p. 133.

17

NEUROLOGICAL PROBLEMS

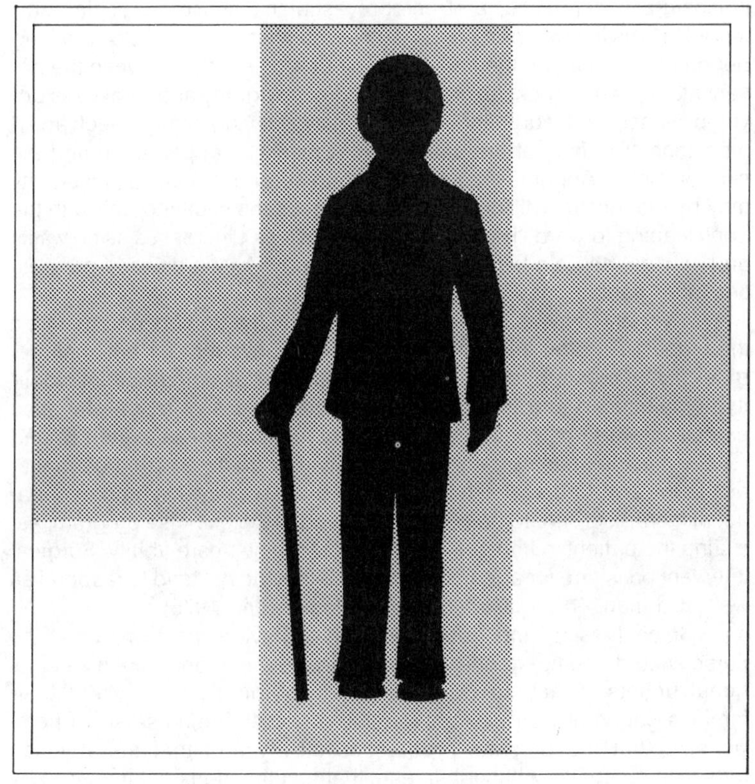

After age 25, there is a gradual but steady loss of neurons, manifested in various ways in each individual. Interestingly, the nervous system does not always demonstrate a correlation between the anatomic changes that occur as an individual ages and the signs and symptoms he or she manifests. Persons with reduced brain substances may be capable of unimpaired performance while those with severe limitations may have no alteration in brain substance. In addition to the aging process, the status of the circulatory system and nutritional factors can also affect neurologic functioning.

DISORDERS AND RELATED CARE PROCEDURES

Parkinson's Disease

Parkinson's disease affects the central nervous system's ability to control body movements. It is most common in males and occurs most frequently in the fifth decade of life. Although the exact cause is unknown, this disease is thought to be associated with a history of metallic poisoning, encephalitis, and cerebrovascular disease—especially arteriosclerosis in aged persons. A faint tremor that progresses over a long period of time may be the first clue. The tremor is reduced when the patient attempts a purposeful movement. Muscle rigidity and weakness develop, witnessed by drooling, difficulty in swallowing, slow speech and a monotone. The face of the patient has a masklike appearance and the skin is moist. Appetite frequently increases and emotional instability may be demonstrated. A characteristic sign is the shuffling gait with the trunk leaning forward. The rate of the patient's gait increases as he walks and may not be able to be stopped voluntarily. As the disease progresses, the patient may be unable to ambulate.

A variety of measures are used to control the tremors and maintain the highest possible level of independence. Levodopa or anticholinergics may be prescribed to decrease the patient's symptoms. Joint mobility is maintained and improved by active and passive range-of-motion exercises; warm baths and massage may facilitate these exercises and relieve muscle spasms caused by rigidity. Contractures are a particular risk to the aged person with Parkinson's disease. Physical and occupational therapists should be actively involved in the exercise program, assisting the patient to find devices that increase self-care ability. Surgical intervention is rare for aged patients since they do not tend to respond as well (Carman, 1968; Carter, 1971; Hodkinson, 1975).

Since tension and frustration will aggravate the symptoms, the nurse should attempt to offer psychological support and minimize emotional upsets. Teaching is beneficial in helping patients and their families gain a realistic insight into the disease. The nurse should emphasize that the disease progresses slowly and that therapy can minimize disability. Although intellectual functioning is not impaired by this disease, the speech problems and helpless appearance of patients may cause others to underestimate their mental ability; this can be extremely frustrating and degrading to the patient, who may react by becoming depressed or irritable. Continuing support by the nurse can help the family maximize the patient's mental capacity and understand personality changes that may occur. Communication and mental stimulation should be encouraged on a level which the patient always enjoyed. As the disease progresses, increased assistance is required by the patient. Skillful nursing assessment is essential to ensure that the demands for assistance are met while the maximum level of patient independence is preserved.

Transient Ischemic Attacks

Transient ischemic attacks, or temporary episodes of central nervous system dysfunction, can be caused by any situation which reduces cerebral circulation. Hyperextension and flexion of the head, such as that which occurs when an individual falls asleep in a chair, can impair cerebral blood flow. Reduced blood pressure resulting from anemia and certain drugs (diuretics and antihypertensives, for example) and cigarette smoking, due to its vasoconstrictive effect, will also decrease cerebral circulation. Hemiparesis, hemianesthesia, aphasia, unilateral loss of vision, diplopia, vertigo, nausea, vomiting, and dysphagia are among the signs which may be manifested with a transient ischemic attack, depending on the location of the ischemic area. These signs can last from minutes to hours, and complete recovery is usual within a day. Treatment may consist of correction of the underlying cause, anticoagulant therapy, or vascular reconstruction. A significant concern regarding transient ischemic attacks is that they increase the patient's risk of cerebral vascular accident.

Cerebral Vascular Accident

Aged persons with hypertension, severe arteriosclerosis, diabetes, gout, anemia, hypothyroidism, silent myocardial infarction, transient ischemic attacks, and dehydration are among the high risk candidates for a cerebral vascular accident, the third leading cause of death in the aged according to the U.S. Bureau of the Census, 1975. Although a ruptured cerebral blood vessel could be responsible for this problem, most cerebral vascular accidents in the aged are caused by partial or complete cerebral thrombosis. Lightheadedness, dizziness, headache, drop attack, and memory and behavioral changes are some of the warning signs of a cerebral vascular accident. A drop attack is a fall caused by a complete muscular flaccidity in the legs but with no alteration in consciousness (Agate, 1971). Patients describing or demonstrating these symptoms should be referred for prompt medical evaluation. Since the nurse is in a key position to learn of these signs, she can be instrumental in helping the patient avoid disability or death from a stroke.

Although the aged have a higher mortality from cerebral vascular accident than the young, those who do survive have a good chance of recovery. Good nursing care can improve the patient's chances of survival and minimize the limitations that impair a full recovery. In the acute phase, nursing efforts have several aims:

1. Maintaining a patent airway
2. Providing adequate nutrition and hydration
3. Monitoring neurologic and vital signs
4. Preventing complications associated with immobility

In addition, unconscious patients need good skin care and frequent turning since they are more susceptible to decubiti formation. If an indwelling catheter is not being utilized, it is important for the nurse to examine the patient for indications of an overdistended bladder and promptly remedy the situation if it should occur. The eyes of the unconscious patient may remain open for a long period of time, risking drying, irritation, and ulceration of the cornea. Corneal damage can be prevented by eye irrigations with a sterile saline solution followed by the use of eyedrops of sterile mineral oil. Eye pads may be used to aid in keeping the lids closed; these are changed daily and frequently checked to make sure the lids are actually closed. Regular mouth care and range-of-motion exercises are also standard measures.

When consciousness is regained and the patient's condition stabilizes, more active efforts can focus on rehabilitation. It may be extremely difficult for patients to understand and participate in their rehabilitation due to speech, behavior, and memory problems. Although these problems vary depending on what side of the brain is affected, some general observations can be noted. Retention span is reduced, and long, complicated directions may be confusing. Memory for old events may be intact, while recent events or explanations are forgotten (a characteristic demonstrated by many aged persons without a history of cerebral vascular accident). Patients may have difficulty transferring information from one situation to another. For example, they may be able to remember the steps in lifting from the bed to the wheelchair but be unable to apply the same principles in moving from the wheelchair to an armchair. Confusion, restlessness, and irritability may be present due to sensory deprivation. Emotional lability may also be a problem.

To minimize the limitations imposed by these problems, the nurse may find the following helpful:

1. Talk to the patient during routine care activities.

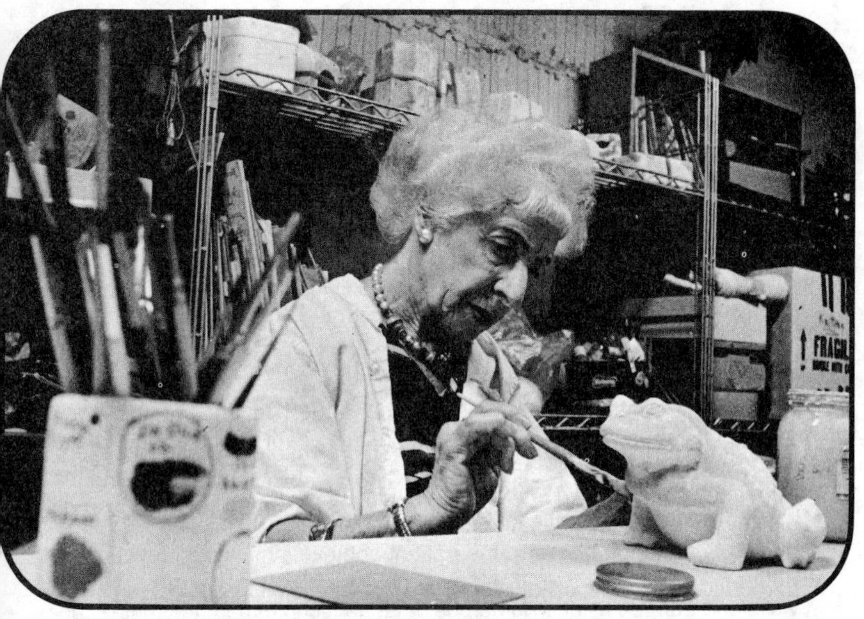

2. Explain in brief form the basics of what has occurred, the procedures being performed, and the activities to expect.
3. Speak distinctly but do not shout.
4. Devise an easy means of communication, such as a picture chart to which one can point.
5. Minimize environmental confusion, noise, and clutter.
6. Aim toward consistency—of those providing care and of the activities.
7. Use objects familiar to patients—their own clothing, clock, etc.
8. Keep a calendar and/or sign in the room showing the day and date.
9. Supply sensory stimulation through conversation, radio, television, wall decorations, and objects for patients to handle.
10. Provide frequent positive feedback; even a minor task may be a major achievement for the patient.
11. Expect and accept errors and failures.

The reader is advised to consult general medical-surgical textbooks for more detailed guidance in the care of patients with stroke. Local chapters of the American Heart Association also provide much useful material for the nurse, the patient, and the family on the topic of stroke.

Brain Tumors

Although brain tumors are not of high incidence in the aged, the resemblance of their symptoms to those commonly attributed to senility often results in delayed diagnoses. For instance, poor memory, confusion, personality change, headache, visual difficulties, poor coordination, and sensory-motor changes may be associated with arteriosclerosis or a multitude of other age-related problems. If these signs are not evaluated thoroughly in an early stage, valuable and potentially successful treatment time may be lost. It is important for the nurse to be aware of the general course of the patient's symptoms and facilitate their prompt evaluation.

NURSING CONSIDERATIONS

A few general statements can be added to the nursing considerations already presented throughout this chapter. The aged patient with a neurological problem may have a greater problem maintaining independence, not only due to the limitations imposed by the disease, but also as a result of those related to the aging process. Skillful and creative nursing assistance can help the patient achieve a maximum level of independence. Some of the self-help devices mentioned—rails in hallways and bathrooms and numerous other household modifications—can promote independent living in the individual's home environment. It is reassuring for the patient to know that assistance is available should the need arise. Periodic home visits by the nurse, regular contact with a family member or friend, and a daily call from a local telephone reassurance program can help the patient feel confident and protected, which also encourages independence. Although patients may perform tasks slowly and awkwardly, family members need to understand that allowing them to function independently is physically and psychologically more beneficial then doing the tasks for them. Continuing patience, reassurance, and encouragement are essential in maximizing the patient's capacity for independence.

Personality changes frequently accompany neurological problems. Patients may become depressed as the realization of their limitations is experienced or frustrated by their need to be dependent on others. Their reactions may be displaced and evidenced as irritability to others. Family members and those caring for the patient may need help in understanding the reasons for the patient's reactions and in learning ways to deal therapeutically with such behavior. Getting offended or angry at such patients may upset or frustrate them further. Understanding, patience, and tolerance are needed to accept any personality changes.

Protecting the patient from hazards is particularly important in nursing the neurologic patient. Uncoordinated movements, weakness, and dizziness are among the problems that cause these patients to have a high risk of accidents. Whether in an institutional setting or a home, the nurse should actively scrutinize the environment for potential sources of mishaps, such as loose carpeting, poorly lit stairwells, clutter, ill-functioning appliances, and for a lack of safeguards such as fire warning systems, fire escapes, and rails and a slip-proof surface in bathtubs. Safety considerations should also include prevention of contractures, decubiti, and other hazards to the structure and function of the body which neurologic patients are more prone to develop. It is an injustice to the patient for preventable complications to hamper progress and compound disability.

REFERENCES

Agate, J. "Common Symptoms and Complaints." In Rossman, I., *Clinical Geriatrics.* Lippincott, Philadelphia, 1971, p. 365.

Carman, J. B. "Anatomic Basis of Surgical Treatment of Parkinson's Disease." *New England Journal of Medicine,* 279:919, 1968.

Carter, A. B. "The Neurologic Aspects of Aging." In Rossman, I. (ed.), *Clinical Geriatrics.* Lippincott, Philadelphia, 1971, p. 138.

Hodkinson, H. M. *An Outline of Geriatrics.* Academic Press, New York, 1975, p. 123.

U.S. Bureau of the Census: *Statistical Abstract of the United States: 1975,* 96th ed., Washington, D.C., 1975, p. 61, No. 86.

18

DERMATOLOGICAL PROBLEMS

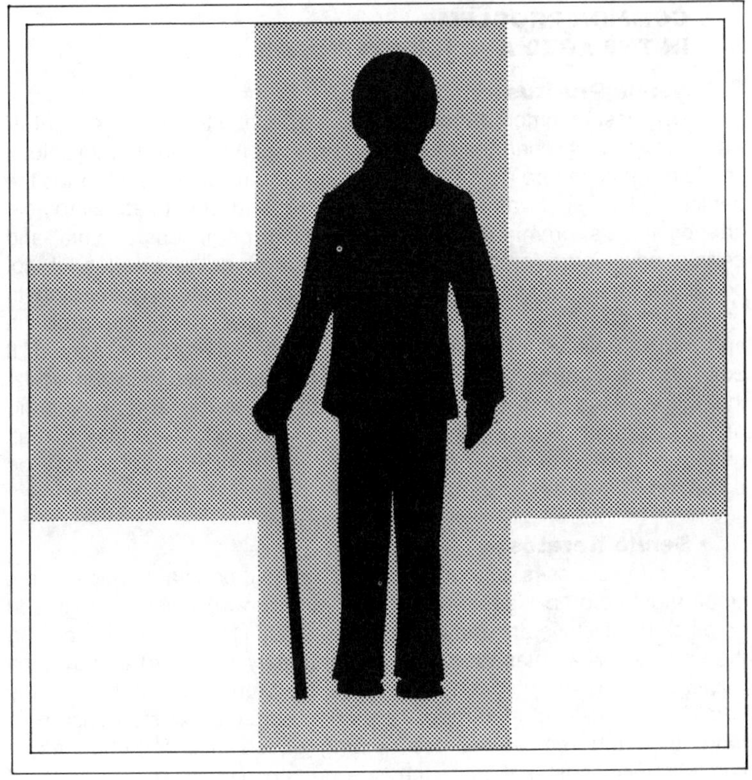

Perhaps the most obvious and most scorned effects of the aging process are those involving the integumentary system. Wrinkles, lines, and drooping eyelids gradually develop due to a loss of elasticity; the skin may appear a gray or pale yellow color; skin pigmentation occurs on hands and other frequently exposed areas; skin resistance is lessened as the skin becomes more dry and thin; the nails become dry and brittle, occasionally to the extent that they may peel. The rate of these changes varies according to the person's activity and to individual nutritional, emotional, biochemical, environmental, and genetic factors. Although the aged can experience the dermatological problems of any other age group, normal aging changes in the integumentary system, impaired circulation, and a generally greater susceptibility to infection contribute to dermatological problems in the older adult. These disorders can also result from irritation, poor hygiene, dietary deficiencies, stress, allergic reactions, and certain diseases.

COMMON PROBLEMS IN THE AGED AND RELATED CARE

Senile Pruritus

The most common dermatological problem in the aged is pruritus. Although atrophic changes alone may be responsible for this problem, senile pruritus can be precipitated by any circumstance which dries the person's skin, such as excessive bathing and dry heat. Diabetes, arteriosclerosis, uremia, liver disease, cancer, pernicious anemia, and certain psychiatric problems can also contribute to pruritus. If not corrected, the itching may cause traumatizing scratching, leading to breakage and infection of the skin. Prompt recognition of this problem and implementation of corrective measures are therefore essential. If possible, the underlying cause should be corrected. Bath oils, moisturizing lotions, and massage are beneficial in treating and preventing pruritus. Vitamin supplements may be recommended, as may a high quality, vitamin-rich diet. Antihistamines and topical steroids may be prescribed for relief.

Senile Keratoses

Senile keratoses, also referred to as actinic or solar keratoses, are small, light-colored lesions (usually gray or brown) found on exposed areas of the skin. Keratin may be accumulated in these lesions, causing the formation of a cutaneous horn with a slightly reddened and swollen base. Freezing agents and acids can be employed to destroy the keratotic lesions, but electrodesiccation or surgical excision ensures a more thorough removal. Close nursing observation for changes in keratotic lesions is vital since they are precancerous.

Seborrheic Keratoses

It is not uncommon for aged persons to have several dark, wartlike projections on various parts of their bodies. These lesions, called seborrheic keratoses, may be as small as a pinhead or as large as a quarter. They tend to increase in size and number with age. In the sebaceous areas of the trunk, face, and neck and in persons with oily skin, these lesions appear dark and oily; in less sebaceous areas they are dry in appearance and of a light color. Normally, seborrheic keratoses will not have swelling or redness around their base. Sometimes abrasive activity with a gauze pad containing oil will remove small seborrheic keratoses. Larger, raised lesions can be removed by freezing agents or by a currettage and cauterization procedure. Although these lesions are benign, medical evaluation is important in order to differentiate them from precancerous lesions. In addition, the cosmetic benefit of removing them should not be overlooked for the aged patient.

Stasis Dermatitis

Poor venous return can cause edema of the lower extremities, which leads to poor tissue nutrition. As the poorly nourished legs accumulate debris, inadequately carried away with the venous return, the legs gain a pigmented, cracked, and exudative appearance. Subsequent scratching, irritation, or other trauma can then easily result in the formation of a leg ulcer. Stasis ulcers need special attention to facilitate healing. Infection must be controlled, and necrotic tissue removed, before healing will take place. Good nutrition is an important component of the therapy, and a diet high in vitamins and protein is recommended. Once healing has occurred, concern should be given to avoiding situations that promote stasis dermatitis. The patient may need instruction regarding a diet for weight reduction or the planning of high-quality meals. Venous return can be enhanced by elevating the legs several times a day and by preventing interferences to circulation such as standing for long periods of time, sitting with legs crossed, and wearing garters. Some patients may require ligation and stripping of the veins to prevent further episodes of stasis dermatitis.

Decubitus Ulcers

Tissue anoxia and ischemia resulting from pressure can cause the necrosis, sloughing, and ulceration of tissue commonly known as a decubitus ulcer. Any part of the body can develop a decubitus ulcer, but the most common sites are the sacrum, greater trochanter, and ischial tuberosities. The aged are high risk candidates for several reasons:

1. Their skin is more fragile and is damaged more easily.
2. They often are in a poor nutritional state.

3. They have reduced sensation of pressure and pain.
4. They are more frequently affected by immobile and edematous conditions, which contribute to skin breakdown.

Prevention. In addition to developing more easily in the aged, decubitus ulcers require a longer period to heal in older persons. As mentioned earlier, it has been estimated that wounds taking 31 days to heal in a 20-year-old, take 55 days in a 40-year-old and 100 days in a 60-year-old (Manney, 1975). Therefore, the most important nursing measure is to prevent their formation, and to do this, it is essential to prevent pressure. Encouraging activity or turning the patient who can't move independently at least every two hours is necessary. Shearing forces which cause two layers of tissue to move across each other should be prevented by not elevating the head of the bed more than 30 degrees, by not allowing patients to slide in bed, and by lifting instead of pulling patients when moving them. Pillows, flotation pads, alternating pressure mattresses, and water beds can be used to disperse pressure from bony prominences. It must be emphasized that these devices do not eliminate the need for frequent position changes. While sitting in a chair, patients should be urged and assisted with shifting their weight at certain intervals. Lamb's wool and heel protectors are useful in preventing irritation to bony prominences. Sheets should be kept wrinkle free and the bed should be checked frequently for foreign objects such as syringes and utensils which the patient may be lying on unknowingly.

A high-protein, vitamin-rich diet to maintain and improve tissue health is essential in avoiding decubitus ulcer formation. Good skin care is another essential ingredient in decubiti prevention. Skin should be kept clean and dry, and blotting the patient dry will avoid irritation from rubbing the skin with a towel. Bath oils and lotions, used prophylactically, will help keep the skin soft and intact. Massage of bony prominences and range-of-motion exercises promote circulation and assist in keeping the tissue well nourished. The incontinent patient should be thoroughly cleansed with soap and water and dried after each episode to avoid skin breakdown from irritating excreta.

Techniques to treat decubiti. Special nursing attention is warranted to promote healing and prevent complications. A variety of techniques are employed in treating the ulcer, including the topical application of granulated sugar, Karaya, antacids, chemical debriding agents, and wet to dry dressings. Cleansing of the ulcer and debriding of necrotic tissue are required for the regeneration of epithelium. Gentle massage to the tissue around the decubitus ulcer will promote circulation and decrease edema. Topical antibiotics may be used to control infection. The nursing measures discussed above regarding decubiti prevention will also benefit the patient who has developed an ulcer. For severe ulcers, surgery may be required. The various techniques used to treat decutiti are described below. More detail regarding these procedures can be obtained by exploring some of the literature cited in the bibliography.

Chemical debriding: Elase (a fibrinolytic enzyme) or Santyl (a collagenase) can be applied to a cleansed wound and dressed with a dry bandage or gauze. Specific instructions and frequency vary according to the agent. These agents facilitate the removal of necrotic tissue, allowing granulation and epithelization of tissue to occur.

Gelfoam with flotation therapy: The compressed or powder form of Gelfoam is implanted in the tissue of a clean wound to promote the growth of new cells. The dressing is left undisturbed for from three to seven days; tissue granulation is better when the dressing is allowed to remain in place longer. A nonpurulent discharge may occur, but it is no cause for alarm. Flotation pads are used to displace weight.

Insulin: After cleansing and irrigation of the wound, ten units of U-40 regular insulin are dropped on the wound. The ulcer is then exposed to air to dry, with no dressing applied. This procedure is performed twice daily.

Karaya: After cleansing the wound with pHisohex and irrigation with a hydrogen peroxide solution, the edges of the wound are massaged. A Karaya ring is then fitted around the wound and Karaya powder sprinkled directly into the wound. Reston is sometimes used to relieve pressure on the wound. A piece of plastic wrap is attached to the Reston to cover the wound while allowing view of it. This window is changed and additional powder added every eight hours.

Maalox or sugar: After cleansing and irrigation of the wound, Maalox or sugar is applied to promote granulation. Irrigation and reapplication of the substance is repeated every eight hours.

Surgical debriding: Necrotic tissue can be removed surgically to promote faster debridment and new tissue growth.

Wet to dry dressings: Following cleansing of the ulcer, gauze dressing soaked in normal saline or other prescribed solutions is placed on the wound for from six to eight hours (or as specified) and allowed to dry. Some debridment occurs as the dry dressing is removed.

General measures: Techniques to treat decubiti including the following general procedures: (1) frequent turning to prevent reduced circulation from blocked capillaries; (2) the use of flotation pads, alternating pressure matresses, water beds, and heel protectors to displace body weight; (3) the use of sheepskin to prevent irritation to the skin and to promote evaporation of skin moisture; (4) using a turn sheet to allow greater weight distribution when lifting or turning the patient and to prevent friction to the skin during these activities; (5) providing a high-protein, high-vitamin diet to promote a positive nitrogen balance and tissue growth.

NURSING CONSIDERATIONS

Some general measures are employed to prevent and manage dermatological problems in the aged. It is important to avoid drying agents, rough clothing, highly starched linens, and other items irritating to the skin. Good skin nutrition and hydration can be promoted by activity, bath oils, lotions, and massages. Although skin cleanliness is important, excessive bathing may be hazardous to the skin; daily partial sponge baths and complete baths every third or fourth day are sufficient for the average aged person. Early attention to and treatment of pruritus and skin lesions is advisable in preventing irritation, infection, and other problems.

Psychological support can be especially important to the patient with a dermatological problem. Unlike respiratory, cardiac, and other disorders, dermatological problems are often visibly unpleasant—to the patient and others. Visitors and staff may unnecessarily avoid touching and being with the patient in reaction to the skin problems they see. The nurse can reassure visitors regarding the safety of contact with the patient and provide instruction for any special precautions that must be followed. The most important fact to emphasize is that the patient is still normal, with normal needs and feelings, and will appreciate normal interactions and contact.

All persons should be encouraged to look their best and make the most of their appearance. However, efforts to avoid the normal outcomes of the aging process are for the most part fruitless and frustrating. Money which could be applied to more basic needs is sometimes invested on attempts to defy reality. The nurse should emphasize to persons young and old that no cream, lotion, or miracle drug will remove wrinkles and lines or return youthful skin. While clarifying misconceptions regarding rejuvenating products, the nurse can encourage cosmetic use for the purpose of protecting the skin and maintaining an attractive appearance—from which many benefits may be derived. Perhaps, as society achieves a greater acceptance and understanding of the aging process, cosmetic use will be replaced by an appreciation for the natural beauty of age.

REFERENCE

Manney, J. R. *Aging in American Society.* Univ. of Michigan Press, Wayne State University, Ann Arbor, Mich., 1975, p. 27.

19

SENSORY DEFICITS

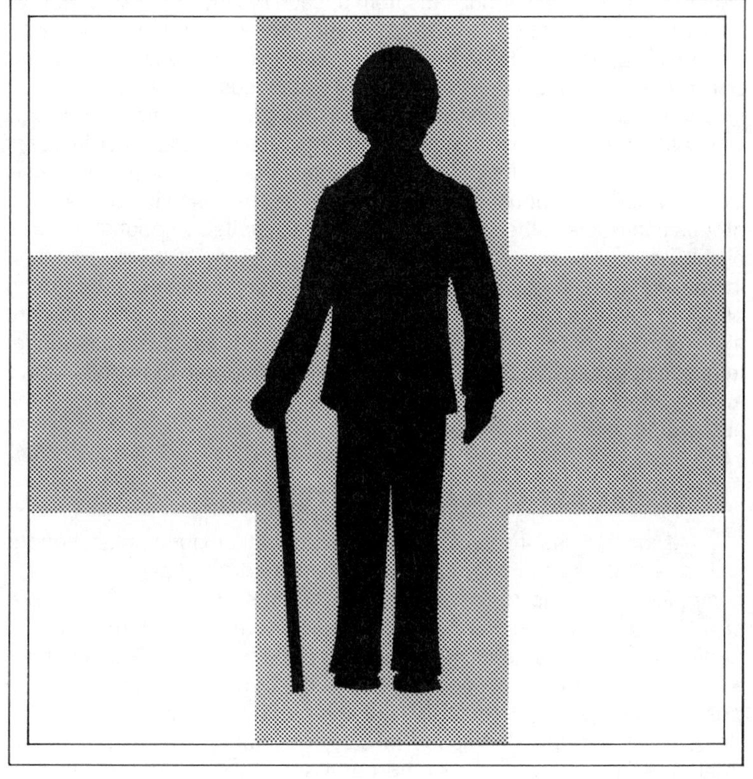

Good sensory function is an extremely valuable asset, one which is often taken for granted. Intact senses facilitate accurate perception of the environment. People are better able to protect themselves from harm when they can see, hear, smell, touch, and verbalize danger; and the beauties of the earth are more fully appreciated when the senses are functioning at their optimum level. In addition, communication, the sharing of experiences, and the exchange of feelings are more complete when all the senses can participate. Imagine with what distortion the environment is perceived when sensory function is impaired. People might suspect they are being talked about if they are unable to hear the conversation of those around them. Common everyday experiences, such as reading the newspaper and recognizing a familiar face on the street, can be hampered by poor eyesight. Food tastes bland without properly functioning taste buds; and freshly cut flowers lose their fragrances to poor olfactory functioning.

The reduced ability to protect oneself from hazards due to sensory deficits can result in serious falls from unseen obstacles; missed alarms and warnings; ingestion of hazardous substances from not recognizing their taste; an inability to detect the odor of smoke or gas; and burns and skin breakdown because of decreased cutaneous sensation of excessive temperature and pressure. And as though the multiple problems which affect the elderly aren't enough, they are also the most frequent victims of these sensory deficits. Alterations during the aging process, excessive use and abuse, and the disease processes that affect all age groups contribute to their problems. Sensory deficits compound the other problems which threaten the health and well-being of the aged—their increased vulnerability to accidents, their social isolation and declining physical function, and their many other limitations regarding self-care activities. Since it is the rare older individual who does not also suffer from sensory deficit, it behooves the nurse working with the aged to have a sound knowledge of the sensory problems affecting them and of the associated assistive techniques.

VISUAL DEFICITS AND RELATED CARE

As the eye undergoes a variety of structural and functional changes with age, the lids become thinner and wrinkled, displaying skin folds commonly known as "bags" (Figure 19-1). Ptosis, inversion, and eversion of the lid are common. The conjunctiva, easily irritated by dust particles and air pollutants, is thinner and more fragile. The cornea gains a smoky appearance, being less translucent and more spherical. Deposits of fat over the cornea and grayish plaques on the sclera may be detected. The pupil decreases in size, becoming less responsive to light, and there is sclerosis of the pupil sphincter. Peripheral vision is

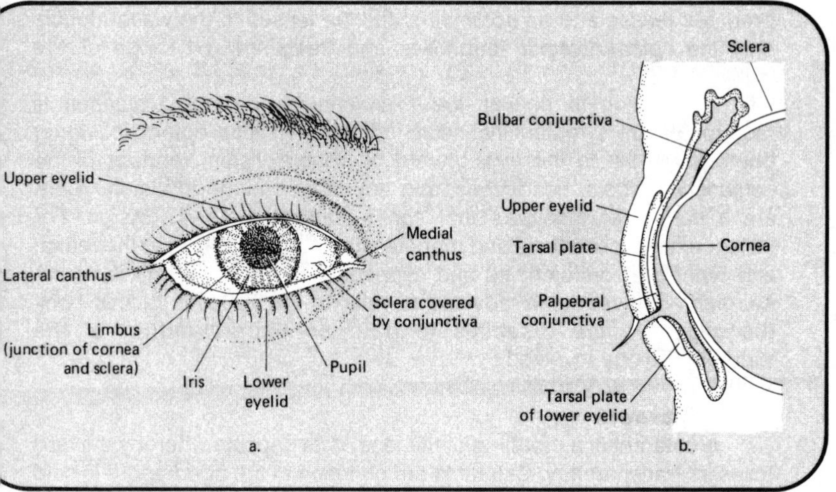

Figure 19-1. Gross anatomy of the eye. (a) Anterior view. (b) Cross-sectional view. (Source: Barbara Bates. *A Guide to Physical Examination,* Lippincott. Philadelphia. 1974.)

more difficult as the visual field narrows, and vision at night and in dimly lit areas is a greater problem due to the increase in the threshold of light perception. Yellowing of the lens makes vision for low-tone colors (blues and greens) more difficult. Visual acuity is reduced, and there is a slower adaptation to dark. Defective accommodation due to loss of elasticity in the lens of the eye (presbyopia) is common. The eyes have slower responses, fewer secretions, and a lower tissue resistance, predisposing the aged person to eye irritation and trauma. There may be a liquefaction of vitreous humor, accompanied by the release of supporting tissue, and cholesterol crystals may develop, causing bothersome but harmless spots before the aged individual's eyes.

In spite of these changes, a majority of older persons have sufficient visual capacity to meet normal self-care demands with the assistance of corrective lenses. Serious visual problems can develop, however, and should be recognized early to prevent significant visual damage. Routine eye examinations by an *ophthalmologist* are important in detecting and treating eye problems early. Frequently, people postpone eye examinations because their present corrective lenses are still functional or because there seems to be no apparent need or because they have limited finances. The gerontological nurse can be instrumental in ensuring appropriate visual care by emphasizing that beyond the need for corrective lenses, eye examinations are important in detecting other problems. It is important to inform people that while an *optician* prepares lenses and an *optometrist* fits the lenses to the visual deficit, only the *opthalmologist* diagnoses and treats the full range of eye diseases.

In addition to annual eye examinations, prompt evaluation is required for any symptom that could indicate a visual problem, including burning or pain in the eye, blurred or double vision, redness of the conjunctiva, spots, headaches, and any other change in vision. There are a variety of disorders that can threaten the aged's vision. For instance, arteriosclerosis and diabetes can cause damage to the retina, and nutritional deficiencies and hypertension can result in visual impairment. The reader is advised to refer to the sections of this book discussing these diseases to gain an understanding of the pathophysiology involved.

Cataracts

A cataract is a clouding of the lens or its capsule whereby the lens loses its transparency. Cataracts are common in the aged and it is said that everyone would develop cataracts if they lived long enough. Most aged persons do have some degree of lens opacity with or without the presence of other eye disorders. There is no discomfort or pain associated with cataracts. At first, vision is distorted and objects appear blurred. The opacification continues, and eventually there is complete lens opacity and complete loss of vision. Glare from sunlight and bright lights is extremely bothersome to the affected person. Nuclear sclerosis develops; with this the lens of the eye becomes yellow or yellow-brown, and eventually the color of the pupil changes from black to a cloudy white.

Surgery to remove the lens is the only cure for a cataract. Patients with a single cataract may not necessarily undergo surgery if vision in the other eye is good, and these individuals should concentrate on strengthening their existing visual capacity, reducing their limitations, and employing the safety measures applicable to any visually impaired person (Figure 19-2). Sunglasses, sheer curtains over windows, furniture placed away from bright light, and several soft lights instead of a single

Figure 19-2. Compensating for visual deficits in the aged: (a) Face person when speaking. (b) Use several soft indirect lights instead of a single glaring one. (c) Avoid glare from windows by using sheer curtains or stained windows. (d) Use large-print reading material. (e) Have frequently used items within visual field. (f) Avoid use of low-tone colors and attempt to use bright ones. (g) Use contrasting colors on doorways, stairs, and for changes in levels. (h) Identify personal belongings and differentiate room and wheelchair with a unique design rather than by letters or numbers.

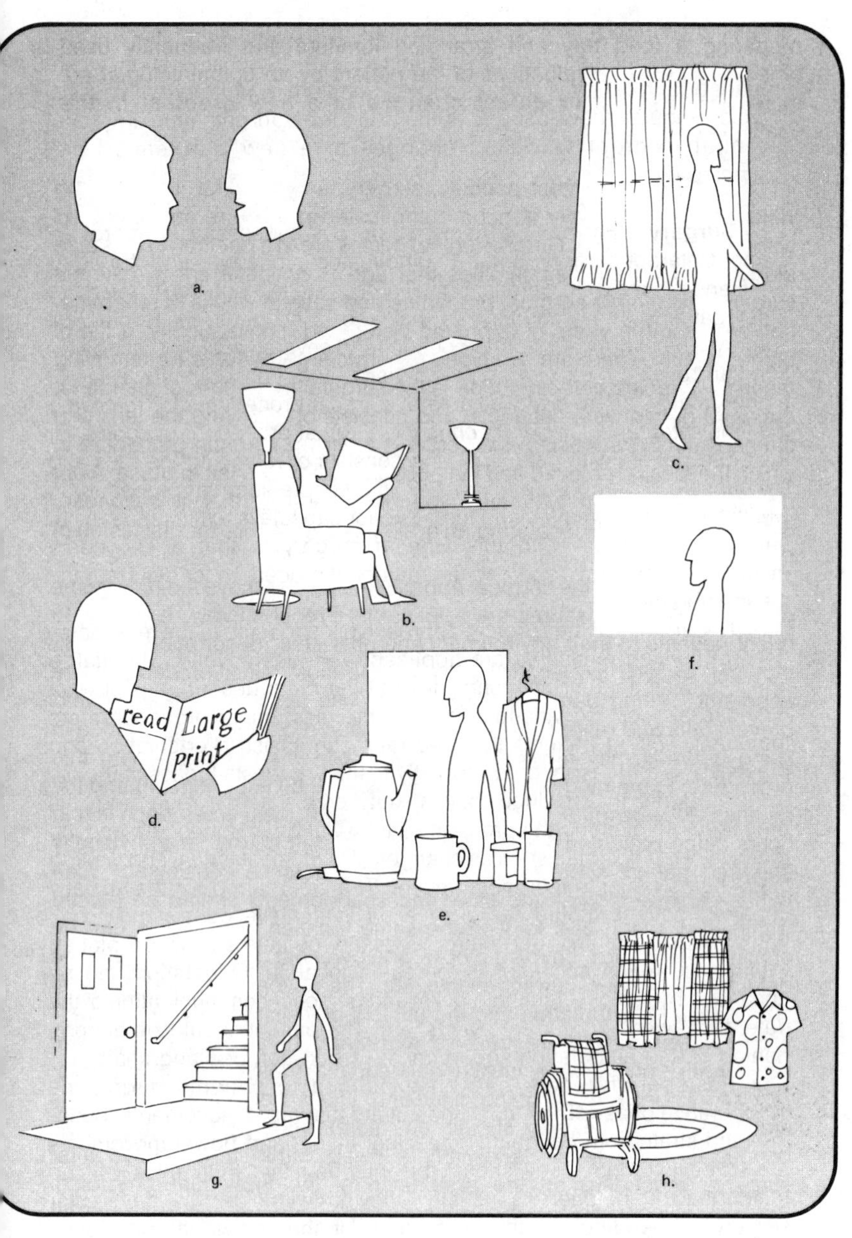
a.
c.
b.
f.
read
Large
print
d.
e.
g.
h.

bright light minimize annoyance from glare. It is beneficial to place items within the visual field of the unaffected eye, a consideration when preparing a food tray and arranging furniture and frequently used objects. Regular reevaluations of the patient by an opthalmologist are essential in order to detect changes or a new problem in the unaffected eye.

Surgery. For most patients, surgery is successful in improving vision. Cataract surgery is not a complicated procedure and the aged withstand it quite well. Gerontological nurses are in a position to reassure older patients and their families that age is no deterrent to cataract surgery. The simple surgical procedure and several weeks of rehabilitation can result in years of improved vision and, consequently, a life of higher quality. There are two types of surgical procedures for removing the lens. *Intracapsular extraction* is the surgical procedure of choice for the aged patient with cataracts, and consists of removing the lens and the capsule. *Extracapsular extraction* is a simple surgical procedure in which the lens is removed and the posterior capsule is left in place. A not uncommon problem with this type of surgery is that a secondary membrane may form, requiring an additional procedure for discission of the membrane.

Regardless of the surgical approach used to remove the lens, some general nursing measures are applicable. Preoperatively, it is vital to orient patients to their environment and offer clear descriptions of what they can expect. Explanations of even the most minor procedures are important. Telling patients that bed rails can assist in orientation and prevent falls and responding promptly to their requests for assistance in using bedrails may reduce their anxiety or resistance regarding this procedure. Explaining the procedures they will be experiencing and the routines of the hospital, such as changes of shift, meal times, and visiting hours helps patients feel more secure. The staff caring for the visually impaired patient should make an effort to achieve consistency. Call lights, bedside tables, and other necessary objects should be placed within easy reach and kept in the same location. Orientation can be enhanced by radios, chiming clocks, and personal communication of the date, time, weather, current events, etc. The patient should be accompanied during ambulation and in transfers between bed and chair.

Postoperative care can be explained to patients during the preoperative phase. They must understand that rapid movements, bending, and strain from coughing, sneezing, lifting, and bowel movements are to be avoided. They should be informed that their eyes will be bandaged. Ambulation is usually allowed within a few days after surgery, depending on the preference of the individual physician. Because of poor vision and weakness, assistance is necessary for all

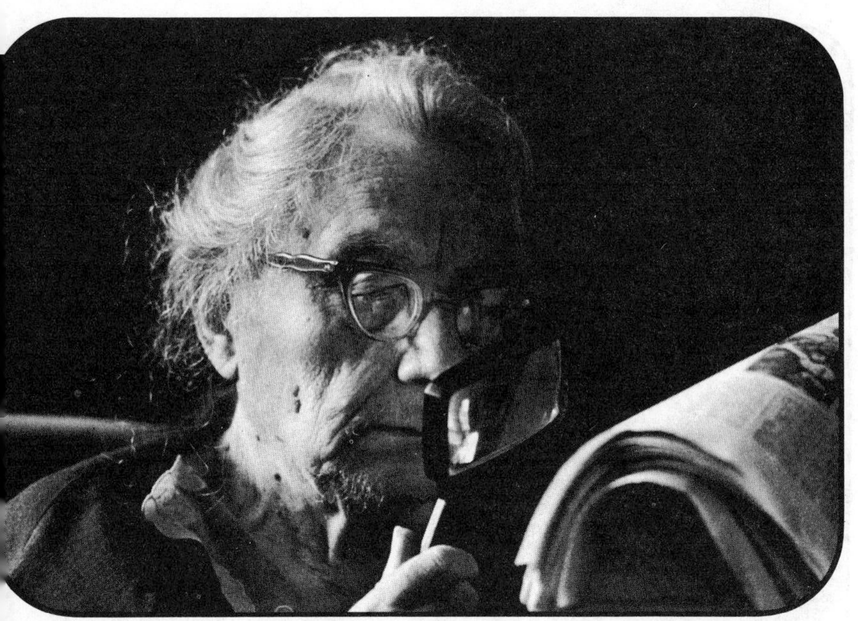

activities performed out of bed. While minimal pain is usually controlled by analgesics, severe pain indicates a complication requiring the immediate attention of the surgeon. After several weeks, the patient will receive temporary corrective lenses. A true adjustment to these requires time and practice. Permanent lenses are usually prescribed two months after surgery. Contact lenses are being used increasingly for patients who have had cataract surgery. Some patients are unable to use them but those who can tend to make a more rapid adjustment to their new vision.

Glaucoma

Glaucoma ranks after cataracts as a major eye problem in the aged, tending to have a high incidence between the ages of 40 and 65 and declining in incidence in old age. Ten percent of all blindness in the United States is a result of glaucoma. Although the exact cause is unknown, glaucoma can be associated with an increased size of the lens and with iritis, allergy, endocrine imbalance, emotional instability, and a family history of this disorder. An increase in intraocular pressure occurs rapidly in acute glaucoma and gradually in chronic glaucoma.

Acute glaucoma. With acute glaucoma, the patient experiences severe eye pain, nausea, and vomiting. In addition to the increased

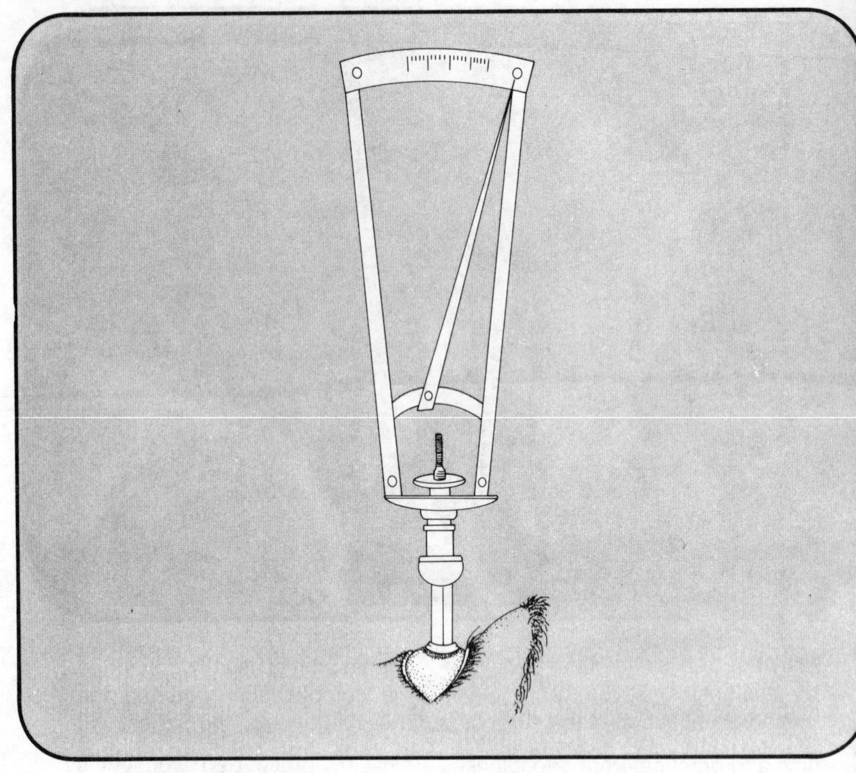

Figure 19-3. Measuring intraocular pressure by use of a tonometer.

tension within the eyeball, there is edema of the ciliary body and dilation of the pupil. Vision becomes blurred, and blindness will result if this problem is not corrected within a day. Diagnosis is confirmed by placing a tonometer on the anesthetized cornea to measure the intraocular pressure (Figure 19-3). The normal pressure is within 20 mmHg. A reading of from 20 to 25 mmHg is considered potential glaucoma. Another diagnostic test (gonioscopy) uses a contact lens and a binocular microscope to allow direct examination of the anterior chamber and differentiate angle-closure from open-angle glaucoma. In the past, if intraocular pressure did not decline within 24 hours, there would be surgical intervention. However, medications are now effective in treating the acute attack: carbonic anhydrase inhibitors, which reduce the formation of aqueous solution; and mannitol, urea, or glycerin, which reduce fluid due to their ability to increase osmotic tension in the circulating blood. An iridectomy may be performed after the acute attack to prevent future episodes of acute glaucoma.

Chronic glaucoma. Chronic glaucoma is the more common type. It often occurs so gradually that affected individuals are unaware that they have a visual problem. Peripheral vision becomes increasingly impaired so slowly that people may not realize for a long time why they bump or knock over items at their side. As the impairment progresses, central vision is affected. People may complain of a tired feeling in their eyes or of headaches or misty vision or of seeing halos around lights—symptoms which tend to be more pronounced in the morning. The cornea may have a cloudy appearance and the iris may be fixed and dilated. Although this condition usually involves one eye, both eyes can become affected if treatment is not sought. The same diagnostic procedures as mentioned with acute glaucoma are used to determine this problem. Treatment, aimed toward reducing the intraocular pressure, may consist of a combination of a miotic and a carbonic anhydrous inhibitor or of surgery to establish a channel to filter the aqueous fluid (e.g., iridectomy, iridencleisis, cyclodialysis, and corneoscleral trephining.)

Care and prevention. The vision lost due to glaucoma is not able to be restored. However, additional damage can be prevented by avoiding any situation or activity which increases intraocular pressure. Physical straining should be prevented, as should emotional stress. Mydriatics, stimulants, and agents which elevate the blood pressure must not be administered. It may benefit patients to carry a card or wear a bracelet indicating their problem to prevent administration of these medications in situations where they may be unconscious or otherwise unable to communicate. Abuse and overuse of the eyes must also be prevented. Periodic evaluation by an ophthalmologist is an essential part of the continued care of the patient with glaucoma.

Detached Retina

The aged may experience detachment of the retina, a forward displacement of the retina from its normal position against the choroid. The symptoms, which can be gradual or sudden, include the perception of spots moving across the eye, blurred vision, flashes of light, and the feeling that a coating is developing over the eye. There are blank areas of vision, progressing to complete loss of vision. The severity of the symptoms depends on the degree of retinal detachment. Prompt treatment is required to prevent continued damage and eventual blindness. Initial measures most likely to be prescribed are bedrest and the use of bilateral eye patches. The latter can be most frightening to the aged patient, who may react with confusion and unusual behavior. The patient should be made to feel as secure as possible; frequent checks and communication, easy access to a call light or other means of assistance, and full, honest explanations will help provide a sense of well-being. After time has been allowed for the maximum amount of "reattachment" of the retina to occur, surgery may be planned.

Several surgical techniques are used in the treatment of detached retina. Electrodiathermy and cyrosurgery cause the retina to adhere to its original attachment; scleral buckling and photocoagulation decrease the size of the vitreous space. Eye patches remain on the patient for several days after surgery. Specific routines vary according to the type of surgery performed. The patient needs frequent verbal stimuli to minimize anxiety and enhance psychological comfort. Physical and emotional stress must be avoided. Approximately two weeks after surgery, the success of the operation can be evaluated. A minority of patients must undergo a second surgery. It is important for the patient to understand that periodic examination is important, especially since some patients later suffer a detached retina in the other eye.

Corneal Ulcers

Inflammation of the cornea, accompanied by a loss of substance, causes the development of a corneal ulcer. Febrile states, irritation, dietary deficiencies, lowered resistance, and cerebral vascular accident tend to predispose the individual to this problem. Corneal ulcers, which are extremely difficult to treat in the aged, may scar or perforate, leading to destruction of the cornea and blindness. This problem is responsible for 10 percent of all blindness. The affected eye may appear bloodshot on inspection and show increased lacrimation. Pain and photophobia are also present. Nurses should advise clients to seek assistance promptly for any irritation, suspected infection, or other difficulty with the cornea as soon as it is identified. Early care is often effective in preventing the development of a corneal ulcer and preserving visual capacity. Cycloplegics, sedatives, antibiotics, and heat may be prescribed to treat a corneal ulcer. Sunglasses will ease the discomfort associated with photophobia. It is important that the underlying cause be treated—be it an infection, abrasion, or presence of a foreign body. Corneal transplants are occasionally done for more advanced corneal ulcers.

HEARING DEFICITS

Hearing deficits can result from changes to the ear which occur with aging (Figure 19-4). The external ear does not undergo significant change, although cerumen secretion is somewhat altered. Cerumen,

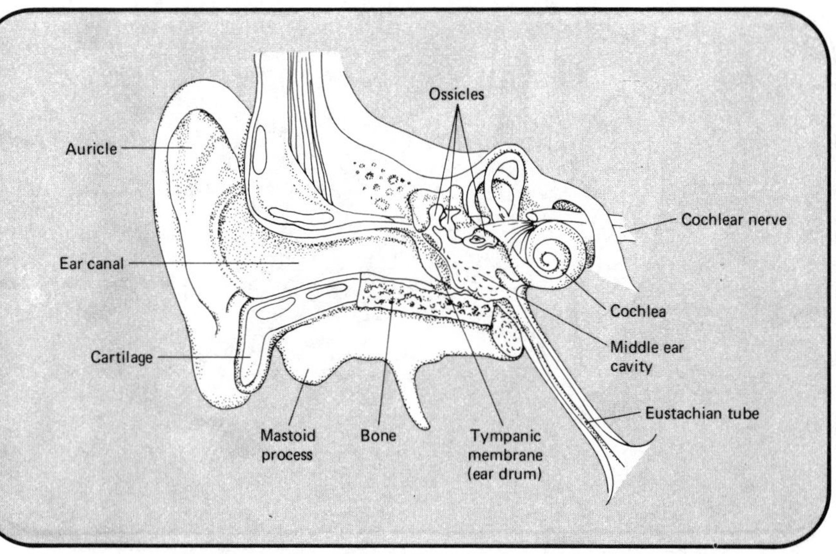

Figure 19-4. Anatomy of the ear. (Source: Barbara Bates, *A Guide to Physical Examination*, Lippincott, Philadelphia, 1974.)

secreted in lesser amounts, contains a greater amount of keratin in the aged which makes it harder and easily impacted. The middle ear may experience atrophy or sclerosis of the tympanic membrane. The inner ear and retrocochlear lose their efficiency, and there is a degeneration of the cells at the base of the cochlea. The changes affecting the inner ear are demonstrated first by a loss in the ability to hear high-frequency sounds; this is followed by a loss of middle and then low frequencies as well. *Presbycusis* is the commonly used term to describe this progressive hearing loss associated with aging.

Causes and Types of Deficits

Most aged have some degree of hearing loss, resulting from a variety of factors aside from aging. Exposure to noise, such as that of jets, traffic, and guns cause cell injury and loss. (The higher incidence of hearing loss in men may be associated with the fact that they are more often employed in occupations which subject them to loud noises, e.g., truck driving, construction, and heavy factory work.) Recurrent otitis media can damage hearing, as can trauma to the ear. Certain drugs may be ototoxic, including aspirin, streptomycin, neomycin, and karomycin; the delayed excretion of these drugs in many older persons may promote this effect. Diabetes, tumors of the nasopharynx, other disease pro-

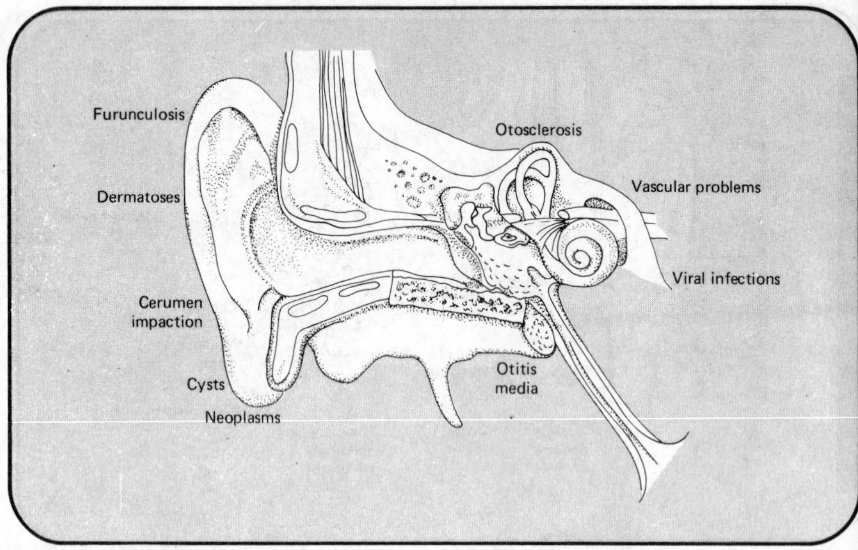

Figure 19-5. Problems affecting the ears of aged people.

cesses, and psychogenic factors can also contribute to hearing impairment.

There are particular problems which affect the aged ear (Figure 19-5). Vascular problems, viral infections and, as mentioned, presbycusis are often causes of inner ear damage. In otosclerosis an osseous growth causes fixation of the footplate of the stapes in the oval window of the cochlea. This may be a middle ear problem; it is a disorder, more common among women, that can progress to complete deafness. Middle ear infections are less common in older individuals; they usually accompany more serious disorders, such as tumors and diabetes. The external ear can be affected by dermatoses, furunculosis, cerumen impaction, cysts, and neoplasms.

The diagram below briefly outlines the normal transmission of sound through the ear. Interference with the transmission of the physical sound waves causes *conduction deafness*. Conduction deafness may be due to an easily correctable problem, such as infection or cerumen accumulation. *Perception deafness* is the term used to describe a problem with the nerve endings registering the electrical signals. Degeneration of the auditory nerve with age may be a factor in this form of deafness. The aged may have both conduction and perception deafness.

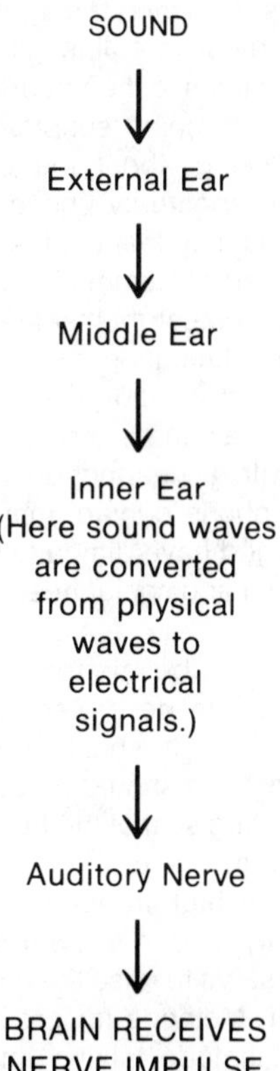

Methods of Care

The first measure to employ in caring for someone with a hearing deficit is to encourage audiometric examination. Hearing impairment should not be assumed a normal consequence of aging and ignored. It would be most sad and negligent if the cause of the hearing problem was easily correctable (e.g., removal of cerumen or a cyst) but was allowed to unnecessarily limit the life of the affected individual. The aged should be advised not to purchase a hearing aid without a complete audiometric evaluation. Many older persons invest money for a hearing aid from their limited budget just to discover that their particular hearing deficit can't be improved by this means.

Sometimes the underlying cause of the hearing problem can be corrected. Frequently, however, the aged must learn to live with varying degrees of hearing deficits. Assisting the aged to live with these deficits is a challenge in gerontological care. It is not unusual for the impaired to demonstrate emotional reactions to their hearing deficits. Unable to hear conversation, patients may become suspicious of those around them and accuse people of talking about them. Anger, impatience, and frustration can result from repeatedly unsuccessful attempts to understand conversation. Patients may feel confused or react inappropriately upon receiving distorted verbal communications. Being limited in the ability to hear danger and protect themselves, they may feel insecure. Being self-conscious of their limitation, they may avoid social contact to escape embarrassment and frustration.

Social isolation can be a serious threat because people sometimes avoid the aged person with a hearing deficit due to the difficulty in communication. Even telephone contact may be threatened. (Approximately 10 percent of the aged have difficulty hearing telephone conversations.) Physical, emotional and social health can be seriously affected by this deficit.

Someone nearby should be alerted to the individual's hearing problem so that he or she can be protected in an emergency. In an institutional setting, such patients should be located near the nurse's station. People with hearing loss should be advised to request explanations and instructions in writing so that the full content is received. Those working with the aged can minimize the limitations caused by hearing deficits. To individuals with high-frequency hearing loss the speaker should talk slowly, distinctly, and in a low-frequency voice. Raising the voice or shouting will only serve to raise the high-frequency sounds more and compound the deficit. Methods for promoting more accurate and complete communication include talking into the least impaired ear; facing the individual when talking; using visual speech—sign language, gestures, and facial expressions; allowing the person to lipread; using flash cards, word lists, and other similar aids and devices.

Hearing Aids. The otologist can determine if a hearing aid would be valuable for the given individual and recommend the particular aid best suited for his or her needs. The nurse is in a key position to educate the aged individual on the importance of consulting an otologist before purchasing a hearing aid (Figure 19-6). Patients must understand that even with a hearing aid their problems will not be solved. Hearing will not return to "normal"; speech may sound distorted through the aid because when speech is amplified, so are all environmental noises, and this can be most uncomfortable and disturbing to the individual. Sounds may be particularly annoying in areas where reverberation can easily occur (such as a church or a large hall). Some persons never make the

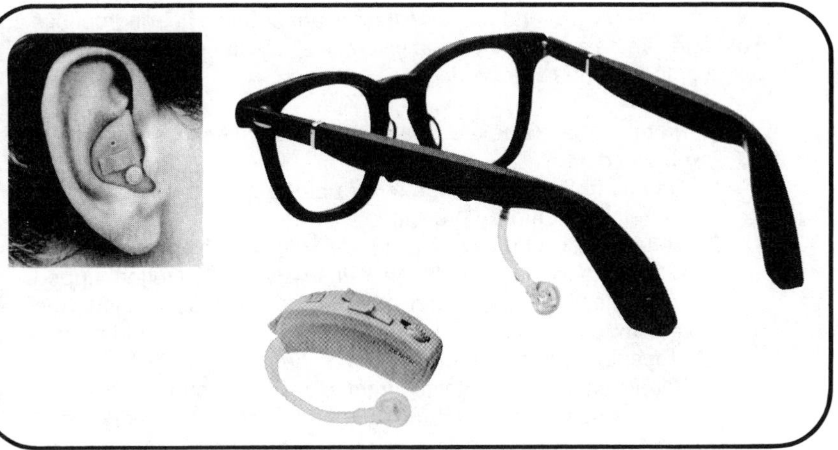

Figure 19-6. Types of hearing aids: (a) In-the-ear model. (b) Behind-the-ear model. (c) Eyeglass model. (Courtesy Zenetron, Manufacturer of Zenith Hearing Aids.)

adjustment to a hearing aid and choose not to wear the appliance rather than to tolerate these disturbances and distortions.

To facilitate adjustment to a hearing aid, an initial period should be provided for experimentation with the controls. This will help the wearer find the most beneficial setting. It may be useful for the person to wear the hearing aid for short periods of time at first, increasing the length of time as adjustment is made. To reduce the disturbances, the individual may find it useful to sit in the front rows of churches and meeting halls, where there is less reverberation. Lowering the amplification in a noisy environment—such as a train station, airplane terminal, or stadium—may also reduce annoyance and discomfort.

Like any fine instrument, the hearing aid must be well cared for. The ear mold can be separated from the receiver for daily washing with soap and water. The cannula should be checked for patency, since cerumen can accumulate in it and interfere with the function of the hearing aid. A pipe cleaner will effectively remove any particles from the cannula. The batteries should be periodically checked; it may not be a bad idea to install new batteries prior to the time the old ones are expected to wear out. The wearer may find it useful to carry extra batteries in a pocketbook or pocket. Prompt repair is advisable when damaged cords or faulty functioning are detected.

Prevention. Gerontological nurses have a responsibility to help aging persons protect and preserve their hearing. Some hearing deficits in old age can be avoided by good care of the ears throughout life. Such care should include the following:

1. Prompt and complete treatment of ear infections should be obtained.
2. Trauma to the ear—from a severe blow, a foreign object in the ear, etc.—should be prevented.
3. Cerumen or particles should be removed by irrigating the external auditory canal rather than by using cotton tipped applicators, hairpins, and other similar devices. It should be remembered that a forceful stream of solution during this procedure can cause perforation of the eardrum.
4. People should be protected from exposure to loud noises, such as those associated with factory and construction work, vehicles, loud music, and explosions. Earplugs or other sound-reducing devices should be used when exposure is unavoidable.
5. Regular audiometric examinations should be scheduled.

Local chapters of hearing and speech associations and organizations serving the deaf can provide assistance and educational materials to those affected by and interested in hearing problems.

OTHER SENSORY DEFICITS AND RELATED CARE

Sight and hearing are not the only senses affected by the aging process; other sensations are also reduced with age. The number of functioning taste buds may be significantly decreased, most obviously by the reduced ability to taste sweet and salty flavors. Pain and pressure are not as easily sensed by the aged. Age-related effects on tactile sensation may also be noted by the difficulty some aged persons have in discriminating different temperatures. Some loss of olfactory function may be noted.

To compensate for the multiple sensory deficits the aged may be experiencing, special attention may be paid to stimulation of all the senses during part of daily living activities. The diet can be planned to include a variety of flavors and colors. Perfumes, fresh flowers and scented candles (safely used) can provide interesting fragrances to smell. In an institutional setting, having a pot brewing fresh coffee in the patients' area can provide a pleasant and familiar aroma during the early morning hours; likewise, a tabletop oven can allow for cookie baking and other cooking activities in the patients' area, providing a variety of stimuli. Different textures can be used in upholstery and clothing fabrics. Clocks that chime, music boxes, and windchimes can vary the environmental sounds which are heard. The design of facilities for the aged should take into consideration the use of different shapes and colors. Intellectual stimulation—through conversation, music, and books, for instance—is also vital.

Touch is not only a means of sensory stimulation, but also an expression of warmth and caring. Too frequently, the nurse may inadvertently only touch the patient during specified procedures, when doing *to* the patient. It is easy for this patient to begin to feel that others perceive him only in terms of tasks rather than as a total human being. How often are patients referred to as "a complete bath," "a foley irrigation," or "a feed"? How often are these labels nonverbally communicated to the patient when the nurse's only encounters with him are for the sake of these activities? To hold a hand, rub a cheek, and pat a shoulder, basic as they may seem, can convey a message to the patient that he is still perceived as a human being. Acceptance of the patient's efforts to touch is also important. The universal language of touch can often communicate a friendship, warmth, and caring which overcomes the most severe sensory deficit.

20

SURGICAL CARE

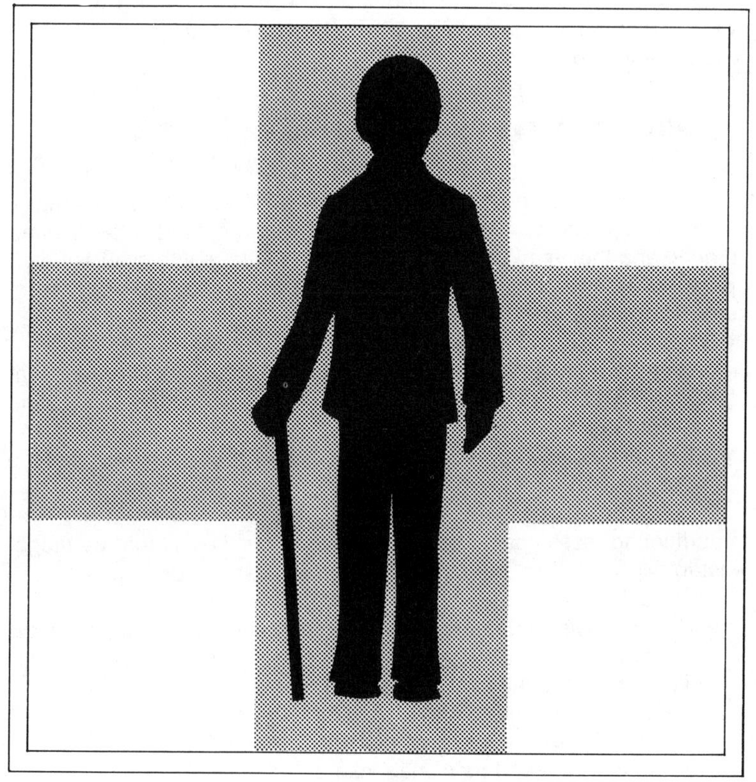

The improvement of surgical procedures and the increased numbers of persons living to old age account for the fact that nurses are now confronted with many more aged surgical patients. People are no longer denied the benefit of surgery based on their age alone. Surgical intervention has provided many of our aged people not only with more years to their lives, but with more functional years. Successful surgical management of an older person's health problems is dependent on the nurse's understanding of the age-related factors that alter normal surgical procedures.

In general, the aged have a smaller margin of physiological reserve and are less able to compensate for and adapt to physiological changes. Infection, hemorrhage, anemia, blood pressure changes, and fluid and electrolyte imbalances are more problematic for the aged. Unfortunately, inelasticity of blood vessels, malnourishment, increased susceptibility to infection, and reduced cardiac, respiratory, and renal reserves cause complications to occur more frequently in the aged, especially during emergency or complicated surgical procedures. By strengthening their capacities preoperatively, maintaining these capacities postoperatively, and being alert to early signs of complications, the nurse can help reduce the risk of problems.

PREOPERATIVE PROCEDURES

The gerontological nurse must be sensitive to the fears many older patients have concerning surgery. Throughout their lifetimes, the aged may have witnessed severe disability or death in older persons having surgery, and they may be concerned about similar outcomes from their operation. Reassurance should emphasize the increased success of surgical procedures:

- Better diagnostic tools facilitating earlier diagnosis and treatment
- Improved therapeutic measures, including surgical techniques and antibiotics
- Increased knowledge concerning the unique characteristics of the aged

In addition to reassurance, patients and their families should be taught what to expect before, during, and after the operative procedure:

- Preoperative preparation—scrubs, medications, and nothing to eat by mouth
- Types of reactions expected to anesthesia
- Length of the surgery and a brief description
- Routine recovery room procedures
- Expected pain and its management

Turning, coughing, and deep-breathing exercises
Rationale for and frequency of dressing changes, suctioning, oxygen, catheters, and other anticipated procedures

Explanations given by the nurse should be communicated to others responsible for care through documentation in the patient's record. Concerns, questions, and fears should be identified by the nurse during assessment and preoperative preparation, and the physician should be made aware of these findings.

It is advisable for the nurse to review with the physician the medications the patient is receiving to determine those which must be continued throughout the hospitalization. Medications which the patient usually takes may need to be administered in spite of NPO restrictions. Sudden interruption of steroid therapy, for instance, can cause cardiovascular collapse and must be prevented. The nurse may learn that the patient has been taking antihypertensive, tranquilizing, or other medications prior to hospitalization. Occasionally, patients forget or are reluctant to tell the physician about these drugs. Since cardiac and pulmonary functions can be altered by certain drugs, it is important to make sure this information is communicated to the physician.

Due to the direct nature of the care she gives, the nurse may be the only person to recognize certain problems. She may discover loose teeth in an aged patient, and they can become dislodged and aspirated during the surgical procedure, causing unnecessary complications. This problem should be brought to the physician's attention in an effort to ensure preoperative dental correction. Another precaution during preparation for surgery is to pad the bony prominences of aged patients to protect them from the pressure of lying on a hard operating room table and subsequent skin breakdown.

OPERATIVE AND POSTOPERATIVE PROCEDURES

Since anesthesia produces depression of the already compromised functions of the cardiovascular and respiratory systems of the aged patient, it must be carefully selected. Close monitoring by the anesthesiologist during the surgery can detect and prevent difficulties in the patient's vital functions. Prolonged surgery for the aged patient is discouraged. Rough, frequent handling of the tissue during surgery is usually avoided since this stimulates reflex activity, increasing the demand for anesthesia. If inhaled agents are used for anesthesia, the nurse should be aware that the patient may remain anesthesized for a longer period of time due to the slower elimination of these agents; turning and deep breathing will facilitate a faster elimination of inhaled agents.

Frequent, close observation and monitoring is extremely important postoperatively. The decreased ability of the aged to manage stress reinforces the need to detect and treat symptoms of shock and hemorrhage promptly. While not being fully conscious from surgery, the aged patient may demonstrate restlessness as the primary symptom of hypoxia. It is important that this restlessness not be mistaken for pain; administration of a narcotic could deplete the body's oxygen supply even more. Prophylactic administration of oxygen may be a beneficial component of the postoperative therapy. Blood loss should be accurately measured, and if excessive, promptly corrected. Frequent checking of urinary output can help reveal the onset of serious complications. Fluid and electrolyte imbalances can be avoided and detected through strict recording of intake and output. (Output should include drainage, bleeding, vomitus, and all other sources of fluid loss.)

Routine care in the recovery phase of older patients is similar to that for all other adults. Activity is vital postoperatively; the benefits of surgery will be diminished if the patient becomes debilitated from the complications arising from immobility. Since the aged patient has a greater risk of developing infections, strict attention must be paid to caring for wounds and changing dressings. A good nutritional status is beneficial to tissue healing and should be encouraged. To conserve the patient's energy and provide comfort, relief of pain is essential. Maintaining regular bowel and bladder elimination, keeping joints mobile and assisting the patient in achieving a comfortable position can assist in pain control. If medications are employed for pain relief, attention should be paid to the reduced activity that may result and to the prevention of the ill effects of such immobilization. It is vital to observe the patient for respiratory depression if narcotic analgesics are administered.

There are several postoperative complications to which aged patients are particularly subject (Glenn, 1974; Mason, Gau, and Byrne, 1976). Respiratory complications include atelectasis, pulmonary emboli, and pneumonia. If pneumonia develops in an aged patient, it is more problematic than it would be for a younger adult and it requires a longer period for recovery. Cardiovascular complications include embolus, thrombus, myocardial infarction, and arrhythmias. Cerebrovascular accident and coronary occlusion occur, but less commonly. Reduced activity and lowered resistance can cause decubiti to develop easily. Paralytic ileus, accompanied by fever, dehydration, abdominal tenderness, and distention, is also a postoperative complication which the aged may experience.

It is not unusual for the positioning on the operating room table and the pulling and moving while unconscious to cause soreness of the aged patient's muscles and bones for several days postoperatively. The nurse should be aware that this is a normal consequence and should take steps to provide comfort. The nurse is in a key position to assist the geriatric patient in achieving maximum benefit from surgery. The most sophisticated surgical procedure in the world performed by the most skillful surgeon is of little value if poor rehabilitative care causes disability or death from avoidable complications. To combine the principles and practices of surgical nursing with the unique characteristics of the aged patient is an immense challenge to the gerontological nurse. To see the increased capacity and more meaningful life many aged persons derive from the benefits of surgery is an immense satisfaction.

REFERENCES

Mason, J. H., Gau, F. C., and **Byrne, M. P.** "General Surgery." In Steinberg, F. U. (ed.), *Cowdry's, The Care of the Geriatric Patient,* 5th ed. Mosby, St. Louis, 1976, pp. 236–244.

Glenn, F. "Surgical Principles for the Aged Patient." In Chinn, A. B. (ed.), *Working with Older People,* Vol. IV. U.S. Dept. of Health, Education, and Welfare, 1974, pp. 259–262.

21

MENTAL ILLNESS AND ILLNESS IN OLD AGE

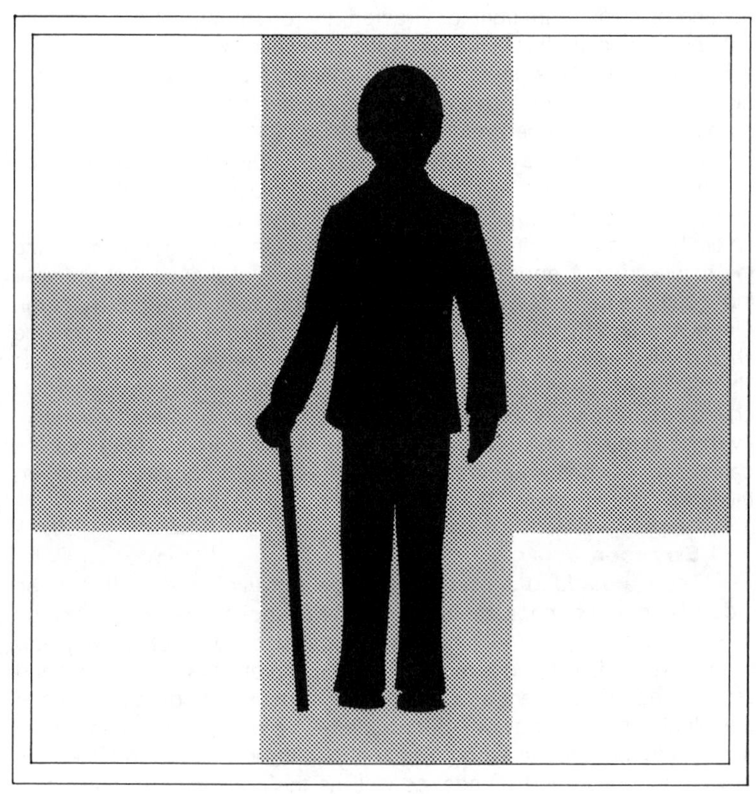

Mental health in old age indicates a capacity to cope with and manage life's stresses in an effort to achieve a state of emotional homeostasis. The aged have an advantage over other age groups in that they have probably had more experience with coping, problem solving, and stress management by virtue of the years they have lived. Most older persons have no delusion regarding what they are or what they are going to be. They have integrity—knowing where they've been, what they've accomplished, and who they really are. Immigrating to a new country, fighting in a world war, and surviving the Great Depression may be among the multitudinous stresses that today's aged have managed to overcome. Such experiences have provided them with a unique emotional strength which should not be underestimated.

RECOGNIZING THE PROBLEMS

Many myths have prevailed regarding mental health and the aged. For instance, there has been a popular belief that with age there is a decline of mental functioning. Granted, there is a loss of neurons with age, but there actually is little correlation between the number of neurons lost and impaired mental function. Another myth propagated has had to do with personality changes with age. Statements have been made that as one grows old, one becomes "more rigid," "childlike," or "senile." These descriptions have been so widely accepted that when an aged person demonstrates these characteristics, it is often considered normal and no attempt is made to explore or treat the underlying cause; some reversible conditions are ignored for this reason. The aged experience the same organic and functional forms of mental illness that younger individuals experience, and they require the same prompt, thorough diagnostic and therapeutic actions employed for the young. At no time should the signs of mental illness be interpreted or accepted as "normal" for the aged. Aging alone does not necessitate a significant change in personality, and several studies have demonstrated personality to be stable over a lifetime (Birren, 1964; Neugarten, 1968). Nurses can promote a better understanding of the aging process by clarifying these misconceptions to the public and to professional persons.

Stresses

There are added stresses in old age, however, that challenge the elderly's coping capacities. Physiological changes may reduce energy reserves, impose physical limitations, and cause the onset of many new symptoms. Bodily changes may result in an alteration in body image and self-concept. Retirement and the independence of children are among the situations in old age which can alter roles and positions. Independence may be threatened by a loss of health or reduced income. The deaths of spouse and friends, as well as the realization of one's own mortality must be faced. Health problems may also produce emotional wear and tear. These stresses are above and beyond the usual stresses of daily living, such as managing a household, marketing, and meeting self-care demands.

Most aged persons cope with these stresses remarkably well; more are interested in working through their problems than surrendering to them. There are situations, however, when the aged individual is more vulnerable to these stresses and mental health can be threatened: illness and hospitalization; death of family, friends, or pets; loss of family or friends for reasons other than death; the illness of a spouse and other added burdens; a reduction in income or an increase in expenses; a change of environment.

The various types of therapeutic assistance that can benefit the aged individual in these situations include crisis intervention, counseling, diversional therapy, health care, psychotherapy, medications, and supplemental income. The most appropriate solution to the problem presented should always be sought. For example, let us say that an elderly man is depressed, and that in exploring the situation it is learned that he is depressed because he lost his part-time job and can't meet his expenses. Antidepressant medications may assist him, but the most appropriate solution would be to obtain financial assistance for him. This action may reestablish his emotional homeostasis and preserve his mental health. It must be remembered that no one approach or technique can be effective for all problems.

Grief. Grief as a result of a loss can occur at any age. Sighing, choking, tightness of the throat, weakness, and gastrointestinal symptoms may occur in the grieving process. Although grief is most often associated with death, individuals can grieve at virtually any significant loss. Such losses may involve bodily function, appearance, a house, or a pet. It is important for the nurse to appreciate the impact of all losses to the aged and to understand the natural grieving process. (Grief is discussed further in Chapter 24.)

Signs of Mental Illness

Since nurses have close contact with the elderly and are often in a key position to detect changes in mental function, they need to be aware of the general signs of mental illness which the aged may demonstrate.

- Disinterested in self-care activities
  - Inattention to hygienic practices
  - Not changing clothing
  - Poor eating habits
- Inappropriate behavior or speech

Deterioration of intellect
Poor judgment
Suspiciousness
Withdrawal

Careful, accurate documentation of specific changes observed by the nurse can facilitate diagnosis and treatment. It is essential, however, to assess the behaviors the individual demonstrates that are suggestive of mental illness. Is an elderly man suspicious because he can't hear what those around him are saying? Is the older woman withdrawn because the high-crime district in which she lives makes it unsafe for her to leave her apartment at night? If a person wears a coat on a warm July afternoon, is it because of poor judgment or because lower body temperature actually necessitates the added warmth? Is the individual's disinterest in self-care activities and inattention to hygienic practices due to the fact that the bathroom is unheated and it is too cold to shower or bathe? Quite frequently, the peculiar behaviors observed in aged persons make a great deal of sense if their origin is explored.

Diagnosis and Treatment

Increased interest is being shown in the relationship of physiological problems to mental illness. Among the factors that can cause an alteration in mental function or a manifestation of emotional disorders are hypotensive states, which decrease cerebral circulation; respiratory diseases, which interfere with full oxygenation of the blood; infections; fluid and electrolyte imbalances; uremia; compromised liver function; sensory deficits; arteriosclerosis; metabolic disorders; and certain medications. This emphasizes the necessity of a thorough physical examination whenever mental dysfunction is detected. Unfortunately, acceptance of mental dysfunction as "normal" for aged individuals often causes delayed or missed diagnosis and treatment of the correctable physiological problems that are at the root of the emotional problem—a profound disservice to the aged and a discredit to the helping professions!

Once detected, the mental illness should be specifically diagnosed in the aged. *Senility is not a diagnosis.* The term senility has served as a catch-all for any sign the aged display reflecting a decline in mental function. It has been used so indiscriminately that it is meaningless in communicating an exact, accurate description of the given individual. It has also been used carelessly at times, implying a decline in mental function as an anticipated outcome of the normal aging process. Senility is not unique to the aged, nor is it a normal state. Those working with other persons must be careful not to accept as normal levels of mental dysfunction which would prompt aggressive therapeutic action if noted in other age groups. The aged can be found to have any of the mental illnesses occurring in other age groups. Some people have been affected by an illness for a major portion of their life span; some have problems that first become apparent in old age. Only through an accurate differential diagnosis can effective therapeutic actions be determined.

Just as the aged have a right to the full diagnostic measures utilized for younger adults, they also have a right to the full range of treatment measures. In the past, medications and institutionalization have been the major approaches employed for the mentally ill aged. Psychotherapy has been used with the aged to a significantly lesser degree than with younger adults. The aged comprised a small minority of the private practice of psychiatrists (Butler, 1975). Community-based mental health programs concern themselves with only a small number of the aged in need of their services. Although approximately 30 percent of the persons in psychiatric hospitals are aged, only slightly more than 2 percent are in community-based programs. The aged can and do benefit from many different approaches. Creativity and variety should be used in the treatment of the mentally ill aged.

COMMON MENTAL HEALTH PROBLEMS OF OLD AGE AND RELATED NURSING ACTIONS

Depression

Depression is the most frequent problem psychiatrists treat in the elderly, and it increases in incidence with age (Butler, 1971a). Although depressive episodes may have been a problem for certain individuals throughout their lifespan, it is not uncommon for depression to be a new problem in old age. When one considers the adjustments and losses the aged face, often concurrently, it is not surprising that depression may occur, e.g., the independence of one's children; the reality of retirement; significant changes or losses of roles; reduced income restricting the pursuit of satisfying leisure activities and limiting the ability to meet basic needs; decreasing efficiency of the body; a changing self-image; the deaths of family members and friends, reinforcing the reality of one's own shrinking lifespan; and overt and covert messages from society that one's worth is inversely proportional to one's age. Under these circumstances, it is understandable that many persons slump into an emotional valley in old age.

Depression can be demonstrated in a variety of ways in older persons. "Vegetative symptoms" are the most common manifestations of this problem, including insomnia, weight loss, anorexia, and constipation. Apathy, self-depreciation, inertia, and remorse, often attributed to "growing old," can also indicate depression. Mental confusion resulting

TABLE 21-1: SUICIDE
RATES PER 100,000 POPULATION

Age	Males	Females
15–24	17.0	4.3
25–44	21.9	9.5
45–64	28.5	12.0
65 and over	38.1	7.8

Source: National Center for Health Statistics, *Vital Statistics of the United States, 1973.*

from malnutrition may have depression as its root. The nurse must remember that depressions do not assume a typical picture in the aged, although they do tend to last longer in aged persons. Therapy can help improve this condition quickly, and treatment includes any of the approaches utilized for other age groups. Psychotherapy and medications are successful in almost half of all depressions in aged persons. Treatment should not be withheld because the depression is assumed to be associated with a physical illness; alleviating the depression may help the individual better cope with and manage any other existing problem. It is essential to realize that physical health can be significantly threatened by untreated depression.

Suicidal impulses are sometimes associated with depression. The suicide rate increases with age and is particularly high in aged Caucasian males (Table 21-1). All suicidal threats in the aged should be taken seriously. In addition to recognizing obvious suicidal attempts, the gerontological nurse must learn to recognize those that are more subtle but equally destructive. Medication misuse, either in the form of overdosages or omission of dosages, may be a suicidal gesture. Starvation may be another sign. Engaging in activities that oppose a therapeutic need or threaten a medical problem—such as ignoring dietary restrictions or refusing a particular therapy—may indicate a desire to die. Walking through a dangerous area, driving while intoxicated, and subjecting oneself to other risks can also be signals of suicidal desires.

The suicidal aged need close observation, careful protection, and prompt therapy. The nurse can compliment other therapeutic measures by providing opportunities to increase the individual's self-worth and by offering activities from which satisfaction can be derived. It is important to recognize and comment favorably on a person's clothing, jewelry, hairstyle, or smile; and even the simplest arts and crafts creation should be complimented. The nurse can demonstrate sensitivity and reflect interest in the individual by remembering past and future satisfactions and events. Although aged individuals may feel that their life is meaning-

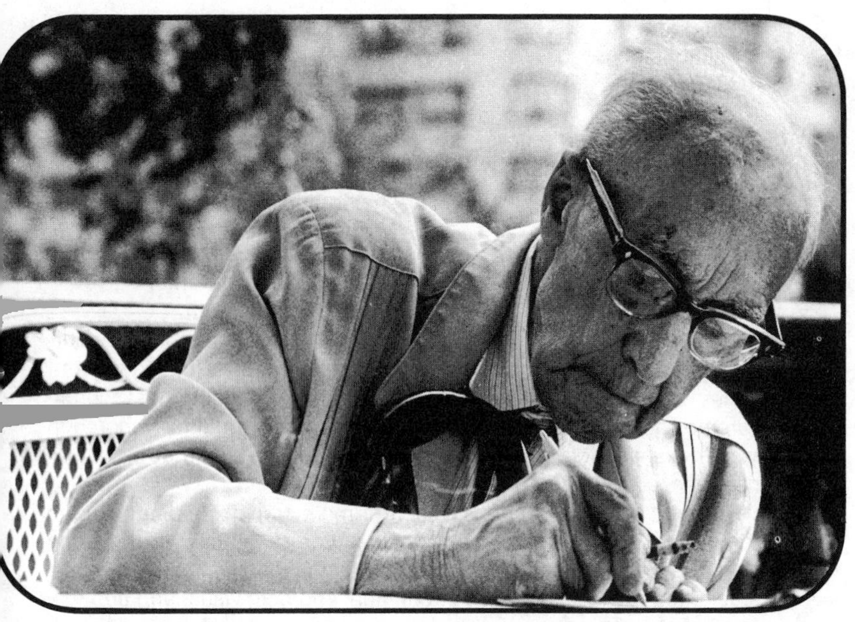

less at a given moment, commenting on how much they helped others at some previous time or on how much everyone is looking forward to some future action can balance the current negative feelings with the more positive feelings associated with other times. Gerontological nurses need to identify even the most minor positive behaviors which can be reinforced. While helping the aged face and manage the many problems which can cause stress and depression, the nurse can instill and help the aged maintain a faith and hope in the future.

Organic Brain Syndrome

Organic brain syndromes are among the most common form of mental illness in the aged. Associated with some impairment of brain tissue function, this disorder affects intellect, memory, judgment, orientation, comprehension, and general emotional stability. *Acute brain syndrome* usually has a rapid onset. Restlessness, night confusion, and a fluctuating level of awareness are demonstrated. There can be a misidentification of people. For instance, affected individuals may believe that their nurse is their sister, or they may not be able to recognize their children. If hallucinations are present, they tend to be visual rather than auditory. The causes of acute syndrome are multiple and include the following:

- Fluid and electrolyte imbalances
- Malnutrition
- Anemias
- Congestive heart failure
- Hormonal imbalances
- Hypotension
- Infection
- Trauma
- Decreased cardiac function
- Decreased respiratory function
- Decreased renal function
- Ingestion of toxic substances
- Hyper- and hypo-glycemia
- Hyper- and hypo-thyroidism
- Medications (e.g. barbiturates, diuretics, L-Dopa, and steroids)

Fortunately, acute brain syndrome is reversible. Treatment of the underlying cause frequently results in rapid and marked improvement. Families of aged persons who demonstrate signs of organic brain syndrome should be urged to take the affected individual for a thorough physical examination and not merely accept these signs as a natural consequence of the aging process.

Chronic brain syndrome, a disorder more commonly diagnosed in elderly women, involves a loss or malfunction of neurons in the brain cortex. The individual may demonstrate disorientation, memory deficits, misidentification, delusions, confabulation, and both visual and auditory hallucinations. There is a progressive change in behavior, although social behavior may not be affected. This degenerative brain disease usually has many causes. If cerebral arteriosclerosis is the underlying cause, there may be occasional improvements in the individual's mental function due to periodic improvements in cerebral circulation. Along with a history of symptoms, electroencephalography, echoencephalography, and brain scanning are among the diagnostic procedures employed to confirm this problem.

Unlike acute brain syndrome, chronic brain syndrome is irreversible. Medications and other therapeutic measures may be used to promote a limited degree of improvement. Affected individuals will need continued reevaluation of their changing capacity to meet self-care demands. As this disorder progresses and increased limitations develop, the nurse can plan interventions which promote health and safety and prevent threats to well-being. The difficulty family members and friends may have observing the progressive mental deterioration of this individual should be recognized, and appropriate support should be offered. It can be terribly painful for a husband to hear his wife tell a jumbled tale of how imaginary people appear in her room at night, or for a child not be recognized by his parent. Realistic explanations coupled with sensitive reassurance can help to ease the agonizing feelings of those involved with the impaired individual.

Anxiety

New problems and the adjustments to physical, emotional, and socioeconomic limitations in old age add to the variety of causes for anxiety. Anxiety reactions, not uncommon in aged persons, can be manifested in various ways, including somatic complaints, rigidity in thinking and behavior, insomnia, fatigue, hostility, restlessness, chain smoking, pacing, fantasizing, confusion, and increased dependency. There may be an increase in pulse, blood pressure, and the frequency of urination. Anxious individuals may excessively handle their clothing, jewelry, or utensils. They may become intensely involved with a minor task, such as folding a piece of linen, and may attempt to focus on an activity outside the one with which they are involved, such as watching the activity in another area while they are being interviewed.

Nurses can assist the anxious person by simplifying the environment through measures such as the following:

- Allowing adequate time for conversations, procedures, and other activities
- Preparing the individual for anticipated activities
- Providing thorough, honest, and basic explanations
- Controlling the number and variety of persons with whom the individual must interact
- Preventing overstimulation of the senses by reducing noise, using soft lights, maintaining stable temperature, etc.
- Keeping and using familiar objects

Paranoia

Paranoid states frequently occur in aged persons, especially in aged women (Butler, 1971b). Considering the realities of old age, it is not surprising that sensory losses, so common among the aged, can easily cause the environment to be misperceived; that illness, disability, living alone, a limited budget, and the regular encounters with ageism do not contribute feelings of security. Old people's mistrust of the environment may actually be quite a sensible and normal reaction to the fact that they are common victims of crime. It is difficult to say whether paranoia is a sign of a mental illness or a safe defense against the realities one faces in old age.

The initial consideration in working with paranoid aged individuals is to explore mechanisms which could reduce insecurity and misperception. Corrective lenses, hearing aides, supplemental income, new housing, and a stable environment are valuable improvements. Psychotherapy and medications can be employed when improvement is not achieved through other techniques. The nurse should be aware that these states can threaten individuals with self-imposed isolation and that appropriate measures are needed to prevent and manage such a situation.

Hypochondriasis

Hypochondriasis, a problem frequently found among aged persons, is commonly associated with depression. However, it may be demonstrated for certain purposes. For some persons, it may be an attention getting mechanism. Often, health professionals reinforce this behavior by reacting to physical complaints but not recognizing or rewarding periods of health and good function. Some people may find hypochondriasis an effective means to control a spouse or children. Older people may use it as a means of socialization; if they do not have travels, professions, or interests they can share with others they can count on most of their peers appreciating or experiencing one ailment or another. Providing alternative interests and not reinforcing the associated behavior may assist individuals with hypochondriasis more than efforts to convince them that there is no physical cause for their symptoms.

NURSING CONSIDERATIONS

Mental health in old age implies a satisfaction and interest in life. This can be displayed in a variety of ways, ranging from quiet reflection to zealous activity. The quiet individual who stays at home does not necessarily have less mental health than the gregarious person who is actively involved in every senior citizen program. It is important to realize that there is no singular mold for the mentally healthy aged and that attempts to assess an older individual's mental status based on any given stereotype are to be avoided.

Good mental health practices throughout an individual's lifetime promote good mental health in old age. To preserve mental health, individuals need to maintain the activities and interests which they find satisfying. They need opportunities to prove their value as a member of society and to have their self-worth reinforced. Security through the provision of adequate income, safe housing, the means to meet basic human needs, and support and assistance through stressful situations will promote mental health. A basic ingredient in the preservation and promotion of mental health which must not be underestimated is optimum physical health.

The nurse must recognize that there are times in everyone's life when disturbances occur, altering the capacity to manage stress. The same techniques that would be employed in the presence of a physical problem should be employed by the nurse in an effort to restore emotional homeostasis:

1. Strengthen the individual's capacity to manage the problem.
2. Minimize or eliminate the limitations imposed by the problem.
3. Act for or do for the individual when necessary.

Efforts which strengthen the individual's capacity to manage an emotional problem include improvement of physical health, a good diet, thorough explanations, meaningful activity, income supplements, and socialization. Efforts which minimize or eliminate the limitations imposed by an emotional problem include providing consistency in care, not fostering hallucinations, reality orientation, and correction of physical problems. Efforts involving acting for or doing for the individual include choosing an adequate diet, bathing, managing finances, directing activities, and keeping the individual in a protective environment. These examples are by no means all inclusive and do not imply that an action which involves "acting for" can't also be used to "strengthen capacity" or "minimize a limitation."

Drugs may be used in the treatment of mental illness. As has been discussed in other chapters, drug therapy in the aged requires close monitoring and extreme caution. The nurse should observe for the effectiveness of the drug and the changes it may cause in the patient. Toxic effects must be observed for, and frequent evaluation to determine the patient's continued need for the drug is essential. Although drugs can be a beneficial compliment to other forms of therapy, they are not to be utilized as a singular means of treatment. The aged can benefit from psychiatric help. They, like any other age group, should be provided a fair opportunity to solve problems and work through their crises. As advocates for the aged, nurses can encourage the establishment of available, accessible, and affordable mental health services—in nursing homes, communities, and all geriatric care settings.

REFERENCES

Birren, J. E. *The Psychology of Aging.* Prentice-Hall, Englewood Cliffs, N.J., 1964.

Butler, R. N. "Clinical Psychiatry in Late Life." In Rossman, I. (ed.), *Clinical Geriatrics.* Lippincott, Philadelphia, 1971. (a) p. 442; (b) p. 446.

——— *Why Survive? Being Old in America.* Harper & Row, New York, 1975, pp. 233–234.

Neugarten, B. L. (ed.). *Middle Age and Aging.* Univ. of Chicago Press, 1968.

22

GERIATRIC PHARMACOLOGY

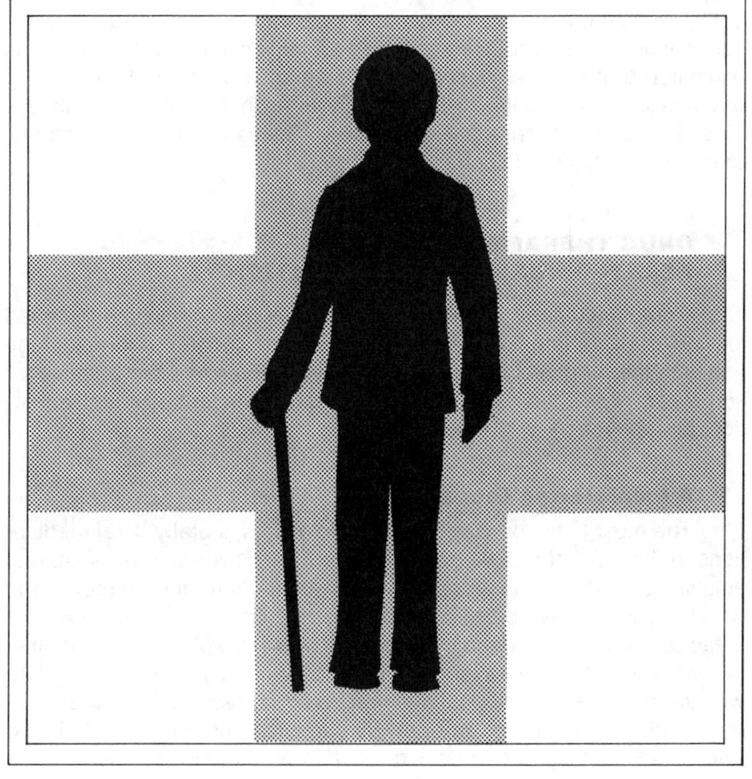

Because of their many health problems, the elderly are likely to receive a greater quantity and variety of medications. Although they account for only 10 percent of the total population, 25 percent of all prescription medications ordered are for the elderly. In addition, they may self-medicate with over-the-counter drugs such as analgesics, antacids, antihistamines, and laxative preparations, in an attempt to manage the health problems they face. The risk of adverse reactions to medications always increases as the quantity increases, and since alterations during the aging process decrease the efficiency of the body, drug therapy is further complicated for the aged.

Investigators claim that adverse drug reactions are responsible for from 3 to 5 percent of all hospital admissions (Caranasos, Stewart, and Cluff, 1974; Hurwitz, 1969) and that there is a higher proportion among the aged. Studies report incidences of drug reactions in hospitalized individuals ranging anywhere from 10 to 30 percent (Hoddinott, 1967; Seidl et al., 1966). One study, involving 1160 patients in Belfast hospitals, reported an incidence of 10.2 percent (Hurwitz and Wade, 1969)—interestingly, only 6.3 percent were patients under age 60 while 15.4 percent were over 60, more than double (Hurwitz, 1969). It has been estimated that on one-seventh of all hospital days some type of drug reaction occurs, costing approximately three million dollars annually (Task Force on Prescription Drugs, 1969). This is in addition, of course, to the disability and discomfort that may result.

DRUG THERAPY AND RELATED NURSING CONSIDERATIONS

Complications associated with drug therapy emphasize the need for nurses to be familiar with the principles of geriatric pharmacology and with the relationship between these principles and the administration of drugs and their absorption, distribution, metabolism, detoxification, and excretion by the body.

Administering Drugs

The most common way to administer drugs is orally. Oral medications in the form of tablets, capsules, liquids, powders, elixers, spirits, emulsions, mixtures, and magmas are used either for their direct action on the mucous membrane of the digestive tract, as in the case of antacids, or for their systemic effects, as with antibiotics and tranquilizers. Although administration is simple, certain problems can interfere with the process. Dry mucous membrane of the oral cavity, not uncommon in older individuals, can prevent capsules and tablets from being swallowed. If they are then expelled from the mouth, there is no therapeutic value; if they dissolve in the mouth, they can irritate the mucous membrane. Proper oral hygiene, ample fluids for assistance with swallowing and mobility, proper positioning, and an examination of the oral cavity after administration will ensure the medication of the full benefit of travel through the gastrointestinal system. Some elderly may not even be aware that a tablet is stuck to the roof of their dentures or under their tongue.

Large tablets, generally difficult for an older person to swallow, should be crushed and mixed with a small amount of soft food, such as applesauce or gelatin. As a rule, capsules should not be broken open and mixed. Medications are put into capsule form so that unpleasant tastes will be masked or so that the coating will dissolve when it comes into contact with specific gastrointestinal secretions. Breaking the capsule defies the purposes of using it, and perhaps another form of the drug should be prescribed if there is a swallowing problem. Some vitamin, mineral, and electrolyte preparations are bitter in taste, and even more so for older persons, whose taste buds for sweetness are lost long before those for sourness and bitterness. Combining the medication with foods and drinks such as applesauce and juices can make them more palatable and also prevent gastric irritation. Individuals should always be made aware that the food or drink they are ingesting contains a medication. Oral hygiene after the administration of oral drugs will prevent an unpleasant aftertaste.

Drugs prescribed in suppository form for local or systemic action are administered by insertion into various body cavities. They act either by melting from body heat or dissolving in body fluids. Because circulation to the lower bowel and vagina is decreased and the general body temperature reduced in older individuals, a prolonged period may be required for the suppository to melt. If there is no alternative route which can be utilized and the suppository form must be given, the nurse should try to remain with the individual until the suppository is thoroughly melted in order to prevent drug loss through expulsion.

Intramuscular and subcutaneous administration of drugs are necessary when immediate results are sought or when other routes aren't possible, either due to the nature of the drug or the status of the individual. The upper, outer quadrant of the buttocks is the best site for intramuscular injections, and the outer portion of the upper arm for subcutaneous injections. Frequently, the older person will bleed or ooze after the injection because of the decreased tissue elasticity; a small bandage with pressure may be helpful. Alternating the injection site will help reduce discomfort. Special attention should be paid to injecting a medication in an immobile limb because inactivity of the limb will reduce the rate of absorption. A person receiving frequent injections should be checked for signs of infection at the injection site; reduced cutaneous sensation in the aged or lack of sensation, as in a stroke patient, may prevent the individual from being aware of a complication.

Occasionally, intravenous administration of drugs is essential. In addition to observing the effects of this medication, the nurse needs to be alert to the amount of fluid in which the drug is administered. Declining cardiac and renal function make the aged not only more susceptible to dehydration, but also to overhydration. Signs of circulatory overload must be closely observed for, including elevated blood pressure, increased respirations, coughing, shortness of breath, and symptoms associated with pulmonary edema. Intake and output balance, body weight, and specific gravity should be monitored by the nurse. Of course, the complications associated with intravenous therapy in any age group—infiltration, air embolism, thrombophlebitis, pyrogenic reactions, etc.—are also observed for in the aged. Decreased sensation may mask any of these potential complications, emphasizing the necessity for close nursing observation.

Assessment. When administering medications to older individuals, the nurse should assess certain factors:

1. Ascertain whether the correct dosage has been prescribed—not only the normal dosage range but the *lowest dose* required for effectiveness. Generally, lower dosages are required for the elderly.
2. Ascertain whether the most effective route of administration is being utilized.
3. Determine whether the drug continues to be required.
4. Determine whether the drug continues to have a therapeutic effect.
5. Make sure adverse reactions to the drug aren't present. These sometimes develop suddenly from medications taken over a long period. Since they sometimes do not appear when expected they must be watched for. Side effects may not be similar in all individuals; what may cause a rash in one individual could cause mental confusion in another.

The nurse should reflect her continued assessment of these items in written documentation. If problems are detected or if there is any question as to the appropriateness of the drug's administration, the drug should be withheld until the physician can be consulted.

Safeguards. Special nursing action is warranted when older individuals are expected to administer medications themselves. A detailed description—verbal and written—should be given to the per-

Breakfast:

- Ampicillin, 1 capsule
- Digoxin, 1 tablet: REMEMBER TO TAKE PULSE
- Multivitamins, 1 capsule
- Ferrous sulfate, 1 tablet

Lunch:

- Ampicillin, 1 capsule
- Ferrous sulfate, 1 tablet

Dinner:

- Ampicillin, 1 capsule
- Ferrous sulfate, 1 tablet

Bedtime:

- Ampicillin, 1 capsule

Each medicine bottle is coded as follows:

Code	Medication	Amount prescribed:
	Ferrous sulfate	300 mg TID (3 times a day)
	Multiple vitamins	1 capsule qAM (every morning)
	Ampicillin	250 mg QID (1 capsule) (4 times a day)
	Digoxin	250 mcg qAM (1 tablet)

Figure 22-1. Color-coded schedule of medication dosage for aged patients who are visually impaired or illiterate.

son, outlining the drug name, dosage schedule, route of administration, action, special precautions, and adverse reactions. Other drugs or foods incompatible with a given prescribed drug should be mentioned. A color-coded dosage schedule can be developed to assist persons who have visual deficits or who are illiterate (Figure 22-1). Medication labels with large print and caps that can be easily removed by weak or arthritic hands should be provided. The nurse should review the medication schedule and explore any new symptoms at every patient-nurse encounter. A variety of potential medication errors can be prevented or corrected by close monitoring. Several studies have revealed some common self-medication errors to guard against—errors in dosage administered, noncompliance due to misunderstanding, discontinuation or unnecessary continuation of drugs without a physician's advice, and using medications prescribed for previous illnesses (Boyd et al., 1974; Brady, 1973, Schwartz et al., 1962).

Absorption and Distribution by the Body

Absorption. Generally older people have less of a problem with the absorption of medications than with their administration, detoxification, and excretion. However, a variety of factors will alter the absorption of drugs. For instance, the general decrease in the number and function of cells with increased age can reduce the rate at which drugs are absorbed because of reductions in the following:

1. Cellular and intracellular fluid
2. Oxygen uptake and utilization
3. Cardiac output and circulation
4. Glomerular filtration rate
5. Gastric acid secretion
6. Thyroid activity
7. Mechanisms that regulate temperature

Although the nurses cannot permanently correct these changes, they can use measures to facilitate absorption. Exercise will stimulate circulation and should be encouraged, as should an adequate fluid intake. Hypotension, which can reduce blood flow, should be avoided. Preparations that neutralize the gastric secretions will have to be avoided if an acidic gastric environment is necessary for a particular drug's absorption. Body temperature could be monitored to prevent hypothermia. It is possible to avoid using drugs that inhibit the effect of each other, such as tetracycline preparations and magnesium antacids, and foods that interfere with drug action, as with processed cheeses and monamine oxidase (MAO) inhibitors. When urinary tract antibiotics that require an acidic urine pH are prescribed, the nurse can offer juices and foods rich in vitamin C. One form of administration may prove to have greater absorption potential than another, and the nurse should bring this suggestion to the physician's attention. There is some thought that there is less efficient absorption of drugs through the gastrointestinal tract with advanced age, including substances such as fat, thiamine, glucose, iron, and 3-methylglucose (Bender, 1968).

Distribution. Although it is difficult to predict how drug distribution will differ among aged individuals, it is known that changes in circulation, membrane permeability, body temperature, and tissue structure can modify this process. As mentioned in earlier chapters, adipose tissue does replace other tissues with age; medications which accumulate in adipose tissue, such as certain barbiturates, can be of longer duration due to the slower distribution throughout the body.

Metabolism, Detoxification, and Excretion

The renal system is primarily responsible for the body's excretory functions, and among its activities is the excretion of drugs. Drugs filtered through the kidneys follow a process similar to that for most of the constituents of urine. After systemic circulation, the drug filters through the walls of glomerular capillaries into Bowman's capsule. It continues down the tubule, where substances beneficial to the body will be reabsorbed into the bloodstream through proximal convoluted tubules, and where waste substances that are excreted through urine will flow into the pelvis of the kidney. Capillaries surrounding the tubules reabsorb the filtered blood and join to form the renal vein. It is estimated that almost ten times more blood circulates through the kidneys, as compared with similar sized body organs, to promote this filtration process.

The reduced efficiency of body organs with advanced age affects the kidneys as well, complicating drug excretion in the elderly. The number of nephron units are decreased in number (Rossman, 1971) and as much as 64 percent of the nephrons can be nonfunctional in very old individuals (Hoffman, 1970). The glomerular filtration rate is reduced 46 percent between the ages of 20 and 90 (Davies and Shock, 1950), along with a reduction in tubular reabsorption (Miller, McDonald, and Shock, 1952). Decreasing cardiac function contributes to the almost 50 percent reduction in blood flow to the kidneys (Hoffman, 1970). The implications of the reduced kidney efficiency are important. Drugs are not as quickly filtered out of the blood stream and are present in the body longer. The biological half-life, or the time for one half of the drug to be excreted, can increase up to 40 percent. These factors can lead to an increased risk of adverse reactions.

The liver also has many important functions that influence drug detoxification and excretion. Carbohydrate metabolism in the liver converts glucose into glycogen and releases it into the bloodstream when needed. Protein metabolism in the parenchymal cells of the liver are responsible for the loss of the amine groups from amino acids, which aid in the formation of new plasma proteins, such as prothrombin and fibrinogen as well as in the conversion of some poisonous nitrogenous by-products into nontoxic substances, such as the conversion of ammonia into urea. Fatty acids and ketone bodies are metabolized in the liver to prepare essential substances such as vitamin B-12. Also important is the liver's formation of bile, which serves to break down fats through enzymatic action and to remove substances such as bilirubin from the blood. Although no significant effects have been reported, the liver's decrease in size and function with age might interfere with the formation of certain necessary body substances, such as prothrombin, albumin, and vitamins A, D, and B-12.

Certain enzymes may not be secreted, interfering with the metabolism of drugs requiring enzymatic activity. Most importantly, the detoxification and conjugation of drugs can be significantly reduced, so that the drug stays longer in the bloodstream. There is some evidence indicating larger drug concentrations at administration sites in aged individuals (Wade, 1972).

Adverse Reactions

The higher risk of adverse reactions to drugs in the elderly has already been discussed. Certain general factors related to adverse reactions should be kept in mind by the nurse:

1. The signs and symptoms of an adverse reaction to a given drug may differ in older individuals.
2. A prolonged period of time may be required for an adverse reaction to become apparent in older individuals.
3. An adverse reaction to a drug may be demonstrated even after a drug has been discontinued.
4. Adverse reactions to a drug that has been administered over a long period without problems can develop suddenly.

Varying degrees of mental dysfunction are often early symptoms of an adverse reaction to such commonly prescribed medications for the elderly as codeine, digitalis, lidocaine, methyldopa, phenobarbital, L-Dopa, valium, librium, and various diuretics. Any medication that can promote hypoglycemia, acidosis, fluid and electrolyte imbalances, temperature elevations, increased intracranial pressure, and reduced cerebral circulation can also produce mental disturbances. The nurse should be alert to changes in mental status and should consult with the physician regarding medications that could be responsible. The aged may easily be victims of drug-induced senility. Unfortunately, mental dysfunction in the aged is sometimes treated symptomatically; that is, with medications but without full exploration of the etiology. This will not correct an original drug-related problem, and it will predispose the individual to additional complications from the new drug.

COMMONLY USED DRUGS, REACTIONS, AND RELATED PROCEDURES

The nurse should be thoroughly knowledgeable about the drugs commonly prescribed for the elderly, including the actions of such drugs, the necessary precautions, and the adverse reactions. To supplement the material presented in the following pages, it is advisable for the nurse to obtain more complete information from the pharmacology literature.

Analgesics

For the relief of rheumatic pain and similar discomforts that are common with aged people, various analgesics can be employed. Aspirin remains a major drug used by the aged, having antipyretic and anti-inflammatory actions in addition to its analgesic effects. When used for arthritic conditions, aspirin reduces pain and swelling, which promotes joint mobility. Aspirin's effectiveness and relatively low cost make it quite popular. Of the various side effects of this drug, gastrointestinal bleeding is one of the most serious. Iron deficiency anemia in an older individual should suggest an assessment of aspirin consumption to explore the existence of gastrointestinal hemorrhage. Using buffered or enteric-coated aspirin preparations and avoiding aspirin ingestion on an empty stomach are helpful measures in preventing gastrointestinal irritation and bleeding. Since older persons are very likely to prescribe and take aspirin on their own nurses should caution them on several points.

Aspirin should not be used for persons on anticoagulants unless it is closely monitored by a physician.

Probenecid has an antagonistic action with salicylates and should not be administered concurrently.

Sodium bicarbonate increases the rate of urinary excretion of salicylates, diminishing their action; therefore, older patients taking salicylates should be discouraged from using baking soda to relieve indigestion.

Since people can develop a tolerance for aspirin, the patient should discuss the need for a dosage increase with a physician and not increase the dosage independently.

Occasionally, disturbances of the central nervous system develop when individuals with decreased renal function use salicylates. Since renal function may be reduced in some older persons, symptoms of central nervous system problems should be observed for, including changes in mental status (most commonly, confusion), dizziness, tinnitus, and deafness. Acetaminophen may bring older persons relief. This drug is a nonsalicylate antipyretic and analgesic, with rare incidents of adverse reactions.

Codeine is sometimes prescribed as a mild analgesic. Two effects of this drug are of significance to the aged. First, codeine therapy may result in drowsiness, predisposing an elderly person to accidents. The nurse should caution the person about this effect and advise against driving, climbing a ladder, or any other activity which could pose a risk. Second, constipation sometimes occurs when a person is taking codeine. Due to reduced peristalsis and an often limited intake of bulk foods, constipation is already a not uncommon problem for the aged; thus the probability of constipation while on codeine therapy is fairly high. The nurse should encourage the ingestion of fruit juices and bulk foods as a prevention and closely observe and record bowel elimination patterns to detect constipation early.

Narcotic analgesics are prescribed for the aged to relieve severe pain of short duration, such as occurs postoperatively or with a myocardial infarction, and to provide relief from pain during the terminal phase of an illness when analgesics of lesser potency aren't effective. These drugs must be used with extreme caution in the aged. Morphine sulfate, an opium derivative, is used for the relief of severe pain. In addition to its analgesic effect, it acts to produce euphoria and mild disorientation, reduce peristalsis, slow respirations, increase sphincter muscle tone, and reduce the heartbeat slightly while increasing the force of the beat. Since morphine sulfate can dull sensations and depress respirations, it should be used with extreme caution in older individuals. There is some belief that a lower dose of this drug should be prescribed for the aged, who tend to react more to its depressant effects; it is recommended that aged individuals should receive one-half the usual adult dosage and that morphine be avoided in persons 70 years of age or older.

Meperidine is a narcotic analgesic for mild to severe pain with actions similar to morphine but without the severe problems associated with morphine. Unlike morphine, meperidine does not produce deep sedation or respiratory depression; however,these effects will be seen if the drug is administered with other central nervous system depressants. In the aged especially, meperidine is known to cause hypotension, dizziness, nausea, and impaired mental and physical functioning. Precautions must be taken if the patient is receiving phenothiazines because these drugs will potentiate the action of meperidine. This drug should not be administered if the individual is receiving MAO inhibitors or has received them within the previous two weeks.

Nurses should employ alternative measures to relieve pain before resorting to analgesics. Sometimes, position changes, warm baths, back rubs, conversations, or diversional activity can make the intensity of pain less severe. Only after other measures are no longer able to relieve discomfort should drugs be used. Narcotic analgesics must always be used cautiously and selectively in the aged. The continued requirement for an analgesic should be frequently assessed. No patient should be denied the benefit of an analgesic on the basis of age alone. Instead, the goal of analgesic therapy in the aged is to provide the greatest possible comfort with the least possible number of adverse reactions.

Antianginal Drugs

Nitroglycerin and the long-acting organic nitrates are prescribed for acute angina pectoris episodes in patients with coronary insufficiency, coronary heart disease, coronary occlusion, and subacute myocardial infarction. Since it is not uncommon for many elderly individuals to use nitroglycerin outside of a health care facility, the nurse should include these points when educating the patient about this drug:

1. Nitroglycerin is administered and absorbed sublingually; its purpose is to provide relief in several minutes.
2. Persons should sit or lie down for a short period following administration of nitroglycerin as dizziness, flushing, and cranial throbbing are common reactions.
3. Nitroglycerin tablets should be stored in a closed dark container, away from heat, and not used if over six months old since potency is reduced over time.
4. Nitroglycerin should be used only when necessary since tolerance can develop.
5. If several nitroglycerin tablets do not relieve the attack, the nurse or physician should be promptly contacted.

Some of the adverse reactions to antianginal drugs of particular significance to the aged are irregular and rapid pulse, dizziness, hypotension, decreased respirations, rise in intraocular pressure, blurred vision, muscular weakness, and mental confusion.

Antiarrhythmic Drugs

Procainamide may be used to treat arrhythmias from a variety of conditions. It is known to produce a rapid hypotensive action, and close monitoring is warranted when it is administered to older persons. A reduced dose is recommended for the aged. *Lidocaine,* which does not produce the degree of hypotension that procainamide does, is used to treat multiple ectopic beats associated with acute infarction. This drug is administered parenterally. Particular adverse reactions demonstrated in the aged include mild hypotension, drowsiness, dizziness, and blurred vision. *Propranolol,* a beta-receptor blocking agent, is used to control atrial tachycardia. It is also used in the management of digitalis intoxication and postanesthesia arrhythmias. For hypertensive elderly individuals who have had difficulty with methyldopa, guanethidine, or bethanidine therapy, propranolol is often an effective hypotensive agent.

Bradycardia, depression, fatigue, gastrointestinal disturbances, and dizziness are some of the adverse reactions to this drug. *Quinidine* may be used for controlling ventricular ectopic beats and, prophylactically, for paroxysmal arrhythmias. It is recommended that a lower dose be administered to older persons. Adverse reactions include ringing in ears, headache, dizziness, and gastric upset.

Antibiotics

Similar principles guiding the use of antibiotics in other age groups apply to their use in the aged. Liquid forms of certain antibiotics may prove beneficial to older persons who frequently have difficulty swallowing large capsules. The intramuscular dosages for antibiotic drugs may have to be lowered since the aged obtain higher blood levels of these drugs. Altered tissue structure in aged persons warrants care in the intramuscular injection of these drugs to make sure accidental subcutaneous or intravenous injection doesn't occur. Adverse reactions should be closely observed for because reduced kidney efficiency may promote the accumulation of toxic levels of these drugs.

There are some special considerations for the nurse to remember when an aged person is receiving antibiotic therapy. The oral form of ampicillin remains stable in the presence of gastric acid; the nurse should advise older patients that the use of antacids may change the acidity of the gastric contents, thus threatening the potency of this drug. The excretion of ampicillin can be slowed if the patient is receiving probenecid, and if penicillin is being administered, ampicillin will be totally inactivated. Klebsiella infections may develop following ampicillin therapy and symptoms of this problem should be closely observed for. Gentamicin has a high potential for toxicity and should be used with caution in the elderly, especially in those with impaired renal function. As vestibular and auditory ototoxicity may be caused by gentamicin, it should be avoided for use in patients receiving potent diuretics because many of these agents contribute to ototoxicity as well. The aged are also especially subject to the ototoxic effects of streptomycin. The incidence of adverse reactions is significant in elderly persons receiving the long-acting sulfonamide drugs which are commonly prescribed for the treatment of urinary tract infections.

Tetracycline can depress plasma prothrombin activity, necessitating adjustment if the patient is also receiving anticoagulant therapy. Excessive accumulation and possible liver toxicity can occur in patients with impaired renal function. Signs of hepatic and renal damage—potential complications of tetracycline therapy—should be closely observed for, especially during intravenous administration of this drug. Antacids containing aluminum, calcium, or magnesium will impair the absorption of tetracycline, as will certain foods and dairy products; the nurse should caution patients about this problem and recommend that the drug be administered from one to two hours before or after meals.

Oral forms of penicillin must be administered at regular intervals to maintain a constant blood level of the drug. This may be of particular problem to the aged who must self-administer the drug and remember how and when to do so. A medication calendar or assistance from a family member can compensate for poor memory and increase the likelihood of accurate and regular administration of the drug. If penicillin is to be administered intramuscularly, it is essential that the site of injection be rotated each time; reduced muscle tissue in the aged contributes to poor absorption and pain from injection of this drug. Accidental subcutaneous injection of penicillin may cause a "sterile abscess," and accidental intravenous injection can be extremely dangerous. It should be remembered that although an elderly person might not have experienced a problem with penicillin in the past, an allergic reaction can develop suddenly; close nursing observation is essential.

Anticoagulants

Anticoagulants are used with caution in the aged due to the higher risk of anticoagulant bleeding. There is a greater possibility of a lowered prothrombin time being produced in atherosclerotic individuals, many of whom are in the geriatric population. Some physicians discourage anticoagulant therapy in persons over age 70, while others believe the cautious utilization of these agents may be of great benefit to the aged.

Heparin is usually prescribed for rapid anticoagulation, followed by a coumarin drug for prolonged results. Heparin does not dissolve existing clots but rather inhibits the formation of clots by preventing the conversion of fibrinogen to fibrin. The same general principles applied to heparin therapy in the general population are also applied with the aged. Aspirin should be avoided or given with extreme caution because acetylsalicylic acid can interfere with platelet aggregation and cause bleeding. Digitalis, antihistamines, nicotine, and tetracyclines will partially counteract the effects of heparin. Higher dosages of this drug are required when the patient is febrile, emphasizing the importance of nursing observation and communication regarding vital signs. Heparin will also block the eosinophilic response to ACTH (adrenocorticotropic hormone) adrenocorticosteroids, and insulin. Osteoporosis and spontaneous fractures are known to occur when heparin has been used over a long period of time. Older females should be carefully observed during heparin therapy as they tend to have a higher incidence of bleeding.

Warfarin may also be prescribed for anticoagulant therapy. It inhibits fibrin clotting but has no effect on established thrombus, nor does it reverse ischemic tissue damage. Caution is necessary when this drug is administered in the presence of infectious disease, trauma, an indwelling catheter, hypertension, and moderate to severe hepatic or renal insufficiency. Alcohol, antibiotics, MAO inhibitors, phenothiazines, salicylates, sulfonamides, and thyroxine are some of the drugs that increase warfarin's sensitivity; barbiturates, corticosteroids, diuretics, and multivitamins can decrease its sensitivity. As several of these drugs are regularly used by older individuals, it is essential that a complete assessment of all medications the individual is taking be performed to prevent interference with anticoagulant therapy. For outpatients, the capacity of the individual to use an anticoagulant accurately and to detect side effects readily should be carefully assessed in order to avoid serious errors and consequent threats to health status.

Anticonvulsants

Seizure disorders in the aged are sometimes a reflection of a lifelong history of epilepsy and sometimes a result of cerebral arteriosclerosis, hemiplegia, or other disease processes. Anticonvulsant drugs are used, singularly or in combination, to sustain a blood level that is able to control seizures with the least amount of adverse reactions. Phenobarbital is not as popular in treating the aged as it is with younger adults because it can cause emotional disturbance, delirium, disorientation, ataxia, and coma. Mysoline, of lesser toxicity, is the drug of choice for long-term anticonvulsant therapy in the aged. Dilantin is widely used to control seizure disorders; a common side effect of this drug is gingival hyperplasia, which can be minimized and controlled by regular, thorough oral hygiene.

Other drugs, such as sulthiame and carbamazepine, may also be prescribed for anticonvulsant therapy in the aged. Most oral anticonvulsants are known to cause some degree of gastric irritation. Administering these drugs with food or immediately after a meal may reduce this problem. Blurred vision and diplopia should be noted because these visual disturbances may indicate the need for a dosage adjustment. Fatigue, easy bruising, sore throat, pallor, and unusual bleeding may indicate the development of blood dyscrasias, frequently associated with this drug group; routine urinalyses and blood sample evaluation should be performed.

Antihistamines

Since the aged more frequently experience side effects such as dizziness, disturbed coordination, sedation, and hypotension from antihistamines, these drugs are used with care. Patients should be advised to monitor activities and not subject themselves to situations which could threaten their safety, such as working with a power tool or driving an automobile. These drugs are available without prescription, and self-medication may be a problem. Older persons especially should consult with their nurse or physician before using them. Misuse of antihistamines can produce a tolerance which lessens the effectiveness necessary of other drugs the patient may be taking and can mask symptoms of disease, which delays diagnosis.

Antihypertensive Drugs

As mentioned in earlier chapters, a rise in blood pressure normally occurs with advanced age and that which may be a hypertensive level for a younger adult may be normal for an elderly person. Higher blood pressure levels are often necessary to compensate for the blood flow resistance resulting from arteriosclerosis. Thus, a high blood pressure alone does not warrant the use of antihypertensive drugs. When antihypertensive drugs are indicated, aggressive therapy is discouraged. Thiazide diuretics are commonly used for the management of hypertension in the aged. These drugs work by interfering with the renal tubular mechanism of electrolyte reabsorption. There is an increase in the excretion of sodium and chloride and, to a lesser extent, of potassium, magnesium, and bicarbonate. The excretion of calcium and ammonia, on the other hand, is reduced. The increased excretion of ammonia may increase the concentration of blood ammonia. Other antihypertensive drugs may be potentiated by the thiazides.

Elderly people are at a greater risk of developing a fluid and electrolyte imbalance, and diuretics increase this risk considerably. The nurse should attempt to prevent this by recognizing the signs of an imbalance early and by employing prompt measures to correct it. Signs include dryness of the mouth, mental confusion, thirst, weakness, lethargy, drowsiness, restlessness, muscle cramps, muscular fatigue, hypotension, oliguria, nausea, vomiting, slow pulse rate, and gastrointestinal disturbances. Potassium depletion can be prevented by potassium supplements and citrus juices. Hypokalemia could sensitize the heart to the toxic effects of digitalis, which is a significant consideration for the patient being given both digitalis and diuretics. Thiazides may increase blood glucose levels, and the nurse should be aware that insulin requirements for the diabetic patient may need adjusting if the patient is receiving these drugs. Symptoms of diabetic complications should be closely observed for. Latent diabetes mellitus could be manifested during thiazide therapy.

As the onset of action is rapid and frequent voiding is expected, these drugs should be given in the morning. Bedtime administration may predispose the older person to falls while attempting to reach the bathroom or embarrassing bed-wetting incidents. It is helpful for the nurse to offer the bedpan at least every two hours and to plan activities so that easy access and availability of a toilet is provided. Fear of incontinence or absence of a bathroom facility can discourage the older person from engaging in social activities. The nurse should note whether patients are decreasing their fluid intake to avoid the annoying need for frequent voiding and should help them understand the importance of maintaining a good fluid intake.

Reserpine can either be combined with a thiazide diuretic or used alone in the management of mild hypertension. This drug produces tranquilizing effects, in addition to lowering the blood pressure, and frequently causes mental depression. Since the risk is greater with advanced age, close monitoring of aged patients receiving this drug is important. The nurse should be alert to the most subtle indications of depression, closely noting any withdrawal, agitation, lack of interest in activities or self-care, new questions or conversations about death, and suicidal behaviors.

Methyldopa may be prescribed for moderate to severe hypertension in the aged. Frequent evaluation of hematocrit and hemoglobin should be done, since hemolytic anemia may develop in patients receiving this drug. The breakdown of methyldopa or its metabolites may cause the urine to darken when exposed to air; it is helpful for the nurse to prepare the patient, the family and those providing care for the patient to expect this condition. Close observation of individuals with angina pectoris is required because methyldopa may aggravate this problem. Tolerance to methyldopa may develop when used for several months, emphasizing the necessity of continued nursing evaluation of this drug's effectiveness.

Occasionally, monoamine oxidase (MAO) inhibitors are prescribed for moderate to severe hypertension in the aged; they are also employed as antidepressants. MAO inhibitors must be used with extreme caution in the aged. The nursing staff and patient should be taught that certain foods must be avoided during therapy with these drugs, including chocolate, yeast extract, avocado, pickled herring, pods of broad beans, chicken livers, and processed or aged cheeses. No food or drink requiring the action of bacteria or molds for preparation or preservation, such as alcoholic beverages, can be ingested. Cream cheese, ricotta, and cottage cheese are acceptable. MAO inhibitors are not administered to patients who are receiving methyldopa, dopamine, meperidine, centrally acting sympathomimetic amines (such as the amphetamines), or peripherally acting sympathomimetics (such as ephedrine, frequently contained in cold remedies), or to patients who have received L-Dopa within a one-month period prior to initiating MAO inhibitors. Antihistamines, hypnotics, caffeine, sedatives, tranquilizers, and narcotics must be used carefully in combination with MAO inhibitors and in lower dosages. Febrile illness can potentiate the actions of these drugs. MAO inhibitors can also cause orthostatic hypotension, and induce hypoglycemia and increase symptoms of parkinsonism.

Close monitoring of older patients on antihypertensive therapy is essential. A severe reduction in blood pressure may decrease cerebral circulation, threatening mental functioning; frequent evaluation of blood pressure—preferably in lying, sitting, and standing positions—is necessary. Patients should be advised against rising from a sitting or lying position rapidly, so as to prevent falls resulting from orthostatic hypotension. The nurse should be familiar with the side effects of drugs in this group and facilitate their prompt correction if they occur.

Anti-inflammatory Drugs

Of the musculoskeletal problems in the aged for which anti-inflammatory drugs are used, arthritic conditions are the most common. The salicylates (discussed above under analgesics) are the most popularly chosen anti-inflammatory drugs. For more severe problems, steroids and other potent drugs may be used, but with extreme caution due to the many serious effects they produce. The steroids have profound metabolic effects, modifying the body's immune response. Resistance to infection may be reduced and symptoms of infection masked. Sodium and fluid retention tends to occur, and nursing attention should be given to daily weights, limited sodium intake, monitoring of fluid intake and output, evaluation of blood pressure, and observation for edema. A demineralization of the bones may occur during steroid therapy, predisposing the older person to pathologic fractures. Patients with ocular herpes simplex who receive prednisone may experience corneal perforation; prolonged use of prednisone can cause glaucoma, with possible damage to the optic nerve, and posterior subcapsular cataracts.

Phenylbutazone and indomethacin are potent nonsteroids that are effective for relief in arthritic conditions. Phenylbutazone commonly produces side effects, the incidence of which increases with age. These include nausea, epigastric pain, stomatitis, gastrointestinal bleeding (especially when the patient has had a peptic ulcer in the past), sodium and fluid retention, agranulocytosis, and a variety of other blood dyscrasias. Administration of this drug with meals or with milk reduces the amount of gastric irritation. Nursing observations for the patient receiving phenylbutazone should focus on the development of a sore throat, temperature elevation, mouth lesions, weight gain, change in blood pressure, and the passage of black and tarry stools. Frequent blood evaluations are essential, and it is recommended that phenylbutazone be used selectively, and for short periods of time. Although indomethacin is of lesser toxicity than phenylbutazone, it is not without serious side effects, and it should also be used cautiously in the aged. Adverse reactions to this drug include headache, nausea, gastric irritation, abdominal pain, diarrhea, and gastrointestinal bleeding in patients who have a history of peptic ulcers. The suppository form of this drug is beneficial in alleviating gastric intolerance. The nursing observations and considerations necessary in the use of phenylbutazone are applicable with indomethacin.

Antiparkinsonism Drugs

No drugs are presently available to alter the course of Parkinson's disease. Those that will diminish the symptoms and limitations of the disease include: trihexyphenidyl (Artane), methylphenidate hydrochloride (Ritalin), and amantadine hydrochloride (Symmetrel). Most of these drugs reduce muscular rigidity to improve coordination, posture, and balance; tremor is less effectively helped by drug therapy. While they may be valuable, these drugs are likely to produce side effects in older individuals. Common side effects are dryness of the mouth, nausea, vomiting, epigastric distress, and blurred vision. Administering these drugs during or after meals may reduce gastric discomfort; and providing fluids, hard candy, and frequent oral hygiene may reduce dryness of the mouth. Urinary retention and altered mental function, including confusion, dizziness, excitement, and drowsiness, are symptoms which should be particularly observed for in the aged. These drugs should not be administered to patients with glaucoma, mental confusion, tachycardia, or urinary retention. (The aged are more subject to the atropinelike effect that many of these drugs have on the eye and bladder.) In antiparkinsonism drug therapy, the beginning dosage should be low and increases should be gradual; the dosage should be gradually tapered when the drugs are discontinued in order to prevent a Parkinsonian crisis.

Larodopa (L-Dopa) is increasingly successful for relief of the symptoms of Parkinson's disease. It is used selectively in patients with severe cardiovascular or respiratory disease, bronchial asthma, glaucoma, and renal, hepatic, and endocrine disease; it is contraindicated in patients with a history of organic brain disease or psychosis. MAO inhibitors must be discontinued at least two weeks prior to initiating larodopa—these two drugs cannot be administered concurrently. Patients having a peptic ulcer are in greater risk of upper gastrointestinal hemorrhage when given larodopa. Symptoms of depression and suicidal tendencies should be closely observed for by the nurse when this drug is used.

Debriding Agents

Enzymes are sometimes applied to decubiti to assist in debridement efforts. Elase is a fibrinolytic enzyme which acts on the denatured proteins in necrotic decubiti. Santyl is a collagenase ointment which dissolves the collagen matter attaching the necrotic tissue to the wound. The objective of these agents is to remove the necrotic tissue which allows granulation and epithelization to occur, facilitating wound healing. Neither of these agents affects living cells. The nurse should closely observe the patient who has wounds being debrided for signs of infection. Specific directions, precautions, and adverse reactions accompany these agents.

Digitalis

Digitalis preparations are used in the treatment of congestive heart failure, atrial flutter and fibrillation, supraventricular tachycardia, and extrasystoles, to increase the force of myocardial contraction through direct action on the heart muscle. The resulting improvement in circulation helps to reduce edema as well. These drugs are absorbed from the intestinal tract within 2 hours after administration, reaching their peak in from 1 to 12 hours. The most popularly used drug from this group is digoxin. The biological half-life of digoxin is normally 34 hours but may be as long as 45 hours in the elderly. This implies the need for a lower dose of this drug in the aged and indicates that the risk of adverse reactions may be greater. Continued administration of digoxin can cause a heart block because of the slowing effect this drug has on the heart. Anorexia may develop, followed by nausea and vomiting several days later. Excessive and copious salivation may occur, as may diarrhea.

Other signs of toxicity include headache, fatigue, malaise, drowsiness, neuralgic pain, blurred vision, aphasia, and hallucination. Confusion, vision problems, and disorientation are the most common adverse reactions in the aged; and it is here that keen nursing assessment and communication with the physician can correct drug-induced senility. When potassium is lost, which sensitizes the heart to the toxic effects of digoxin, digitalis toxicity is promoted. Offering potassium-rich foods or supplements may prevent this problem. In order to reduce gastric discomfort, digoxin can be administered with meals. Digitalis preparations are quite irritating to the tissues and should not be given subcutaneously. Intramuscular forms should be given deep into the gluteal muscles and used only when absolutely necessary, due to the discomfort, the possible development of sterile abscesses, and the uncertainty regarding absorption.

In addition to observing for adverse reactions, an important nursing measure is checking the pulse rate prior to the administration of digoxin. Apical pulse is recommended, and when the apical pulse rate is lower than 60, the drug should be withheld until the physician is consulted and makes a decision. If patients are being prescribed digoxin on an outpatient basis, careful instruction is required. Older persons must be able to find and take their radial pulse and must have the visual capacity to see the second hand on a clock in order to count a minute. Confusion or memory problems can interfere with the accurate counting of the pulse rate, and it is wise to obtain a periodic return demonstration from other individuals to evaluate their capacity for this skill. Families can assist with this procedure and they should receive instruction and be made aware of the signs of toxicity.

General Anesthetics, Hypnotics, and Sedatives

The aged respond differently to general anesthesia. Absorption, distribution, and elimination are delayed, and older persons frequently remain anesthetized longer than desired. Since the risk of respiratory and cardiovascular depression is high, a significantly reduced dose of the anesthetic has to be used. The nurse should evaluate vital signs frequently and promote activity in all body systems.

The aged are often prescribed hypnotics and sedatives for the treatment of insomnia, nocturnal restlessness, anxiety, acute confused states, and related disorders. The drug serves as either a hypnotic or sedative, depending on the dose prescribed. Unlike sedatives, hypnotics do not suppress mental activity, limit attention span, or diminish the ability to concentrate. Since a tolerance to sedatives can develop after several weeks of use, continued evaluation of their effectiveness is required. Nurses should be aware that restlessness, insomnia, and nightmares may occur after sedatives are discontinued. Some aged persons, especially those with some degree of mental impairment, demonstrate residual effects of these drugs for days after they are administered. The nurse should observe for limitations in cognitive functioning on the day following the administration of a sleeping medication; it is unwise to forfeit daytime awareness or independent functioning solely for a full night's sleep, especially since the lack of daytime activity and stimulation may be the cause of insomnia in the first place. As the aged are more vulnerable to the many hazards of immobility, the nurse should note reductions in body movements when these drugs are used. Many of these drugs produce hypotension, drowsiness, and impaired coordination, and nurses should provide assistive measures and educate patients regarding safety considerations.

Chloral hydrate is an effective sedative and hypnotic used in the aged. This drug tends to produce less toxicity and fewer residual effects than many other similar drugs. Usually, chloral hydrate is not prescribed for patients with cardiac disease because it has a depressant action on the heart. The nurse should monitor vital signs and carefully observe for signs of decreased cardiac function. Chloral hydrate is avoided or cautiously used with patients receiving anticoagulant therapy.

Barbiturates. Since an older person reacts more sensitively to barbiturates, they are used carefully. Barbiturates are stored in adipose tissue, and the increased proportion of adipose tissue in an aged person's body can result in an accumulation of these drugs. Since barbiturates are detoxified in the liver, they should be used cautiously if a patient's liver functioning is impaired. Their depressant action warrants caution if a patient has respiratory difficulties. Barbiturates should not be given if other depressants to the central nervous system are being used. Nurses should be aware that barbiturates lower the basal metabolic rate, blood pressure, and mental activity, and that care has to be adjusted accordingly, allowing ample time for activities. Since barbiturates will reduce peristalsis, predisposing the patient to constipation, the nurse should also observe bowel patterns.

A dependence on these drugs can cause symptoms of barbiturate poisoning, including decreased physical and mental function, anxiety, insomnia, amnesia, and cardiac and gastrointestinal disorders. Acute barbiturate poisoning can cause respiratory depression, apnea, severe central nervous system depression, and circulatory collapse. Less severe but important adverse reactions include lethargy, nausea, vomiting, bronchospasm, residual sedation, and general allergic reactions. Barbiturates may decrease the potency of anticoagulant therapy, which could subject the individual to other health threats as well. If a tolerance to these drugs develops with prolonged use, there may be a tendency for the individual to increase the dosage; this can produce adverse reactions and should be discouraged.

Barbiturates are serious drugs and must be used selectively and cautiously, especially with the elderly, whose functioning is already declined and who may be more susceptible to adverse reactions. Nurses should attempt to find alternative means to relax the older individual, with back rubs, warm milk, a quiet environment, etc., using barbiturates only when absolutely necessary and not as a routine measure. Glutethimide is sometimes employed as a barbiturate substitute, producing beneficial and less toxic effects. Paraldehyde and bromides are rarely used as hynotics or sedatives in the aged.

Insulin and Oral Hypoglycemic Agents

Hypoglycemia is a more probable and serious problem than ketosis in older diabetics. Unfortunately, the classic signs and symptoms of hypoglycemia are sometimes replaced by other ones in the aged. Instead of restlessness, tachycardia, and profuse perspiration, symptoms may include speech disorders, confusion, and disorientation; these may be easily mistaken for "senility" in the aged. Keen nursing observation and thorough education for patient and family are essential. Some medications—such as antibacterial sulfonamides, phenylbutazone, salicylates, propranolol, probenecid, dicoumarol, and MAO inhibitors—are capable of potentiating a hypoglycemic reaction. The action of barbiturates and alcohol may be prolonged by some oral hypoglycemics.

For a more thorough discussion of these drugs, see Chapter 12.

Laxatives

A reduction of peristalsis, activity, and bulk and fluids in the diet are among the causes of constipation in the aged. Add to these factors the belief of many aged persons that a daily bowel movement is essential, and it is easy to understand why laxatives are so widely used, and abused, in the older population. Measures to promote bowel elimination without the use of laxatives (discussed in Chapter 7) should be implemented before resorting to medications. When laxatives are necessary, they should be selectively chosen and used. Diocytyl sodium sulfosuccinate (Colace) is a stool softener often prescribed for older persons. It is not irritating to the intestinal tract and usually promotes a bowel movement in from one to three days after administration of the initial dose. Peri-Colace has the stool softening action of Colace but adds a mild stimulant which provides gentle peristalsis. A bowel movement usually results in from 8 to 12 hours following the administration of Peri-Colace.

Bisacodyl (Dulcolax) stimulates peristalsis and is available in tablet or suppository form; the oral form is effective in approximately 6 hours, and the suppository form in from 15 to 60 minutes. Supportive measures, such as exercise, drinking plenty of fluids, and ingesting bulk foods, are beneficial. The nurse should observe for the effectiveness of these agents and consult with the physician if results are not obtained within a reasonable time. Mineral oil should be discouraged as a laxative for the aged because it interferes with the absorption of fat-soluble vitamins. Bulk laxatives are also not advised because many of them require chewing of a pellet form, a difficult activity for most older individuals. Magnesium preparations should be used carefully; they may reduce the already reduced acidity of the gastric environment and interfere with the digestive process or the effectiveness of medications requiring gastric acidity for action.

General Principles

There are many risks associated with drug therapy in the aged. On the other hand, there are many benefits derived by the aged from the use of medications. The benefits must be weighed with the problems in assessing whether or not a given drug is advantageous. If an older individual is able to maintain an active life style as a result of the relief aspirin provides his arthritic joints, he may be willing to tolerate the slight gastric discomfort from the drug. However, he may not be willing to tolerate dulled mental activity throughout the day to benefit from a sedative which provides a full night's sleep.

At no time should a valuable drug be withheld due to an individual's age. The aged should have the same opportunity as the young to benefit from drug therapy and achieve their optimum level of well-being. Rather than fearing or completely discouraging drug use in the aged, those providing care should use drugs discreetly, selectively, and intelligently.

REFERENCES

Bender, A. D. "Effect of Age on Intestinal Absorption: Implications for Drug Absorption in the Elderly." *Journal of the American Geriatrics Society,* 16:1331, 1968.

Boyd, J. R., Covington, T. R., Stanaszek, W. F., and **Coussons, R. T.** "Drug Defaulting, II: Analysis of Noncompliance Patterns." *American Journal of Hospital Pharmacy,* 31:485–491, 1974.

Brady, E. S. "Drugs and the Elderly." In Davis, R. S. (ed.), *Drugs and the Elderly.* Andrus Gerontology Center, Univ. of Southern Calif. Los Angeles, 1973, pp. 2–3.

Caranasos, G. J., Stewart, R. B., and **Cluff, L. E.** "Drug Induced Illness Leading to Hospitalization." *Journal of the American Medical Assoc.,* 228:713–717, 1974.

Davies, D. E., and **Shock, N. W.** "Age Changes in Glomerular Filtration Rate. Effective Renal Plasma Flow and Tubular Excretory Capacity in Adult Males." *Journal of Clinical Investigation,* 29:496, 1950.

Hoddinott, B. C., Gowdey, C. W., Coulter, W. K., and **Parker, J. M.** "Drug Reactions and Errors in Administration on a Medical Ward." *Canadian Medical Assoc. Journal,* 97:1001–1006, 1967.

Hoffman, A. M. (ed.). *The Daily Needs and Interests of Older People.* Thomas, Springfield, Ill., 1970, pp. 200–201.

Hurwitz, N. "Admissions to Hospital Due to Drugs." *British Medical Journal,* 1:539–540, 1969.

——— and **Wade, O. L.** "Intensive Hospital Monitoring of Adverse Reactions to Drugs." *British Medical Journal,* 1:531–536, 1969.

Miller, J. H., McDonald, R. K., and **Shock, N. W.** "Age Changes in the Maximal Rate of Renal Tubule Reabsorption of Glucose." *Journal of Gerontology,* 7:196, 1952.

Rossman, Isadore (ed.). *Clinical Geriatrics.* Lippincott, Philadelphia, 1971, p. 24.

Schwartz, D., Wang, M., Zeitz, L., and **Goss, M. E. W.** "Medication Errors Made by Elderly, Chronically Ill Patients." *American Journal of Public Health,* 52:2018–2029, 1962.

Seidl, L. G., **Thornton**, G. F., **Smith**, J. W., and **Cluff**, L. E. "Studies on the Epidemiology of Adverse Drug Reactions, III. Reactions in Patients on a General Medical Service." *Johns Hopkins Hospital Bulletin*, 119:229–315, 1966.

Task Force on Prescription Drugs. *Final Report.* U.S. Dept. of Health, Education, and Welfare, 1969.

Wade, O. L. "Drug Therapy in the Elderly." *Age and Ageing*, 1:65, 1972.

23

SEXUALITY

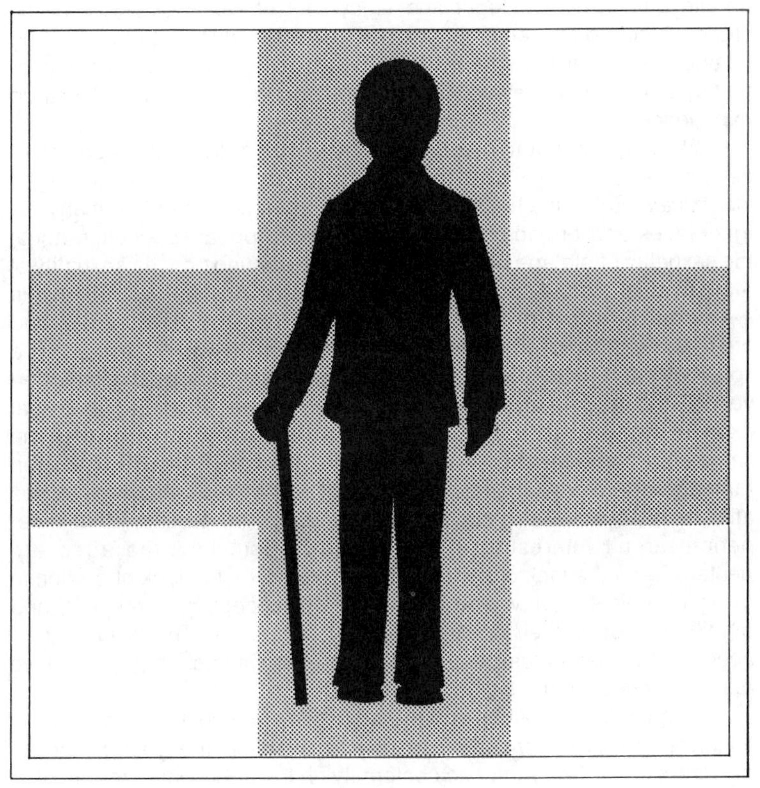

For many years, sex was a major conversational taboo in our country. Discussion and education concerning this natural, normal process was discouraged and avoided in most circles. Literature on the subject was minimal and usually secured under lock and key. An interest in sex was considered sinful and highly improper. There was an awareness that sexual intercourse had more than a procreative function, but the other benefits of this activity were seldom openly shared and sexual expression outside of wedlock was viewed as disgraceful and indecent. The reluctance to accept and intelligently confront human sexuality led to the propagation of numerous myths, the persistence of ignorance and prejudice, and the relegation of sex to a vulgar status.

Fortunately, attitudes have changed over the years, and sexuality has come to be increasingly understood, and accepted as natural and pleasurable. Education has helped erase the mysteries of sex for both adults and children, and magazines and books on the topic flourish. Sex courses, workshops, and counselors throughout the country are helping people gain greater insight and enjoyment of sex. Not only has the stigma attached to premarital sex been greatly reduced, but increasing numbers of unmarried couples are living together with society's acceptance. Sex is now viewed as a natural, good, and beautiful shared experience.

Natural, good, and *beautiful* for the varied individuals in society—seldom are these terms used to describe the sexual experiences of *aged individuals.* When the topic of sex and the aged is confronted, many old ignorances and prejudices concerning sex reappear. Education about the sexuality of old age is minimal; literature abounds on the sexuality of all individuals in the society *except the elderly.* Any signs of interest in sex or open discussions of sex by older persons are discouraged, and often labeled as lecherous. The same criteria which would make a man a "playboy" at age 30 makes him a "dirty old man" at age 70. Unmarried young and middle-aged adults who engage in pleasurable sexual experiences are accepted—but widowed grandparents seeking the same enjoyment are often viewed with disbelief and disgust. Myths run rampant. How many times do we hear that women lose all desire for sex after menopause, that older men can't achieve an erection, that older people aren't interested in sex anyhow? Somehow the aged are neutered—by the lack of privacy afforded them, by the lack of credence given to their sexuality, and by the lack of acceptance, respect, and dignity granted to their continued sexual expression. The myths, ignorance, and vulgar status previously associated with sex in general have been conferred on the sexuality of the aged.

Such misconceptions and prejudices are an injustice to persons of all ages. They reinforce any fears and aversion the young have to growing old, and they impose conformity on the aged which require that they either forfeit warm and meaningful sexual experiences or suffer feelings of guilt and abnormality. Nurses can play a significant role in educating and counseling about sexuality and the aged; they can encourage attitudinal changes by their own example. A good perspective regarding sexuality is required because sexuality encompasses much more than a physical sexual act. It includes the love, warmth, caring, and sharing between people; a seeing beyond the gray hair, wrinkles, and other manifestations of aging; an exchange of words and touches by sexual human beings. Feeling important to someone else and wanted by him or her promotes security, comfort, and emotional well-being. With the multiple losses of roles and functions that the aged experience, the comfort and satisfaction derived from a meaningful relationship are especially significant.

Sexuality also includes expressing oneself and being perceived as man or woman, although many persons are currently attempting to eliminate masculine and feminine stereotypes. Today's aged were socialized into masculine and feminine roles—the aged have had a lifetime of experience with the understanding that men are to be aggressive, independent, and strong and that women are to be pretty, dainty, and dependent on their male counterparts. It is difficult and just as unfair to try to alter the roles of aged persons as it is to try to convince today's liberated woman that she is limited to the roles of wife and mother. The socialization of today's older population and their role expectations must be recognized and respected. Yet nurses may witness subtle or blatant violations of respect to the aged's sexual identity. Examples of such a lack of respect are not hard to find:

- Belittling the aged's interest in clothing, cosmetics, and hairstyles
- Dressing men and women residents of an institution in similar and asexual clothing
- Denying a woman's request for a female aide to bathe her
- Forgetting to button, zip, or fasten clothing when dressing the elderly
- Unnecessarily exposing aged individuals during examination or care activities
- Discussing incontinent episodes when the involved individual's peers are present
- Ignoring a man's desire to be cleaned and shaved before his female friend visits
- Not recognizing attempts by the aged to look attractive
- Joking about two aged persons' interest in and flirtation with each other

Why is it so difficult to understand that a recognition of sexual identity is important to the aged? It is not unusual for a 30-year-old to be interested in the latest fashions, for two 35-year-old's to be dating, or for a 20-year-old female to prefer a gynecologist who is a woman. Most any younger woman would panic if a new date saw her before she had time to adjust her cosmetics, hair, and clothing. Chances are that no care provider would walk into the room of a 25-year-old in traction and precede to undress and bathe him in full view of other patients in the room. The aged require the same dignity and respect and appreciate the same recognition as sexual human beings that is afforded to persons of other ages. The aging process does not negate one's sex or alter the significance of sexual identity.

SEXUAL INTERCOURSE

With the exception of the outstanding work done by Pearl in 1925, Kinsey in 1934, and Masters and Johnson in 1966, there has been minimal exploration into the realities of sex in old age. Research has primarily involved small numbers of persons, and valid data are scarce. Possibly contributing to the lack of research and information are the following factors:

1. The acceptance and expansion of sexology has been relatively recent.
2. Impropriety was formerly associated with open discussions of sex.
3. There is a misconception on the part of professionals, the aged, and the general public that the aged are neither interested in nor capable of sex.
4. Practitioners lack experience in, and do not have an inclination for, discussing sex with any age group. Even today, medical and nursing assessments frequently do not reflect inquiry into sexual history and activity.

Nurses should be aware of recent interest and research in the area of sex in old age and communicate these research findings to colleagues and clients in an effort to promote a more realistic understanding of the aged's sexuality. Research has disproven the belief that aged persons are not interested in, or capable of, engaging in sex; older individuals can enjoy the pleasures of sexual foreplay and intercourse. Since the general pattern of sexual behavior is found to be basically consistent throughout life, individuals who were disinterested in sex and had infrequent intercourse throughout their lifetime will not usually develop a sudden insatiable desire for sex in old age. On the other hand, a couple who has maintained an interest in sex and continued regular coitus throughout their adult life will most likely not forfeit this activity at any particular age. Homosexuality, masturbation, a desire for a variety of sexual partners, and other sexual patterns also continue into old age. Sexual styles, interests and expression must be placed in the perspective of a total life experience.

Although clinical data is minimal and additional research is necessary, some general statements can be made about sex in the later years. According to Masters and Johnson (1966a), there tends to be a decrease in sexual responsiveness and a reduction in the frequency of orgasm. Older males are slower to erect, mount, and ejaculate, and older females may experience dyspareunia as a result of less lubrication and a decreased distensibility and thinning of the vaginal walls. Many older females gain a new interest in sex, possibly because they no longer have to fear an unwanted pregnancy or because they have more time and privacy with their children grown and gone. While there are individual differences in the intensity and duration of sexual response in older people, for both sexes, regular sexual expression is important in promoting sexual capacity and maintaining sexual function. With good health and the availability of a partner, sexual activity can continue well into the seventh and eighth decades.

The findings from Masters and Johnson's clinical investigations into the sexual responses of older persons are presented in their fine book *Human Sexual Response*. Since only a brief summary is be presented in this text, the nurse is encouraged to review their work for more specific information. The sexual response cycle was divided arbitrarily into four phases to provide a means of description:

1. ***Excitement phase*** The initial excitement phase results from stimulation from any source.
2. ***Plateau phase*** Sexual tensions are intensified during the plateau phase, and if they reach an extreme, orgasm will be well achieved; if the tension level drops, the individual will enter the resolution phase.
3. ***Orgasmic phase*** In the orgasmic phase, which lasts a few seconds, sexual stimuli are released. Although the entire body is involved to varying degrees, the orgasm is primarily concentrated in the clitoris, vagina, and uterus of the female and in the penis, prostate, and seminal vesicles of the male.
4. ***Resolution phase*** Sexual tensions are lost during the resolution phase; the female is capable of additional orgasms if stimulated during this period.

Using these phases as a framework, some of the changes in the sexual cycle of the aged can be discussed.

The Aged Female

During the excitement phase, older women experience clitoral response and nipple erection similar to that of younger women. Sex flush, caused by superficial vasocongestive skin response, does not occur as frequently, and there is less muscle tension elevation in response to sexual stimuli. Whereas the labia majoris separates, flattens, and elevates in response to sexual tensions in younger women, these responses do not occur in older women. The reactions of the labia minoris are also reduced. The secretory activity of the Bartholin's gland is reduced, and to a greater degree, so is vaginal lubrication. The vaginal wall expansion of the excitement phase occurs to a lesser degree.

As with all phases of the sexual cycle, the intensity of the plateau phase is also reduced. The older female does not demonstrate the intensity of areolae engorgement that a younger female does. During the orgasmic phase, the older woman has vaginal contractions in the same fashion as the young woman; these contractions are of lesser duration in the aged female. As in the younger woman, there is a small degree of involuntary distension of the external urinary meatus. In the resolution phase, nipple erection continues to exist, possibly for hours after the orgasm. The older female may experience urinary frequency, urgency, and burning for several hours after intercourse.

The Aged Male

The aged male may require more direct stimulation to achieve an erection than the younger male. During the excitment phase, it may take two to three times longer to achieve full penile erection, although once achieved, it can be maintained for a longer period of time before ejaculation. There is a significant reduction in the scrotal vasocongestive response to sexual tension. Like the older female, the older male experiences a sex flush less frequently. The plateau phase tends to be slower in the older male, and it is possible that a full erection will not occur until just before ejaculation. Although the physiologic response during orgasm is similar to that of the younger male, the older male does have a slower orgasmic phase. During ejaculation there may be more of a seepage of semen rather than a forceful emission; the entire ejaculatory process may be less forceful. Orgasm may not occur during every intercourse, especially if there is frequent intercourse. The most significant difference in the resolution phase of the older male is that it is of longer duration.

In general, it can be stated that "if elevated levels of sexual activity are maintained from earlier years and neither acute nor chronic physical incapacity intervenes, aging males usually are able to continue some form of active sexual expression into the 70- and even 80-year age

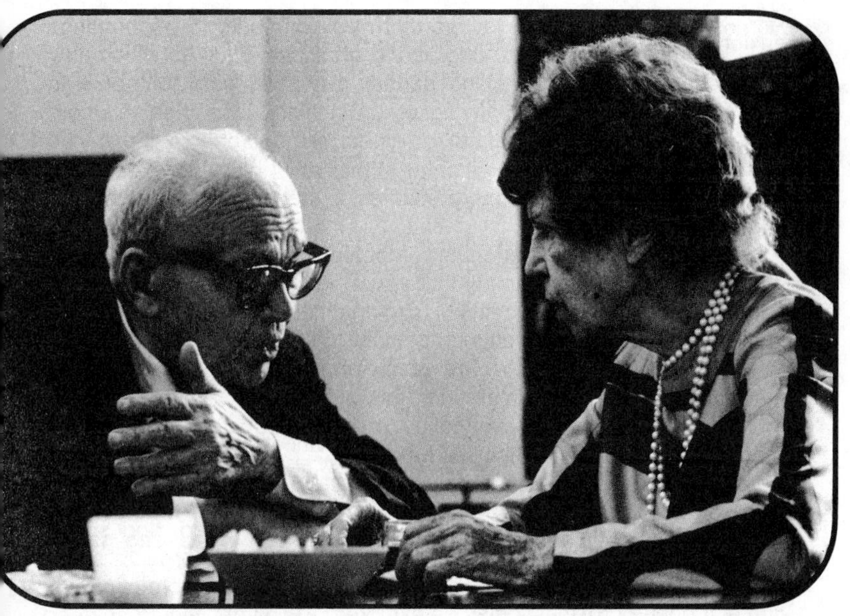

groups" (Masters and Johnson, 1966b). When there is a problem in the aged male's sexual functioning, the causes generally fall into one of six categories (Masters and Johnson, 1966c):

1. Monotony of a repetitious sexual relationship
2. Preoccupation with career or economic pursuits
3. Mental or physical fatigue
4. Overindulgence in food or drink
5. Physical or mental infirmities of either partner
6. Fear of performance associated with or resulting from any of the above

SEXUAL PROBLEMS

Impotence

The greatest sexual problem for males at any age is impotency. Although older males more frequently have organic causes for their impotency, psychological factors are most commonly responsible for this problem in males of all ages. Slower sexual response, less frequent and less forceful ejaculations, and irregular patterns of orgasms with intercourse are among the factors that may contribute to performance anxiety in the older male. A long period of disuse, such as which may occur when there has been no partner available, can contribute to impotency when an opportunity for sexual activity does arise. A single impotent experience may alarm or embarrass the aged male to the degree that he is discouraged from further attempts; this experience may also erroneously be interpreted as a signal of ceasing sexual function due to "old age."

The older male experiencing impotency needs reassurance that this does not necessarily imply that sexual function is lost forever. This male and his partner need realistic explanations regarding the possible causes of impotency and encouragement to continue their efforts. The partner should be made aware of the importance of patience and sensitivity in helping the male with this problem. The value of sexual counselors must not be overlooked in helping the aged male with impotency. Coupled with the need for reassurance, the aged male who is impotent can benefit from a thorough physical examination. Neurological disorders, undiagnosed diabetes, obesity, alcoholism, medications, and other organic causes for impotency can be treated, and sexual functioning can be improved in some situations. If the organic cause results in impotency which cannot be improved, the possible implantation of a penile prosthesis may be explored. At no time should an aged male's impotency be written off to "old age" or regarded as something which isn't really important to an older person.

Prostate problems are discussed in Chapter 16 and will not be repeated here. However, it is important to emphasize that a prostatectomy does not have to result in impotency. Some change in the pattern of ejaculation may be noted, but in most cases satisfying intercourse is possible. The male undergoing a prostatectomy needs reassurance and a realistic understanding regarding the effects of this surgery on his sexual performance. While understanding that his sexual capacity will not necessarily be destroyed, he must also be aware that he will not have a sudden or drastic improvement of sexual functioning following this surgery.

Physical and Mental Barriers

There are some factors which can interfere with sexual performance in both sexes. Drugs, such as many of the antihypertensives and tranquilizers, and alcohol can depress sexual capacity. Malnutrition, anemia, diabetes, and other physical disorders can interfere with sexual function, as can physical and emotional stress. Misconceptions, such as beliefs that intercourse is not possible after a hysterectomy or prostatectomy or that sexual activity is harmful to a cardiac disorder, may discourage sexual enjoyment. A practical problem, particularly common among women who traditionally marry older men and consequently are left widowed, is lack of a partner. Another barrier to sexual expression is the lack of privacy. In addition, the impact of concerns over how others will perceive one's interest in sex may significantly interfere with sexual performance.

Whenever possible, health problems should be identified and corrected; poor health can interfere with sexual interest and capacity at any age. Older persons may benefit from counseling regarding the effects of poor diet and alcohol on sexual capacity—factors they may not have considered as related to sex at all. Specific information concerning capacities and limitations of sexual activity in the light of any existing health problem is an important component of patient education. The nurse can help aged individuals by demonstrating an understanding, acceptance, and respect for them as sexually active human beings.

NURSING CONSIDERATIONS

There are a variety of ways in which the nurse can foster sexuality in the aged, some of which have already been discussed. Basic education can help the aged understand the effects of the aging process on sexuality by providing a realistic framework of sexual functioning. A willingness on the nurse's part to discuss sex openly with the aged demonstrates acceptance and respect for their sexuality. Physical, emotional, and social threats to the aged's sexuality should be recognized, and solutions should be sought for problems—whether caused by the disfigurement of surgery, obesity, depression, poor self-concepts, fatigue, or having no lock on a bedroom door to guarantee privacy.

Consideration must be given to the sexual needs of older persons in institutional settings. Too often, couples admitted to the same facility are not able to share a double bed, and frequently they aren't even able to share the same room if they are evaluated as requiring different levels of care. How unnatural, unreal, inhumane, and unfair to be forced to travel to another wing of a building to visit a person who has intimately shared 40, 50, or 60 years of one's lifetime. Where in most institutional settings can two such individuals find a place where they will not be interrupted or in full view of others? The aged in institutional settings have a right to privacy. They should be able to close and lock a door, feeling secure that this action will be honored. They should not be made to feel guilty or foolish by their expressions of love and sexuality. They should not have to have their sexuality sanctioned, screened, or severed by any other person.

There have been recommendations for "petting rooms" in institutional settings to provide an area for couples to have privacy. Although the value of such rooms in providing privacy is positive, their artificiality must be examined. How many young couples could relax and thoroughly enjoy sex in a room specifically labeled for such a purpose? Is privacy really provided when curious minds realize a couple is in this room and fantasize about the activities behind the closed doors? Perhaps it would be more natural and beneficial to respect the aged's privacy in their bedrooms and to designate periods of the day when residents know that they will not be disturbed unless an emergency develops. Nursing staff in such facilities should not overlook the basic courtesy of knocking on a person's door before entering a room.

Masturbation is often beneficial in releasing sexual tensions and maintaining continued function of the genitalia. The nurse can convey her acceptance and understanding of the value of this activity. The nurse's approving attitude and open view can help eliminate feelings of guilt or abnormality related to masturbation activities.

As mentioned throughout this chapter, it is vital for the nurse to be aware of, respect, and encourage the aged's sexuality. The nurse, as a role model, can foster a positive attitude regarding sex and the aged. Improved understanding, increased sensitivity, and humane attitudes can help today's and tomorrow's aged population realize the full potential of sexuality in the later years.

REFERENCES

Masters, W. H., and **Johnson, V. E.** *Human Sexual Response.* Little, Brown, Boston, 1966. (a) pp. 223–270; (b) p. 264; (c) p. 261.

24

THE DYING PROCESS

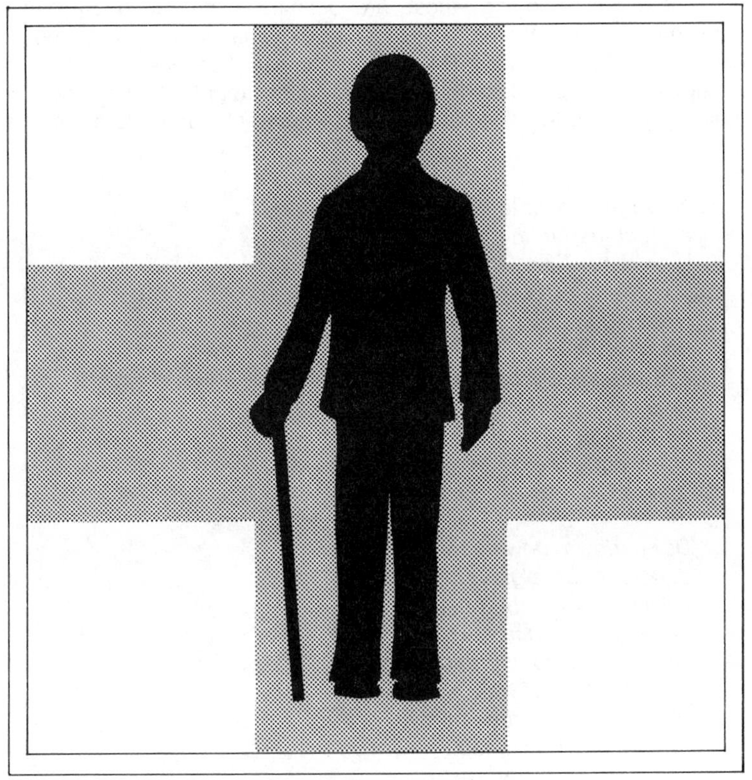

Death is an inevitable, unequivocal, and universal experience, common to all humanity. It is difficult for human beings to face, perhaps the most difficult and painful reality of all. Although a certainty, the cessation of life is often dealt with in terms of fury, fear, and flight. So reluctant are mortals to accept their mortality. . . .

It is difficult for the gerontological nurse to avoid facing the reality of death since over 80 percent of all who die are aged (Schultz, 1976). But it is not only the final event of death the gerontological nurse must learn to deal with; it is the entire dying process—the complex of experiences which dying individuals, their family, their friends, and all others involved with them must go through. It is far from easy to work with this complicated process, and it requires a fine blend of sensitivity, insight, and knowledge of the vast topic of death.

WHAT IS DEATH?

The final termination of life . . . the cessation of all vital functions . . . the act or fact of dying—these are definitions the dictionary offers concerning death, attempts at succinct explanations of this complex experience (McKechnie, 1974). But we humans are often reluctant to accept such simple descriptions of this inescapable thief of life. For example, the world of literature reflects many eloquent words on the topic:

Now I am about to take my last voyage,
a great leap in the dark.
THOMAS HOBBS

Do not go gentle into that
good night,
Old age should burn and
rave at close of day;
Rage, rage against the dying
of the light.
DYLAN THOMAS

Down, down, down into the
darkness of the grave,
Gently they go, the beautiful,
the tender, the kind;
Quietly they go, the intelligent,
the witty, the brave.
I know. But I do not approve.
And I am not resigned.
EDNA ST. VINCENT MILLAY

Death hath this also, that it
openeth the gate to good fame,
and extinguisheth envy.
FRANCIS BACON

Each person is born to one
possession which outvalues
all the others—his last breath.
MARK TWAIN

The night comes on that
knows not morn,
When I shall cease to be
all alone,
To live forgotten, and love forlorn.
TENNYSON

For so the game is ended
That should not have begun.
A. E. HOUSMAN

For as we well wot, that
a young man may dye
soon: so be we very sure
that an olde man cannot
live long.
SIR THOMAS MORE

Thou shalt come to thy grave
in a full age, like as a shock
of corn cometh in his season
JOB 5:26

The silence of that dreamless sleep
I now envy too much to weep.
BYRON

Death is fortunate for the
child, bitter to the youth,
too late to the old.
PUBLILIUS SYRUS

Death is the mother of beauty.
WALLACE STEVENS

Throughout Shakespeare's voluminous works there is a recurrent mention of death:

. . . death—
The undiscover'd country, from
whose bourne
No traveller returns.
HAMLET

The stroke of death is as
a lover's pinch,
Which hurts, and is desir'd.
ANTONY AND CLEOPATRA

A man can die but once:
We owe God a death.
HENRY IV

Dramatic, or amusing, the descriptions of death offered in popular literature have done little to enhance our knowledge of its true meaning. Current scientific literature does not provide much more in the way of specific, definite definitions of death. There is the United Nations Vital Statistics definition that death is the permanent disappearance of every vital sign. But then there are terms such as *brain death,* death of brain cells determined by a flat electroencephalograph reading; *somatic death* determined by the absence of cardiac and pulmonary functions; and *molecular death,* determined by the cessation of cellular function. The controversy lies in deciding at which level of death a person is considered dead. There are situations in which an individual with a flat EEG still has cardiac and respiratory functions; could this individual be said to be dead? There are also situations in which individuals with flat EEGs and no cardiopulmonary functions still have living cells that permit their organs to be transplanted; are individuals really dead if they possess living cells? The answers to these questions are not easy or simple. Much current thought and investigation is focused on the need for a single criterion in the determination of death.

THE REALIZATION OF MORTALITY

There was a time when most births and deaths occurred in the home. In extended family living, more older persons were part of the household and could be naturally observed as they grew old and died. Direct contact with births and the dying process was not uncommon. Viewed as natural processes, these events were managed by familiar

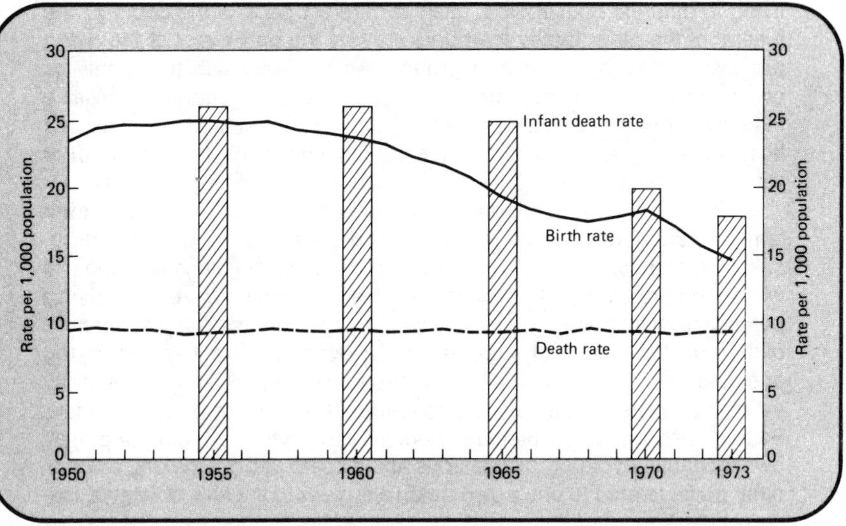

Figure 24-1. Changes in birth and death rates from 1950 to 1973. (Source: U.S. Bureau of the Census, *Statistical Abstract of the United States, 1975,* p. 52.)

faces in familiar surroundings. Intimate encounters with the beginning and end of life were rich experiences that provided insights and helped foster understanding of these realities. Perhaps the family felt a certain comfort and closeness by being with and doing for the life about to begin or end. And who can determine the benefit to the infant or the dying individual of being comforted and cared for by close loved ones? A high mortality rate also made experiences with the dying process more common in days past (Figure 24-1). Not only were living conditions poor, health care facilities inadequate, disease control techniques limited, and technologies to fight and control nature's elements unheard of, but there were fewer numbers of hospitals and other institutions in which people could die.

As Figure 24-1 indicates, the mortality rate has decreased over the years. Health and medical care are now more available and accessible, and new medications and therapeutic interventions increase the possibility of surviving an illness. Sophisticated and widespread life-saving technologies and improved standards of living have also lowered the number of deaths in the population. The declining mortality rate is one of several factors that have limited our experience with the dying process. Another factor is that our more mobile nuclear families are frequently comprised of young members, with older parents and grandparents living in different households, often in different parts of the country. The funeral of the older family members may be the only event of the dying process shared by other age groups. Aged persons in the family or community will most likely not die in their familiar environment. With a majority of deaths occurring in an institutional setting, and over half in a hospital setting, rarely do family and friends remain with the individual or witness the dying process (Butler, 1975a).

The separation of individuals from their loved ones and their familiar surroundings during the dying process seems discomforting, stressful, and unjust. "The final indignity in hospitals is to isolate the old when they are dying" (Butler, 1975b). How inhumane to remove dying persons from intimate involvement with their support systems at the time of their greatest need for support. As our direct experiences with dying and death are lessened, death becomes a more impersonal and unusual event. Its reality is difficult to internalize; it is held at arm's distance. Perhaps this explains why many persons have difficulty accepting their own mortality. Avoiding discussions about death and not making a will or other plans related to one's own death are clues to the lack of internalization of one's mortality. Although the topic of death can be confronted on an intellectual level, it is often this internalization of life's finiteness that remains difficult.

In order to assist the dying and their families effectively, nurses should analyze their own attitudes toward death. Denying their own mortality or feeling angry about it, nurses may tend to avoid dying persons or discourage their efforts to deal realistically with their death or instill false hopes in them and their families. The difficult process of confronting and realizing one's own mortality need not be viewed as depressing by the nurse; it can provide a fuller appreciation of life and the impetus for making the most of every living day. Nurses who understand their own mortality are more comfortable helping individuals through their dying process. A very special book that may be helpful to nurses is *Gramps,* which depicts an aged man's dying experience narratively and photographically (Jury and Jury, 1976). With honesty and sensitivity, the family supports this dying man in his familiar surroundings as his life is declining. The children, grandchildren, and great-grandchildren who share Gramp's dying experience do so with extraordinary warmth, love, and naturalness. One cannot help but marvel at how these individuals learn to accept their own mortality by sharing this process.

SUPPORTING THE DYING INDIVIDUAL

For a long time nurses were more prepared to deal with the care of a dead body than with the dynamics involved with the dying process. Not only was open discussion of an individual's impending death rare, but it was not unusual for the dying person to be moved to a separate and often isolated location during the last few hours of life. If the family was present, they were frequently left alone with the dying person, without benefit of a professional person. Rather than planning for additional staff support for the dying person and his family, nurses were concerned with whether a patient would live until their next shift and require postmortem care. When death did occur, the body was removed from the unit in secrecy so that other patients wouldn't be aware of the event. Nurses were discouraged from "showing emotion" when a patient died. A detached objectivity was promoted as part of nursing the dying patient.

Nursing has now moved toward a more humanistic approach to caring for the dying patient. Emphasis on meeting the total needs of the patient has stimulated greater concern for the psychosocial care of the dying. There is now recognition that family and "significant others" play a vital role in the dying process, and must be considered by the nurse. Knowledge has increased in the field of thanatology (the study of death and dying), and more nurses are exposed to this body of knowledge. The nursing profession has come to realize that professionalism does not negate human emotions in the nurse-patient relationship. These factors have contributed to increased nursing involvement with the dying individual. Since the dying process is unique for every human being, individualized nursing intervention is required. Previous experiences with death, religious beliefs, philosophy of life, age, and health status are among the multitude of complex ingredients affecting the dying process. The nurse must carefully assess the particular experiences, attitudes, beliefs, and values that all individuals bring to their dying process. Only through this assessment can the most therapeutic and individualized support be given to the dying person.

Coping Mechanisms and Related Nursing Intervention

Although the dying process varies in each individual, common reactions that have been observed to occur provide a basis for generalizations. Elizabeth Kubler-Ross, after several years of experiences with dying patients, developed a conceptual framework outlining the coping mechanisms of dying in terms of five stages (1969). It behooves the nurse to be familiar with these stages and to understand the most therapeutic nursing interventions during each stage. Not all dying persons will progress through these stages in an orderly sequence. Neither will every dying person experience all of these stages. However, an awareness of Kubler-Ross' conceptual framework can assist the nurse in supporting dying individuals as their many complex reactions to death are demonstrated. A brief description of these stages is provided below, along with pertinent nursing considerations.

Denial and isolation. Upon becoming aware of their impending death, most individuals initially react by denying the reality of the situation. "It isn't true" and "there must be some mistake" and "they're wrong, not me" are among the comments reflective of this denial. Patients sometimes "shop" for a physician who will suggest a different diagnosis or invest in healers and fads that promise a more favorable outcome. Denial serves several useful purposes for the dying person: it is a shock absorber after learning the difficult and shocking news that one has a terminal condition; it provides an opportunity for people to test the certainty of this information; it allows people time to internalize this information and mobilize their defenses.

Although the need is strongest during the early stages, dying persons may use denial at various times throughout their illness. They may fluctuate between wanting to discuss their impending death and denying its reality. The nurse must be sensitive to the person's need for defenses while also being ready to participate in dialogues on death when the person needs to do so. Contradictions may occur, and although these can be confusing, the nurse should try to accept the dying person's use of defenses rather than focus on the conflicting messages. People's individual life philosophy, their unique coping mechanisms, and the knowledge of their condition will determine when denial will be replaced for less radical defense mechanisms. Perhaps the most important nursing action during this stage is to accept the dying individual's reactions and provide an open door for honest dialogue.

Anger. The stage of denial is gradually replaced, and the "No, not me" reaction is substituted for one of "Why me?" The second stage, anger, is often extremely difficult for individuals surrounding the dying person since they are frequently the victims of displaced anger. In this stage, the dying person expresses the feeling that nothing is right. Nurses don't answer the call lights soon enough; the food tastes awful; the doctors don't know what they're doing; and visitors either stay too long or not long enough. Seen through the eyes of the dying person, this anger is understandable. Why wouldn't people resent not having what they want when they want it when they won't be wanting it very much longer? Why wouldn't they be envious of those who will enjoy a future they will never see? Their unfulfilled desires and the unfinished business of their life may cause outrage. Perhaps their complaints and demands are used to remind those around them that they are still living beings.

During this time, the family may feel guilt, embarrassment, grief, and anger as a result of the dying person's anger. They may not understand why their intentions are misunderstood or their actions unappreciated. It is not unusual for them to question whether they are doing things correctly. The nurse can help the family gain insight into

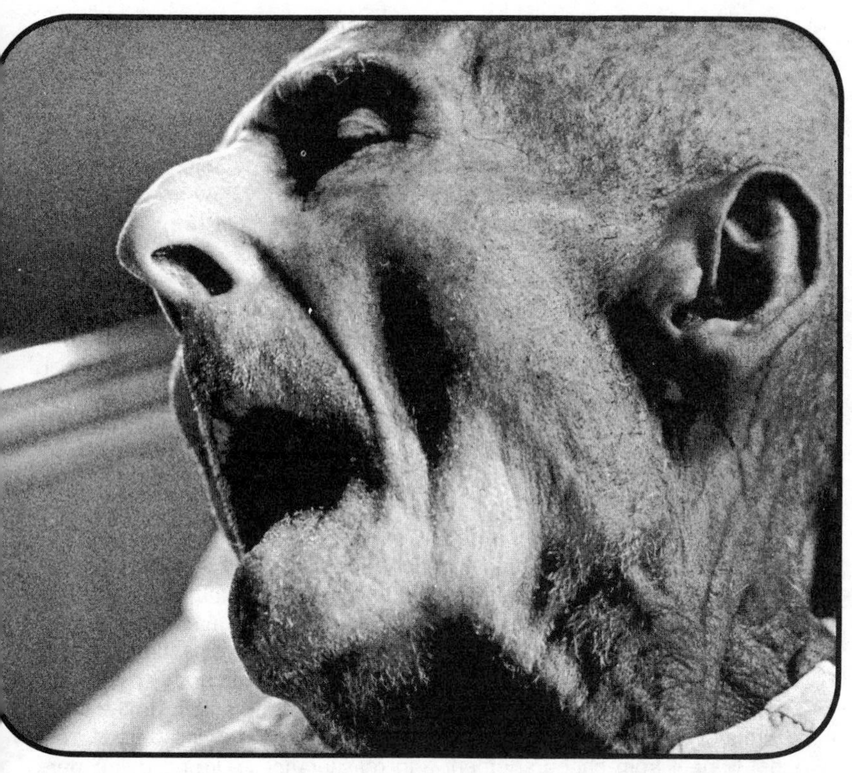

the individual's behavior which will relieve their discomfort and, thereby, create a more beneficial environment for the dying person. If the family can be brought to a realization that the person is reacting to impending death and not to them personally, it may facilitate a supportive relationship and prevent guilt feelings.

The nurse should also guard against responding to the dying person's anger as a personal affront. The best nursing efforts may receive criticism for not being good enough; cheerful overtures may be received with scorn; the call light goes on the minute the nurse leaves the room. It is important that the nurse assess such behavior and understand that it may reflect the anger of the second stage of the dying process. Instead of responding to the anger, the nurse should be accepting, implying to the dying person that it is all right to vent these feelings. Anticipating needs, remembering favorite things, and maintaining a pleasant attitude can counterbalance the anticipated losses that are becoming more apparent to the dying individual. It may be useful for the nurse to discuss her feelings about the patient's anger with an objective colleague who can serve as a sounding board; and to validate that the relationship continues to be therapeutic.

Bargaining. After recognizing that denying and being angry don't change the reality of impending death, dying persons may attempt to negotiate a postponement of the inevitable. They may agree to be a better Christian if God lets them live through one more Christmas; they may promise to help themselves more if the physician initiates aggressive therapy to prolong life; they may promise anything in return for an extension of life. Most bargains are made with God and usually kept a secret. Sometimes such agreements are shared with clergymen. The nurse should be aware that dying persons may feel disappointed at not having their bargain honored or guilty over the fact that having gained time, they want an additional extension of life, even though they agreed that the request would be their last. It is important that these often covert feelings be explored with the dying person.

Depression. When a patient is hospitalized with increasing frequency and has a declining functional capacity and a greater prevalence of symptoms, the reality of the dying process is emphasized. The aged patient may already have had many losses and experienced depression. Not only may lifetime savings, pleasurable pastimes, and a normal lifestyle be gone, but bodily functions and even bodily parts may be lost. All this quite understandably leads to depression. Unlike other forms of depression, however, the depression of the dying person may not benefit from encouragement and reassurances. Urging dying persons to cheer up and look at the sunny side of things implies that they shouldn't contemplate their impending death. It is unrealistic to believe that since most of us normally grieve the loss of a significant person or object, dying people shouldn't be deeply saddened by the most significant loss of all—their life.

The depression of the dying person is usually a silent one. It is important for the nurse to understand that cheerful words may be far less meaningful to dying individuals than holding their hand or silently sitting with them. Being with this person as he openly or silently contemplates his future is a significant nursing action during this stage. The nurse may also have to help the family understand this depression, explaining that their efforts to cheer the dying person can hinder his or her emotional preparation rather than enhance it. The family may require reassurance for the helplessness they feel at this time. The nurse might emphasize that this type of depression is necessary in order for the individual to be able to approach death in a stage of acceptance and peace. An interest in prayer and a desire for visits from a clergyman are commonly seen during this stage. The nurse should be particularly sensitive to the dying person's religious needs and facilitate the clergy-client relationship in every way possible.

Acceptance. For many dying persons, there comes a time when the struggling ends and relief ensues. It is as though a final rest is being taken to gain the strength for a long journey. This acceptance should not be mistaken for a happy state; it implies that the individual has come to terms with his or her death and found a special peace. During this stage, patients may benefit more from nonverbal than verbal communication. It is important that their silence and withdrawal not result in isolation from human contact. Touching, comforting, and being near the person are valuable nursing actions. An effort to simplify the environment may be required as the dying person's circle of interests gradually shrinks. It is not unusual for the family to need a great deal of assistance in learning to understand and support their loved one during this stage.

Hope during the five stages of dying. Significantly, hope commonly permeates all the stages of the dying process. Hope can be used as a temporary but necessary form of denial; as a rationalization for enduring unpleasant therapies; and as a source of motivation. It may provide a sense of having a special mission to comfort an individual through the last days. A realistic confrontation of impending death does not negate the presence of hope. In Cicero's succinct words, "While there's life, there's hope."

SUPPORTING FAMILY AND FRIENDS

Thomas Mann's comment that "a man's dying is more the survivors' affair than his own" is a reminder that the family and friends of the dying person should be considered in the nursing care of that person. They too may have needs requiring therapeutic intervention during the dying process of their loved one. Offering the appropriate support throughout this process may prevent unnecessary stress and provide immense comfort to those involved with the dying person. Just as dying persons experience different reactions as they cope with the reality of their impending death, so may the family and friends pass through the stages of denial, anger, bargaining, and depression before they are ready to accept the fact that a very special person in their lives is going to die. The reactions described below may be demonstrated by family and friends.

Denial and isolation This stage may involve discouraging patients from talking or thinking about death; visiting patients less frequently; stating that patients will be better as soon as they return home, start eating, have their intravenous tube removed, etc.; and "shopping" for a doctor or hospital who will have a special "cure" for the terminal illness.

Anger Reactions may include criticizing staff for the care they are giving; reproaching a family member for not paying attention to the patient's problem earlier; and questioning why someone who has led such a good life should have this happen.

Bargaining People may tell the staff that if they could take patients home they know they could improve their condition. Through prayers or open expression they may agree to take better care of the patient if given another chance. They may consent to take some particular action (go to church regularly, volunteer for good causes, give up drinking) if only the patient could live to a particular time.

Depression Family and friends may become more dependent on the staff. They may begin crying and limiting contact with the patient.

Acceptance In this stage people may react by wanting to spend a great deal of time with the dying person; telling the staff of the good experiences they've had with the patient and how they're going to miss him or her. They may request the staff to do special things for the patient (arrange for favorite foods, eliminate certain procedures, provide additional comfort measures). They may frequently remind the staff to be sure to contact them when "the time comes." They may begin making specific arrangements for their own lives without the patient (change of housing, plans for property, strengthen other relationships for support).

Obviously the type of nursing support will vary depending on the stage a family member or friend is assessed to be in. While the nursing actions described for the dying individual during each stage may be applicable for family and friends, the stages experienced by those involved with the dying person may not coincide with the patient's own timetable for these stages. For instance, patients may have already worked through the different stages, come to accept the reality of death, and be ready to openly discuss the impact of their death and make plans for their survivors. However, family members and friends may be at very different stages and not be able to deal with the patient's acceptance. The nurse must be aware of these discrepancies in stages and provide individualized therapeutic interventions. While providing appropriate support to family and friends as they pass through the stages, the nurse can offer opportunities for dying persons to discuss their death openly with a receptive party.

Helping the Family After a Death

When patients die, the nurse should be available to provide any needed support to the family. Some people wish to have several minutes in private with deceased patients to view and touch them. Others want the nurse to accompany them as they visit the deceased. Still others may not want to enter the room at all. The personal desires of the family and friends must be respected; nurses should be careful not to make value judgments of the family's reaction based on their own attitudes and beliefs. It is beneficial to encourage the family and friends to express their grief openly. Crying and shouting may help people cope with and work through their feelings about the death more than suppressing their feelings to achieve a calm composure. (Unfortunately, public figures have often been presented as reacting in a composed and stoical manner to a death, thus providing poor role models.)

Funeral and burial arrangements may require guidance by a professional also. The survivors of the deceased may be experiencing grief, guilt, or other reactions which place them in a very vulnerable position. At this time they are especially susceptible to sales pitches equating their love for the deceased to the cost of the funeral. Funerals may be arranged costing thousands of dollars more than survivors can actually afford, either depleting any existing savings or leaving a debt which will take years to repay. The family may need to have the extravagant plans presented by a funeral director counterbalanced by realistic questions concerning the financial impact of such a funeral. Someone must take the role of reminding the family that life does go on, and that their future welfare must be considered. Whether it be the nurse, a clergyman, or a neighbor, it is valuable to identify some person who can be an advocate for the family at this difficult time, and prevent them from being taken advantage of. (Rather than waiting for a death to occur before thinking through reasonable funeral plans, people should be encouraged to learn about the funeral industry and plan in advance for funeral arrangements.) In addition to books on the topic (e.g., Morgan, 1973), there are a number of memorial societies which can assist individuals in their planning.*

In addition to assisting the family through the funeral, someone should be available to check on family members several weeks after the death. After the excitement of the funeral has diminished and fewer visitors are calling to pay their respects, the full impact of the death may first be realized. Gorer (1965) has described the three stages of mourning as (1) a period of shock during the first few days following the

* More information on memorial societies can be obtained by contacting the Continental Association of Funeral and Memorial Societies, 59 East Van Buren Street, Chicago 60605.

death; (2) a period of intense grief lasting six to eight weeks; and (3) a period of reawakening of interest in life. As can be noted, intense grief occurs during that letdown period when fewer resources may be available to provide support. Several studies have revealed higher mortality rates in widowers, especially during the first year following the death (Glick et al., 1974; Hobson, 1964; Maddison and Viola, 1968; Parkes, 1976; Parkes and Brown, 1972). Since there are potential threats to the mourning individual's well-being, planned interventions may prove valuable. The gerontological nurse can arrange for a visiting nurse, a church member, a social worker, or some other resource to contact the family members several weeks following the death to make sure they are not experiencing any crisis. Widow-to-widow and similar groups support individuals through their grieving process. It may also be beneficial to provide the phone number of a person who the family can contact if assistance is required.

Edwin Schneidman, who has done considerable "postventive" work with survivors, offers some concise guidance in working with the family and friends of the deceased (Shneidman, 1976):

1. Total care of a dying person needs to include contact and rapport with the survivors-to-be.
2. In working with survivor-victims of dire deaths, it is best to begin as soon as possible after the tragedy; within the first seventy-two hours if possible.
3. Remarkably little resistance is met from survivor-victims; most are willing to talk to a professional person, especially one who has no ax to grind and no pitch to make.
4. The role of negative emotions toward the deceased—irritation, anger, envy, guilt—needs to be explored, but not at the very beginning.
5. The professional plays the important role of reality tester. . . not so much the echo of conscience as the quiet voice of reason.
6. Medical evaluation of the survivors is crucial. One should be alert for possible decline in physical health and in overall mental well-being.

SUPPORTING THE NURSE

The staff working with the dying individual have their own set of feelings regarding this significant experience. It may be extremely difficult for nurses, not only to accept a particular patient's death, but to come to terms with the whole issue of death. As was discussed earlier in this chapter, some nurses share the difficulty many persons have realizing their own mortality. Nurses' experiences with death may be limited, as may their exposure to the subject through formal education. In a health profession where the emphasis is primarily on "curing," death may be viewed as a dissatisfying failure. Nurses may feel powerless as they realize that their best efforts can do little to overcome the reality of impending death.

It is not unusual for a nurse who is involved with a dying patient to also experience the stages of the dying process described by Elizabeth Kubler-Ross. Nurses are commonly observed to avoid contact with dying patients, tell a patient to "cheer up" and not think about death, continue to practice "heroic" measures although a patient is nearing death, and grieve at the death of a patient. Nurses may be limited in their ability to support patients and their families if they are at a different stage from them. For example, the nurse may be unable to accept that the patient is dying, and avoidance of the topic and unrealistic plans for the patient's future reflect this denial. The patient, however, may be at the point of accepting the reality of the dying process and may want to discuss personal feelings. Recognizing that the nurse is still denying, the patient may avoid an open discussion of death and be deprived of an important therapeutic activity.

The nurse working with a dying patient requires a great deal of support. Colleagues should help nurses explore their own reactions to dying patients and recognize when those reactions interfere with a therapeutic nurse-patient relationship. The attitude of colleagues and the climate of the environment should be such that nurses can retreat from a situation which is not therapeutic either for them or the patient. To encourage the nurse to cry or show emotions in other forms may be extremely beneficial. The utilization of thanatologists and other resource people may also be valuable in providing support to nurses as they assist an individual through the dying process.

REFERENCES

Butler, R. N. *Why Survive? Being Old in America.* Harper & Row, New York, 1975. (a) p. 218; (b) p. 191.

Glick, I. O., Weiss, R. S., and **Parkes, C. M.** *The First Years of Bereavement.* Wiley, New York, 1974.

Gorer, G. *Death, Grief and Mourning.* Doubleday (Anchor Books), New York, 1965.

Hobson, C. J. "Widows of Blackton." *New Society,* September 14, 1964.

Jury, Mark, and **Jury, Dan.** *Gramp.* Grossman, New York, 1976.

Kubler-Ross, E. *On Death and Dying.* Macmillan, New York, 1969.

Maddison, D., and **Viola, A.** "The Health of Widows in the Year Following Bereavement." *Journal of Psychosomatic Research,* 12:297, 1968.

Marris, P. *Widows and Their Families.* Routledge, London, 1958.

McKechnie, J. L. (ed.). *Webster's New Twentieth Century Dictionary of the*

English Language, Unabridged, 2nd ed. World Publishing Co., New York, 1974.

Morgan, E. *A Manual of Death Education and Simple Burial.* Celo Press, Chicago, 1973.

Parkes, C. M. "The Broken Heart." In Shneidman, E. S. (ed.), *Death: Current Perspectives.* Aronson Jason, New York, 1976, pp. 333–347.

——— and **Brown, R. J.** "Health After Bereavement: A Controlled Study of Young Boston Widows and Widowers." *Psychosomatic Medicine,* 34:449–461, 1972.

Schultz, R. "Meeting the Three Major Needs of the Dying Patient." *Geriatrics,* 31(6):132, June 1976.

Shneidman, E. S. "Postvention and the Survivor-Victim." In Shneidman, E. S. (ed.), *Death: Current Perspectives.* Aronson Jason, New York, 1976.

25

SERVICES FOR THE AGED

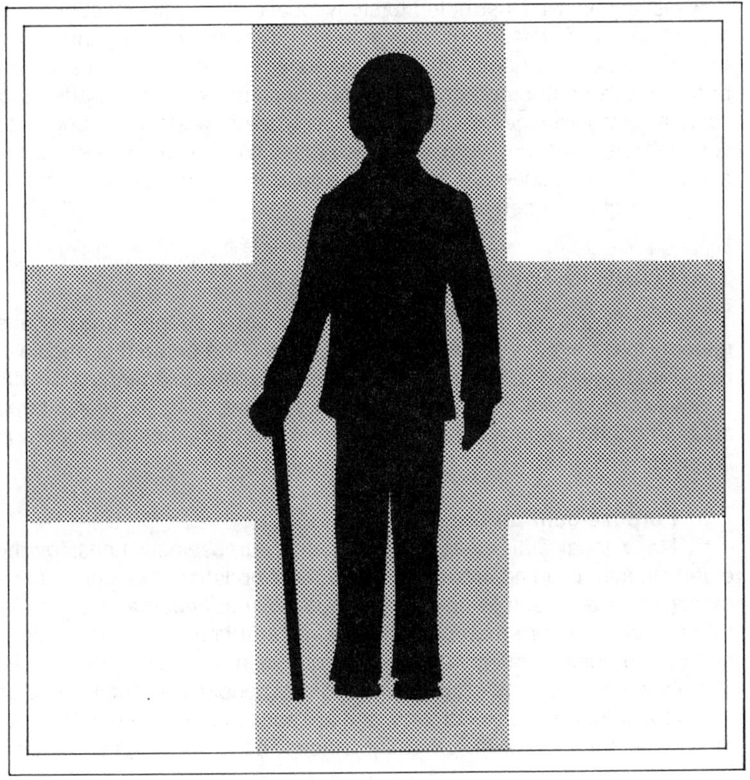

The Department of Health and Social Services, together with many voluntary and charitable organizations, endeavors to provide a comprehensive service for the aging population. Many of these services have evolved because of the social changes which have created new problems for the elderly. In the first half of this century the elderly often faced hardship and deprivation, but, with their families living close by, they did not face these problems alone. Now families are much more scattered, many women are working and do not devote all their time to the family. Slum clearance has broken up the old communities. Motorways, increased car ownership, and commuting have increased personal mobility, and have contributed to the break-up of the family unit. Elderly people are often left far from caring relatives. Solutions to the new problems have been seriously considered, some have been tried and tested, and, while it is by no means complete, a structure has been formed to deal with the new difficulties faced by the aged.

The Social Science Research Unit, set up in 1973 by the DHSS and now disbanded, was instructed to study local authority social services in the state of development. Voluntary and charitable organizations, through their vigilance and their understanding of the needs of old people, have contributed greatly to the constantly changing patterns of service. Many services for the aged which are now statutory began as voluntary services, but were soon seen to be indispensable. Even so, we are still short of a coherent policy in the organized services to minister to the needs of our elderly citizens.

LIVING IN THE COMMUNITY

This is a very desirable option for elderly people, and for the majority in Britain this is their way of life. Ninety-five percent of people of retirement age live in the community, either in their own homes or with relatives or companions; 2½ percent live in homes, hostels, or sheltered accommodation; and another 2½ percent are permanently resident in hospitals.

Purpose-built units

Many local authorities have included purpose-built units for the elderly in their building programs. The accommodation is designed to be managed by a person living alone who is likely to become less mobile. When such units are incorporated in a general housing estate, elderly people are, ideally, integrated into the community, finding interest and stimulation in other age groups. Units for old people are usually sited on the ground floor of a block of flats, and are specially designed for the use of elderly tenants, with carefully placed handrails, higher electric sockets, sensibly planned kitchens giving easy access to cupboards and heating apparatus, and centrally heated at an adequate and constant temperature.

Continuing to live in one's own home

This is a natural choice, but the premises may be difficult to manage, or even dangerous. Ill-lit passages, awkward stairs, or uneven floor surfaces may become more difficult as the person grows older. A visiting nurse or health visitor could advise on hazards likely to cause accidents, and how these hazards may be minimized. A visit from an occupational therapist should be requested, to consider the home as a whole and to recommend and implement the necessary changes needed for safety and comfort. Changes to be considered might include the installation of handrails on stairways and by baths and toilets, ramps to replace awkward steps, or even simply the rearrangement of furniture to make storage cupboards accessible without unnecessary bending, or worse, standing on chairs. Floor coverings, lighting, heating arrangements, and kitchen facilities can all be studied and probably improved.

Living with relatives

Caring for one's aged parents is by no means considered conventional today. However, many families in Britain do care for elderly relatives by incorporating them into the family home. This is done with varying degrees of success and mutual satisfaction.

Sheltered accommodation

This terms is used to describe a group of dwellings (flats or bungalows) which have a resident warden living within the group. Sheltered accommodation is an ideal home for an elderly person who is not completely able to manage alone, but who is unwilling to surrender independence to an institution. There is a call system, bell, or intercom to summon the warden in case of emergency or illness. Wardens also visit each unit regularly, once or twice weekly, depending on the need. The warden only takes on emergency duties, such as calling a doctor or nurse, and is not expected to carry out any nursing duties to the bed-fast. Sheltered accommodation allows the elderly freedom and complete independence, while giving them the extra confidence of an intermediary link with medical help. There is usually a commonroom for social gatherings, for those who need social contact.

Almshouses

There are about 2,000 almshouse trusts spread over the country. These trusts are registered charities, with ancient charters, and were set up originally by charitable groups of guilds, such as the goldsmiths. It is not surprising, therefore, that the buildings owned by the trusts are themselves very old. Nevertheless, most have been kept in good repair and are often quite picturesque. Over the years they have been modernized by the addition of central heating and bathrooms, these additions not detracting from the often charming exteriors.

Eligibility for the tenancy of an almshouse varies, depending on the conditions decided by each trust. Usually people who have been connected with the trade which the trust represents, or who were born in the area, are considered eligible. Application to live in an almshouse is made direct to the trustees, and the names and addresses can usually be obtained from the local old people's welfare organization. Like sheltered accommodation, the almshouse is a single self-contained unit, with an independent occupant. Some, but not all, have a warden living on the premises. Almshouses were probably the forerunner of sheltered accommodation.

Residential homes for the elderly

1. Local authority

Like many other aspects of gerontology, the planning and setting up of homes is developing with each new purpose-built establishment and is gradually improving. Residential accommodation varies greatly from place to place, depending on the age of the building, and the degree of enlightened information in the planning. It is the duty of all concerned with the care of the aged to make sure that the planners know what kind of structure is needed. Probably the best source of information on the ideal home for the aged is the consumers themselves.

Most of the newer homes accommodate between 20-40 people, largely in single rooms, but with a smaller number of double rooms. They have communal dining rooms and a commonroom for social activities. In addition to these newly built homes, some local authorities have adapted large private houses, which, while having some charm and character, may be situated in the country, away from shops and other urban facilities. They may be two-story buildings without lifts, and rooms may have to be shared. It is an advantage that such variations exist, provided the physical and emotional needs of the people are considered.

Admission to any local authority home is by application to the social services department which is responsible for their management. An application form is filled in after a visit by a social worker, who will discuss the needs and capabilities of the prospective resident. The social worker will find out if assistance is needed with bathing or dressing, if stairs can be managed safely, and if attention is required at night. An inquiry will be made about finance, and the charge for accommodation will be set according to the resident's ability to pay. The need for residential accommodation in homes is greater than the number of places available. If waiting is likely to cause hardship, arrangements can be made for residence in a private home, the fees being met jointly by the family and from public money, the respective amounts being negotiated by a social worker. Local authorities are authorized to provide this type of help, although in practice not all have the financial resources to do so.

2. Private homes

Accommodation in a privately run home is usually more readily available. The prices vary appreciably, depending on the locality and on the services offered. Choice may be limited by the price (which may vary from £30 to £100 per week). A social worker, who is familiar with the homes in the area, will advise if asked, and may arrange visits to a selection of homes to assist the prospective resident in making the right choice.

3. Homes run by voluntary organizations

Some registered charities run residential homes. These include religious bodies, professional and trade organizations. Some cater for specific handicaps, such as deafness or blindness. Application for admission is made to the head office. Here, too, the social worker or health visitor can advise on the suitability of someone seeking this type of accommodation.

TABLE 25.1 SOME ORGANIZATIONS WITH RESIDENTIAL HOMES

name and address of head office	no. of homes	
The Abbeyfield Society 35a High Street Potters Bar, Herts EN6 5DL	640	single lonely elderly; 8 to 10 residents with a housekeeper providing 2 meals a day; unfurnished rooms
The British Red Cross Society, 9 Grosvenor Crescent, London SW1X 7EJ	20	also 3 short-stay homes and 5 holiday homes (1 in Harrogate open all year)

The Church Army Sunset and Anchorage Homes, CSC House, North Circular Road, London NW10 7UG	13	2 for men only, 7 for women only; 1 short-stay home; mostly cubicled bedrooms; also hostels
Church of England Committee for Social Work and Social Services, Room 247, Church House, Dean's Yard, London SW1P 3NZ		can provide names and addresses of religious communities caring for elderly women and of homes specifically for members of C of E
The Civil Service Benevolent Fund, Watermead House, Sutton Court Road, Sutton, Surrey SM1 4TF	8	3 for seven residents only; 1 for disabled of all ages
Distressed Gentlefolks' Aid Association, Vicarage Gate House, Kensington, London W8 4AQ	10	elderly gentlefolk in reduced circumstances; 7 nursing homes; also flatlets
The Friends of the Elderly and Gentlefolk's Help, 42 Ebury Street, London SW1W 0LZ	12	3 for women only; over age of 70; single rooms, unfurnished
Jewish Welfare Board, 315–317 Ballards Lane, London N12 8LP	12	for those of Jewish faith; also some unfurnished sheltered flatlets in London and Herts
Methodist Homes for the Aged, 1 Central Buildings, London SW1H 9NS	34	primarily for Methodists; over age of 70

Mutual Households Associations, Cornhill House, 41 Kingsway, London WC2B 6UB	9	unfurnished apartments in country houses of historic or architectural interest; residents make capital loan on entry, then pay weekly
The Religious Society of Friends, Friends House, Euston Road, London NW1 2BJ	8	also some unfurnished flatlets with some meals provided and warden or housekeeper
The Royal British Legion, Pall Mall, London SW1Y 5JY	5	for ex-servicemen/women
Royal United Kingdom Beneficent Association, 6 Avonmore Road, London W14 8RL	24	3 run by RUKBA for women only. nomination rights in others; annuitants of RUKBA (gentlefolk with income below £1200; £1920 if married couple); also sheltered flatlets in London and Bexhill
The Salvation Army women's social services, 280 Mare Street, Hackney, London E8 1HE men's social services, 110–112 Middlesex Street, London E1 7HZ	40	eventide residences: 2 for men only, some for women only; over age of 70; ambulant
The SOS Society, 14 Culford Gardens, London SW3 2SU	5	2 for women only
Women's Royal Voluntary Service, 17 Old Park Lane, London W1Y 4AJ	23	average 25 residents; income less than about £2000 pa; also unfurnished flatlets with two meals provided and house manager

THE ELDERLY IN HOSPITAL

Any person, regardless of their age, can be admitted to a medical, psychiatric, or specialist surgical ward. In most cases, this is initiated by the GP, via a referral to a consultant in an out-patients' clinic. Alternatively, the patient may be admitted as an emergency directly to hospital, or through an accident and emergency department.

The older patient, who may have domestic problems and minor medical ailments, may remain longer in the general ward. His specific needs are often not catered for, making it difficult to discharge him, and blocking the bed for acute admissions. The recent policy trend has been to establish Geriatric Units or Departments, which deal specifically with the broad spectrum of the needs of the elderly. Newly-built district general hospitals usually incorporate such a facility.

The team approach to geriatric care

The team is led by a consultant in geriatric medicine, who understands the aging process and the illnesses and social predicaments prevalent among the old. A GP may make a request for the geriatrician to do a domiciliary visit, to assess the total medical and social needs of the individual. When an elderly patient is admitted to the Geriatric Unit, it may be necessary for the doctor to seek the advice of a specialist surgeon or physician. If treatment is needed, the patient may be transferred to his care temporarily, although remaining under the auspices of the geriatrician.

All grades of staff will contribute to the comprehensive nursing care. Ideally, some will have completed the JBCNS course in geriatric nursing. While occupational therapy and physiotherapy are important in the treatment of the disabled of all ages, a great deal of this type of work concerns the rehabilitation of the elderly. Often, treatment is started while the patient is still in hospital, the main emphasis being on personal care. Dressing, undressing, toileting, and eating can seem impossible tasks to a patient who has recently lost the use of one or more limbs, following a stroke or an injury.

At the request of the geriatric consultant, treatment is started as early as possible, and aims to restore the affected parts to as near normal as possible, by encouraging their use with apparatus or aids; teaching the patient to use the unaffected limb to exercise the affected ones; and teaching the use of special aids, designed for maximum mobility and to facilitate independence. A social worker attached to the department can assess home conditions and financial circumstances and can apply for financial benefits and home aids to help the discharged patient and his family.

Some departments have a health visitor, who is able to liaise between home and hospital. She can perform a vital function by maintaining contact with discharged patients. She is able to keep an eye on their progress and monitor any points of incapacity or stress. Her task is also important in regard to health education, giving advice on heating, hygiene, and diet.

Other professional workers may visit on a sessional basis, such as a speech therapist, dietician, optician, dentist, and chiropodist. Volunteer helpers play an immense part in providing to in-patients the small services and comforts which enrich their sheltered lives. They may read or write letters, arrange flowers, get some shopping, and generally keep the patient in touch with the outside world. Youth clubs, schools, and women's organizations may arrange for members to visit and help patients. These links with the community are valuable in increasing public awareness of the needs of the aged. The Women's Royal Voluntary Service (WRVS) is organized in many hospitals to provide a shopping trolley and mobile library which go to the wards. Sometimes a Hospital League of Friends is established, which is active in the hospital and forms strong links with the community for fund-raising events. This enables the hospital to provide extra amenities and entertainments, particularly for the continuing care of psycho-geriatric patients. Ministers of religion are particularly welcomed by the older patients, to provide spiritual comfort and friendship. The hospital staff should welcome the patient's relatives as part of the team. All help and encouragement should be given when a relative is willing to look after or assist a patient after discharge. Many families feel frightened and unsupported when left to care for an infirm relative. Knowing that staff will be willing to offer advice or assistance could give them confidence to tackle the situation.

If the unit offers short-term admission for emergency or holiday relief, this also allows the family to get a well-earned rest and gives them security if a crisis occurs.

Special consideration and help will probably be needed for the elderly of immigrant families. They may become increasingly isolated from the community at large, owing to language and cultural barriers.

Types of care

Within the unit, different wards will cater for different degrees of ill-health and varying degrees of disability. With progressive care, the patient may be able to move to wards for the less dependent as he improves.

Acute or assessment ward

New admissions are received into this ward, where they are treated for acutely presenting illness. The consultant geriatrician will then consider and assess the prognosis for rehabilitation, and decide upon the course of treatment required.

Short-term rehabilitation ward

Short-term rehabilitation is advised to assist recovery following diseases which have not caused severe disability. Mobilization and rehabilitation is started as early as possible.

Long-term rehabilitation ward

Stay in a long-term ward is recommended when treatment and rehabilitation are likely to be long and slow, due, for instance, to more severe disability following illness or an accident.

The self-care unit

This caters for those who need practice in skills required for total self-care prior to discharge. The patient is supervised by an occupational therapist who can assess if the person will be able to manage safely at home. The unit is a simulation of the home environment, including a bath, toilet, kitchen stove, and utensils. The patient regains confidence and competence with home chores and personal caring, so vital if he or she is living alone.

Continuing care

Transfer to a long-stay ward takes place after all attempts at rehabiiitation have failed to produce a satisfactory and safe result. The object is at least to maintain any level of improvement already achieved, and to progress slowly, if possible. Nursing care will be concentrated on preventing the physical and mental complications which commonly occur to patients who remain hospitalized or bed-bound for a long time. This ward may also be the last home for the patient who is dying.

Psycho-geriatric ward

This special ward is for the aged mentally sick. Treatment is given according to the ability of the patient to comprehend instructions and interpret them correctly; this treatment is social and diversional, and is intended to prevent regression. In a psychiatric hospital, there will be acute psycho-geriatric wards to deal with those who are likely to respond to treatment and recover. This includes those suffering from acute brain syndrome (toxic confusional state) depression, anxiety, and paranoid states. Long-term care is available for those with irreversible brain damage from the dementing process.

Day hospitals

These operate five days a week. The patients are brought in and taken home by ambulance, hospital car, or by private car with a relative or friend. The day hospital has five main functions:

1. To ensure an early discharge from hospital, thus vacating a bed for a more acutely ill patient.
2. Continuation of treatment and rehabilitation on a regular basis after leaving hospital, thus preventing regression and relapse and ensuring maximum mobility and independence in the patient's normal daily life.
3. To check the decline in the condition of the patient, before admission becomes necessary.
4. To keep patients in their own homes for as long as possible, and to encourage greater independence, thereby relieving the strain on caring relatives.
5. Prevention or delay of disability from crippling diseases, such as arthritis, thus avoiding admission to hospital.

Suitable patients for a day hospital are selected by a consultant geriatrician, and are either transferred from a ward after discharge, or recommended following a domiciliary visit by the consultant, at the request of a general practitioner. A complete examination is made on the first day, following the same procedures which would be taken on admission to a general hospital. This includes blood tests, EKG, X-rays, urine test, weight, BP, and TPR. Previous medical records are obtained, and current medication, if any, considered. When investigations are complete the consultant decides on treatment and the number of visits needed each week.

The treatment in a day hospital is as intensive as that received by in-patients. The staff consist of doctors, nurses, physiotherapists, and occupational therapists, with special sessional visits from audiologists, oculists, dentists, speech therapists, chiropodists, and social workers. At some day hospitals there is a liaison officer whose function is to create a link between the hospital and the community services. Follow-up and supervision are needed when treatment is completed, and is carried out by a health visitor or community nurse. The day hospital has proved to be of great value in the treatment and care of the increasing numbers of geriatric patients. More day hospitals are now being attached to geriatric units.

The day center

This provides day care in a pleasant environment, supervised by qualified personnel. Although the function of the day center is primarily social, efforts are made to maintain any degree of independence which the patient may have. Meals are supplied, as well as essential nursing care; games and diversional therapy are included in the daily program. The change of environment offered by the day center is invaluable to the lonely person. There may also be a visiting hairdresser to provide a service at reduced rates. This is useful for many elderly people who would find the task of washing their hair very difficult to manage alone. Modern centers also have shower or sit-in bath units, to enable staff to offer clients a bath in the warm, clean surroundings. A chiropodist may visit to attend to foot inspections and treatment. Coach outings and visits to places of interest in the neighborhood can make a welcome change in the summer months. Some day centers provide light industrial work, which offers some small remuneration.

An increasing number of day centers cater solely for psychogeriatric patients who, with some supervision, are able to remain in the community. Nurses at the center will ideally be trained psychiatric nurses, or will have some experience of the aged mentally ill. They can undertake to give depot injections and will be able to detect early signs of mental stress. The contact with the staff at the center is very beneficial to the clients.

The benefits of the day care center are not confined to the patient. Relatives, caring for a severely handicapped person at home, can be under great strain. A break from responsibility, even if only for a few hours once or twice a week, can be such a relief as to tip the balance between continued care at home with the family and admission to a long-stay geriatric ward.

COMMUNITY PERSONNEL

The general practitioner

The GP provides the primary medical care, often working at a health center or in group practice. He usually has first contact with the patient, keeps a record of the medical history, and is in a position to know something of the domestic situation. He can treat the minor ailments of old age and he can refer the patient to a consultant colleague for a specialist opinion. The GP may be instrumental in applying to the courts for compulsory removal of an old person who refuses to go to a hospital or similar institution. This statute applies to people who are incapacitated, living in insanitary conditions, and who are unable to care for themselves or to get help from others. The GP can also be required to sign an order for compulsory admission to a psychiatric hospital, under a section of the Mental Health Act (1959).

The community nurse

The community nurse may also be called a district or home nurse. They carry out procedures at the request of the general practitioner, or continue care after the patient's discharge from hospital at the request of the consultant geriatrician. In recent years the number of people requiring home nursing has risen sharply. This pressure on the service has made it necessary to consider how to make the best use of special nursing skills. In 1965 the ministry set up a subcommittee and a report was commended to the local authorities, suggesting that there was scope for wider use of ancillary staff. Routine work, such as bathing or helping with bathing, was delegated to the ancillary staff under the supervision of the trained nurse, allowing the nurse to concentrate on the more skilled attention required by very sick or terminally ill patients.

Working closely with the general practitioner, the nurse is able to supervise prescribed medication, to ensure the correct use of drugs, and to report any side-effects which may become evident. Discontinued or out-of-date drugs may accumulate in the home, and are a potential danger. The visiting nurse will take the responsibility for removing and disposing of the excess drugs, by returning them to the doctor or chemist (with the patient's permission, as he is legally the owner of the drugs).

Health visitors

Health visitors are usually attached to a health center or to a general practice. Some now specialize in geriatrics, and can be attached to a geriatric unit and/or day hospital. This liaison creates a most effective follow-up system between hospital and home.

Routine visits to the elderly in the community are invaluable. People living alone often suffer from seemingly minor irritations and discomfort, which they consider too trivial to mention to a doctor. A little swelling of the feet, loss of hair or weight, or undue thirst are often dismissed as signs of "growing old." To the health visitor, however, "growing old" is not a disease, and natural aging processes are distinguishable from early symptoms of a developing abnormality. The health visitor will report to the doctor, causing investigations to be made and treatment started where necessary. Heating arrangements are carefully studied during a visit, and corrected if inadequate. The elderly on low incomes often economize on fuel, and unwittingly put themselves at risk of hypothermia, which can be fatal. The seriousness of a deficient heating system is of great concern to the health visitor, who can, if necessary, arrange for financial assistance with the cost of heating.

The health visitor will advise on a manageable and well-balanced diet, particularly important for old people living alone, and can arrange for the delivery of a main meal on some days. The number of days per week when a meal is supplied will depend on the Meals-on-Wheels service available in the area. Social activities in the neighborhood will be well known to the health visitor, who, understanding the emotional and physical needs of the patient, is able to arrange diversional outings where the need arises.

The occupational therapist

Working in the community, the occupational therapist can be asked to visit the home and to advise on or implement adaptations or changes necessary for the safe and easy management of the home. Individual requirements vary greatly, from a ramp constructed to make for easy passage over an awkward step, to a simple gadget for picking up a fallen object. Many such problems can be solved by ingenuity and improvisation, making the home safer and easy to manage. Adaptations to the home, including telephone installation, may be provided free or at reduced rates by the local authority.

The social worker

Before 1970, social workers used to deal with one specific section of people needing help: they would be employed to concentrate their attentions on either the physically handicapped, the mentally disordered, the elderly, or children. Following the recommendations of the Seebohm Report, these specialties were integrated into the comprehensive social services department within the local authority. Social workers now receive an integrated training, which equips them to deal with a family case-load, which may include various social problems. The social worker can advise the elderly person on financial entitlements, and provide information about borough facilities. She may also be a supportive visitor, especially in times of grief, depression, and despair.

Home helps

An application can be made to the social services department of the local authority, for the services of a home help. This service enables elderly people to continue living at home, even when the simplest household tasks are beyond their abilities. It is preferable if the recommendation for a home help is made by a social worker, GP, or health visitor. The local organizer will then call to discuss with the applicant the sort of help which is required. This may include cleaning the floors, cleaning out the fire grate, ironing, or shopping – in fact, any reasonable routine household tasks necessary to maintain a good standard of cleanliness in the home. In order to assess the elderly person's ability to contribute toward the cost of the home helps service, an inquiry is made about financial circumstances. Payment is not made direct to the home help, but to the local authority. Payment is made on an hourly basis, and a signature is required to confirm that the agreed hours have been worked.

Good neighbor scheme

Local authorities are increasingly using reliable neighbors to keep an eye on a lonely person. The neighbor will receive an honorarium (small fee) for making regular calls on one person, and giving a hand with small tasks such as collecting the pension, doing a little shopping or light housework, or making a snack meal.

Laundry service

This is available in some areas for incontinent people, if their relatives are unable to cope with the amount of laundering required. Sheets are collected regularly and replaced with clean linen. Disposable incontinence pads may also be supplied.

Holiday beds

Holidays are not only desirable but essential for a person who cares for an elderly relative at home. The much-needed break from responsibility may be arranged by the temporary admission of the old person to a geriatric hospital or old people's home, for two or three weeks a year. If the patient is a suitable case for an old peoples' home, the arrangements are made by the social worker. If more nursing care is needed than is possible in a home, the GP will arrange temporary hospital admission in consultation with the hospital's consultant geriatrician.

Holidays

Holiday schemes for the elderly are organized by the local authorities, or by voluntary services on behalf of the local authorities. Some voluntary organizations independently sponsor their own holidays for elderly and handicapped people. There are four main ways in which local authorities provide holidays:

By providing their own purpose-built holiday accommodation, or by using some of the beds in ordinary residential accommodation for holiday purposes.

Using accommodation provided by voluntary organizations, or using voluntary organizations on an agency basis, giving financial support.

Using commercial organizations, usually for group holidays.

Sponsoring individuals to take their own holiday. (See Tables 25.2 and 25.3.)

In 1973, the DHSS Social Science Research Unit published a study on holiday schemes for the elderly and physically handicapped. This wide-ranging report covers the legislative background, homes, voluntary bodies, hotels and boarding houses, and commercial holiday camps.

TABLE 25:2 CHOICE OF SCHEMES BY LOCAL AUTHORITIES: PROPORTIONS OF ALL AUTHORITIES BY TYPE WHICH OPERATE SCHEMES OF DIFFERENT TYPES

Type of authority	Total number of authorities	*Percentage of each type of scheme using			
		Local Authority Holiday Homes	Voluntary Centres	Commercial Centres	Other
London Boroughs	30	23	90	100	47
English County Councils	41	15	46	66	54
English County Boroughs	73	12	42	64	37
Wales‡	14	—	—	—	—
Total	158				

*Some authorities use more than one scheme therefore the rows do not sum to 100%.

‡The numbers are too small to warrant the use of percentages.

From: *Local authority holidays for the elderly and physically handicapped.* HMSO, 1973, Crown Copyright.

TABLE 25:3 TYPES OF SCHEMES: LOCAL AUTHORITIES IN DIFFERENT REGIONS PROVIDING DIFFERENT TYPES OF SCHEME

	Number of authorities				
	Total number of authorities	Type of scheme using			
		Local Authority Holiday Homes	Voluntary Centres	Commercial Centres	Other
Region					
London and South eastern	39	7	34	35	19
Wales	14	—	6	12	3
Northern	14	3	7	7	9
East and West Ridings	12	3	5	8	5
Northwest	13	5	6	8	4
North Midland	13	1	4	10	5
Midland	17	1	3	16	5
Eastern	16	—	8	6	7
Southern	8	—	5	6	3
Southwestern	12	2	6	8	6
Total	158	22	83	116	66

From: *Local authority holidays for the elderly and physically handicapped.* HMSO, 1973, Crown Copyright.

Day or night sitters

Local authorities or voluntary organizations may be able to provide a responsible "sitter" for an elderly person needing constant supervision. This gives the family a break for a day out, or for an undisturbed night's rest.

Meals on Wheels

If a person is unable to prepare a main meal of the day, they may ask the social services department to arrange for the delivery of a mid-day meal. The food may be delivered hot in packs from a heated container or may need to be heated up. The service varies in each area, but is usually available between two to five days a week. Some services may provide meals at weekends or during emergencies. A small charge is usually made for each meal. The delivery of meals ensures a varied and balanced diet, and provides another contact for the housebound. Without this service, nutritional diseases and vitamin deficiencies would occur much more frequently, because of the tendency of people living alone to subsist on convenience foods – largely carbohydrate, with little mineral or vitamin content.

Lunch clubs

In some areas the social services department or old people's welfare organizations have arranged lunch clubs. Mid-day meals are served at the club two or three times a week, for the ambulant retired person. In addition to the obvious nutritional value of attending a lunch club, there is the advantage of making social contact. Transport is not usually provided, but special arrangements might be made by a social worker if really necessary.

Pop-in parlor

This is a kind of subsidized teashop/resting place, run by voluntary helpers. It provides cheap snacks and the chance of company and warm surroundings. Some also have armchairs and reading matter.

VOLUNTEER ORGANIZATIONS AND CHARITIES

The proliferation of volunteer agencies and self-help groups is an encouraging sign of social concern for the well-being of less able minorities. There is no doubt that the increasing corps of volunteer helpers in the community provides an important reinforcement to the heavy workload of the statutory personnel. With their friendly visits and help in awkward tasks, a lifeline is offered to old folk who might otherwise be overlooked and isolated within a busy community. In an effort to make the maximum use of the voluntary help available, some areas employ a volunteer organizer. This person acts as an intermediary between the voluntary agencies or individuals and the local health and social services departments. This ensures that the right kind of help will be deployed when and where it is most needed.

Youth clubs, women's groups, schools, and university students arrange to make visits to local people and to help with shopping, gardening, or decorating. Task Force and Lions International organize volunteers to embark on helpful projects for the aged in the community.

The British Red Cross Society and Women's Royal Voluntary Service are concerned with maintaining links with needy people in the community. One very important facility is transport, provided to take the elderly to clinic appointments or to visit relatives in hospital. Clergymen keep a check on their housebound parishioners and other members of the congregation may offer to visit the elderly. Many organizations exist for the welfare of the elderly; among them are Help the Aged, Contact, Cruse, RUKBA and the Pre-retirement Association, and Age Concern, the vigorous campaigning organization. The manual ***Help, I Need Somebody*** lists organizations and the type of help they offer. Many old people often prefer the help and companionship of an unpaid worker; they may be unwilling to take the time to "worry" a busy professional. Many are extremely proud and refuse what they regard as state charity. A considerable number of volunteers are pensioners themselves, and are often strong contributors to the body of helpers.

Libraries

In some areas the local library runs a mobile service for the handicapped, and some carry books with extra-large print for people with failing eyesight. The Women's Royal Voluntary Service organize a Books-on-Wheels service in some areas where no mobile library service exists.

Public transport

Fare concessions are offered by British Rail to men and women over 65. A "Railcard" may be obtained by showing a pension book. Most local authorities offer cheaper or free bus services for pensioners. Conditions and fares vary from place to place, and some areas offer no concessions at all. Information about reduced-price travel can be obtained from local council offices.

The government has laid down statutory requirements which are binding on local authorities, but services available go beyond legislation, because of the efforts of voluntary organizations. In recent years, Age Concern has campaigned strongly on behalf of the elderly. Information on services in an area can be obtained from Age Concern, or from the welfare department at council offices.

Department of Health & Social Security	Alexander Fleming House, Elephant & Castle, London SE1. This is the head office dealing with national insurance and supplementary benefits.
Scotland:	3 Lady Lawson Street, Edinburgh EH3 9SH
Wales:	Government Buildings, Gabalfa, Cardiff CF4 4YJ
N. Ireland:	Dundonald House, Upper Newtownards Road, Belfast BT4 3SF
Age Concern	
England:	Bernard Sunley House, 60 Pitcairn Road, Mitcham (01-640-5431) Provides information, publications, and addresses of local Age Concern groups.
Scotland:	33 Castle Street, Edinburgh (031-225 5000)
Wales:	Crescent Road, Caerphilly, Mid Glamorgan CF8 (0222 869224)
N. Ireland:	2 Annadale Avenue, Belfast BT7 3JH (0232 640011)

REFERENCES

Age Concern. *Your Rights for Pensioners*. 1977.

Comfort, Alex. *A Good Age.* Mitchell Beazley, 1977.

Consumers Association. *Where to Live After Retirement*. 1977.

Gladden. *British Public Service Administration.* Staples Press, 1961.

Hepworth, N.P. *The Finance of Local Government*. Allen & Unwin, 1970.

H.M.S.O. *Research and development work on equipment for the disabled.* 1972.

H.M.S.O. *Health & Welfare: the development of community care.* 1975.

H.M.S.O. *Local Authority holidays for the elderly and physically-handicapped.* 1973.

Knight, S. *Help! I Need Somebody.* Herts. Library Service, 1977.

DEFINITION OF TERMS

AGED	Used as an adjective to mean old. As a noun to mean old people.
AGING	Continuous process of maturation, beginning at birth and terminating at death.
GERIATRICS	Concerned with the diseases of old age.
GERONTOLOGY	Study of the normal aging process
INCIDENCE	Number of new cases of a condition occurring during a specific period of time.
LIFE EXPECTANCY	Average number of years that an organism is capable of living.
OLD AGE	Conventionally accepted as being the period of life beyond the age of 65.
PREVALENCE	Number of cases of a condition existing at a given time.
SENESCENCE	Period of life in which changes relating to the aging process are evident.

GLOSSARY

The American way of spelling words in common usage occurs throughout the text. While this is of no great importance, the English spelling of technical words is listed in this glossary to avoid confusion.

AMERICAN	ENGLISH
Anemia	Anaemia
Anesthetic	Anaesthetic
Diarrhea	Diarrhoea
Dyspnea	Dyspnoea
Edema	Oedema
Esophagus	Oesophagus
Estrogen	Oestrogen
Fecal	Faecal
Gynecology	Gynaecology
Hemorrhoid	Haemorrhoid
Hemorrhage	Haemorrhage
Hypoalbuminemia	Hypoalbuminaemia
Hypokalemia	Hypokalaemia
Hyperglycemia	Hyperglycaemia
Hypoglycemia	Hypoglycaemia
Hematuria	Haematuria
Ischemia	Ischaemia
Leukemia	Léukaemia
Myxedema	Myxoedema
Orthopnea	Orthopnoea
Seborrheic	Seborrhoeic
Tumor	Tumour
Uremia	Uraemia
EKG (abbrev)	ECG (abbrev) (electrocardiogram)
Fibers	Fibres
Disks	Discs
Cecum	Caecum
Orchiectomy	Orchidectomy
Anesthesiologist	Anaesthetist

Bibliography

CHAPTER 2:
Theories of Aging

Andrew, Warren. *The Anatomy of Aging in Man and Animals.* Grune & Stratton, New York, 1971.

Birren, James E. *The Psychology of Aging.* Prentice-Hall, Englewood Cliffs, N.J., 1964.

Birren, James E. (ed.). Handbook of Aging and the Individual. Univ. of Chicago Press, 1959.

Botwinick, Jack. *Aging and Behavior.* Springer, New York, 1973.

Clark, Margaret, and **Anderson, Barbara G.** *Culture and Aging.* Thomas, Springfield, Ill. 1967.

Comfort, A. *Aging: The Biology of Senescence.* Holt, Rinehart and Winston, New York, 1964.

Curtis, H. J. *Biological Mechanisms of Aging.* Thomas, Springfield, Ill., 1966.

Kastenbaum, Robert (ed.). *Contributions to the Psychology of Aging.* Springer, New York, 1965.

Kent, Donald P. "The Elderly in Minority Groups: Variant Patterns of Aging." *Gerontologist,* 11:(1) 26–29, 1971.

Krohn, Peter L. (ed.). *Symposium on Topics in the Biology of Aging.* Wiley, 1966.

Miller, Stephen J. "The Social Dilemma of the Aging Leisure Participant." In Rose, A. and Peterson, W. (eds.), *Older People and Their Social World,* Davis, Philadelphia, 1965, pp. 77–92.

Neugarten, Bernice L. *Middle Age and Aging,* Univ. of Chicago Press, 1968.

Shock, Nathan W. (ed.). *Aging: Some Social and Biological Aspects.* American Association for the Advancement of Science. Horn-Shafer, Baltimore, 1960.

Tibbitts, Clark (ed.). Handbook of Social Gerontology. Univ. of Chicago Press, 1960.

Tibbitts, Clark, and **Donahue, Wilma** (eds.). *Social and Psychological Aspects of Aging.* Columbia Univ. Press, New York, 1962.
Walford, R. L. "Immunologic Theory of Aging." *Gerontologist,* 4:195–197, 1964.
Woolhouse, H. W. (ed.). *Aspects of the Biology of Aging.* Academic Press, New York, 1967.

CHAPTER 3: Adjustments in Aging

Barrett, J. *Gerontological Psychology.* Thomas, Springfield, Ill. 1972.
Birren, James E. *The Psychology of Aging.* Prentice-Hall, Englewood Cliffs, N.J., 1964.
Blau, Zena. *Old Age in a Changing Society.* New Viewpoints, New York, 1973.
Burnside, Irene M. "Accountrements of Aging." *Nursing Clinics of North America,* 7(2):291–301, June 1972.
Cameron, P., et al. "Consciousness of Death Across the Life Span." *Journal of Gerontology,* 28(1):92–95, January 1973.
Cavan, R. "Family Tensions Between the Old and Middle-Aged." In Vedder, C. (ed.), *Problems of the Middle Aged.* Thomas, Springfield, Ill., 1965.
Clark, M., and **Anderson, B.** *Culture and Aging: An Anthropological Study of Older Americans.* Thomas, Springfield, Ill., 1967.
Conti, Mary Louise. "The Loneliness of Old Age." *Nursing Outlook,* 18:28–30, August 1970.
Curtin, Sharon. *Nobody Ever Died of Old Age.* Little, Brown, Boston, 1972.
de Beauvoir, Simone. *The Coming of Age.* Warner Paperback Library, New York, 1973.
Erikson, Erik. *Childhood and Society,* 2nd ed. Norton, New York, 1950.
Geist, H. *The Psychological Aspects of the Aging Process.* Warren H. Green, St. Louis, 1968.
Golden, H. "The Dysfunctional Effects of Modern Technology on the Adaptability of the Aging." *Gerontologist,* 13:136, Summer 1973.
Havighurst, R., and **Glasser, R.** "An Exploratory Study of Reminiscence." *Journal of Gerontology,* 72(2):245–253, 1972.
Heilbrun, Alfred B., Jr., and **Lais, Charles V.** "Decreased Role Consistency in the Aged." *Journal of Gerontology,* 19:325–329, 1964.
Jury, Mark, and **Jury, Don.** *Gramp.* Grossman, New York, 1976.
Kopelke, Charlotte E. "Retirement As A Nursing Concern." *Journal of Gerontological Nursing,* 4:13–19, 1975.
"The Middle Years," *American Journal of Nursing.* 75:993–1024, June 1975.
Morrison, Esther. "Old, Aged, or Elderly . . . What's In A Name?" *Journal of Gerontological Nursing,* 2:25–27, 1975.
Neugarten, Bernice (ed.). *Middle Age and Aging.* Univ. of Chicago Press, 1968.
Neugarten, Bernice, et al. *Personality in Middle and Late Life.* Atherton Press, New York, 1964.
Reichard, S., et al. *Aging and Personality.* Wiley, New York, 1962.
Rosow, Irving. "Old Age: One Moral Dilemma of an Affluent Society." *Gerontologist,* 2:182–191, 1962.
Rosow, Irving. *Social Integration of the Aged.* Free Press, New York, 1967.
Schonfield, D. "Future Commitments and Successful Aging." *Journal of Gerontology,* 28(2):189–196, April 1973.
Soddy, K., and **Kidson, M.** *Men In Middle Life.* Lippincott, Philadelphia, 1967.
Stone, Virginia. "Give the Older Person Time." *American Journal of Nursing,* 69:2124–2127, October 1969.

Tibbitts, Clark (ed.). *Handbook of Social Gerontology*. Univ. of Chicago Press, 1960.

Walters, Dolores. "Life Is Beautiful at 87." *Journal of Gerontological Nursing*, 2:23–24, 1975.

CHAPTER 4: Changes Associated with the Aging Process

Agate, J. N. *The Practice of Geriatric Medicine*, 2nd ed. Heinemann Medical, London, 1970.

Brocklehurst, J. C. (ed.). *Textbook of Geriatric Medicine and Gerontology*. Churchill Livingstone, Edinburgh and London, 1973.

Clark, M., and **Anderson, B. G.** *Culture and Aging*. Thomas, Springfield, Ill., 1967.

Eisdorfer, C. "Verbal Learning and Response Time in the Aged." *Journal of Genetic Psychology*. 107:15, 1965.

Kastenbaum, R. *Contributions to the Psychology of Aging*. Springer, New York, 1965.

Lansing, Albert (ed.). *Cowdry's Problems of Aging*. Williams & Wilkens, St. Louis, 1952.

Loether, H. J. *Problems of Aging*. Dickenson, Belmont, Calif., 1967.

Neugarten, B. L. (ed.). *Personality in Middle and Late Life*. Atherton Press, New York, 1964.

Shanas, E., Townsend, P., Wedderburn, D., Friis, H., Milhj, P., and **Stehouwer, J.** *Old People in Three Industrial Societies*. Atherton Press, New York, 1968.

Tibbitts, C., and **Donahue, W.** (eds.). *Social and Psychological Aspects of Aging*. Columbia Univ. Press, New York, 1962.

Williams, R. H., Tibbitts C., and **Donahue, W.** (eds.). *Processes of Aging*, Vols. I and II. Atherton Press, New York, 1963.

CHAPTER 6: The Nursing Process

Birren, J. E. *The Psychology of Aging*. Prentice-Hall, Englewood Cliffs, N.J., 1964.

Blainey, Carol Gohrke. "Site Selection in Taking Body Temperature." *American Journal of Nursing*, 74(10):1859–1861, October 1974.

Burnside, Irene. "Interviewing the Aged." In Burnside, Irene (ed.), *Psychosocial Nursing Care of the Aged*. McGraw-Hill, New York, 1973.

Caird, F. I., and **Judge, T. G.** *Assessment of the Elderly Patient*. Pitman Medical Publishing Co., New York, 1974.

Carrieri, Virginia K., and **Sitzman, Judith.** "Components of the Nursing Process." *Nursing Clinics of North America*, 6(1):115–124, March, 1971.

Carter, J. H., et al. *Standards of Nursing Care: A Guide for Evaluation*. Springer, New York, 1972.

Cowdry, E. V., and **Steinberg, Franz U.** (eds.) *The Care of the Geriatric Patient*. Mosby, St. Louis, 1971.

Donabedian, Avedis. Part 1: "Some Issues in Evaluating the Quality of Nursing Care." *American Journal of Public Health*, 59:1833–1836, October 1969.

Evans, D. M. "Haematological Aspects of Iron Deficiency in the Elderly." *Gerontologia Clinica*, 13:12–20, 1971.

Gaitz, C. M., and **Baer, P. E.** "Diagnostic Assessment of the Elderly: A Multifunctional Model." *Gerontologist*, 10:47–52, 1970.

Knowles, Lois N. (ed). "Symposium on Putting Geriatric Nursing Standards Into Practice." *Nursing Clinics of North America,* 7(2):201–309, June 1972.

Little, Dolores E., and **Carnevali, Doris.** *Nursing Care Planning.* Lippincott, Philadelphia, 1969.

Mann, George V. "Relationship of Age to Nutrient Requirements." *American Journal of Clinical Nutrition,* 26:1096–1097, October 1973.

Moses, D. F. "Assessing Behavior in the Elderly." *Nursing Clinics of North America,* 7(2):225–233, June 1972.

Neugarten, Bernice. *Middle Age and Aging.* Univ. of Chicago Press, 1972.

Nichols, Glennodee A. "Taking Adult Temperatures—Rectal Measurements." *American Journal of Nursing,* 72(6):1092–1093, June 1972.

——— et al. "Oral, Axillary and Rectal Temperature Determinations and Relationships." *Nursing Research,* 15:307–310, Fall 1966.

——— and **Kucha, Delores H.** "Taking Adult Temperatures—Oral Measurements." *American Journal of Nursing,* 72(6):1091–1092, June 1972.

Orem, Dorothea E. *Nursing: Concepts of Practice.* McGraw-Hill, New York, 1971.

Phaneuf, M. C. *The Nursing Audit: Profile for Excellence.* Prentice-Hall (Appleton), Englewood Cliffs, N.J., 1972.

Rossman, Isadore (ed.). *Clinical Geriatrics.* Lippincott, Philadelphia, 1971.

Shock, N. W., and **Yiengst, M. J.** "Age Changes in the Acid-Base Equilibrium of the Blood of Males." *Journal of Gerontology,* 5:1–4, 1950.

Taylor, Joyce W. "Measuring the Outcomes of Nursing Care." *Nursing Clinics of North America,* 9(2):337–348, June 1974.

Yura, Helen, and **Walsh, Mary B.** *The Nursing Process: Assessing, Planning, Implementing and Evaluating,* 2nd ed. Prentice-Hall (Appleton), Englewood Cliffs, N.J., 1973.

Wandelt, M. S., and **Phaneuf, M. C.** "Three Instruments for Measuring the Quality of Nursing Care." *Hospital Topics,* 50:20–29, August 1972.

CHAPTER 7: Assisting the Aged with Universal Self-Care Demands

Barrows, C. H. "Nutrition, Aging and Genetic Program." *American Journal of Clinical Nutrition,* pp. 829–833, August 1972.

Bates, J. F. et al. "Studies Relating Mastication and Nutrition in the Elderly." *Gerontologica Clinica,* 13:227–232, 1971.

Birren, J. E. *The Psychology of Aging.* Prentice-Hall, Englewood Cliffs, N.J., 1964.

DeWalt, Evelyn M. "Effect of Timed Hygienic Measures on Oral Mucosa in a Group of Elderly Subjects." *Nursing Research,* 24(2):104–108, 1975.

Exton-Smith, A. N. "Physiological Aspects of Aging: Relationship to Nutrition." *American Journal of Clinical Nutrition,* 25:853–859, August 1972.

Fisher, Seymour, and **Cleveland, Sidney E.** *Body Image and Personality.* Dover, New York, 1968.

Fuerst, Elinor V., and **Wolff, Lu Verne.** *Fundamentals of Nursing,* 3rd ed. Lippincott, Philadelphia, 1964.

Greenberg, Barbara. "Reaction Time in the Elderly." *American Journal of Nursing,* 73:2056–2058, December 1973.

Jaeger, Dorothea, and **Simmons, Leo W.** *The Aged Ill.* Prentice-Hall (Appleton), Englewood Cliffs, N.J., 1970.

Jennings, Muriel, Nordstrom, Margene J., and **Shumake, Norine.** "Physiological Functioning in the Elderly." *Nursing Clinics of North America,* 7(2):237–251, June 1972.

Kornzweig, Abraham L. "The Eye in Old Age." In Rossman, Isadore (ed.), *Clinical Geriatrics,* Lippincott, 1971.

Leonard, B. J. "Body Image Changes in Chronic Illness." *Nursing Clinics of North America,* 7(4):687–695, December 1972.

Lofholm, Paul. "Self-Medication by the Elderly." In Davis, Richard H. (ed.), *Drugs and the Elderly.* Andries Gerontology Center, Univ. of Southern California, Los Angeles, 1973.

Masters, W. H., and **Johnson, V.** *Human Sexual Response.* Little, Brown, Boston, 1966.

Orem, Dorothea E. *Nursing: Concepts of Practice.* McGraw-Hill, New York, 1971.

Rao, Dodda. "Problems of Nutrition in the Aged." *Journal of the American Geriatrics Society,* 21:362, August 1973.

Rossman, Isadore (ed.). *Clinical Geriatrics.* Lippincott, Philadelphia, 1971.

"Symposium on Nutrition." *Geriatrics,* 29, May 1974.

Wylie, Ruth C. *The Self Concept.* Univ. of Nebraska Press, 1961.

CHAPTER 8: Cardiovascular Problems

Adatto, I. J., Poske, R. M., Pouget, J. M., Pilz, C. G. and **Montgomery, M. M.** "Rheumatic Fever in the Adult." *Journal of the American Medical Assoc.,* 194:1043, 1965.

Agate, J. A. (ed.). *Medicine in Old Age.* Lippincott, Philadelphia, 1966.

Anderson, W. F. *Practical Management of the Elderly.* Davis, Philadelphia, 1967.

Bedford, P. D., and **Caird, F. I.** *Valvular Disease of the Heart in Old Age.* Little, Brown, Boston, 1960.

Beland, Irene L. *Clinical Nursing: Pathophysiological and Psychosocial Approaches,* 3rd ed. Macmillan, New York, 1975.

Bell, William R. "Reaching the Correct Diagnosis of Pulmonary Thromboembolism." *Geriatrics,* 30:49–53, September 1975.

Brunner, Lillian S., and **Suddarth, Doris S.** *Textbook of Medical-Surgical Nursing,* 3rd ed. Lippincott, Philadelphia, 1975.

——— *The Lippincott Manual of Nursing Practice.* Lippincott, Philadelphia, 1974.

Chobanian, Aram V. "Hypertension: Major Risk Factor for Cardiovascular Complications." *Geriatrics,* 31:87–95, January 1976.

Dall, J. L. C. "Digitalis Toxicity in Elderly Patients." *Lancet,* 1:194, 1965.

Dock, W. "How Some Hearts Age." *Journal of the American Medical Assoc.,* 195:442, 1966.

Fisch, C., Genovese, P. D., Dyke, R. W., Laramore, W., and **Marvel, R. J.** "The Electrocardiogram in Persons Over 70." *Geriatrics,* 12:616, 1957.

Fowler, N. O. "Chronic Cor Pulmonale." *Geriatrics,* 22:156, 1967.

Freeman, J. T. (ed.). *Clinical Features of the Older Patient.* Thomas, Springfield, Ill., 1965.

Harris, R. "Special Features of Heart Disease in the Elderly Patient." In Chinn, A. B. (ed.), *Working with Older People,* Vol. IV. U.S. Dept. of Health, Education, and Welfare, 1974, pp. 81–102.

——— *The Management of Geriatric Cardiovascular Diseases.* Lippincott, Philadelphia, 1970.

Henry, James P. "Understanding the Early Pathophysiology of Essential Hypertension." *Geriatrics,* 31:59–72, January 1976.

Landowne, M., Brandfonbrener, M. and **Shock, V. W.** "Relation of Age to

Certain Measures of the Performance of the Heart and Circulation." *Circulation,* 12:567, 1955.

Librach, G., Schadel, M., Seltzer, M., and **Hart, A.** "Assessing Incidence and Risk Factors in Myocardial Infarction." *Geriatrics,* 30:79–93, September 1975.

McMillan, J., and **Leo, H.** "The Aging Heart, II: The Valves." *Journal of Gerontology,* 19:1, 1964.

Moidel, Harriet C., Giblin, Elizabeth C., and **Wagner, Berniece M.** (eds.). *Nursing Care of the Patient with Medical-Surgical Disorders,* 2nd ed. McGraw-Hill, New York, 1976.

Pathy, M. S. "Clinical Presentation of Myocardial Infarction in the Elderly." *British Heart Journal,* 29:190, 1967.

Perloff, Dorothee. "Diagnostic Assessment of the Patient with Hypertension." *Geriatrics,* 31:77–83, January 1976.

Remington, Richard D. "Blood Pressure: The Population Burden." *Geriatrics,* 31:48–54, January 1976.

Rodstein, Manuel. "Heart Disease in the Aged." In Rossman, Isadore (ed.), *Clinical Geriatrics,* Lippincott, Philadelphia, 1971.

Shafer, Kathleen N., et al. *Medical-Surgical Nursing,* 5th ed. Mosby, St. Louis, 1971.

Syzek, Barbara J. "Cardiovascular Changes in Aging: Implications for Nursing." *Journal of Gerontological Nursing,* 2(1):28, 1976.

White, Paul D. "Cardiovascular Disorders." In Cowdry, E. V., and Steinberg, F. U. (eds.), *The Care of the Geriatric Patient.* Mosby, St. Louis, 1971.

CHAPTER 9:
Peripheral Vascular Disease

Beland, Irene L. *Clinical Nursing: Pathophysiological and Psychosocial Approaches,* 3rd ed. Macmillan, New York, 1975.

Blumenthal, Herman T. "Aging and Peripheral Vascular Disease." In Chinn, Austin B., *Working with Older People. A Guide to Practice,* Vol. IV. U.S. Dept. of Health, Education, and Welfare, Rockville, Md., 1974 pp. 103–112.

Brunner, Lillian S., and **Suddarth, Doris S.** *Textbook of Medical-Surgical Nursing,* 3rd ed. Lippincott, Philadelphia, 1975.

——— *The Lippincott Manual of Nursing Practice.* Lippincott, Philadelphia, 1974.

Cobey, James C., and **Cobey, Janet H.** "Chronic Leg Ulcers." *American Journal of Nursing,* 74:258–259, February 1974.

Compere, C. L. "Early Fitting of Prosthesis Following Amputation." *Surgical Clinic of North America,* 48:215, 1968.

Haimovici, Henry. "The Peripheral Vascular System." In Rossman, Isadore, *Clinical Geriatrics.* Lippincott, Philadelphia, 1971, pp. 165–181.

Harris, P., et al. "The Fate of Elderly Amputees." *British Journal of Surgery,* 61:665–668, 1974.

Kerstein, M. D., Zimmer H., Dugdale, F. E., and **Lerner, E.** "What Influence Does Age Have on Rehabilitation of Amputees?" *Geriatrics,* 30:67–71, December 1975.

Lofgren, Eric P., and **Lofgren, Karl A.** "Alternatives in the Management of Varices." *Geriatrics* 30:111–113, September 1975.

Moidel, Harriet C., Giblin, Elizabeth C., and **Wagner, Berniece M.** (eds.). *Nursing Care of the Patient with Medical-Surgical Disorders,* 2nd ed. McGraw-Hill, New York, 1976.

Rose, Mary Ann. "Home Care After Peripheral Vascular Surgery." *American Journal of Nursing,* 74:260–262, February 1974.
Shafer, Kathleen N., et al. *Medical-Surgical Nursing,* 5th ed. Mosby, St. Louis, 1971.

CHAPTER 10: Cancer

Beland, Irene L. *Clinical Nursing: Pathophysiological and Psychosocial Approaches,* 3rd ed. Macmillan, New York, 1975.
Bouchard, Rosemary, et al. *Nursing Care of the Cancer Patient.* Mosby, St. Louis, 1972.
Browning, Mary, and Lewis, Edith P. (eds.). "The Nurse and the Cancer Patient." *American Journal of Nursing,* New York, 1973.
Brunner, Lillian S., and Suddarth, Doris S. *Textbook of Medical-Surgical Nursing,* 3rd ed. Lippincott, Philadelphia, 1975.
——— *The Lippincott Manual of Nursing Practice.* Lippincott, Philadelphia, 1974.
Clifford, G. O. "Hematologic Problems in the Elderly." In Rossman, Isadore (ed.), *Clinical Geriatrics.* Lippincott, Philadelphia, 1971, pp. 261–264.
Donovan, C. "What's New in Cancer Control." *American Journal of Nursing,* 76(6):962, June 1976.
Exton-Smith, A. N., and Windsor, A. C. M. "Principles of Drug Treatment in the Aged." In Rossman, Isadore (ed.), *Clinical Geriatrics.* Lippincott, Philadelphia, 1971, pp. 383–384.
Jarvik, L. "Genetic Aspects of Aging." In Rossman, Isadore (ed.), *Clinical Geriatrics.* Lippincott, Philadelphia, 1971, pp. 99–100.
Moidel, Harriet C., Giblin, Elizabeth C., and Wagner, Berniece M. (eds.). *Nursing Care of the Patient with Medical-Surgical Disorders,* 2nd ed. McGraw-Hill, New York, 1976.
Ostfield, A. M., and Gibson, D. C. (eds.). *Epidemiology of Aging.* U.S. Dept. of Health, Education, and Welfare, Publication (NIH) 75–711, Bethesda, Md., 1972.
Pelner, L. "Specific Aspects of Malignancy in the Older Body." In Freeman, Joseph (ed.), *Clinical Features of the Older Patient.* Thomas, Springfield, Ill., 1965, pp. 345–352.
Rinear Eileen. "Helping the Survivors of Expected Death." *Nursing,* 75, 3:60–65, March 1975.
Shafer, Kathleen N., et al. *Medical-Surgical Nursing,* 5th ed. Mosby, St. Louis, 1971.
Zippin, Calvin, et al. "Identification of High Risk Groups in Breast Cancer." *Cancer,* 1381–1387, December 1971.

CHAPTER 11: Respiratory Problems

Beland, Irene L. *Clinical Nursing: Pathophysiological and Psychosocial Approaches,* 3rd ed. Macmillan, New York, 1975.
Brunner, Lillian S., and Suddarth, Doris S. *Textbook of Medical-Surgical Nursing,* 3rd ed. Lippincott, Philadelphia, 1975.
——— *The Lippincott Manual of Nursing Practice.* Lippincott, Philadelphia, 1974.
Henshaw, H. C. *Diseases of the Chest.* Saunders, Philadelphia, 1969.

Moidel, Harriet C., Giblin, Elizabeth C., and **Wagner, Berniece M.** (eds.). *Nursing Care of the Patient with Medical-Surgical Disorders,* 2nd ed. McGraw-Hill, New York, 1976.

Report of the Surgeon General. The Health Consequences of Smoking. U.S. Government Printing Office, Washington, D.C., 1972.

Rodman, T., and **Sterling, F. H.** *Pulmonary Emphysema and Related Lung Diseases.* Mosby, St. Louis, 1969.

Schwaid, M. C. "The Impact of Emphysema." *American Journal of Nursing,* 70:1247–1250, June 1970.

Sedlock, Stephanie A. "Detection of Chronic Pulmonary Disease." *American Journal of Nursing,* 72(8):1407–1411, August 1972.

Shafer, Kathleen N. et al. *Medical-Surgical Nursing,* 5th ed. Mosby, St. Louis, 1971.

Stolley, Paul D. "Asthma Mortality." *American Review of Respiratory Disease,* 105:883–890, 1972.

Ungvarski, P. "Mechanical Stimulation of Coughing." *American Journal of Nursing,* 71:2358–2361, December 1971.

CHAPTER 12: Diabetes

American Diabetes Association. *Diabetes Mellitus: Diagnosis and Treatment,* Vol. 3. New York, 1971.

Davies, D. "Advances Toward Understanding Diabetes Mellitus." *Geriatrics,* 30(11):79–83, November 1975.

Ellenberg, M. "Diabetes in the Older Age Group." *Geriatrics,* 19:47, 1964.

Gitman, Leo. "Diabetes Mellitus in the Aged." In Chinn, A. B., *Working with Older People: A Guide to Practice,* Vol. IV. U.S. Dept. of Health Education, and Welfare, Rockville, Md. 1974, p. 219.

Marble, A., et al. (eds.). *Joslin's Diabetes Mellitus,* 11th ed. Lea and Febiger, Philadelphia, 1971.

Rafkin, H., and **Ross, H.** "Diabetes in the Elderly." In Rossman, I. (ed.), *Clinical Geriatrics.* Lippincott, Philadelphia, 1971, pp. 391–403.

CHAPTER 13: Musculoskeletal Problems

Avioli, L. V. "Aging, Bone, and Osteoporosis." In Steinberg, F. U. (ed.), *Cowdry's, The Care of the Geriatric Patient,* 5th ed. Mosby, St. Louis, 1976, pp. 119–132.

Ball, B. "Helping Patients Adjust to Rheumatoid Arthritis." *Nursing,* 72(2)11–17, October 1972.

Beckenbaugh, R. D. "Reconstructing the Crippled Arthritic Hand." *Geriatrics,* 31(3):89–93, March 1976.

Beland, Irene L. *Clinical Nursing: Pathophysiological and Psychosocial Approaches,* 3rd ed. Macmillan, New York, 1975.

Bennage, B. A., and **Cummings, M. E.** "Nursing the Patient Undergoing Total Hip Arthroplasty." *Nursing Clinics of North America,* 8:107–116, March 1973.

Brewerton, D. A. "Rheumatic Disorders." In Rossman, I. (ed.), *Clinical Geriatrics.* Lippincott, Philadelphia, 1971, pp. 301–307.

Brunner, Lillian S., and **Suddarth, Doris S.** *Textbook of Medical-Surgical Nursing,* 3rd ed. Lippincott, Philadelphia, 1975.

——— *The Lippincott Manual of Nursing Practice.* Lippincott, Philadelphia, 1974.

Cabanela, M. E. "Superiority of Total Hip Replacement Arthroplasty." *Geriatrics,* 31(3):61–66, March 1976.

Chamberlin, G. W. "Bone: Radiological and Clinical Aspects." In Freeman, J. T. (ed.), *Clinical Features of the Older Patient.* Thomas, Springfield, Ill., 1965, pp. 359–376.

Chao, E. Y. S. "The Biomechanics of Total Joint Replacement Surgery." *Geriatrics,* 31(3):48–57, March 1976.

Devas, M. "Orthopedics." In Steinberg, F. U. (ed.), *Cowdry's, Care of the Geriatric Patient,* 5th ed. Mosby, St. Louis, 1976, pp. 258–274.

Ford, L. T. "Orthopedic Surgery." In Cowdry, E. V., and Steinberg, F. U. (eds.), *The Care of the Geriatric Patient.* Mosby, St. Louis, 1971.

Freehafer, A. A. "Injuries to the Skeletal System of Older Persons." In Chinn, A. B. (ed.), *Working with Older People,* Vol. IV. U.S. Dept. of Health, Education, and Welfare, Rockville, Md., 1974, pp. 180–193.

Grob, D. "Common Disorders of Muscles in the Aged." In Chinn, A. B. (ed.), *Working with Older People,* Vol. IV. U.S. Dept. of Health, Education, and Welfare, Rockville, Md., 1974, pp. 156–162.

——— "Prevalent Joint Diseases in Older Persons." In Chinn, A. B. (ed.), *Working with Older People,* Vol. IV. U.S. Dept. of Health, Education, and Welfare, Rockville, Md., 1974, pp. 163–171.

Habermann, Edward T. "Orthopedic Aspects of the Lower Extremities." In Rossman, I. (ed.). *Clinical Geriatrics.* Lippincott, Philadelphia, 1971, pp. 309–325.

Hahn, B. H. "Arthritis, Bursitis, and Bone Disease." In Steinberg, F. U. (ed.), *Cowdry's, The Care of the Geriatric Patient,* 5th ed. Mosby, St. Louis, 1976, pp. 11–34.

Henderson, E. D. "Putting the Pieces Together." *Geriatrics,* 31(3):46–47, March 1976.

Howell, T. H. *A Student's Guide to Geriatrics.* Staples, London, 1970, pp. 135–150.

Johnson, K. A. "When Total Knee Arthroplasty is Indicated." *Geriatrics,* 31(3):71–75, March 1976.

Larson, C. B., and **Gould, M. L.** *Calderwood's Orthopedic Nursing,* 7th ed. Mosby, St. Louis, 1970.

Loxley, A. K. "The Emotional Toll of Crippling Deformity." *American Journal of Nursing,* 72:1839–40, October 1972.

Lutwak, L. "Metabolic Disorders of the Skeleton in Aging." In Chinn, A. B. (ed.), *Working with Older People,* Vol. IV. U.S. Dept. of Health, Education, and Welfare, Rockville, Md., 1974, pp. 172–179.

Marmor, L. "Surgery for Osteoarthritis." *Geriatrics,* 27:89–95, February 1972.

Moidel, Harriet C., Giblin, Elizabeth C., and **Wagner, Berniece M.** (eds.). *Nursing Care of the Patient with Medical-Surgical Disorders,* 2nd ed. McGraw-Hill, New York, 1976.

Shafer, Kathleen N., et al. *Medical-Surgical Nursing,* 5th ed. Mosby, St. Louis, 1971.

Shoemaker, R. R. "Total Knee Replacement." *Nursing Clinics of North America,* 8:117–125, March 1973.

Sorka, C. "Combating Osteoporosis." *American Journal of Nursing,* 73:1193–1197, July 1973.

Spencer, H., Baladad, J., and **Lewin, I.** "The Skeletal System." In Rossman, I. (ed.), *Clinical Geriatrics.* Lippincott, Philadelphia, 1971, pp. 289–300.

Stauffer, R. U. "Total Ankle Joint Replacement as an Alternative to Arthrodesis." *Geriatrics,* 31(3):79–85, March 1976.

Thewlis, M. W. *The Care of the Aged,* 6th ed. Mosby, St. Louis, 1954, pp. 599–642.

Trueta, J. *Studies of the Development and Decay of the Human Frame.* Saunders, Philadelphia, 1968.

CHAPTER 14: Hematologic Problems

Beland, Irene L. *Clinical Nursing: Pathophysiological and Psychosocial Approaches,* 3rd ed. Macmillan, New York, 1975.

Brunner, Lillian S., and **Suddarth, Doris S.** *Textbook of Medical-Surgical Nursing,* 3rd ed. Lippincott, Philadelphia, 1975.

——— *The Lippincott Manual of Nursing Practice.* Lippincott, Philadelphia, 1974.

Clifford, G. O. "Hematologic Problems in the Elderly." In Rossman, I. (ed.), *Clinical Geriatrics.* Lippincott, Philadelphia, 1971, pp. 253–266.

Craytor, J. K. "Talking with Persons Who Have Cancer." *American Journal of Nursing,* 69:744–748, April 1969.

Hugos, R. "Living with Leukemia." *American Journal of Nursing,* 72:2185–2188, December 1972.

Maekawa, T. "Hematologic Diseases." In Steinberg, F. U. (ed.). *Cowdry's, The Care of the Geriatric Patient,* 5th ed. Mosby, St. Louis, 1976, pp. 152–166.

Moidel, Harriet C., Giblin, Elizabeth C., and **Wagner, Berniece M.** (eds.). *Nursing Care of the Patient with Medical-Surgical Disorders,* 2nd ed. McGraw-Hill, New York, 1976.

Shafer, Kathleen N., et al. *Medical-Surgical Nursing,* 5th ed. Mosby, St. Louis, 1971.

Wilson, P. "Iron-Deficiency Anemia." *American Journal of Nursing,* 72:502–504, March 1972.

CHAPTER 15: Gastrointestinal Problems

Amberg, J. R., and **Zboralske, F. F.** "Gallstones After Seventy." *Geriatrics,* 20:539, 1965.

Bargen, J. Arnold. "Gastroenterologic Disorders." In Cowdry, E. V., and Steinberg, F. U., *The Care of the Geriatric Patient.* Mosby, St. Louis, 1971, pp. 80–104.

Becker, G. H., Meyer, J., and **Necheles, H.** "Fat Absorption in Young and Old Age." *Gastroenterology,* 14:80–92, January 1950.

Beland, Irene L. *Clinical Nursing: Pathophysiological and Psychosocial Approaches,* 3rd ed. Macmillan, New York, 1975.

Berman, P. M., and **Kirsner, J. B.** "Gastrointestinal Problems." In Steinberg, F. U. (ed.). *Cowdry's The Care of the Geriatric Patient,* 5th ed. Mosby, St. Louis, 1976, pp. 93–118.

Bertolini, A. M. *Gerontologic Metabolism.* Thomas, Springfield, Ill. 1969.

Bhaskar, S. N. "Oral Lesions in the Aged Population." *Geriatrics,* 23:137–149, October 1968.

Brunner, Lillian S., and **Suddarth, Doris S.** *Textbook of Medical-Surgical Nursing,* 3rd ed. Lippincott, Philadelphia, 1975.

——— *The Lippincott Manual of Nursing Practice.* Lippincott, Philadelphia, 1974.

Davidoff, A., Winkler, S., and **Lee, M.** *Dentistry for the Special Patient: The Aged, Chronically Ill and Handicapped.* Saunders, Philadelphia, 1972.

Elfenbaum, A. "Dentistry for the Elderly in Health and Illness." In Chinn, A. B. (ed.), *Working with Older People,* Vol. IV. U.S. Dept. of Health, Education, and Welfare, Rockville, Md., 1974, pp. 337–358.

——— "Newer Problems of Older Patients—an Introduction to Geriatric Dentistry. In *Dental Clinics of North America.* Saunders, Philadelphia, 1968.

Greenwood, A. H. "Dental Care for the Elderly Poses Special Problems." *Geriatrics,* 31(5):103, May 1976.

McGinty, M. D. "Hiatal Hernia." *Hospital Medicine,* 7:133–143, April 1971.

Moidel, Harriet C., Giblin, Elizabeth C., and **Wagner, Berniece M.** (eds.). *Nursing Care of the Patient with Medical-Surgical Disorders,* 2nd ed. McGraw-Hill, New York, 1976.

Painter, Neil S. "Diverticular Disease of the Colon: A Bane of the Elderly." *Geriatrics,* 31(2):53–58, February 1976.

Rowe, Nathaniel H. "Dental Surgery." In Steinberg, F. U. (ed), *Cowdry's, The Care of the Geriatric Patient,* 5th ed. Mosby, St. Louis, 1974, pp. 300–309.

Salter, R. H. "Some Aspects of Diverticular Disease of the Colon." *Age and Aging.* 2:225–229, November 1973.

Shafer, Kathleen N., et al. *Medical-Surgical Nursing,* 5th ed. Mosby, St. Louis, 1971.

Silverman, S. I. *Principles and Practices of Dental Care for the Chronically Ill, Handicapped and the Aged.* Symposium, New York University, May 1975.

Sklear, Manuel. "Gastrointestinal Diseases in the Aged." In: Chinn, A. B., *Working with Older People,* Vol. IV. U.S. Dept. of Health, Education, and Welfare, Rockville, Md., 1974, pp. 124–131.

Straus, Bernard. "Disorders of the Digestive System." In Rossman, Isadore, *Clinical Geriatrics,* Lippincott, Philadelphia, 1971, pp. 183–202.

Unger, James L., and **McGregor, Douglas H.** "When Esophageal Carcinoma Is Obscured by Other Factors." *Geriatrics,* 31(2):53–58, February 1976.

CHAPTER 16: Genitourinary Problems

Alvarez, W. C. "Will a Prostate Operation Produce Impotence?" *Geriatrics,* 20:996, 1965.

Beland, Irene L. *Clinical Nursing: Pathophysiological and Psychosocial Approaches,* 3rd ed. Macmillan, New York, 1975.

Birnbaum, S. J. "Geriatric Gynecology." In Chinn, A. B. (ed.), *Working with Older People,* Vol. IV. U.S. Dept. of Health, Education, and Welfare, Rockville, Md., 1974, pp. 149–155.

Bowles, W. T. "Urologic Surgery." In Steinberg, F. U. (ed.), *Cowdry's, The Care of the Geriatric Patient,* 5th ed. Mosby, St. Louis, 1976, pp. 275–283.

Brocklehurst, J. C. "The Urinary Tract." In Rossman, Isadore (ed.), *Clinical Geriatrics.* Lippincott, Philadelphia, 1971, pp. 219–228.

——— **Dillane, J. B., Griffiths, L.,** and **Fry, J.** "The Prevalence and Symptomatology of Urinary Infection in An Aged Population." *Gerontologica Clinica,* 10:242, 1968.

Brunner, Lillian S., and **Suddarth, Doris S.** *Textbook of Medical-Surgical Nursing,* 3rd ed. Lippincott, Philadelphia, 1975.

——— *The Lippincott Manual of Nursing Practice.* Lippincott, Philadelphia, 1974.

Clark, C. L. "Catheter Care in the Home." *American Journal of Nursing,* 72:922–924, May 1972.

Delehanty, L., and **Stravino, V.** "Achieving Bladder Control." *American Journal of Nursing,* 70:312–316, February 1970.

Gibbs, G. E. "Perineal Care of the Incapacitated Patient." *American Journal of Nursing,* 69:124–125, January 1969.

Grabstald, H. "Management of Tumors of the G.U. Tract in the Geriatric Patient." *Journal of the American Geriatrics Society,* 14:95, 1966.

Jaffe, J. W. "Common Lower Urinary Tract Problems in Older Persons." In Chinn, A. B. (ed.), *Working with Older People,* Vol. IV. U.S. Dept. of Health, Education, and Welfare, Rockville, Md., 1974, pp. 141–148.

Jeffcoate, T. N. A. *Principles of Gynecology,* 3rd ed. Prentice-Hall (Appleton), Englewood Cliffs, N.J., 1967.

Kahn, A. I., and **Snapper, I.** "Medical Renal Diseases in the Aged." In Chinn, A. B. (ed.), *Working with Older People,* Vol. IV. U.S. Dept. of Health, Education, and Welfare, Rockville, Md., 1974, pp. 131–140.

Keuhnelian, J. G., and **Saunders, V. E.** *Urologic Nursing.* Lippincott, Philadelphia, 1971.

Lapides, J., and **Zierdt, D.** "Renal Function with Aging." *Journal of the American Medical Assoc.,* 201:778, 1967.

Moidel, Harriet C., Giblin, Elizabeth C., and **Wagner, Berniece M.** (eds.). *Nursing Care of the Patient with Medical-Surgical Disorders,* 2nd ed. McGraw-Hill, New York, 1976.

Owen, M. L. "Special Care for the Patient Who Has Had a Breast Biopsy or Mastectomy." *Nursing Clinics of North America,* 7:373–382, June 1972.

Rossman, Isadore. "The Anatomy of Aging." In Rossman, Isadore (ed.), *Clinical Geriatrics.* Lippincott, Philadelphia, 1971, p. 9.

Shafer, Kathleen N., et al. *Medical-Surgical Nursing,* 5th ed. Mosby, St. Louis, 1971.

Winter, C. C., and **Barker, M. R.** *Nursing Care of Patients with Urologic Diseases.* Mosby, St. Louis, 1972.

Wright, V. Cecil. "Carcinoma of the Vulva." *Journal of the American Geriatrics Society,* 14(5):232-235, May 1976.

CHAPTER 17: Neurological Problems

Beland, Irene L. *Clinical Nursing: Pathophysiological and Psychosocial Approaches,* 3rd ed. Macmillan, New York, 1975.

Brunner, Lillian S., and **Suddarth, Doris S.** *Textbook of Medical-Surgical Nursing,* 3rd ed. Lippincott, Philadelphia, 1975.

——— *The Lippincott Manual of Nursing Practice.* Lippincott, Philadelphia, 1974.

Carini, E., and **Owens, G.** *Neurological and Neurosurgical Nursing.* Mosby, St. Louis, 1970.

Carter, A. B. "The Neurologic Aspects of Aging." In Rossman, I. (ed.), *Clinical Geriatrics.* Lippincott, Philadelphia, 1971, pp. 123–141.

Cooney, L. M. and **Solitaire, G. B.** "Primary Intracranial Tumors in the Elderly." *Geriatrics,* 27:94–104, January 1972.

Dayhoff, N. "Soft or Hard Devices to Position Hands?" *American Journal of Nursing,* 75(7):1142–1144, July 1975.

Dervitz, H. L. and **Zislis, J. M.** "A Medical Perspective of Physical Therapy and Stroke Rehabilitation." *Geriatrics,* 25:123–132, June 1970.

Dolan, M. B. "Autumn Months, Autumn Years." *American Journal of Nursing,* 75(7):1145–1147, July 1975.

Hardin. W. B. "Neurologic Aspects." In Steinberg, F. U. (ed.), *Cowdry's, The Care of the Geriatric Patient,* 5th ed. Mosby, St. Louis, 1976, pp. 364–379.

Hull, J. T. "The Prevalence and Incidence of Parkinson's Disease." *Geriatrics,* 25:128–133, May 1970.

Jacobansky, A. M. "Stroke." *American Journal of Nursing,* 72:1260–1263, July 1972.

Locke, S. "Cerebrovascular Disorders in Later Life." In Chinn, A. B. (ed.), *Working With Older People: A Guide to Practice,* Vol. IV. U.S. Dept. of Health, Education, and Welfare, Rockville, Md., 1974, pp. 50–59.

——— "Neurological Disorders of the Elderly." In Chinn, A. B. (ed.), *Working With Older People: A Guide to Practice,* Vol. IV. U.S. Dept. of Health, Education, and Welfare, Rockville, Md., 1974, pp. 45–49.

Moidel, Harriet C., Giblin, Elizabeth C., and **Wagner, Berniece M.** (eds.), *Nursing Care of the Patient with Medical-Surgical Disorders,* 2nd ed. McGraw-Hill, New York, 1976.

Shafer, Kathleen N., et al. *Medical-Surgical Nursing,* 5th ed. Mosby, St. Louis, 1971.

Skelly, M. "Aphasic Patients Talk Back." *American Journal of Nursing,* 75(7):1140–1141, July 1975.

CHAPTER 18: Dermatological Problems

Barrett, D., and **Klibanski. A.** "Collagenase Debridement." *American Journal of Nursing,* 73:849–51, May 1973.

Beland, Irene L. *Clinical Nursing: Pathophysiological and Psychosocial Approaches,* 3rd ed. Macmillan, New York 1975.

Blass, M. A. "Improvised Cushions." *American Journal of Nursing,* 70(12):2605, December 1970.

Brunner, Lillian S., and **Suddarth, Doris S.** *Textbook of Medical-Surgical Nursing,* 3rd ed. Lippincott, Philadelphia, 1975.

——— *The Lippincott Manual of Nursing Practice.* Lippincott, Philadelphia, 1974.

Conrad, A. H. "Dermatologic Disorders." In Steinberg, F. U. (ed.), *Cowdry's, The Care of the Geriatric Patient,* 5th ed. Mosby, St. Louis, 1976, pp. 178–190.

Lang, C., and **McGrath, A.** "Gelfoam for Decubitus Ulcers." American Journal of Nursing, 74(3) 460–461, March 1974.

Moidel, Harriet C., Giblin, Elizabeth C., and **Wagner, Berniece M.** (eds.), *Nursing Care of the Patient with Medical-Surgical Disorders,* 2nd ed. McGraw-Hill, New York, 1976.

Pfaudler, M. "Flotation, Displacement and Decubitus Ulcers." *American Journal of Nursing,* 68(11):2351–2355, November 1968.

Shafer, Kathleen N., et al. *Medical-Surgical Nursing,* 5th ed. Mosby, St. Louis, 1971.

Tindall, J. P. "Geriatric Dermatology." In Chinn, A. B. (ed.), *Working with Older People: A Guide to Practice,* Vol. IV. U.S. Dept. of Health, Education, and Welfare, Rockville, Md., 1974, pp. 3–27.

Van Ort, S. R., and **Gerber, R. M.** "Topical Application of Insulin in the Treatment of Decubitus Ulcers: A Pilot Study." *Nursing Research,* 25(1):9–12, January–February 1976.

Vasile, J., and **Chaitin, H.** "Prognostic Factors in Decubitus Ulcers of the Aged." *Geriatrics,* 27:126–129, April 1972.

Wallace, G., and **Hayter, J.** "Karaya for Chronic Skin Ulcers." *American Journal of Nursing,* 74(6):1094–1098, June 1974.

Weinstein, L. D., and **Davidson, B. A.** "Fluid-Support Mattress and Seat for the

Prevention and Treatment of Decubitus Ulcers." *Lancet,* 2:625–626, September 25, 1965.

Young, A. W. "Skin Diseases." In Rossman, I. (ed.), *Clinical Geriatrics.* Lippincott, Philadelphia, 1971, pp. 203–218.

CHAPTER 19: Sensory Deficits

Amburgey, P.I. "Environmental Aids for the Aged Patient." *American Journal of Nursing,* 66:2017–2018, September 1966.

American Foundation for the Blind. *An Introduction to Working with the Aging Person Who Is Visually Handicapped.* New York, 1972.

Brunside, I. M. "Clocks and Calendars." *American Journal of Nursing,* 70:117–119, January 1970.

——— "Touching Is Talking." *American Journal of Nursing.* 73:2060–2063, December 1973.

Chodil, J., and **Williams, B.** "The Concept of Sensory Deprivation." *Nursing Clinics of North America,* 1970. 5:453, Sept, 1970.

Cockerill, E. E. "Reflections on My Nursing Care." *American Journal of Nursing,* 65:83–85, May 1965.

Condl, E. D. "Ophthalmic Nursing: The Gentle Touch." *Nursing Clinics of North America,* 5:467–476, September 1970.

Davis, H., and **Silverman, S. R.** *Hearing and Deafness.* Holt, Rinehart and Winston, New York, 1970.

Downs, F. S. "Bedrest and Sensory Disturbances." *American Journal of Nursing,* 74:434–438, March 1974.

Gordon, D. M. "Eye Problems of the Aged." In Chinn, A. B. (ed.), *Working with Older People,* Vol. IV. U.S. Department of Health, Education, and Welfare, Rockville, Md., 1974, pp. 28–37.

Kornzweig, A. L. "The Eye in Old Age." In Rossman, I. (ed.), *Clinical Geriatrics.* Lippincott, Philadelphia, 1971, pp. 229–246.

Nilo, E. R. "Needs of the Hearing Impaired." *American Journal of Nursing,* 69:114–116, January 1969.

Ohno, M. J. "The Eye-Patched Patient." *American Journal of Nursing,* 71:271–274, February 1971.

Reuben, R. "Aging and Hearing." In Rossman, I. (ed.), *Clinical Geriatrics.* Lippincott, Philadelphia, 1971, pp. 247–252.

Rummerfield, P. S., and **Rummerfield, M. J.** "Noise Induced Hearing Loss." *Occupational Health Nurse,* 17:23–24, November, 1969.

Saunders, W. H., et al. *Nursing Care in Eye, Ear, Nose and Throat Disorders,* 2nd ed. Mosby, St. Louis, 1968.

Seamon, F. W. "Nursing Care of Glaucoma Patients." *Nursing Clinics of North America,* 5:489–496, September 1970.

Senturia, B. H., and **Prince, L. L.** "Otolaryngological Problems in the Geriatric Patient." In Chinn, A. B. (ed.), *Working With Older People,* Vol. IV. U.S. Department of Health, Education, and Welfare, Rockville, Md., 1974, pp. 38–44.

Worrell, J. D. "Nursing Implications in the Care of the Patient Experiencing Sensory Deprivation." In Kintzel, K. C. (ed.), *Advanced Concepts in Clinical Nursing,* Lippincott, Philadelphia, 1971.

CHAPTER 20: Surgical Care

Alexander, S. "Surgical Risk in the Patient with Arteriosclerotic Heart Disease." *Surgical Clinics of North America,* 48:513, 1968.

Dodd, R. B. "Anesthesia." In Steinberg, F. U. (ed.), *Cowdry's, The Care of the Geriatric Patient,* 5th ed. Mosby, St. Louis, 1976, pp. 247–257.

Duncalf, D., and **Kepes, E. R.** "Geriatric Anesthesia." In Rossman, I. (ed.), *Clinical Geriatrics.* Lippincott, Philadelphia, 1971, pp. 421–438.

Glenn, F. "Surgical Principles for the Aged Patient." In Chinn, A. B. (ed.), *Working with Older People,* Vol. IV. U.S. Dept. of Health, Education, and Welfare, Rockville, Md., 1974, pp. 250–266.

——— **Moore, S. W.,** and **Beal, J.** (eds.). *Surgery in the Aged.* McGraw-Hill, New York, 1960.

Mason, J. H., Gau, F. C., and **Byrne, M. P.** "General Surgery." In Steinberg, F. U. (ed.), *Cowdry's, The Care of the Geriatric Patient,* 5th ed. Mosby, St. Louis, 1976, pp. 217–246.

Powers, J. H. (ed.). *Surgery of the Aged and Debilitated Patient.* Saunders, Philadelphia, 1968.

Schein, C. J., and **Dardik, H.** "A Selective Approach to Surgical Problems in the Aged." In Rossman, I. (ed.), *Clinical Geriatrics.* Lippincott, Philadelphia, 1971, pp. 405–420.

CHAPTER 21: Mental Health and Illness in Old Age

Blank, M. L. "Raising the Age Barrier to Psychotherapy." *Geriatrics,* 29(11):141–148, November 1974.

Botwinick, J. *Aging and Behavior.* Springer, New York, 1973, pp. 25–27, 54–59, 60–66, and 309.

Braceland, F. J. "Predicting the Future of Mental Health Care." *Geriatrics,* 29(11):178–186, November 1974.

Brown, B. S. "How Do Mental Health and Aging Affect Each Other? New Center Will Encourage Search for Answers." *Geriatrics,* 31(2):40–44, February 1976.

Buell, D. "Psychiatrists Pay New Heed to Mental Problems of Aged." *National Observer,* January 25, 1975, p. 17.

Burnside, I. M. "Group Work Among the Aged." *Nursing Outlook,* 17(6):68–71, June 1969.

——— (ed). *Psychosocial Nursing Care of the Aged.* McGraw-Hill, New York, 1973.

Busse, E., and **Pfeiffer, E.** *Mental Illness in Later Life.* American Psychiatric Association, Washington, D.C., 1973.

Butler, R. N. "Clinical Psychiatry in Late Life." In Rossman, I. (ed.), *Clinical Geriatrics.* Lippincott, Philadelphia, 1971, pp. 439–460.

——— "Mental Health and Aging: Life Cycle Perspectives." *Geriatrics,* 29(11):59–60, November 1974.

——— "Psychiatry and the Elderly: An Overview." *American Journal of Psychiatry,* 132(9):893–900, September 1975.

——— *Why Survive? Being Old in America.* Harper & Row, New York, 1975, pp. 225–259.

——— and **Lewis, M. I.** *Aging and Mental Health.* Mosby, St. Louis, 1973.

Casady, M. "If You're Active and Savvy at 30, You'll Be Warm and Witty at 70." *Psychology Today,* 9(6):138, November 1970.

Gage, F. "Suicide in the Aged." *American Journal of Nursing,* 71(11):2153–2155, November 1971.

Garetz, F. K. "Breaking the Dangerous Cycle of Depression and Faulty Nutrition." *Geriatrics,* 31(6):73–75, June 1976.

Garnick, S. "Psychological Study in the Management of the Geriatric Patient." In Chinn, A. B. (ed.), *Working With Older People: A Guide To Practice,* Vol. IV. U.S. Dept. of Health, Education, and Welfare, Rockville, Md., 1974, pp. 321–336.

Gordon, S. K. "The Phenomenon of Depression in Old Age." *Gerontologist,* 13(1):100–105, Spring 1973.

Hall, J. E., and **Weaver, B. R.** *Nursing of Families in Crisis.* Lippincott, Philadelphia, 1974.

Harrison, C. "The Institutionally Deprived Elderly." *Nursing Clinics of North America,* 3:697–707, December 1968.

Hoogerbeets, J. D., and **LaWall, J.** "Changing Concepts of Psychiatric Problems in the Aged." *Geriatrics,* 30(8):83–87, August 1975.

Kahn, R. L. "The Mental Health System and the Future Aged." *Gerontologist,* 15(1):24–31, February 1975.

Kastenbaum, R., and **Mishara, B. L.** "Premature Death and Self-injurious Behavior in Old Age." *Geriatrics,* 26(7):70–81, July 1971.

——— ". . . Gone Tomorrow." *Geriatrics,* 29(11):127–134, November 1974.

Kern, R. A. "Emotional Problems in Relation to Aging and Old Age." *Geriatrics,* 26(6):83–93, June 1971.

Libow, L. B. "Pseudo-senility: Acute and Reversible Organic Brain Syndromes." *Journal of American Geriatrics Society,* 21:112–120, March 1973.

Looney, D. S. "Senility Is Also a State of Mind." *National Observer,* March 31, 1973, p. 1.

Neugarten, B. L. (ed.). *Middle Age and Aging.* Univ. of Chicago Press, 1968.

Parker, B., Deibler, S., Feldshub, B., Frosch, W., Laureano, E., and **Sillen, J.** "Finding Medical Reasons for Psychiatric Behavior." *Geriatrics,* 31(6):87–91, June 1976.

Patterson, R. C., Abrahams, R., and **Baker, F.** "Preventing Self-Destructive Behavior." *Geriatrics,* 29(11):115–121, November 1974.

Post, Felix. *The Clinical Psychiatry of Late Life.* Pergamon Press, London, 1965.

Raskind, M. A., Alvarez, C., Pietrzyk, M., Westerlund, K., and **Herlin, S.** "Helping the Elderly Psychiatric Patient in Crisis." *Geriatrics,* 31(6):51–56, June 1976.

Yelom, I., and **Terrazas, F.** "Group Therapy for Psychotic Elderly Patients." *American Journal of Nursing,* 68:1690–1694, 1968.

CHAPTER 22: Geriatric Pharmacology

Ayd, F. J. "Tranquilizers and the Ambulatory Geriatric Patient." *Journal of the American Geriatrics Society,* 8:908, 1960.

Bellville, J. W., Forrest, W. H., Jr., Miller, E., and **Brown, B. W., Jr.** "Influence of Age on Pain Relief from Analgesics." *Journal of the American Medical Assoc.,* 217:1835–1841, 1971.

Bender, A. D. "Pharmacologic Aspects of Aging: A Survey of the Effect of Increasing Age on Drug Activity in Adults." *Journal of the American Geriatrics Society,* 12:114, 1964.

——— "Gerontological Basis for Modifications in Drug Activity with Age." *Journal Pharm. Science,* 54:1225, 1965.

——— "The Effect of Increasing Age on the Distribution of Peripheral Blood Flow in Man." *Journal of the American Geriatrics Society,* 13:192, 1965.

——— "Pharmacologic Aspects of Aging: Additional Literature." *Journal of the American Geriatrics Society,* 15(1):68–74, 1967.

Calloway, N. O., and **Merrill, R. S.** "The Aging Adult Liver, I: Bromsulphalein and Bilirubin Clearances." *Journal of the American Geriatrics Society,* 13:594, 1965.

Davis, L. D., Lawton, A. H., Prouty, R., and **Chow, B. F.** "The Absorption of Oral Vitamin B-12 in an Aged Population." *Journal of Gerontology,* 20:169, 1965.

Davison, W. "Drug Hazards in the Elderly." *Gerontologica Clinica,* 7:257, 1965.

"Drugs and the Elderly Mind." *Lancet,* 2:126, 1972.

Fikry, M. E., and **Aboul-Wafa, M. H.** "Intestinal Absorption in the Old." *Gerontologica Clinica,* 7:171, 1965.

Freeman, J. T. *Clinical Principles and Drugs in the Aging.* Thomas, Springfield, Ill., 1963.

——— "Drug Therapy in Aging Patients." *Geriatrics,* 18:174, 1963.

Friedman, S. A., Raizner, A. E., Rosen, H., Solomon, N. A., and **Sy, W.** "Functional Defects in the Aging Kidney." *Annals of Internal Medicine,* 74:41–45, 1972.

Halford, F. D., and **Mithoefer, J. C.** "The Effect of Morphine and Respiration in the Aged." *Surgical Clinics of North America,* 40:907, 1960.

Hamilton, L. D. "The Aged Brain and the Phenothiazines." *Geriatrics,* 21:131, 1966.

Herrmann, G. R. "Digitoxicity in the Aged: Recognition, Frequency and Management." *Geriatrics,* 21:109, 1966.

Hurley, J. D. "Cancer Chemotherapy." *Journal of the American Geriatrics Society,* 10:1058, 1962.

Hurwitz, U. "Predisposing Factors in Adverse Reactions to Drugs." *British Medical Journal,* 1:536–539, 1969.

Kayne, R. C., Cheung, A., and **McCarron, M. M.** *Monitoring of Drug Therapy of Long Care Patients.* Presented at the Second Annual Scientific Session, Western Division, American Geriatrics Society, Los Angeles, 1973.

Keyes, J. W. "Problems in Drug Management of Cardiovascular Disorders in Geriatric Patients." *Journal of the American Geriatrics Society,* 13:118, 1965.

Lamy, P. O., and **Kitler, M. E.** "Drugs and the Geriatric Patient." *Journal of the American Geriatrics Society,* 19:23, 1971.

Lely, A. H., and **Van Enter, C. H. J.** "Non-Cardiac Symptoms of Digitalis Intoxication." *American Heart Journal,* 83:149–152, 1972.

Nicholson, W. J. "Medicine in Old Age: Disturbances of the Special Senses and Other Functions." *British Medical Journal,* 1:33–35, 1974.

Olson, E. V., Johnson, B. J., Thompson, L. F., McCarthy, J. A., Edmonds, R. E., Schroeder, L. M., and **Wade, M.** "The Hazards of Immobility." *American Journal of Nursing,* 67:781–796, 1967.

Pfeiffer, E. "Use of Drugs which Influence Behavior in the Elderly: Promises, Pitfalls and Perspectives." In Davis, R. H. (ed.), *Drugs and the Elderly.* Andries Gerontology Center, Univ. of South California, Los Angeles, 1973, pp. 43–44.

Rubb, T. U. "Use of Drugs in the Older Age Groups." *Pharmaceutical Journal,* 1:507, 1961.

Schwid, S. A., and **Gifford**, R. W. "The Use and Abuse of Antihypertensive Drugs in the Aged." *Geriatrics, 122:172, 1967.*

Smith, W. N., and **Melmon**, K. L. "Drug Choice in Disease." In Melmon, K. L., and Morrelli, H. F. (eds.), *Clinical Pharmacology: Basic Principles in Therapeutics*. Macmillan, New York, 1972, p. 5.

Stewart, R. B., and **Cluff**, L. E. "A Review of Medication Errors and Compliances in Ambulant Patients." *Clinical Pharmacology and Therapeutics*, 13:463–468, 1972.

CHAPTER 23: Sexuality

Armstrong, E. B. "The Possibility of Sexual Happiness in Old Age." In Beigel, H. G. (ed.), *Advances in Sex Research*. Harper & Row, New York, 1963.

Bengtson, V. L. "Sex in Nursing Homes." *Medical Aspects of Human Sexuality*, 9:21, 1975.

Botwinick, J. "Drives, Expectancies and Emotions." In Birren, J. E. (ed.), *Handbook of Aging and the Individual*. Univ. of Chicago Press, 1960.

——— *Aging and Behavior*. Springer, New York, 1973, pp. 35–49.

Calleja, M. A. "Homosexual Behavior in Older Men." *Sexology*, August 1967, pp. 46–48.

Cameron, P., and **Biber**, H. "Sexual Thought Throughout the Life Span." *Gerontologist*, 13:144–147, Summer 1973.

Christenson, C., and **Gagnon**, J. H. "Sexual Behavior in a Group of Older Women." *Journal of Gerontology*, 20:351–356, 1965.

Comfort, **Alex**. *The Joy of Sex*. Simon & Schuster, New York, 1972.

——— "Sexuality in Old Age." *Journal of the American Geriatrics Society*, 22(10):440–442, October 1974.

Daly, M. J. "Sexual Attitudes in Menopausal and Postmenopausal Women." *Medical Aspects of Human Sexuality*, May 1968, pp. 48–53.

Davis, M. E. "Estrogen and the Aging Process." In *Year Book of Obstetrics and Gynecology*, 1964–1965. Year Book Medical Publishers, Chicago, 1965.

Finkel, A. L. "The Relationship of Sexual Habits to Benign Prostatic Hypertrophy." *Medical Aspects of Human Sexuality*, October 1967, pp. 24–25.

——— "Sex After Prostectomy." *Medical Aspects of Human Sexuality*. March 1968, pp. 40–41.

——— "Sexual Function During Advancing Age." In Rossman, I. (ed.), *Clinical Geriatrics*. Lippincott, Philadelphia, 1971.

——— **Moyers**, T. G., **Tobenkin**, M. I., and **Karg**, S. J. "Sexual Potency in Aging Males: Frequency of Coitus Among Clinic Patients." *Journal of the American Medical Assoc.*, 170:1391–1393, 1959.

Freeman, J. T. "Sexual Capacities in the Aging Male." *Geriatrics*. 16:37–43, 1961.

Goldfarb, A. F., **Daly**, M. J., **Lieberman**, D., and **Reed**, D. M. "Sex and the Menopause." *Medical Aspects of Human Sexuality*, November 1970, pp. 64–89.

Jacobson, L. "Illness and Human Sexuality." *Nursing Outlook*, 22(1):50–53, January 1974.

Kent, S. "Continued Sexual Activity Depends on Health and the Availability of a Partner." *Geriatrics*, 30(11):142–144, November 1975.

Lewis, M. I., and **Butler**, R. N. "Neglected by Women's Lib." *National Observer*, June 29, 1972, p. 20.

Lobsenz, N. M. "Sex and the Senior Citizen." *The New York Times Magazine,* January 20, 1974, pp. 8–28.

Newman, G., and **Nichols, C. R.** "Sexual Activities and Attitudes in Older Persons." *Journal of American Medical Assoc.,* 173:33–35, 1960.

Pfeiffer, E. "Sexuality in the Aging Individual." *Journal of the American Geriatrics Society.* 22(11):481–484, November 1974.

Rubin, H. H., and **Newman, B. W.** *Active Sex After Sixty.* Arco, New York, 1969.

"Sex Behavior of Older Women." *Sexology,* June 1966, p. 734.

Sontag, S. T. "The Double Standard of Aging." *Saturday Review,* September 1972, pp. 29–38.

Verwoerdt, A., Pfeiffer, E., and **Wang, H. S.** "Sexual Behavior in Senescence." *Geriatrics,* 24:137–154, February 1969.

Weinberg, J. "Sexuality in Later Life." *Medical Aspects of Human Sexuality,* April 1971, pp. 216–227.

Whiskin, F. E. "The Geriatric Sex Offender." *Medical Aspects of Human Sexuality.* April 1970, pp. 125–129.

CHAPTER 24: The Dying Process

Allen, B. "Until Death Ensues." *Nursing Clinics of North America,* 7(2):303–308, June 1972.

Becker, Ernest. *The Denial of Death.* Free Press, New York, 1973.

Black, P. McL. "Focusing on Some of the Ethical Problems Associated with Death and Dying." *Geriatrics,* 31(1):138–141, January, 1976.

Cameron, P., et al. "Consciousness of Death Across the Life Span." *Journal of Gerontology,* 28(1):92–95, January 1973.

Davis, Richard H. (ed.). *Dealing with Death.* Andrus Gerontology Center, Univ. of Southern California, Los Angeles, 1973.

Elner, R. "Dying in the U.S.A." *International Journal of Nursing Studies,* 10(3):171–184, August 1973.

Fuchs, Beverly. "On Death and Dying." Unpublished paper presented to Osler Nursing Staff, Johns Hopkins Hospital, Baltimore, November 1976.

Kastenbam, Robert, and **Aisenberg, Ruth.** *The Psychology of Death.* Springer, New York, 1972.

Klass, D., and **Gordon, A.** "Goals in Teaching About Death." *The Maryland Teacher,* 23(3):8–9, 22-24, Spring 1976.

Kutscher, A., and **Goldberg, M.** (eds.). *Caring for the Dying Patient and His Family.* Health Sciences, New York, 1973.

Maguire, Daniel C. *Death By Choice.* Doubleday, New York, 1974.

Mitford, J. *The American Way of Death.* Simon & Schuster, New York, 1963.

Quint, J. C. *The Nurse and the Dying Patient.* Macmillan, New York, 1967.

Schoenberg, B., et al. (eds.). *Psychosocial Aspects of Terminal Care.* Columbia Univ. Press, New York, 1972.

Schultz, R. "Meeting the Three Major Needs of the Dying Patient." *Geriatrics,* 31(6):132–137, June 1976.

Shneidman, E. S. (ed.). *Death: Current Perspectives.* Aronson Jason, New York 1976.

Simms, L. M. "Dignified Death: A Right Not A Privilege." *Journal of Gerontological Nursing,* 1(5):21–25, November–December 1975.

Weisman, A. D. *On Dying and Denying.* Behavior Publications, New York, 1972.

Williams, R. *To Live and To Die: When, Why and How.* Springer-Verlag, New York, 1974.

Index

EMPLOYEE RELATIONS IN CONTEXT

David Farnham

INSTITUTE OF PERSONNEL AND DEVELOPMENT

First published in 1997

An earlier version of this text, *Employee Relations*, was published in 1993 by the Institute of Personnel Management

Phototypeset by The Comp-Room, Aylesbury
and printed in Great Britain
by Short Run Press, Exeter

British Library Cataloguing in Publication Data

A catalogue record for this book is available from the British Library

ISBN 0-85292-680-4

The views expressed in this book are the author's own, and may not necessarily reflect those of the IPD.

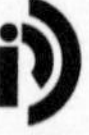

INSTITUTE OF PERSONNEL
AND DEVELOPMENT

IPD House, Camp Road, London SW19 4UX
Tel: 0181 971 9000 Fax: 0181 263 3333
Registered office as above. Registered Charity No. 1038333
A company limited by guarantee. Registered in England No. 2931892

Contents

PART 2 MANAGING EMPLOYEE RELATIONS

List of figures

List of tables

List of exhibits

List of abbreviations

ACAS	Advisory, Conciliation and Arbitration Service
ADST	approved deferred share trust
AEU	Amalgamated Engineering Union
AEEU	Amalgamated Engineering and Electrical Union
AMMA	Assistant Masters and Mistresses Association
APEX	Association of Professional Executive Clerical and Computer Staff
ASB	Amalgamated Society of Boilermakers
ATL	Association of Teachers and Lecturers
BIFU	Banking Insurance and Finance Union
C and P	custom and practice
CAC	Central Arbitration Committee
CBI	Confederation of British Industry
CIR	Commission on Industrial Relations
CO	Certification Officer
COHSE	Confederation of Health Service Employees
CWU	Communication Workers Union
CPAUIA	Commission for Protection Against Unlawful Industrial Action
CPSA	Civil and Public Services Association
CRTUM	Commissioner for the Rights of Trade Union Members
CSC	*Confédération des Syndicats Chrétiens*
DDA 1955	Disability Discrimination Act 1995
DfEE	Department for Education and Employment
DGB	*Deutscher Gewerkschaftsbund*
EA 1980	Employment Act 1980
EA 1982	Employment Act 1982
EA 1988	Employment Act 1988
EA 1989	Employment Act 1989
EA 1990	Employment Act
EU	European Union
EETPU	Electrical Electronic Telecommunications and Plumbing Union
ELM	external labour market
EMU	European monetary union
EPA 1975	Employment Protection Act 1975
EPCA 1978	Employment Protection (Consolidation) Act 1978
EqPA 1970	Equal Pay Act 1970

EqPAR 1983	Equal Pay Amendment Regulations 1983
ERA 1996	Employment Rights Act 1996
ESO	employee share ownership
ETUC	European Trade Union Confederation
EWC	European works council
FBP	fall back position
FGTB	*Fédération Général du Travail de Belgique*
GMB	General Municipal and Boilermakers
GPMU	Graphical Paper and Media Union
HASAWA 1974	Health and Safety at Work etc. Act 1974
HRM	human resources management
ICFTU	International Confederation of Free Trade Unions
ILM	internal labour market
ILO	International Labour Organisation
IPD	Institute of Personnel and Development
IPM	Institute of Personnel Management
IRA 1971	Industrial Relations Act 1971
ISP	ideal settlement point
ISTC	Iron and Steel Trades Confederation
IT	information technology
ITs	industrial tribunals
JCC	joint consultative committee
LO	*Landesorganisationen i Sverige*
LLM	local labour market
MBL 1977	Employee Participation in Decision Making Act 1977
MSFU	Manufacturing Science and Finance Union
NALGO	National and Local Government Officers Union
NAS/UWT	National Association of Schoolmasters/Union of Women Teachers
NFC	National Freight Corporation
NGA	National Graphical Association
NHS	National Health Service
NSAs	new-style agreements
NUCPS	National Union of Civil and Public Servants
NUM	National Union of Mineworkers
NUPE	National Union of Public Employees

NURMTW	National Union of Railway Marine and Transport Workers
NUT	National Union of Teachers
PF	Police Federation
PRB	pay review body
PRP	performance-related pay
PSBR	public sector borrowing requirement
QWA	quality work assured
RCN	Royal College of Nursing of the United Kingdom
RRA 1976	Race Relations Act 1976
RSP	realistic settlement point
SAP	Social Action Programme
SAYE	save as you earn
SC	Social Charter
SCE	Standing Committee of Employment
SCPC	Standing Commission on Pay Comparability
SDA 1975	Sex Discrimination Act 1975
SERPS	State Earnings Related Pension Scheme
SOGAT	Society of Graphical and Allied Trades
TCO	*Tjänstemannens Centralorganisation*
TGWU	Transport and General Workers Union
TQC	total quality control
TQM	total quality management
TUA 1984	Trade Union Act 1984
TUC	Trades Union Congress
TULRA 1974	Trade Union and Labour Relations Act 1974
TULRCA 1992	Trade Unions and Labour Relations (Consolidation) Act 1992
TUPE 1981	Transfer of Undertakings (Protection of Employment) Regulations 1981
TUREA 1993	Trade Union Reform and Employment Rights Act 1993
UCATT	Union of Construction Allied Trades and Technicians
UCW	Union of Communication Workers
UMA	union membership agreement
UN	United Nations
UNICE	Union of Industrial and Employers' Confederations of Europe
USA	United States of America

USDAW	Union of Shop Distributive and Allied Workers
WA 1986	Wages Act 1986
WIRS 1980	Workplace Industrial Relations Survey 1980
WIRS 1984	Workplace Industrial Relations Survey 1984
WIRS 1990	Workplace Industrial Relations Survey 1990

Preface

This book is an updated version of my employee relations book first published in the Management Studies 2 Series. It takes account of significant developments in employee relations over the past few years, especially the political, legal and social contexts, including the likely impact of New Labour's approach to employee relations, the Treaty of Amsterdam and changes in UK and European law. Being an introductory book, it is a study guide on employee relations for students of personnel and development, rather than a conventional textbook. Employee relations is defined as that part of personnel and development that enables competent managers to reconcile, within acceptable limits, the interests of employers as buyers of labour services and those of employees as suppliers of labour services in the labour market and the workplace. Within this framework, the main task of those responsible for managing the employment relationship is to develop appropriate institutions, policies and rules to promote 'good' working relations with those whom they employ, and to prevent conflict between management and employees over those matters in which both parties have mutual, though sometimes diverging, interests.

It differs from related books in the field (Farnham and Pimlott 1995; Bayliss and Kessler 1995; Salamon 1997) in three main respects. First, it focuses on 'employee relations', within their socio-economic contexts, rather than 'industrial relations'. In this sense, the book is written from a managerial perspective and seeks to provide a framework within which students of personnel and development will be able to identify and understand the role of management in employee relations, operationally, strategically and contextually. Compared with other texts, this one also gives more emphasis to the individual facets of the employment relationship, to non-union variants of employee relations and to other aspects of employee relations management.

This does not mean that this book is written from a narrow, prescriptive point of view. It seeks to be analytical, academic and rigorous in its approach but emphasises the contingent nature of employee relations management. Contingency means that there are not only choices and alternative approaches for managements in taking employee relations decisions but also constraints and limitations on managerial discretion.

Second, in line with its managerial thrust, compared with other texts, this book provides far more opportunities for developing competency and skills in personnel and development students by enabling them to apply employee relations knowledge and skills to practical situations. This practical approach to employee relations is underlined not only by the conceptual, theoretical and empirical content of the chapters but also by the assignments at the end of them. These assignments require students to do wider reading, undertake activities and problem-solve issues. Assignments may be done individually or in groups and they may be presented orally, in writing or both. Where an assignment refers to 'your organisation', and the student is not in current employment, this may be interpreted by the reader as meaning 'any organisation with which you are familiar'.

Although this book focuses largely on British experience and practice in employee relations, its third feature is that it incorporates some international comparisons. This is to enable students of personnel and development to understand some of the external trends and alternative approaches in employee relations in countries and national cultures other than their own.

Part 1 focuses on The Components of Employee Relations. This part of the book provides an overview of employee relations concepts, actors, processes, contexts and skills. Chapter 1 explores the elements of employee relations in terms of the interests of the buyers and sellers of labour services, the agreements and rules made by them, the conflict-resolving processes they use and the major external influences on employee relations behaviour. In Chapter 2, the major parties to employee relations – management, management organisations, employee organisations and state agencies – are identified and their roles discussed. Chapter 3 analyses the main processes and outcomes of employee relations. These include: management-led approaches; joint approaches; third-party intervention; industrial sanctions; legal enactment; and worker participation, especially in Europe.

Chapter 4 examines the economic and legal contexts of employee relations management. The topics discussed range from Keynesianism and supply-side economics to the statutory floor of employment protection rights, the law and trade disputes and the 'Social Charter' of the European Union. In Chapter 5, the basic employee relations skills required of managers are reviewed and examined, such as negotiating, handling grievances, dealing with discipline and managing redundancy.

Part 2 of the book focuses on Managing Employee Relations. Chapter 6 analyses the changing economic, technological, social and political environments within which employee relations management takes place and their implications for management strategy. In Chapter 7, the role of the state in employee relations is considered. It discusses the traditional role of the state, the 'Employee Relations Consensus' between 1945 and 1979 and the changing policies of the state in the 1980s and 1990s, including New Labour's policy proposals on employee relations. Chapter 8 focuses on management and trade unions. This includes: developments in union policy, structure and practice; union responses to the changing employee relations environment; the law and union membership; and union recognition.

Chapter 9 focuses on collective bargaining and joint consultation. It examines some of the theoretical issues relating to collective bargaining, the emerging patterns of collective bargaining and the knowledge and skills underpinning negotiating practice. It also considers the nature of joint consultation and some of its variants. In Chapter 10, alternative, largely non-union patterns of employee relations management, other than that of collective bargaining, are considered. These include: employee involvement practices; employee communication; and worker participation. Finally, in Chapter 11, attention is switched to industrial action. The topics addressed here include the forms industrial action takes, the influences on it, international comparisons and the law and industrial action.

In getting this book to press, I would particularly like to acknowledge the efforts of Matthew Reisz and his production colleagues at IPD House. I would also like to thank my colleagues Marjorie Corbridge and Stephen Pilbeam for writing Chapter 5 and Sylvia Horton for writing Chapter 6. Thanks also go to Mike Darton for producing the author and subject indexes. The result is, we believe, a text which is up to date, will be of practical use to students and teachers of employee relations and will make students aware of the complex influences on employee relations management.

David Farnham
August 1997

REFERENCES

BAYLISS, F. *and* KESSLER, S. 1995. *Contemporary Industrial Relations.* Basingstoke: Macmillan.

FARNHAM, D. *and* PIMLOTT, J. 1995. *Understanding Industrial Relations.* London: Cassell.

SALAMON, M. 1997 (forthcoming). *Industrial Relations: Theory and practice.* London: Prentice Hall.

Part 1

THE COMPONENTS OF EMPLOYEE RELATIONS

1 The elements of employee relations: an overview

Employee relations in market economies take place wherever work is exchanged for payment. Therefore, the essence of employee relations is paid employment or the pay–work bargain between employers and employees. An employee is someone who works under a contract of employment, sometimes called 'a contract of service', for an employer. A contract of employment contrasts with 'a contract for services'. These are made between independent contractors and those buying their specialist services, such as fee-paid, self-employed management consultants selling their consultancy skills to companies. To determine whether or not a worker has the legal status of an employee or that of an independent contractor, the courts apply a number of tests. These include the type of work, the nature of the orders given, the method and frequency of payment, the power to dismiss and the understanding between the parties. But the crucial test is that of 'control'. In other words, who has the ultimate right to tell the worker what to do? If one person can tell another what job to do, how it is to be done and when, where and with whom, then that party is the employer in law and the other is an employee.

The pay–work bargain between employer and employee is influenced by a series of factors, including:

- the institutional arrangements by which employment decisions are made
- external factors such as the economic, political and legal contexts of the exchange relationship
- the ideas and values underpinning employment activity.

Organisations, whatever their ownership, size or outputs, employ people to work for them, hiring them for the knowledge, skills and capabilities which individual workers possess, and reward them accordingly. People, in turn, seek paid employment to earn incomes so that they can spend the money they earn, as consumers in the market place. There are also other more complex reasons why people work but the economic imperative is the fundamental one.

Employee relations, therefore, are concerned with the interactions amongst the primary parties who pay for work and those who provide it in the labour market (employers and employees), those acting as secondary parties on their behalf (management or management organisations and trade unions) and those providing a third-party role in employment matters (state agencies and European Union institutions). Employee relations practices in any organisation are a product of a number of factors. The principal ones are:

- the *interests* of the buyers and sellers of labour services (or human resources skills)
- the *agreements and rules* made by them and their agents
- the *conflict-resolving processes* that are used
- the *external influences* affecting the parties making employment decisions.

INTERESTS IN EMPLOYEE RELATIONS

The economic imperatives

Today's employers are normally organisations. As employers, organisations vary widely in their patterns of ownership, size of employment units, numbers of employment units and types of workers employed. Business organisations in the private sector are characterised by being driven by the profit motive and market factors and are found in the primary economic sector (agriculture, mining and fishing), the secondary sector (manufacturing and construction) and the tertiary sector (services). Larger enterprises operate on several sites, employing a wide variety of human resources skills including managerial, professional, technical, administrative and what are traditionally called 'manual' groups of workers. Some private enterprises are heavily unionised, whilst others are non-unionised. Larger firms tend to have well-organised, professional personnel departments; smaller ones do not.

Public sector organisations, other than a few commercial public corporations, are generally driven by welfare or political goals, having been set up by the state to provide a series of services to the general public (Farnham and Horton 1996). These are normally financed by some form of taxation on individuals or corporations but their services are 'free' at the point of consumption by those using them. The public sector is usually classified as consisting of the public corporations, central government, including the National Health Service, and the local authorities (Fleming 1989; Central Statistical Office 1991; Office for National Statistics 1997). Public sector organisations tend to be large, complex enterprises, employing a wide variety of occupational groups and skills, with relatively high levels of union membership and bureaucratically driven personnel policies and departments.

Since business organisations are driven by the profit motive and market values, one of the main aims of those directing them and those responsible for their economic effectiveness is to obtain a financial surplus of revenues over costs at the end of each accounting cycle. Unless they achieve this financial target, businesses cannot, in the medium term at least, survive as viable economic units. At the extremes, firms may be either labour intensive, as in parts of the service sector, or capital intensive, as in hi-tech production industries. In either case, the cost-effective utilisation and managing of human resources is essential to organisational success. Private employers can stay profitable only where:

- total pay and employment costs are kept within planned human resources budgets
- worker productivity per head is increased
- human resources budgets are exceeded, pay is cut or the numbers employed in the enterprise at current pay levels are reduced.

Whilst public sector organisations are not driven by market factors, in that they are 'not for profit' enterprises (Starks 1991), they have to operate as efficiently as possible and provide 'value for money' to their political stewards, in Parliament or local government, and to those who pay for them as taxpayers. Like their private sector counterparts, they also have to utilise and manage their human resources cost-effectively, especially since they tend to be labour intensive organisations where some 70 per cent of their costs are labour costs. If labour costs increase in public sector organisations, a number of governmental and employer responses are possible. These include:

- raising taxes
- increasing public borrowing
- introducing 'charges' for services
- increasing labour productivity
- cutting back public services
- reducing their staffing establishments.

Individual men or women in employment, or those seeking work, in contrast, have their own economic interests when working. They typically want:

- the best pay available to them
- good promotion prospects
- the best fringe benefits such as pensions, medical insurance and job training
- the best working conditions, such as short hours of work, holidays with pay and sick pay
- a safe and healthy working environment
- security of employment.

All these elements of the employment package involve economic costs to employers.

Labour market and managerial relations

With employers buying labour skills and work effort and workers selling these in the labour market, there are potential conflicts of interest in the determination of the pay–work bargain or in the market relations between them. Put crudely, the economic interests of employers are such that they want the lowest possible employment costs commensurate with obtaining and retaining the skills and commitment of their workforce. The economic interests of the workforce, in contrast, are that they want the best possible terms and conditions of employment commensurate with their job security and employment prospects. The more that is paid out in pay or non-pay benefits to employees, the less is available to corporate shareholders or for investment purposes and vice versa. Even in the public sector, the higher the employment costs for hiring and retaining staff, the higher the taxes that are needed or the higher the level of public borrowing required to pay for them. These, then, are the underlying conflicts between employers and employees in the labour market under capitalism.

There are other potential conflicts of interest between employers and employees, once labour has been hired in the workplace. These derive from the managerial relations between the parties arising out of the pay–work bargain (Flanders 1968). Employers generally want employees who are compliant with or committed to employer rules and management decisions. If organisations are to achieve their economic targets of profitability, efficiency, productivity and growth – or, at a minimum, survival – managers, who are responsible for organisational success and effectiveness, want employees who respond willingly and flexibly to managerial decisions and initiatives. Managers want to be free to take and implement decisions in the interests of enterprise efficiency and workplace order, without being constrained by individual or collective employee resistance.

Employees, on the other hand, normally want a say in how their work is organised, how the decisions affecting their working lives are taken and how any complaints and grievances relating to their rewards, working arrangements and job content may be resolved. It is potential conflicts over job control which are at the root of managerial relations between managers and employees in the workplace.

Where conflict between employers and employees remains unresolved, in either their market or managerial relations, industrial conflict can result. Employers may take sanctions against their employees, or the employees and their unions may take sanctions against their employers. The situation then becomes a power struggle, with the stronger side trying to force the weaker side to concede to its demands. The outcome of such conflicts depends on the balance of power between the two sides and on other factors such as the availability of third-party intervention, the law and public opinion.

'Good' employee relations

Since there are heavy economic costs to all parties to the employment relationship if they fail to reach agreements and understandings amongst themselves, employers and employees – the latter through their unions where these are recognised – normally emphasise their common interests in the pay–work bargain, rather than their differences. Employers seek predictable labour costs, a stable workforce and co-operative employees. Employees, and recognised unions, in turn, seek reasonable terms and conditions of employment, continuous employment and fair management decisions. It is to the benefit of both employers and employees to focus on their common interests and the mutuality of the employment relationship – their pay–work bargain and other arrangements between them – by resolving their potential conflicts either constitutionally, to avoid damaging and expensive industrial conflict, or by interpersonal negotiation.

For employers, industrial conflict results in lost revenues and loss of reputation for fair dealings with their employees. For employees, industrial conflict means lost pay and possible job losses if the employer's business prospects are damaged. 'Good' employee relations, from both the employers' and employees' points of view, mean establishing institutional arrangements, engendering trust between them, to reconcile their conflicts of interest, build on their common interests and avoid costly confrontations between them.

The state also has an interest in 'good' employee relations. This is expressed through government policies, the law, the state's employee relations agencies and its role as an employer in its own right. One concern of government, as the ultimate source of power in society, is to ensure that any unresolved conflicts between employers and employees, over either their market or managerial relations, do not degenerate into what it considers to be unacceptable or unlawful behaviour, which might damage the economy or threaten social order. This is a difficult role to fulfil, since if government is seen to intervene in a way which is perceived as being too much in favour of one of the parties, at the expense of the other, then the legitimacy of its actions may be disputed. Second, government seeks to provide a framework of law, including state enforcement agencies, within which the parties to employee relations are expected to conduct themselves. It provides the parties with rights and responsibilities, and the means for adjudicating them (Wedderburn 1986). Third, as an employer, government seeks to provide its own 'good' employment practices, so as to facilitate the effective recruitment and retention of appropriately qualified public servants (Farnham 1993; see also Chapter 7 below).

AGREEMENTS AND RULES

Formal, written agreements and rules in employee relations are the principal means for containing any potential conflicts arising from the pay–work bargain, although unwritten 'understandings' (custom and practice) also provide guidelines to behaviour between the buyers and sellers of labour services in the labour market and the workplace (Brown 1972; Terry 1977).

Employment rules may be made unilaterally, bilaterally or trilaterally. Unilateral rules are made by:

- employers and managers (company or management rules)
- management organisations (policy statements)
- workers (customs and practices)
- trade unions (union rules)

- the state (statute and common law)
- EU (directives and regulations).

Agreements are made bilaterally between:

- employers and employees (contracts of employment)
- employers or employers' associations and trade unions (collective agreements).

Wages councils, organised on a tripartite basis amongst employers, unions and independent persons, determined, until recently, minimum wages for certain low-paid groups of workers (wages regulation orders).

Substantive agreements or substantive rules cover the pay and conditions of employment associated with particular jobs. They include rates of pay, additional payments, overtime pay, hours of work, holiday arrangements, holiday pay, sick pay, maternity pay and so on. By specifying the economic rights and obligations attached to particular jobs, substantive agreements or substantive rules regulate the market relations between the buyers and sellers of labour services. Procedural agreements or procedural rules, such as grievance and disciplinary procedures, adjust any differences between the parties to the pay–work bargain, whether in interpreting existing agreements or rules (conflicts of right) or in making new agreements or rules (conflicts of interest).

Substantive and procedural agreements and rules may be regulated internally or externally. Company and management rules, for example, are internally regulated, as are customs and practices, since changing them does not require the consent of external authorities, such as trade unions, management organisations or the state. All other types of substantive and procedural arrangements – whether policy statements by management organisations, union rules, statute and common law, EU directives and regulations, contracts of employment, collective agreements – are externally regulated. In practice, although each of these methods of determining employment rules shades into the others, differentiating them conceptually is useful for analytical purposes.

The employee relations agreements and rules, outlined above, are made at different decision-making levels. Directives and regulations derive from decisions made in EU institutions, whilst statute and common law stem from Parliament and the courts. Industry-wide collective agreements, the policy statements of management organisations and wages regulation orders are determined at multi-employer level. Apart from departmental customs and practices, and externally generated union rules, all other agreements and employee relations rules are made at employer or site level: ie company rules, contracts of employment, company collective agreements and workplace collective agreements.

CONFLICT-RESOLVING PROCESSES

Unilateral employer regulation – company rules or 'the right to manage' – is only one of several types of employment rules. Given the potentially conflictual nature of the employment relationship, there are a number of institutional arrangements by which conflicts of interest between the primary parties to the pay–work bargain (employers and employees) and the secondary parties (management or management organisations and trade unions) may be resolved. Some are collective processes, others are individual ones. Collective processes are those where employees are represented indirectly in employment decision-making with employers and managers, by either trade unions or similar bodies. Individual processes are those where there are direct, face-to-face contacts between employers or managers and their subordinates.

Both collective and individual processes, in turn, can be subdivided into voluntary or legal methods of conducting employee relations. Voluntary methods are those determined independently and autonomously by the parties to employee relations, such as 'free' or 'voluntary' bargaining between employers and trade unions. Legal methods are those supported by the law, whether derived from common law, statutory or European sources. They provide the parties with legal rights and obligations and are ultimately enforceable by the courts, such as in employment protection, health and safety matters or the regulation of industrial conflict.

Figure 1 **Conflict resolution and employee relations**

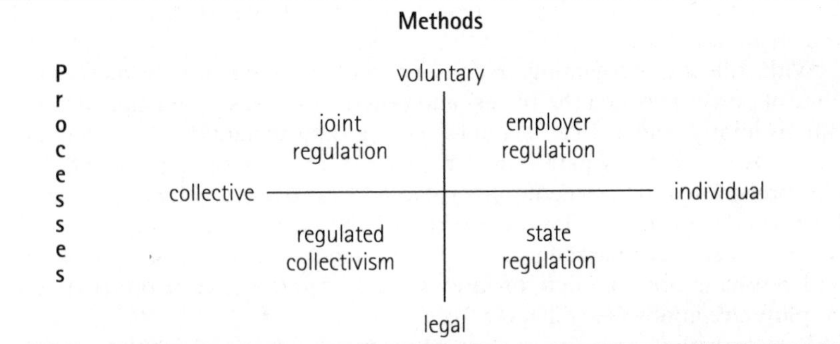

Processes	Methods: voluntary	
	joint regulation	employer regulation
	collective	individual
	regulated collectivism	state regulation
	legal	

Combining collective and individual processes with voluntary and legal methods, as shown in Figure 1, we observe that there are four major approaches to resolving conflict in employee relations. These are:

- joint regulation
- employer regulation
- state regulation
- regulated collectivism.

At any one time, the ways in which the pay–work bargain is determined, interpreted and implemented – within any organisational or national setting – involve, to varying degrees, a combination of these approaches to resolving potential employee relations conflict. But one of them may be the dominant approach.

Joint regulation

This involves a combination of collective processes and voluntary methods and includes:

- collective bargaining
- joint consultation.

Collective bargaining takes place between employer and union representatives and is based on the assumption that both the market and managerial relations between the primary parties to employee relations are power based, with the balance of power weighted in favour of employers and individual managers. This is because any individual employee has a far greater need for a particular job, and the pay–work bargain attached to it, than an employer has for any particular worker (Webb and Webb 1913). Without collective bargaining, individual workers are disadvantaged in the labour market since, where labour supply is plentiful, each worker is competing with others for jobs, enabling pay and conditions to be cut to the lowest possible standards by market-driven employers. Equally, in their managerial relations, without collective bargaining, workers are subject to internal, unilateral employment decisions about their work, over which they have no control.

With collective bargaining, in contrast, there is assumed to be a fairer balance of power between the buyers and sellers of labour, with employers and unions jointly responsible for implementing the substantive and procedural collective agreements determined between them. These terms, conditions and procedures then become incorporated into the individual contracts of employment of the employees covered by the bargaining arrangements. In this way, collective bargaining is a process for identifying, institutionalising and resolving any conflicts of interest or of rights between the parties in employee relations (see Chapter 9).

Joint consultation is the process whereby employer and employee representatives, who may or may not be union representatives, come together, normally at workplace and/or employer levels, to discuss matters of common interest. There are a number of different approaches to joint consultation (Marchington 1989) but the basic distinction between joint consultation and collective bargaining is that it is a collaborative rather than an adversarial process. Joint consultation tends to exclude matters which are subject to negotiation and to focus on matters of a non-controversial nature. It discusses issues prior to management taking a decision, or prior to negotiation, but it does not itself generally involve the taking of decisions. In this sense, the joint consultative process retains the power of management as a group to take and implement decisions, after consultations have been completed (see Chapter 9).

Employer regulation

This involves a combination of individual processes and voluntary methods which are employer and management driven. These include:

- the right to manage
- employee involvement
- profit-sharing
- pay review bodies.

The right to manage is basically concerned with all those decisions, over employment and related issues, which management claim the exclusive right to determine unilaterally. Where trade unions are absent, the employer's freedom to make decisions unilaterally is restricted only by what the law prescribes. Where unions are recognised by the employer, however, management's right to determine and apply employment rules is further restricted. But there are always areas of organisational decision-making, normally incorporated into company or 'works' rules, which remain exclusive to management alone.

There are a number of types of employee involvement. One is team briefing. This is a system of direct communication between line managers and their work teams, based on the principle of cascading information downwards, on a regular and formal basis, from management to employees. It aims to inform employees and work groups of what is happening in their organisation, and why. It also reinforces the role of line managers as leaders of their work teams. Another type of employee involvement is quality circles. These comprise small groups of employees meeting regularly and voluntarily to discuss and solve quality and work-based problems. Quality circles are normally led by first line managers who have been provided with training to improve the effectiveness of quality circles. Quality circles are sometimes monitored by steering committees higher up the organisation (see Chapter 10).

Profit-sharing is also an employer-driven process. It is primarily aimed at emphasising the common, rather than the divergent, interests of employers and employees and at reinforcing this financially. Profit-sharing is where cash bonuses are paid voluntarily by employers to employees out of corporate profits. In practice, these cash bonuses are provided in one of the following ways:

- on a discretionary basis
- as a fixed proportion of profits
- as a proportion above a stated profit threshold
- in relation to dividends paid on share capital.

Profit-sharing does not provide employees with a share in the ownership of an enterprise but simply with an additional monetary claim, over and above their pay and non-pay rewards, based on corporate success (see Chapter 10).

Pay review bodies (PRBs) are appointed by the prime minister for certain groups of public servants. It is a politically driven approach to employee relations. The role of PRBs is to make recommendations to the prime minister about the pay for particular public servants, although the government is not automatically bound by the decisions made. PRBs are established where it is felt that collective forms of pay determination for particular groups – such as top civil servants, doctors and dentists, and the armed services – are inappropriate, although in some cases union evidence is given to the review body, such as for schoolteachers, and this is taken into account in making its recommendations.

State regulation

This combines individual processes with legal methods and includes:

- contracts of employment
- employment protection rights for individual workers
- individual conciliation by the Advisory, Conciliation and Arbitration Service (ACAS)
- union membership rights
- employee share ownership.

Contracts of employment are, in many respects, the focal point of relations between the primary parties to employment – employers and employees, or individual managers and their staff. In essence, a contract of employment is a legal agreement between an employer and an individual employee, whereby the employee undertakes to obey the lawful and reasonable orders of the employer, or its managerial agents, and to take reasonable care in carrying out his or her employment duties, in exchange for remuneration. There is also a duty of fidelity to the employer. The employer, in turn, is bound in duty to pay wages, take reasonable care for the employee's safety and exercise due consideration in dealing with the employee. In practice, many features of the contract of employment are undefined, since they are settled by the courts through the legal device of 'implied terms'. The other main legal sources of the contract of employment include (Lewis 1997):

- statutory statements
- collective agreements
- works rules
- customs and practices.

Employment protection rights for workers are incorporated in legislation which provides a floor of minimum statutory employment rights for individuals, below which no one may fall. These rights include (see also Chapters 3 and 4):

- not to be 'unfairly' dismissed
- minimum periods of notice
- itemised pay statements
- not to be discriminated against on the grounds of gender, nationality or ethnic origin
- not to be made redundant without a minimum payment
- maternity pay and leave.

ACAS is empowered by the Trade Union and Labour Relations (Consolidation) Act (TULRCA) 1992 to provide individual conciliation where employees think that their employment protection rights, such as not to be 'unfairly' dismissed or to statutory maternity pay and leave, have been infringed by an employer. Cases unresolved by ACAS may go to industrial tribunals.

Union membership rights, for individual trade unionists, include: not to be unreasonably excluded or expelled from a trade union; to elect union office holders by secret ballot; to endorse official trade union industrial action by secret ballot; to determine union political funds by secret ballot; and not to be unjustifiably disciplined by the individual's union (see Chapters 4 and 8).

Employee share ownership (ESO), introduced by the Finance Acts 1978 and 1980, provides employees with not only a stake in the ownership of the firm in which they work but also a right to participate in the distribution of its profits. Technically ESO is a legal regulation of an optional, voluntary employee relations practice. It is government- and employer-driven and is aimed at increasing the identification of employees with their employers, making them more conscious of the market pressures on their firms and ensuring they gain financially from corporate profitability. There are certain types of ESO which attract tax advantages such as Approved All Employee Profit Sharing Schemes and Save As You Earn Schemes. Under approved schemes, employees are not liable for income tax on gains in exercising share options.

Regulated collectivism

This involves collective processes, underpinned by the law, and includes:

- wages councils
- conciliation, arbitration and mediation
- trade union rights
- pension fund trustees
- unilateral industrial sanctions
- in the European context, co-determination.

Third-party intervention and trade union rights

Wages councils were established in law to settle the minimum hourly rates of pay and overtime pay in particular industries, where there was no collective bargaining machinery. First set up in 1909, they were abolished in 1993, apart from the 'wages boards' for agricultural workers in England and Wales and in Scotland. They consisted of employer, union and independent representation, including an independent chair. Wages councils determined the pay rates of workers covered by their terms of reference, at regular intervals, and issued wages regulation orders setting out their decisions. These were legally enforceable on all employers in the industries covered by them.

Voluntary conciliation, arbitration and mediation in Britain is provided by ACAS, through the TULRCA 1992, where either a trade dispute is threatened, or negotiations between an employer and a union have broken down. Collective conciliation is the process whereby, with negotiations having broken down, and normally when the agreed procedures to avoid disputes are exhausted, ACAS officers provide assistance to both sides to get them talking again. Their intervention often provides a basis for resolving such conflicts. Arbitration is the process whereby a third party, normally a single arbitrator or a panel of arbitrators, hears the cases of each side, deliberates on their evidence and determines a settlement. Each side agrees in advance to be bound by the decision of the arbitrator and to accept the award. Mediation is the process whereby a third party, normally an individual nominated by ACAS, with the approval of both sides, makes recommendations to the parties which may provide a basis for settling their differences.

Certain legal rights are provided for 'independent' unions having a certificate of independence from the Certification Officer (CO), where they are recognised by employers for collective bargaining purposes. These legal rights include (see also Chapters 3 and 7):

- the appointment of safety representatives and the establishment of safety committees
- consultation on collective redundancies
- information and consultation on business transfers
- secret ballots on employers' premises
- public funds to finance secret postal ballots for specific issues.

Pension fund trustees, whether employee or union representatives, have the right to be consulted where an employer:

- wishes to contract out of the State Earnings Related Pension Scheme (SERPS)
- introduces pension benefits without contracting out of SERPS
- replaces one contracted-out scheme with a new one
- wishes to amend a contracted-out scheme.

Industrial sanctions

Industrial sanctions are normally taken, within a framework established by the law, where there are no alternative conflict resolving processes left. They may be used unilaterally either by employers, management organisations and managers against employees and their unions or by employees and their unions against employers. They are a method of last resort and are used by one party to force the other to concede a demand, often of principle, which cannot be resolved by persuasion, negotiation, compromise or third-party intervention. Industrial sanctions involve the blunt use of employer, union or worker power against the other party. To remain 'constitutional', in other words within the accepted rules of employee relations, they should be taken only after any agreed procedures for avoiding conflict have been used and a 'failure to agree' has been recorded.

Employers use a range of industrial sanctions. These include, in increasing order of severity:

- tight supervision
- harsh discipline
- demotion
- withdrawing overtime
- changing working practices unilaterally
- lockouts
- closing sites or workplaces
- reinvesting in plant and machinery elsewhere.

Formal sanctions by employees and unions against employers and management, in turn, include (see also Chapter 11):

- lax time-keeping
- working inefficiently
- working to rule
- overtime bans
- stoppages of work.

Co-determination

Co-determination, as yet unestablished in Britain, is the process embodied in law whereby employees are enabled to participate in certain areas of managerial decision-making within the business organisations employing them. In Germany, for example, the law provides for the establishment of works councils at plant or site level (Berghahn and Karsten 1987). Works councils are elected by the workforce in all plants or sites where there are five or more employees. They exist to protect the interests of workers in the plant and to ensure that effect is given to legislation, safety regulations and collective agreements affecting employees. They also have the right to participate in certain management decisions relating to the operation of the plant, the conduct of employees and the distribution of working hours. The employer also has to seek the consent of the works council on certain other issues.

Other forms of co-determination by employee representatives in management are provided for by federal law in Germany. These operate at company level. In the mining, iron and steel industries, for example, there is numerical parity of 'capital' and 'labour' representatives on the (upper-tier) supervisory boards of these enterprises. These appoint and dismiss members of the (lower-tier) management board and supervise them. Additionally, the labour director, who is a member of the management board, cannot be appointed against the wishes of the majority of the employee representatives. In limited companies employing more than 2,000 persons, 50 per cent of the supervisory board are shareholder representatives, with the employees' side divided between those employed by the company and external trade union representatives (see Chapters 3 and 10).

EXTERNAL INFLUENCES

Employee relations in the labour market and workplace do not take place in a vacuum. The resolution of potential employment conflict between the buyers and sellers of labour services are affected by a variety of economic and political factors.

The micro-economic level

A major determinant of pay rates and numbers of workers employed by an organisation is the demand for labour relative to its supply. Other things being equal, where labour demand exceeds labour supply, pay rates rise. Where labour supply exceeds labour demand, pay rates fall. There is also the union 'mark-up' differential between union and non-union labour. This is the extent by which unions are able to raise pay rates for their members over and above the market rates for equivalent non-union labour. The union mark-up varies widely across occupations and over time. Stewart (1983), for example, indicates a union mark-up of about 8 per cent in British manufacturing as a whole, with shipbuilding and paper and printing, at that time, having mark-ups of around 18 per cent and 11 per cent respectively. Clearly, the union mark-up varies over time but these figures give some idea of the 'gap' between union and non-union pay.

The determinants of an employer's demand for labour are complex. It depends partly on the structure of the external labour market, its internal labour market and its local labour market, but more particularly on the buoyancy, or not, of its product markets (Brown 1973) or, in the public services, on the ceiling placed on public spending by government (Beaumont 1992). The total supply of labour available to the economy is determined by the size of the population of working age, with the amount supplied being a function of the labour force participation rate, the number of hours that people are willing to work and the amount of effort provided by people at work. From an employer's point of view, the available labour supply is affected by its quality, relative mobility and potential productivity.

A firm's external labour market (ELM) is the numbers of workers that are either available for work or potentially available for new jobs. Within the ELM, pricing and allocating decisions are controlled largely by economic variables, but employer decisions are crucial (Rubery 1989). In practice, because of differences in the quality of labour, in terms of aptitudes, skills and training, the ELM is highly segmented by occupation, industry, geography, gender, race and age (Dex 1989; Jenkins 1989; and Ashton 1989). One theory, the dual labour market hypothesis, is that the ELM is dichotomised into primary and secondary sectors. The primary sector is characterised by 'good' jobs and the secondary sector by 'bad' ones. Good jobs have high pay, high status, excellent promotion prospects, attractive fringe benefits and security of employment. Bad jobs, with the opposite characteristics, are allocated to those excluded from the primary sector, because they lack investment in 'human capital' or are discriminated against. In the secondary sector, where unions are weak or unrecognised, pay rates are established largely by competition and market supply and demand, since with full employment there are sufficient jobs available for all those seeking work at current pay rates, or, in conditions of unemployment, labour supply exceeds labour demand and pay rates fall. Work in the secondary sector is generally low paid, unattractive and unstable.

Internal labour markets (ILMs) are the arrangements by which labour is supplied and demanded within a firm without direct access to the ELM. Employment policies are directed towards those employed in the firm, with most jobs being filled by the promotion or transfer of workers who are already working in the company (Robinson 1970). ILMs, therefore, consist of sets of employment relationships, embodying formal and informal rules, which govern each job and the relationships amongst them. The reasons for ILMs include:

- union pressure for internal promotion, based on seniority
- on-the-job training which makes the jobs unique
- low-cost recruitment
- good employment practice
- more reliable selection
- scarcity of skills in the ELM.

Local labour markets (LLMs) are largely the consequence of the financial and psychological costs and disadvantages, to workers, of extensive time spent travelling to work. These costs further segment a labour force which is already stratified by the characterisitics outlined above. They tend to restrict a firm's labour market to that which is accessible from a limited geographical area, for less skilled occupational groups at least. This definition of LLMs assumes that their key characteristic is that the bulk of an area's working population continually seeks employment there and that local employers recruit most of the labour from the area.

The macro-economy

Government economic policy also affects the buyers and sellers of labour. One approach is Keynesian demand management which dominated British macro-economic policy during the 1940s, 1950s and 1960s (Worswick and Ady 1952; Dow 1964; Worswick and Trevithick 1984). Its focus is on the level of aggregate demand in the economy. This is the total sum spent on goods and services, consisting of consumption, investment, government expenditure and expenditure on exports less imports. With the economy expanding and aggregate demand rising, demand for goods, services and labour increases, unemployment falls and union bargaining power is strengthened. When the economy slows down, because of falls in consumption or investment, demand for goods, services and labour decreases, unemployment rises and union bargaining power is weakened.

Governments using Keynesian demand management techniques seek to influence the level of aggregate demand by counter-cyclical fiscal and monetary policies. These are aimed at trying to slow down the economy when it is booming, because 'full employment' contributes to pay and price inflation, and at trying to boost the economy during recession, because unemployment is rising. Governments cut their spending and raise taxes when the economy is overheating and increase their spending, by public borrowing, and cut taxes when the economy is in recession (see Chapter 4).

The ways in which employers and unions in the private and public sectors react to these policy instruments is crucial in determining whether or not governmental policy succeeds. If pay bargainers fail to respond to the labour market signals given by government, and pay increases rise faster than national productivity, then the 'pay–price' and 'pay–tax/public borrowing' spirals are fuelled, resulting in inflation, low growth and balance of payments problems. If, on the other hand, employers resist 'felt-fair' union pay claims, then increases in trade disputes are likely. For these reasons, Keynesian demand management policies are normally linked with 'prices and incomes' policies, necessitating employer and union co-operation with government, aimed at restraining price and pay rises in line with rises in productivity and efficiency in the corporate sector (Jones 1987; see also Chapter 7 below).

Another approach is where governments focus on 'supply-side' measures, as they have done in Britain and the United States since the mid-1970s. Supply-side economics emphasises that the principal determinant of the rate of growth of an economy, in both the short and long run, is the allocation and efficient use of labour and capital. It is a restatement of neo-classical macro-economic principles. These are based on the notion of 'rational expectations' and a 'natural rate of unemployment' that emerges as a result of efficient market clearing. By this view, the natural rate of unemployment cannot be reduced by raising aggregate demand and attempts to disturb this equilibrium are self-defeating. This is because they will be anticipated and neutralised by economic agents in the market place (Brittan 1988; Green 1989; Levacic 1988).

Supply-side economic policies focus on removing impediments to the supply of and efficient use of the factors of production. They are concerned with the determinants of the natural rate of unemployment, rather than with the level of effective demand in the short run as in Keynesian macro-economics. Amongst these impediments are claimed to be disincentives to work and invest, because of tax structures and tax levels, and institutional barriers, such as trade unions, to the efficient allocation of resources. The policy prescriptions flowing from this analysis are (see also Chapters 4 and 7):

- deregulating labour and product markets, thus making them more competitive and efficient
- privatisation
- cutting public borrowing
- cutting taxes.

The employee relations implications of these supply-side policies are that they result in the strengthening of employer bargaining power in the labour market and managerial rights in the workplace. In the private sector, in order to remain competitive in tight product markets, companies seek increased workforce productivity and efficiency. These are only made possible by reducing unit labour costs and increasing labour flexibility. This results in rising unemployment – unless pay rates fall, new product markets are found or growth rates are high. This weakens union wage bargaining power. In the public sector, there are similar employer pressures to raise efficiency, keep public spending under control and resist union pay claims which are 'not affordable' or not responsive to 'market forces'. The right to manage, in turn, is reinforced at the workplace, because of fear of unemployment and job losses, and union resistance to changes in working practices, new technology and managerial assertiveness is weakened.

Politics, the state and the law

Politics, the state and the law are never neutral in employee relations. The roles of the state – as legislator, manager of the economy, employer or third-party conciliator – its governmental agents, and the courts are crucial in determining the contexts within which employee relations decisions are taken (see Chapter 7).

During the nineteenth century, in the age of classical *laissez-faire*, or the doctrine that economic decisions are best guided by the autonomous decisions of free individuals in the market place, the state's role in employee relations was a minimalist and restrictive one. This reflected the dominant power structures in a society based on landed wealth, a growing entrepreneurial class of manufacturers and merchants and an élitist Parliament and undemocratic political system (Fox 1985). Wide differentials in wealth, class, status and power separated 'master' from 'servant', capitalist from worker, entrepreneur from wage earner and even craftsman from labourer. And common law, described by Kahn-Freund (1983: page 18) as 'a command under the guise of an agreement', dominated the employment contract between the primary parties to the pay–work bargain.

By the early twentieth century, with the slow emergence of trade unionism amongst working people and the gradual democratisation of the parliamentary system, there were three main political and legal legacies of classical *laissez-faire* for employee relations. One was the emergence of a unified 'Labour Movement', linking the now legally emancipated unions with the newly created Labour Party (see Chapter 7). This political alliance was in reaction to the dominance in Parliament of the business and commercial classes and meant that employee relations were now inevitably politicised and dichotomised between those representing the interests of the capitalist and labouring classes respectively (Farnham 1976; 1996). Second, there was a mistrust of the law by working people, especially of the courts, in the ways it affected trade unions, collective bargaining and the regulation of industrial conflict. Their preference was for autonomy in collective bargaining with employers and for non-intervention by the courts and the judges in employee relations. The third legacy was the central importance of the common law in regulating the individual contract of employment.

With the steady growth in the size, power and scope of the state in the twentieth century (White and Chapman 1987), and the continued democratisation of society (Middlemas 1979), it was inevitable that the roles of government and the law would increase in employee relations. Crouch (1979) provides four models of state or public policy on employee relations under advanced capitalism. These are summarised in Figure 2. He describes them as:

- voluntary collective bargaining
- neo-*laissez-faire*
- corporatism
- bargained corporatism.

The model that predominates depends on whether the state is organised on 'corporatist' or 'liberal' principles and whether the position of trade unions within it is 'weak' or 'strong'. A corporatist state is where the economy is largely privately owned but the interests of capitalists, workers and government are integrated and mediated, through centralised institutional mechanisms, to ensure political and economic stability. A liberal state, in contrast, is one based on private enterprise but where the political and economic spheres are disassociated. Economic decisions are decentralised, with businesses, individuals and workers exercising freedom of choice in the market place. A crucial development in economic liberalism is the acceptance of trade unionism, or collectivism. Combination takes place to offset the inequalities between workers as sellers of labour services and capitalists as buyers in the market place, resulting in 'collective' liberalism or collective *laissez-faire*.

Figure 2 **State policies on employee relations**

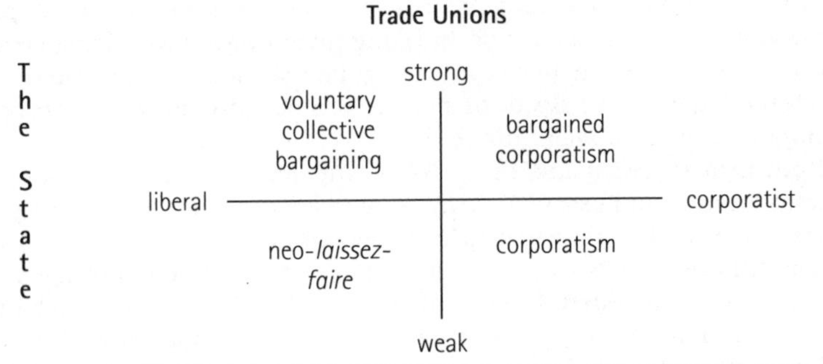

Trade Unions

The State

	liberal	corporatist
strong	voluntary collective bargaining	bargained corporatism
weak	neo-*laissez-faire*	corporatism

Source: Crouch (1979)

Governments, with their economic and legal policy preferences, determine whether employee relations operate in corporatist or liberal contexts and whether trade unions are weak or strong. The centralised, corporate state, with weak trade unions – as in postwar Japan – provides corporatism as the employee relations model. This often comprises a combination of supply-side economic policies, union pay constraint and legal limitations on trade unions. Where unions are strong in a corporate state, the model is described as *bargained corporatism*. This is a situation, as in Britain during the Second World War and in the late 1970s, and in parts of central Europe such as the Federal Republic of Germany, where union leaders accepted politically imposed restraints on 'free collective bargaining' in return for other gains for their members, such as concessions on social policy, laws favourable to union organisation and a share in economic and political decision-making (Crouch 1994).

In the liberal, market-centred state, *voluntary collective bargaining* provides the model for employee relations where unions are strong. This was the dominant model for much of the post-war period in Britain, especially in the 30 years after 1945, apart from 1970–71. It was characterised largely by bipartisan Conservative or Labour governments, with demand management economic policies and legal abstention in employee relations. Where unions are weak in the liberal state, the model is described as neo-*laissez-faire*. This was the case in the interwar period and since the early 1980s. During this period, Conservative governments supported supply-side economic policy and legal intervention in employee relations. These proscribed union activities and industrial action (Moran 1977; Gamble 1988; Farnham 1990; see also Chapter 7 below).

ASSIGNMENTS

(a) Why do people work? What do they get from working? And what are the main implications of employee needs at work for employers and their employee relations policies? Give examples from your own organisation.

(b) Provide examples of employment costs to your organisation for employing various categories of staff, breaking them down into costing classifications. What factors have to be taken into account by the employer in 'costing' the likely effects of a stoppage of work by a key group of employees in the organisation?

(c) Read Brown (1972) and Terry (1977) and analyse what is meant by the term 'custom and practice'. Why do workers use it and why do employers accept it? Looking at your own organisation, identify some current 'customs and practices', indicating management's reaction to them and why they are tolerated. Provide other examples of 'C and P' which management have recently claimed back, how this was done and why.

(d) Interview some managers, including someone in personnel, at least one trade union representative and some employees and ask them to define what they consider to be 'good employee relations'. Comment on and compare their answers and approaches. Rank in order of relative importance the conflict-resolving processes in your organisation used to maintain 'good employee relations', commenting on them as appropriate.

(e) Identify and evaluate the types of labour market from which your employer recruits its employees. How are these labour markets segmented and what are the implications for employee relations?

(f) Read Lewis (1997) and identify the main common law duties of employers and employees under the contract of employment.

(g) Summarise Flanders' analysis of the trade unions' role in politics (1970: pages 24–37). Examine the relevance of his arguments today. Alternatively, discuss his analysis of job regulation and its part in rule making in employee relations (pages 86–94).

(h) Evaluate Kahn-Freund's 'reflections on law and power' in employee relations (1977: pages 1–17). Outline how the role of the law in employee relations has evolved since then and its relevance for management.

REFERENCES

ASHTON, D. 1989. 'Educational institutions, youth and the labour market'. In Gallie, D. (ed.) 1989, *Employment in Britain*, Oxford: Blackwell.

BERGHAHN, V. *and* KARSTEN, D. 1987. *Industrial Relations in West Germany*. Oxford: Berg.

BEAUMONT, P. 1992. *Public Sector Industrial Relations*. London: Routledge.

BRITTAN, S. 1988. *A Restatement of Economic Liberalism*. London: Macmillan.

BROWN, W. 1972. 'A consideration of custom and practice'. *British Journal of Industrial Relations*. X(1), March.

BROWN, W. 1973. *Piecework Bargaining*. London: Heinemann.

CENTRAL STATISTICAL OFFICE. 1991. 'Employment in the public and private sectors'. *Economic Trends*. 458, December.

CROUCH, C. 1979. *The Politics of Industrial Relations*. Glasgow: Fontana.

CROUCH, C. 1994. *Industrial Relations and European State Traditions*. Oxford: Clarendon Press.

DEX, S. 1989. 'Gender and the labour market'. In Gallie, D. (ed.) 1989. *Employment in Britain*, Oxford: Blackwell.

DOW, J. 1964. *The Management of the British Economy 1945 to 1960*. Cambridge: Cambridge University Press.

FARNHAM, D. 1976. 'The Labour Alliance: reality or myth?' *Parliamentary Affairs*. XXIX(1), Winter.

FARNHAM, D. 1983. 'Human resources management and employee relations'. In Farnham, D. and Horton, S. 1993, *Managing the New Public Services*. Basingstoke: Macmillan.

FARNHAM, D. 1990. 'Trade union policy 1979–89: restriction or reform?' In Savage, S. and Robins, L. (eds), *Public Policy under Thatcher*, Basingstoke: Macmillan.

FARNHAM, D, 1996. 'New Labour, new unions and the new labour market' *Parliamentary Affairs*. 49(44), October.

FARNHAM, D *and* GILES, L. 1996. 'Human resources management and employment relations'. In Farnham, D. and Horton, S. (eds) 1996, *Managing the New Public Services*. Basingstoke: Macmillan.

FARNHAM, D. *and* HORTON, S. (eds) 1996. *Managing the New Public Services*. Basingstoke: Macmillan.

FLANDERS, A. 1968. 'Collective bargaining: a theoretical analysis'. In Flanders, A. 1970, *Management and Unions*. London: Faber and Faber.

FLEMING, A. 1989. 'Employment in the public and private sectors'. *Economic Trends*. 434, December.

FOX, A. 1985. *History and Heritage*. London: Allen and Unwin.

GAMBLE, A. 1988. *The Free Economy and the Strong State*. London: Macmillan.

GREEN, F. 1989. *The Restructuring of the British Economy*. London: Harvester.

JONES, R. 1987. *Wages and Employment Policy 1936–85*. London: Allen and Unwin.

JENKINS, R. 1989. 'Discrimination and equal opportunity in employment: ethnicity and race in the United Kingdom'. In Gallie, D. (ed.) 1989, *Employment in Britain*, Oxford: Blackwell.

KAHN-FREUND, O. 1977. *Labour and the Law*. London: Stevens.

KAHN-FREUND, O. 1983. *Labour and the Law*. (3rd edn.) London: Stevens.

LEVACIC, R. 1988. *Supply Side Economics*. Oxford: Heinemann.

LEWIS, D. 1997. *Essentials of Employment Law*. (5th edn) London: IPD.

MARCHINGTON, M. 1989. 'Joint consultation in practice'. In Sisson, K. (ed.) 1989, *Personnel Management in Britain*, Oxford: Blackwell.

MIDDLEMAS, K. 1979. *Politics in Industrial Society*. London: Deutsch.

MORAN, M. 1977. *The Politics of Industrial Relations*. London: Macmillan.

OFFICE FOR NATIONAL STATISTICS 1997. 'Employment in the public and private sectors'. *Economic Trends*. 520, March.

RUBERY, J. 1989. 'Employers and the labour market'. In Gallie, D. (ed.) 1989, *Employment in Britain*, Oxford: Blackwell.

ROBINSON, D. (ed.) 1970. *Local Labour Markets and Wage Structure*. Farnborough: Gower.

STARKS, M. 1991. *Not for Profit Not for Sale*. Bristol: Policy Journals.

STEWART, M. 1983. 'Relative earnings and individual union membership in the UK'. *Economica*.

TERRY, M. 1977. 'The inevitable growth of informality'. *British Journal of Industrial Relations*. 15(1).

WEBB, S. *and* WEBB, B. 1913. *Industrial Democracy*. NY: Longmans.

WEDDERBURN, LORD 1986. *The Worker and the Law*. Harmondsworth: Penguin.

WHITE, G. *and* CHAPMAN, H. 1987. 'Long-term trends in public expenditure'. *Economic Trends*. 408, October.

WORSWICK, D. *and* ADY, P. 1952. *The British Economy 1945–50*. Oxford: Oxford University Press.

WORSWICK, D. *and* TREVITHICK, 1984. *Keynes and the Modern World*. Cambridge University Press.

2 The parties in employee relations

In advanced market economies, employee relations are largely institutionalised. This means that the primary parties to the employment relationship (employers and employees) are bound together by a network of formally agreed rules, agreements and procedures, such as contracts of employment, employment handbooks, grievance, disciplinary and promotion procedures, and by informal customs and practices. These provide both parties with a series of interdependent, individual rights and obligations, emphasising the mutuality of their relationship, which are aimed at reconciling any potential conflicts between them authoritatively and fairly. These rights and obligations between employers and employees are economic, legal and constitutional in character but they are underpinned by a set of normative and moral values associated with fairness, equity and trust in the employment relationship (Hyman and Brough 1975; Fox 1974; Fox 1985).

Another institutional feature of employee relations is the secondary nature of many employment relationships. The secondary parties (management or management organisations and unions) are also bound together by a network of formally agreed rules, agreements and procedures. These include union rules, collective agreements and negotiating and consultative procedures (see Chapters 1, 9 and 10). These link the parties together in a web of mutually independent, collective rights and obligations aimed at reconciling any potential conflicts between them legitimately and peacefully. They are economic and constitutional in character, with their own procedural and substantive, normative order (Flanders and Fox 1969).

The last institutional feature of employee relations is the existence of third parties, normally agents of the state. These bodies are created to influence the decisions of the primary and secondary parties and to ensure either 'fair play' or changes in the balance of power amongst them. The values associated with third-party institutions have varied between those of evenhandedness, balance and legitimacy, on the one side, and of bias, controversy and coercion on the other (see Chapter 7).

MANAGEMENT

The term 'management' is used in two main senses. First, management is the set of activities carried out by those individuals with decision-taking and executive responsibilities in organisations. It focuses on the jobs, tasks and activities which managers do. This definition of management incorporates three aspects of managing: what managers do; how they do it; and how they are grouped in organisations, vertically and horizontally. It recognises that managers are themselves employees who are employed for the knowledge, skills and expertise which they bring into organisations as part of the internal and occupational divisions of labour. Management in this sense focuses on four areas of managing: the nature of managerial work (Mintzberg 1975; Stewart 1982); managerial processes (Fayol 1949; Likert 1961; Peters and Waterman 1982); management levels (Chandler and Daems 1980); and the functional areas of management such as operations, finance, marketing and personnel (Farnham 1990).

The second way in which the term 'management' is used is to describe the group of people in organisations who are collectively responsible for the efficient and effective running of the enterprises they manage. By this view, management is the authority system or the power group which has the responsibility for ensuring the financial viability, organisational success and ultimate accountability of an enterprise to its primary beneficiaries, whether these are shareholders, government ministers or local politicians. Management in this sense focuses on the agency roles of managers in terms of their responsibilities for enterprise effectiveness, corporate efficiency and employee relations. It is this meaning of the term 'management' that is primarily used in this book.

One objective of management collectively is to ensure the profitability and/or efficiency of the organisations in which they work. They have to ensure the most efficient use of enterprise resources and the achievement of enterprise goals. In practice, however, managements also have to take account of the broader social and economic consequences of their decisions, not just the short-term economic ones. In this respect, Brown (1960) amongst others argues that managements have to reconcile a number of conflicting aims and objectives. These include making their enterprises economically viable, whilst at the same time seeking to be responsive to shareholder, customer, supplier and employee interests. Managements, in short, are concerned not only with profits and efficiency, or with 'value for money' in the public sector, but also with being socially responsible to the wider communities with which they interact. They also want good working relations with their employees. This view of management is one most recently revived in the concept of the enterprise as one consisting of a number of interrelated and interdependent 'stakeholders' (Hutton, 1996).

This means that employees are only one of the many stakeholders in organisations and only one of the executive concerns of management. Customers, banks, suppliers and government inspectorates all make demands on management. Employee relations are an important part of the management function but they are only one of management's many organisational roles and corporate responsibilities. This makes the managing of employee relations problematic in any organisation. At one extreme, managements can develop sophisticated employee relations strategies, policies and procedures, which take account of the other, often conflicting, demands made on management. Here the employers' objective is to promote the best employment practices associated with 'model' employing organisations. At the other extreme, managements may act in ways meeting only the minimum employment standards required by the law and local labour market pressures.

Employee relations management

For these and related reasons, medium and larger organisations in both the private and public sectors use employee relations specialists. They are variously described as personnel officers, industrial relations advisers, employee relations managers or, most recently, as human resource managers. It is these members of management who represent the human resource function within the management structure and in its dealings with employee or union representatives, and are the professional managers of the employment contract. In the early 1990s it was estimated that there were some 150,000 people working in the personnel function in Britain, with employee relations accounting for 35 per cent of all personnel activity (Institute of Personnel Management 1992).

The traditional management role in employee relations has been a disinterested, reactive and fire-fighting one. Top management literally did not want to know about employee relations (Winkler 1974). According to Miller (1987), this pattern of reactive, 'non-strategic' employee relations management implies an employee relations function which is characterised by being:

- separate from an organisation's corporate strategy
- short term
- of no interest to the board of directors.

It is also identified with a definition of employee relations focusing principally on unionised groups of manual workers.

Managing collective bargaining

The steady growth of trade unions throughout the first part of the twentieth century, together with employer recognition of trade unions and public policy support for collective bargaining, meant that the joint determination of terms and conditions of employment became the centrepiece of British employee relations by the 1960s (Ministry of Labour 1965). Indeed, the conclusion of the Donovan Commission (1968: page 50) was that 'collective bargaining is the best method of conducting industrial relations'. It added, however, that multi-employer, industry-wide bargaining was no longer capable of imposing its decisions on the participants. The Commission therefore recommended that management should take the initiative and responsibility for reforming collective bargaining at company and plant levels. The means was to be the development of proactive personnel policies, management-led authoritative, collective bargaining machinery, comprehensive procedural agreements and joint arrangements for discussing health and safety at work, within companies or plants. Multi-employer, industry-wide bargaining would deal with those issues, such as overtime premiums, length of working week or holiday periods, which it could most effectively regulate (see Chapter 7).

From the late 1960s, Donovan's recommendations were gradually extended and acted upon in much of the corporate sector, with parallel developments in the public sector. The changes must not be exaggerated, however, as research by Storey (1992: page 259) shows that whilst old-style industrial relations 'fire-fighting' is increasingly being disavowed by managements, there is hardly 'an instance where anything approaching a "strategic" stance towards unions and industrial relations could readily be discerned as having taken its place'. Nevetheless, the outcome has been the steady expansion in numbers of personnel and employee relations specialists to help deal with the workplace issues arising from decentralised collective bargaining, the increasing scope of employment legislation and trade union organisation locally (Millward and Stevens 1986; Millward *et al.* 1992).

In this role, employee relations specialists are a resource from which senior line management can draw advice, expertise and technical know-how. The sorts of tasks in which they are involved include:

- participating in negotiating and joint consultation
- assisting in the drafting of collective agreements
- advising on employment legislation
- advising in grievance and disciplinary cases
- handling redundancies
- providing inputs to personnel policy-making and decision-taking.

It is a role with both advisory and executive functions which typifies this approach to employee relations management.

Human resources management (HRM) and the new industrial relations

Another development, largely since the 1980s, has been the emergence of more strategic approaches to managing employee relations. This has taken place in some larger organisations, especially in the corporate sector, in response to increased product market competition, changes in market structures and technological change. Some of these developments are identified in the debate about HRM (Storey 1989; Storey 1992; Sissons 1989). This debate distinguishes between 'hard' HRM, focusing on human resource strategy and employee utilisation, and 'soft' HRM, with its greater emphasis on the 'human' aspects of management and concern with people in organisations. Whatever the exact nature of HRM, survey evidence reveals a positive picture of strategic HRM by the early 1990s, with 63 per cent of UK organisations surveyed claiming to have personnel or human resource directors, 83 per cent claiming a corporate strategy and 73 per cent claiming a personnel or HRM strategy (Price Waterhouse Cranfield 1990).

Other developments have given rise to a related debate focused on the relationship between the claimed rise of HRM and the apparent decline of trade union power. Bassett (1986) and Wickens (1987), on the basis of limited case study material, proclaim the arrival of a 'new industrial relations' based on single-union, 'no-strike' deals or even no unions at all. Dunn (1990) notes that the rhetoric of industrial relations has changed. From being based on the metaphor of 'trench warfare', it is now based on that of the 'new frontier', which is more consistent with HRM and the notion of a new industrial relations than it is with traditional personnel management.

Models of employee relations management

From this outline analysis, it is clear that the roles and status of employee relations specialists in organisations are now secure but are quite different from what they were when Donovan reported. Employee relations management clearly operates in a variety of modes and at different organisational levels. Some are operating in roles akin to what Tyson (1987) describes as the 'contracts manager' model of the personnel function. This is where employee relations specialists are particularly valued for their capacity to make quick decisions and informal agreements with trade union representatives, and their other activities are largely advisory. Others are operating as what Tyson describes as HRM 'architects'. This is a creative view of personnel and employee relations which aims at contributing to corporate success through explicit human resources policies and integrated systems of labour control between personnel and line managers. The architect model is particularly associated with the management of change, proactive personnel planning and systems of employee involvement (see Chapter 10 on non-union patterns of employee relations).

Managerial approaches to employee relations

In its role as agent of the employer, management has a variety of employment activities to carry out. These include: attracting, recruiting, rewarding, motivating, retaining, directing, disciplining, exiting, negotiating and consulting with employees at work. In undertaking these activities, managements can choose, explicitly or implicitly, from a multiplicity of approaches to employee relations. A critical influence is management style. Management style, according to Purcell (1987: page 535), implies:

> a distinctive set of guiding principles, written or otherwise, which set parameters to and signposts for management action in the way employees are treated and particular events handled. Management style is therefore akin to business policy and its strategic derivatives.

It is management style, in short, which circumscribes the boundaries and direction of acceptable management action in its dealing with employees.

Frames of reference

Some writers suggest that it is management's 'frame of reference' which determines their predominant style of employee relations management. Fox (1966) identifies two major frames of reference, the unitary and the pluralist. The main elements of the unitary view are:

- organisations consist of teams of people, working together for common aims, where there are no conflicts of interest between managers and subordinates
- strong leadership is required from management to achieve common organisational purpose
- trade unions are illegitimate intrusions into the right to manage.

Pluralism, in contrast, emphasises:

- organisations are coalitions of competing interests, where management's role is to mediate amongst different interest groups
- trade unions are legitimate representatives of employee interests
- stability in employee relations results from concessions and compromises between managers and unions in the collective bargaining process.

Fox (1974) develops his analysis further in identifying four 'ideal' typologies of employee relations management. He describes managements as being:

- *traditionalists*, with unitary, anti-union policies
- *sophisticated paternalists*, with unitary, enlightened, employee-centred human resource policies
- *sophisticated moderns*, with pluralist, joint management–union decision-making in defined areas
- *standard moderns*, where unions are recognised but employee relations fire-fighting predominates.

Purcell and Sisson (1983) divide the standard modern management style into 'constitutionalists' and 'consultors'. Constitutionalists codify the limits of collective bargaining, whilst consultors place greater emphasis on joint consultation and joint problem-solving.

Individualism and collectivism

Purcell (1987: pages 535–6) claims that the unitary and pluralist frames of reference are limited in defining management styles. He identifies two main dimensions of management style: individualism and collectivism. Individualism focuses on 'the feelings and sentiments of each employee' and encourages the capacities of individual employees and their roles at work. He distinguishes between 'high' and 'low' degrees of individualism. High individualism emphasises the resource status of employees, with employers wanting to develop and nurture their employees' talents and abilities.

Related employment policies include careful selection, internal labour markets, staff appraisal, merit pay and extensive communication systems, all of which are associated with a 'neo-unitary' approach to employee relations (Farnham and Pimlott 1995). Low individualism emphasises the commodity status of employees, with employers concentrating on the control of both labour costs and the labour process. Profits are the priority and employment policies include recruiting in secondary labour markets, tight workplace discipline and little security of employment. Intermediate between high and low individualism is 'paternalism'. This synthesises caring, welfare employment policies with the subordinate position of lower-level employees in the organisational hierarchy.

Collectivism is the 'extent to which the organisation recognises the right of employees to have a say in those aspects of management decision-making which concern them' (Purcell 1987: page 538). Collectivism is operated through trade union organisation or other forms of employee representative system, thus giving employees a collective voice in organisational decision-making. There are two aspects of collectivism: the levels of employee participation – whether these are 'high' or 'low' – and the degree of legitimacy given to collective organisation by management. High-level employee participation such as co-determination, pension fund trustees and employer-wide collective bargaining, takes place at the corporate level. Low-level employee participation, in contrast, takes place at workgroup, departmental or workplace levels. Management tolerance of collectivism ranges from willing co-operation, at one extreme, to grudging acceptance at the other.

The important point which Purcell makes is that the links between individualism and collectivism in employee relations are complex. Whilst some employers have more individualist management styles, such as most American-owned companies, and some have more collectivist ones, such as many larger British companies, elements of both individualism and collectivism are not incompatible with each other, as in some Japanese-owned and British companies.

> Management styles operate along the two dimensions and . . . action in one area, toward individualism, for example, is not necessarily associated with changes in the collectivism scale (page 541).

In practice, individualist styles of employee relations management tend towards non-unionism, whilst collectivist ones lead to union recognition. Thus whether an employer recognises trade unions for representational, consultative, negotiating or co-determination purposes is a critical and visible expression of management style and approach to employee relations. This does not mean, however, that internal training, promotion ladders and welfare provisions for individual employees are precluded. On the other hand, where trade unions are recognised and employees given a collective voice in employee relations, and the unions are subsequently derecognised, this is clearly an expression of a shift towards a more individualist style of employee relations management (Claydon 1989).

Employee relations policies

It is difficult to define the concept of an 'employee relations policy' with precision. In essence, it represents an employer's intentions and objectives about employment-related and human resource matters and the ways in which these are communicated to managers, employees, the wider community and, where they are recognised, to trade unions and their representatives. In practice, employee relations policies are an amalgam of explicit written statements and implicit unwritten assumptions about how employees are to be treated and managed as individuals and as members of trade unions. They are dynamic, organisationally specific and contingent on the external and internal environments within which organisations operate. Management style is an important determinant of an organisation's employee relations policies but the internal and external contingencies are crucial.

The contingencies acting on management in determining an organisation's employee relations policies include:

- legislation
- other employers' policies
- organisational size, ownership and location
- union power
- prevailing 'good practice'
- most importantly, the links between the organisation's business strategy and its employment and human resources strategy.

Policy choices

One way of analysing management's policy choices in employee relations is outlined in Figure 3. This identifies four potential policy choices for management. First, management can pursue a policy of *worker subordination*. This is based on low degrees of individualism and collectivism, with high levels of management discretion. Policy is operated through firm management control. Second, the policy of *union incorporation* is where there is a relatively high degree of collectivism, a low degree of individualism and policy is operated, in key employment areas, through joint management–union regulation. The third policy choice is *employee commitment* which incorporates a high degree of individualism and a low degree of collectivism, with policy being operated through management-driven programmes of HRM and employee involvement. Fourth, the policy of *worker participation* involves high degrees of both individualism and collectivism, with policy being operated through management–employee co-determination linked, possibly, with employee involvement measures. Indeed worker participation policies are not incompatible with union incorporation and/or employee commitment policies. In practice, of course, managements can adopt different employee relations policies for different groups of workers or different policies for the same group of workers at different times.

Figure 3 **Management policies on employee relations**

		Individualism	
		low	high
Collectivism	low	worker subordination	employee commitment
	high	union incorporation	worker participation

Business strategy and managing personnel

A more sophisticated analysis is that of Thomason (1991). He examines the links between business strategy and management approaches to acquiring and utilising human resources and identifies three historical shifts in business strategy. They are not watertight compartments but are indicative of the main emphases of business strategy in different historical periods, different enterprises over time and some enterprises at any one time. The three approaches are:

- a *product differentiation strategy*, associated with the early industrial revolution
- a *low-cost leadership strategy*, associated with industrial rationalisation which began about 100 years ago
- a *customer/client satisfaction strategy*, associated with 'new wave' rationalisations, in response to global competition and technical change, since the 1960s.

The differentiation strategy depends upon a core skilled workforce, supplemented by peripheral workers recruited for less-skilled work, organised in factories and workshops. The low-cost strategy depends upon the external labour market, where jobs are broken down into small tasks and repetitive activities, in line with the principles of scientific management. In contrast, in organisations seeking special relationships with their customers or clients, emphasis is placed on quality, reliability and product or service delivery and intra-organisational teamwork. This business strategy depends on, first, the development of internal labour markets and job training for existing employees. Second, job tasks and activities are reorganised, with the focus being on flexibility, versatility, multi-skilling and commitment. Third, managements try to create and transmit new corporate cultures to their employees (Anthony 1990), emphasising the primacy of client relationships, quality and teamwork.

Thomason's analysis leads to four possible labour control processes for management. The first stresses the need for quality output and, where recruitment takes place in the external labour market, uses an *employee selection strategy*. The second, which emphasises low-cost production and recruitment in the external labour market, uses an *employee supervision strategy*. This provides a framework of agreed or imposed employment rules and procedures. The third, based on price competition and demand for high-quality products, relies on a *human resources development strategy*, aimed at staff flexibility. The fourth, stressing customer satisfaction and recruitment from the internal labour market, focuses on a *human resources partnership strategy*. This aims at integrating employees into the organisation and at employee commitment.

MANAGEMENT ORGANISATIONS

There are a range of organisations acting on behalf of management interests in employee relations. Some, such as the IPD and the Institute of Directors, are based on individual or personal membership. This section focuses on management organisations that are based on collective or corporate membership and have specific roles in employee relations and related areas.

Employers' associations

An employers' association is defined in law as any organisation of employers, individual proprietors or constituent organisations of employers whose principal purpose includes the regulation of relations between employers and workers or between employers and trade unions. Employers' associations recruit member firms vertically, on an industry-wide basis.

Objectives, functions and ideology

The idea of employers within an industry combining together for employee relations purposes is not a new one. The first such bodies were formed in the nineteenth century in response to trade union organisation. Their central objective was to protect employer interests collectively in dealings with the unions (Clegg 1979). However, unlike in the USA (where, despite anti-trust laws, there have been powerful producer cartels), there has always been a much stronger ideological reluctance by British companies to combine amongst themselves for business purposes. Companies have generally jealously guarded their 'trade secrets' and corporate independence in commercial matters, with the result that membership of employers' associations has often been resisted by some British companies. In recent years, the national collective bargaining function and protective role of employers' associations have diminished, as decentralised bargaining has grown and union power weakened.

One of the main traditional roles of employers' associations has been to bargain collectively for their members, with the trade unions, on a multi-employer or industry-wide basis. The theory underlying this is that multi-employer collective agreements on pay and conditions take labour costs out of competition for all employers in the industry, thus allowing companies to compete in product markets other than by undercutting their competitors' employment costs. A corollary to this is that combination amongst employers also protects individual employers against being 'picked off', one by one, by the union(s) during a trade dispute.

At the end of 1996, the Certification Officer, who is required by law to maintain a list of employers' associations under Section 2 of the Trade Union and Labour Relations (Consolidation) Act 1992, listed 110 such organisations, with another 115 bodies that were unlisted. This compares with 131 listed and 146 unlisted associations in 1992, 148 listed and 187 unlisted associations in 1986, and 196 listed and 280 unlisted associations in 1977 (Certification Office 1997; 1992; 1987; 1978). Despite the reduction in the numbers of employers' associations operating in Britain since the late 1970s, employers' associations continue to have a role in employee relations, especially in industries where labour costs are a high proportion of total costs, or where the industry is dominated by a large number of relatively small companies in competitive product markets, such as electrical contracting, building construction, and printing. Here two-tier bargaining is the norm, with multi-employer bargaining – through such organisations as the Electrical Contractors Association and British Printing Industries Federation – setting a floor of terms and conditions for the industry.

Current activities

In these and similar cases, employers' associations continue to provide a number of services to member firms. These include:

- employer representation in industry-wide bargaining
- intelligence, information and data collection
- assistance in operating procedures to avoid disputes
- policy guidelines and advice on employee relations
- consultancy and training for managements
- representing employers at industrial tribunals
- protection for employers taking part in trade disputes against the trade unions in their industry.

In acting as specialist centres of employee relations knowledge and expertise, employers' associations, like trade unions, are serviced by a cadre of full-time officers who work closely with elected representatives from member companies in determining policy, representing employer interests and fire-fighting on behalf of employers when necessary (Watson 1988).

A main reason why there has been a decline in the absolute numbers and the relative importance of employers' associations in the last decade is the declining importance of multi-employer pay bargaining arrangements in the private sector (Brown and Walsh 1991). Further, the traditional reluctance to combine by private employers has been reinforced by recent changes in business structure, especially decentralised cost centres (Marginson *et al.* 1988), increased product market competition and devolved employee relations policies. In these circumstances, companies, and sometimes plants within multi-site companies, are less inclined to join employers' associations for employee relations purposes. They prefer the autonomy of determining their own employment policies, reward structures and decentralised bargaining arrangements for dealing with trade unions. Indeed, some writers argue that decentralised bargaining provides distinct advantages to managements by keeping local union officials and full-time officers away from strategic decision-making (Kinnie 1987). In some cases, employers have even opted for union derecognition and no bargaining at all (Gregg and Yates 1991).

Another reason for the relative decline in importance of employers' associations is political. Since the late 1970s, governments have adopted market-centred economic policies rather than corporatist ones (see Chapters 1, 4 and 7). Apart from special cases such as the National Farmers' Union, this has generally diminished the role of employers' associations as pressure groups representing the interests of employers nationally in discussions in Whitehall, and government departments. Moreover, with shifts towards greater EU integration and a single European market for labour, capital, goods and services, the role of industry-wide employers' associations is further weakened. The political role of employers' associations is now more effectively carried out by central organisations such as the Confederation of British Industry (CBI), which recruits horizontally and vertically, and supranational ones such as the Union of Industrial and Employers' Confederations of Europe (UNICE) (see below), than by industry-based ones.

The Confederation of British Industry (CBI)

Unlike some of its European counterparts, such as in Germany, Ireland and the Netherlands, the CBI – ever since its formation in 1965 – has been ambivalent about taking on a corporatist role in employee relations in collaboration with unions and government at central level. In recent years, its activities have mainly focused on 'speaking up' for British business. The CBI has an Employment Policy Committee – comprising an Employee Relations Panel, Employment Relocation Panel and Equal Opportunities Panel – and an Education and Training Affairs Committee but it is, as a management organisation, only indirectly involved in employee relations and then only in so far as these affect corporate efficiency, productivity and competitiveness.

The CBI's mission is to 'help create and sustain the conditions in which businesses in the UK can compete and prosper' (Confederation of British Industry 1995: page 9) and its objectives are:

- to provide the means for British industry to influence economic and related policy
- to develop the contribution of British industry to the national economy
- to encourage economic efficiency
- to provide advice and services to its members.

CBI policy prescriptions on employee relations are limited but direct. First, since the 1980s, the CBI has continually expressed its opposition to a tightly regulated labour market and has been strongly opposed to harmonised EU employment legislation and minimum standards of employment protection. Its arguments are that this would adversely affect business competitiveness and restrict the necessary flexibility of the labour market and it continues to support the UK opt-out from the Social Chapter. Second, CBI actions on employment affairs have concentrated on helping its members protect labour cost competitiveness and labour flexibility. The CBI has continually argued the case for linking employee pay to corporate performance and productivity growth. It has also taken part in the public debate about the merits of decentralised pay bargaining (Confederation of British Industry 1991).

The CBI has recently identified its most important economic, European, education and training, employment policy and international activities and those policy changes by government where it considers its influence has been most felt. These include (Confederation of British Industry 1996a):

- working on the private finance initiative with government
- encouraging the Labour party in a more pro-business direction
- keeping European business issues on the political agenda
- contributing to a more dispassionate debate about European monetary union
- lobbying Brussels for action on competitiveness and related business issues
- publishing regional business agendas; focusing on competitiveness
- shifting the Labour party away from statutory training levies towards individual learning accounts
- raising business concerns on how the quality of UK skills base might be addressed
- developing a strong small and medium enterprise agenda, oriented towards growth companies
- supporting full implementation of the Uruguay Round Agreements in World Trade Organisation discussions.

The CBI also published an agenda aimed at the incoming Labour government, elected in May 1997, setting out policies needed 'for sustained wealth creation' in the UK (Confederation of British Industry 1996b: page 3). It set out the features of the global context and the resultant challenges that business and government would have to address jointly. These included:

- meeting the challenges and opportunities of a changing world

- maintaining economic stability
- building a Europe that works
- investing to grow
- focusing on making markets work
- working together effectively
- developing skilled and flexible people.

In the latter context, the CBI wanted an education and training system supporting lifelong learning; employment practices focusing on investment in people as individuals; and labour market legislation supporting flexibility and responsiveness which 'doesn't stand in the way of job creation' (page 10). The CBI therefore supported:

- further improvements in Britain's education and training system
- the attainment of agreed national education and training targets
- a unified and respected qualifications structure for 16–19-year-olds
- tax-incentivised learning accounts for individuals
- Investors in People being made available to small and medium-sized enterprises
- pay linked to performance.

On the other hand the CBI opposed:

- legislative imposition of specific forms of employee relations
- a statutory enforced minimum wage
- a UK opt-in to the Social Protocol at Maastricht.

The CBI claims to represent the interests of more than 250,000 member organisations embracing all sectors of industry and commerce and more than 200 trade associations. Many of its members are multinational businesses or parent companies with subsidiaries, but over 90 per cent of its members are firms with under 200 employees. This means that the CBI recruits both horizontally across industries and vertically within them. To fulfil its tasks, it has a President's Committee, a council, a National Manufacturing Council and 15 standing committees. These bodies are serviced by seven directorates, and a chief economic adviser, comprising: membership and commercial; small and medium-sized enterprises; finance; business environment; European affairs; human resources; and manufacturing and international markets. The CBI is also active in Europe though UNICE.

The Union of Industrial and Employers' Confederations of Europe (UNICE)

UNICE is the official voice of European business and industry in contact with European institutions and was established in 1958. It is composed of 33 central industry and employers' federations from 25 European countries, with a permanent secretariat based in Brussels. Its purposes include (Union of Industrial and Employers' Confederations of Europe 1997);

- to keep abreast of issues that interest its members by maintaining permanent contacts with all the European institutions
- to provide a framework which enables industry and employers to examine European policies and proposed legislation and prepare joint position papers
- to promote its policies and positions at European and national level and persuade European legislators to take them into account
- to represent its members in the dialogue between social partners provided for in European treaties.

UNICE's main priorities are:

- improving European competitiveness leading to growth and the creation of lasting jobs
- completing all aspects of the Single Market
- progressing towards economic and monetary union, with a European system of central banks and a single currency
- pursuing economic and social cohesion in the EU
- developing social policies compatible with competitiveness and economic growth
- supporting the restructuring and economic development of central and eastern Europe
- liberalising world trade on the principles of the GATT Uruguay Round Agreement
- promoting European technology, research and development
- protecting the environment based on sustainable development.

UNICE's principal contacts are with the Commission of the European Communities, the European Parliament, the Council of Ministers and Economic and Social Committee. It also works with other European-level governmental organisations and international non-governmental organisations such as the European Trade Union Confederation (ETUC). It operates through its Council of Presidents, an Executive Committee, a permanent Secretariat in Brussels and a series of policy committees which assist in policy formulation, suggest actions to be taken and implement UNICE decisions (Union of Industrial and Employers' Confederations of Europe 1997).

EMPLOYEE ORGANISATIONS

Trade unions

A trade union is any organisation of workers, or constituent or affiliated organisations, whose principal purposes include the regulation of relations between its members and their employers, managements or employers' associations. The CO listed 245 unions in Britain in December 1996, with a total of 8 million members, although some 80 per cent of this membership was concentrated in the 16 largest unions with 100,000 members or more. This compares with 287 listed unions in 1992, with a total of 9.8 million members, 375 listed unions with 10.8 million members in 1986 and 485 listed unions with 12.1 million members in 1977 (Certification Office 1997; 1992; 1987; 1978).

Objectives, functions and ideology

Trade unions organise by occupation or industry. Where they are occupationally based, unions recruit horizontally across industries and vertically within them. Where they are industrially based, they recruit vertically within an industry, as in Germany's 17 *Industriegewerkschaften* or industrial unions. Because of their deep historical roots, the complex structures of British industry and the variegated patterns of union mergers and amalgamations, British trade unions are rarely based on occupational or industrial lines alone. They tend to recruit both across and within industries, resulting in union membership competition and multi-union representation structures with employers (see Chapter 8 below; Coates and Topham 1988).

Like employers' associations, trade unions exist to protect the interests of their members. The essential rationale of trade unions therefore is to defend and extend their members' individual employment interests, in both their market relations and managerial relations with employers, through collective organisation and strength. Trade union organisation, in other words, is based on an ideology of collectivism, or worker solidarity, summed up in the slogan 'Unity is Strength'. The industrial objectives of trade unions include participating in:

- the determination of pay and conditions
- the maintenance and improvement of health and safety standards within the workplace
- how work and job tasks are organised
- agreed employee relations procedures for resolving grievances, disciplinary and related issues
- 'fair' dealings with management
- improving security of employment in the workplace.

Many unions also have political objectives since, as organisations, they want to influence political decision-making when it affects the interests of their members as employees and citizens, and the interests of unions as employee interest groups. To these ends, the unions seek to influence, first, government economic policies, such as those covering the labour market, the training of human resources, union bargaining power, taxation and public spending. Second, unions are also interested in government legal policy and the ways that it affects individual employment rights and union collective rights to organise, to be recognised by employers and to take industrial action against employers. Third, they want to influence government social policies, in terms of pensions, state benefits and the 'social wage'. Unions also play an international role by seeking links with unions in other countries. They want to influence international labour policy and protest when brother and sister unionists overseas are persecuted or discriminated against by employers or the political authorities (see Chapter 8).

Current activities

Unions use a variety of methods to further their industrial objectives as the collective agents of employee participation in employee relations. These include unilateral regulation, collective bargaining, joint consultation and industrial action. In parts of Europe, such as in Sweden, Germany and Denmark, unions also participate with management in co-determination systems, which provide legal rights for employee representatives in enterprise decision-making (Incomes Data Services 1991).

In furthering their political objectives, unions in Britain use a number of methods. These include lobbying governments, seeking consultations with ministers and maintaining close links with the Labour Party (McIlroy 1988). The political role of the unions is made possible through the device of 'political funds' and the 'political levy'. Under the TULRCA 1992, unions can include the furtherance of political objects amongst their aims and adopt political fund rules. These provide for union expenditure on political objects but any payments made in furthering them must come out of a separate political fund. Union members not wishing to pay the political levy may 'contract out' of paying it. The main uses of union political funds include:

- to affiliate union members to the Labour Party, thereby enabling unions to influence Labour Party policy
- to support Labour Members in Parliament
- to conduct political campaigns on behalf of their members.

In 1995, 47 unions had political funds, with some 5 million members contributing to them, compared with 1990, when 54 unions had political funds, with 6.1 million members contributing to them (Certification Office 1997; 1992).

Trade unions are voluntaristic and democratic bodies, with all the strengths and weaknesses associated with these characteristics. With the closed shop unlawful, individuals generally join the trade union of their choice, according to their occupation, where they work and what unions are recognised. Once recruited, members are allocated to a union branch which is the basic unit of trade union organisation. Branches are linked to regions or divisions which, in turn, are linked to national union headquarters (Farnham and Pimlott 1995).

Unions are democratic bodies in the sense that decisions at workplace, divisional and national levels are taken only after membership debate and by majority voting. Every member is entitled to stand for union office, in accordance with the union rule book and the law, and to participate on an equal basis in union decision-making procedures. In workplaces, shop stewards, workplace representatives and health and safety representatives are elected to speak on behalf of their members with management. Workplaces, branches and divisions, in turn, are serviced and supported by full-time, professional union officers.

Staff associations and professional bodies

The term 'staff associations' is difficult to define with precision but in essence they have three main characteristics:

- their membership is confined to employees of a single employer, where the employees are almost always in non-manual white-collar work
- they do not normally regard themselves as 'trade unions' in the accepted meaning of the term
- they are generally found in the private sector rather than in public sector employment, especially in the financial services such as banks, insurance and building societies.

Staff associations are sometimes encouraged by employers and managements in order to keep unions out of their businesses. Such organisations, confined to a single employer, are rarely effective negotiating bodies. They lack adequate financial resources, find it difficult to bargain on equal terms with the employer and, though operating at low cost, are poorly protected against unexpected hostility from a paternalist or benevolent employer (Certification Office 1981). On the other hand, it is sometimes the employees themselves who, in seeking collective representation with the employer, are reluctant to join a union for ideological, political or social reasons. With their relatively low membership subscriptions and lack of militancy, staff associations sometimes provide an acceptable alternative to trade unions for certain types of white-collar employee (Farnham and Giles 1995).

Professional bodies are not primarily employee relations agencies. They normally seek to:

- control the education and training of new members to the 'profession', acting as 'qualifying associations'
- maintain professional standards amongst members
- advance the standing and status of the profession in the wider community (see Millerson 1964).

Where professional bodies take on a dual function, in seeking to protect and improve their members' employment interests, such as in pay determination or collective bargaining, this is more likely to happen in the public sector rather than the private sector. In the education and the health services, for example, there are groups of professional employees who use their professional bodies in this dual capacity, such as amongst nurses, midwives and teachers.

The Trades Union Congress (TUC)

The TUC is 'the unions' union'. It is a long-established body, formed in 1868, and is the sole central co-ordinating body of the British trade union movement. In comparison with most other European countries, this is fairly unusual since in Europe there are often rival central trade union centres, representing different political, confessional and occupational interests. The TUC is an autonomous body composed of individually affiliated union organisations which pay an annual affiliation fee, based on their membership size. In 1996, the TUC had 74 affiliated unions, representing 6.8 million members, which accounted for 85 per cent of total union membership in the UK at that time. This compares with 74 affiliated unions, with 8.2 million members, in 1991; 89 affiliated unions, with 9.6 million members, in 1986; and 108 affiliated unions, with 11.6 million members, in 1981 (Trades Union Congress 1997; 1991; 1986; 1981).

The general aims of the TUC are:

- to promote the interests of all or any of its affiliated organisations
- to improve the economic and social conditions of workers in all parts of the world
- to affiliate to or assist any organisation having similar objectives to the TUC
- to assist in the complete organisation of all workers eligible for union membership
- to assist in settling disputes between members of affiliated organisations and their employers, between affiliated organisations and their members, and between affiliated organisations themselves.

The TUC also has a series of targeted, workplace objectives which are set out in its Employment Charter for a World Class Britain (Trades Union Congress 1997). It is these objectives which affiliated unions seek to deliver on behalf of their members, underpinned by the belief that all working people should be entitled to them:

- a safe and healthy working environment
- equal treatment at work regardless of sex, race, disability, sexuality or age
- a clear written statement from their employer of the key rights provided by their contract of employment
- lifelong access to education and training
- equivalent treatment whether full-time, part-time, temporary, self-employed or working at home
- provision to help parents and carers combine work and domestic responsibilities

- fair pay, working hours, holidays, pensions and sick pay arrangements
- information and consultation on all matters affecting their security of employment
- fair treatment when disciplinary action is taken against them
- fair treatment in cases of redundancy, including levels of compensation which fully reflect their earnings
- proper protection in cases of business transfers, takeovers, mergers and insolvency
- provision to join and be represented by an independent trade union with proper facilities and fair treatment for union representatives.

The TUC's priorities in the late 1990s were to continue championing the cause of working people and their rights at work, through promoting a 'decent platform' of rights 'as a prerequisite for economic growth and a fair society' (page 2). These included:

- continuing to work on the national minimum wage and the wider challenge of building a successful economy
- mounting a campaign for fair employment rights
- pursuing a 'new unionism' project concentrating on organisation and recruitment
- advancing the TUC agenda in Europe
- raising the profile of the TUC and its affiliates around training issues.

The TUC gives effect to these aims, objectives and priorities in a number of ways. These include:

- developing policies on industrial, economic and social matters and campaigning actively for them
- assisting unions in dispute
- regulating relations between affiliated unions and promoting inter-union co-operation
- providing services to affiliated unions
- nominating representatives on statutory and consultative bodies
- participating in international trade union organisations.

The TUC's policy-making congress meets annually in the first week of September and is attended by more than 800 delegates. The General Council, which governs the TUC between congresses, is elected by congress and has an executive committee, four task groups and six joint committees, covering a very wide range of sub-areas such as economic affairs, employment law, equality issues, health and safety, and public services. The main committees are:

- representation at work
- full employment
- monitoring group on European social dialogue

- organising and recruitment
- pensioners
- race relations
- TUC regions
- trades councils
- women's issues
- youth forum.

These committees and their activities are serviced by seven permanent TUC departments:

- secretary's
- economic and social affairs
- equal rights
- international
- management services and administration
- campaigns and communications
- organisation and services.

The European Trade Union Confederation (ETUC)

The ETUC was founded in 1973 and, in 1997, represented 58 national trade union centres from 14 European countries and 14 industry federations totalling more than 53 million members. With its headquarters located in Brussels, the ETUC is the voice of organised labour throughout Europe, being by far the most representative all-industry trade union federation within the EU. It is the only general trade union organisation recognised as a 'social partner' by the European Commission. It has the following membership:

- unitary trade unions confederations, such as the TUC in the UK, Irish Congress of Trade Unions (ICTU), Czech Moravian Chamber of Trade Unions (CMK OS), Confederation of Trade Unions of the Slovak Republic (KOZ SR) and *Deutscher Gewerkschaftsbund* (DGB) in Germany
- those which are predominantly blue-collar or white-collar union groups, such as the *Landesorganisationen i Sverige* (LO) and the *Tjänstemannens Centralorganisation* (TCO) in Sweden, *Landsorganisasjonen i Norge* (LO-N) and *Akademikernes Felleorganisasjon* (AF) in Norway and *Landesorganisationen i Danmark* (LO) and *Akademikernes Centralorganisation* (AC) in Denmark
- union federations with particular ideological or political tendencies, such as the socialist *Fédération Générale du Travail de Belgique* (FGTB), the Christian *Confédération des Syndicats Chrétiens* (CSC) in Belgium and *Christelijk National Vakverbond* (CNV) in the Netherlands
- 14 European industry Federations, drawn from affiliated unions in particular sectors, such as metal, telecommunications, agriculture, public services, textiles and journalists.

The ETUC has a wide remit and works throughout Europe to promote a variety of economic, political and social objectives on behalf of working people and their families (European Trade Union Confederation 1997). These include:

- the extension and consolidation of political liberties and democracy
- respect for human and trade union rights
- the elimination of all forms of discrimination based on sex, age, colour, race, sexual orientation, nationality, religious or political beliefs and political opinions
- equal opportunities and equal treatment for men and women
- geographically balanced and environmentally sound economic and social development
- freely chosen and productive employment for all
- the development, improvement and enhancement of education and training for all
- the democratisation of the economy
- a steady improvement in living and working conditions
- a society free of exclusion, based on the principles of freedom, justice and solidarity.

The ETUC has the task of carrying out, with the highest degree of cohesion, trade union initiatives at European level so as to attain its goals as part of the process of European integration. To this purpose, the ETUC directs its activities towards (page 1):

- the EU, calls for the deepening of its social, political and democratic aspects, in step with that of its economic and monetary dimensions, for its enlargement to other European countries, and for its active commitment to promoting peace, development and social justice in the world
- the Council of Europe, EFTA and other European institutions which promote co-operation on matters affecting working people's interests
- the European employers' organisations, with a view to establishing solid labour relations at European level via the Social Dialogue and negotiations.

The International Confederation of Free Trade Unions (ICFTU)

The ICFTU was formed in 1949. It now has 141 affiliated organisations in some 97 countries on five continents, with a membership of about 86 million. It is a confederation of national trade union centres, with a secretariat in Brussels and permanent offices in Geneva and New York. Its motto is 'Bread, Peace and Freedom' (International Confederation of Free Trade Unions 1988). The objectives of the ICFTU include:

- promoting the interests of working people throughout the world
- working for rising living standards, full employment and social security

- reducing the gap between the rich and poor
- working for international understanding, disarmament and world peace
- helping workers to organise themselves and secure the recognition of their organisations as free bargaining agents
- fighting against oppression, dictatorship and discrimination of any kind
- defending fundamental human and trade union rights.

The ICFTU helps to defend workers' rights, fight poverty, reduce international tensions and promote peace. It also has very close relations with the International Labour Organisation (ILO), which is the only international body made up of government, employer and worker representatives. Because of ICFTU representation, the ILO has established many international standards to protect workers' rights and denounce violations of trade union rights by governments. The ICFTU insists that all countries should respect basic trade union rights such as freedom of association, free collective bargaining and the right to strike. The ICFTU represents the trade union movement at international conferences, in the United Nations (UN) and in various specialised UN agencies. Finally, the ICFTU maintains close relations with the International Trade Secretariats associated with it, such as the International Metal Workers' Federation and the International Transport Workers' Federation.

STATE AGENCIES

Industrial tribunals (ITs) and the Employment Appeal Tribunal (EAT)

ITs are independent judicial bodies set up to hear matters of dispute in employee relations, quickly, informally and cheaply. ITs have a legally qualified chair, with two other members each of whom are drawn from panels appointed by the Secretary of State for Education and Employment – one after consultation with employee organisations, the other after consultation with employers' organisations. Anyone can present cases at ITs, which deal with a variety of appeals, applications and complaints. ITs also determine questions of compensation delegated to them. About 50 ITs sit daily in England and Wales, with the number of hearings now over 20,000 per year.

The jurisdiction of ITs derives from a series of employment laws and EU regulations, enacted on a piecemeal basis since the mid-1970s. The legal rights stemming from them are largely directed at individual workers and individual trade unionists. The principal legislative provisions include:

- Equal Pay Act 1970 and Equal Pay Amendment Regulations 1983
- Health and Safety at Work etc. Act 1974 and Safety Committees Regulations 1977
- Sex Discrimination Act 1975
- Race Relations Act 1976

- Transfer of Undertakings (Protection of Employment) Regulations 1981
- Wages Act 1986
- Trade Union and Labour Relations (Consolidation) Act 1992
- Trade Union Reform and Employment Rights Act 1993
- Disability Discrimination Act 1995
- Employment Rights Act 1996.

Although the matters that may be considered by ITs are wide-ranging (Department of Employment 1991; Dickens and Cockburn 1986), about 60 per cent relate to claims of unfair dismissal. The other main applications relate to the Wages Act 1986 (16 per cent), redundancy payments (13 per cent), race discrimination (2 per cent), sex discrimination (2 per cent), equal pay (1 per cent), with all other items under 1 per cent each (Central Office of Industrial Tribunals 1995).

The EAT was established by Sections 86 and 87 of the Employment Protection Act (EPA) 1975. It sits regularly in London and Edinburgh and consists of appointed judges and lay members, with special knowledge or experience of employee relations as employer or worker representatives. It hears appeals from the decisions of ITs on questions of law only. It is not the function of the EAT to re-hear the facts of the case as they were put to an IT. Nor does the EAT have power to interfere with the judgement reached by ITs on those facts. Any appeal to the EAT must show that in reaching its decision the tribunal made an error in its interpretation or application of the law. As in tribunals, any person may appear before the EAT, including employer and union representatives. The EAT hears several hundred cases each year.

The Advisory, Conciliation and Arbitration Service (ACAS)

ACAS was created by the Employment Protection Act (EPA) 1975. Its prime statutory duty, now incorporated in the Trade Union and Labour Relations (Consolidation) Act (TULRCA) 1992, is to promote 'the improvement of industrial relations' (Section 209). Until 1993, this duty had included the particular role 'of encouraging the extension of collective bargaining and the development and, where necessary, reform of collective bargaining machinery.' This is now no longer the case. Clearly, ACAS's role is now less circumscribed by legislation than it was in the past. ACAS is independent of government, employers and trade unions but its governing council is drawn from employers, employee organisations and independent experts in employee relations.

In carrying out its statutory duties, ACAS undertakes four main activities:

- preventing and resolving disputes
- providing conciliation services in actual and potential complaints to ITs
- giving advice, assistance and information on industrial relations and employment issues
- promoting good employment practices.

In 1995, ACAS received 1,321 requests for collective conciliation, with 1,229 cases being completed and 1,082 cases resulting in a settlement or progress towards a settlement, and it dealt with 136 cases which were referred to arbitration and dispute mediation. It also received 91,568 cases for conciliating in actual and potential claims to ITs, which was the highest ever total. Of these, 86,252 cases were completed. These consisted of 32,798 settlements, 28,643 withdrawn and 24,991 going to ITs. ACAS's network of Public Enquiry Points was also kept busy, with over 538,000 enquiries (Advisory Conciliation and Arbitration Service 1996).

ACAS's role in resolving disputes is through collective conciliation, arbitration and mediation (see Chapter 3). Collective conciliation is the process whereby employers and trade unions are helped to reach mutually acceptable settlements of disputes through neutral, third-party intervention by an ACAS conciliation officer. It is voluntary, and agreements reached in conciliation are determined by the parties themselves, normally only after agreed procedures are exhausted or when both sides agree that there are overriding considerations requiring it. In 1995, ACAS's completed conciliations consisted of: pay and conditions of employment (48 per cent), followed by redundancy (17 per cent), discipline and dismissal (12 per cent), union recognition (9 per cent), other trade union matters (7 per cent), changes in working practices (3 per cent) and other issues (4 per cent). This compares with 1991, when ACAS's completed conciliations consisted of pay and conditions of employment (41 per cent), followed by redundancy (19 per cent), union recognition (14 per cent), dismissal and discipline (12 per cent), other union matters (7 per cent) and changes in working practices (4 per cent).

Voluntary arbitration is provided where the parties in dispute invite one or more impartial persons to make a decision which both parties agree in advance to accept. It is normally regarded as a means of last resort for determining a peaceful settlement, where disputes cannot be resolved by other methods. In accordance with the TULRCA 1992, ACAS has to ensure that:

- the consent of both parties is obtained
- conciliation is considered
- any agreed procedures have been used and a failure to agree recorded.

Arbitration may proceed, however, where ACAS believes there to be special circumstances for using it. In 1995, the issues referred to arbitration and mediation were: grading (43 per cent), discipline and dismissal (22 per cent), annual pay (17 per cent) and other pay and conditions of employment (14 per cent). In 1991, by contrast, the issues referred to ACAS arbitrators (and mediators) were discipline and dismissal (35 per cent), other pay and conditions of employment (22 per cent), grading (22 per cent) and annual pay (17 per cent).

Mediation is where a third party, appointed by ACAS, assists the parties to reach their own negotiated settlement, by making appropriate suggestions to both sides. These recommendations are similar to those of an arbitrator's award but the parties do not agree in advance to accept them. Mediation tends to constrain the parties more than conciliation does but is more flexible and decisive.

ACAS also has a statutory duty to promote settlements of complaints, by individuals, which have been or could be made to an IT. The largest part of ACAS's workload concerns unfair dismissal. This is followed by claims under the Wages Act 1986, sex discrimination, and racial discrimination.

The advisory and information services provided by ACAS complement its conciliation services. The key areas where ACAS focuses its advisory services are:

- orderly, dispute-free collective bargaining
- the orderly and voluntary resolution of individual employment issues
- effective and felt-fair payment and reward systems
- improved communication, consultation and employee involvement practices
- the effective use of human resources at work, including participative approaches to change.

It is also ACAS's belief, in the ongoing search for competitiveness, that organisations 'must' (Advisory Conciliation and Arbitration Service 1996, page 27):

> develop a positive approach not only to change in the workplace but also to the conduct of industrial relations. In particular we emphasise the need to:
>
> - involve all interested parties in a partnership approach and turn away from an adversarial style of industrial relations
> - seek change though co-operation rather than conflict by recognising the importance for employees and their representatives of being informed, consulted and fully involved in all aspects of change
> - understand the importance of people and the benefits of developing them to their full potential.

The Central Arbitration Committee (CAC)

The CAC is a standing, independent arbitration body, working nationally in employee relations. It was set up as 'the Industrial Court' in 1919 and its current status and constitution are embodied in the TULRCA 1992. The CAC has three panels, one consisting of the independent chair and deputy chairs and two of members with experience as employers and employees. Cases are normally heard by a committee of three, with one member from each panel. The CAC deals with issues relating to national disputes, a single employer or a particular employee group. It provides voluntary arbitration in trade disputes at the request of one party, but with the agreement of the other. It also determines claims by trade unions for disclosure of information for collective bargaining purposes. Its workload tends to be light, with most claims referring to disclosure of information.

The Certification Officer (CO)

The CO, originally established under Section 3 of the EPA 1975, has six main functions, now stemming from the TULRCA 1992 (Certification Office 1997):

- maintaining a list of trade unions and determining their independence
- dealing with complaints by members that a union has failed to maintain an accurate register of members; seeing that unions keep proper accounting records; investigating the financial affairs of unions; and ensuring that the statutory requirements regarding members' superannuation schemes are observed
- dealing with complaints by members that a union has failed to comply with the legal provisions regarding secret postal ballots in union elections for executive committees, presidents and general secretaries
- ensuring observance of the statutory procedures governing political funds for trade unions and dealing with complaints about breaches of political fund rules
- seeing that the statutory procedures for amalgamations and transfer of engagements between unions are complied with and dealing with complaints by members about the conduct of merger ballots
- maintaining a list of employers' associations and ensuring their compliance with the statutory requirements relating to accounting records, annual returns, political funds and transfers of engagements and amalgamations.

The Commissioner for the Rights of Trade Union Members (CRTUM)

The CRTUM was created under the Employment Act 1988 and her duties are now incoporated in the TULRCA 1992. She has two sets of powers, which overlap with the duties of the CO. The first is to grant assistance to union members contemplating or taking legal action against a union or an official or a trustee arising out of an alleged or threatened breach of a member's statutory union membership rights. These include where a union:

- has without the support of a properly conducted secret ballot called for industrial action by its members
- has not observed the statutory requirements relating to union elections and membership registers
- has applied its funds for electoral or party political purposes without a properly constituted political fund
- has failed to comply with the rules approved by the CO in any ballot on a political resolution
- has failed to bring proceedings to recover union property applied to pay or indemnify an individual for a penalty imposed for an offence or contempt of court

- has denied members their statutory right of access to its accounting records
- has failed to secure that certain offenders do not hold a position in a union to which they are not legally authorised
- has not stopped its trustees permitting an unlawful application of the union's property or are proposing to comply with an unlawful direction.

Second, the CRTUM may also grant assistance when a union member complains that a union has failed to observe the requirements of its own rule book. Typical areas of complaint include:

- the appointment, election or removal of persons from union office
- union disciplinary proceedings
- authorising or endorsing industrial action
- balloting members
- imposing, collecting or distributing levies for industrial action
- the application of a union's funds or property
- the constitution or proceedings of any conferences or committees.

The means by which individual union members can enforce these rights are through the courts, ITs or the CO, depending on the unlawful act. In general, the Commissioner has wide discretion in deciding whether to grant assistance or not. Assistance includes paying for legal advice or legal representation, or making arrangements for such advice or representation to be provided.

Commissioner for Protection Against Unlawful Industrial Action (CPAUIA)

The CPAUIA was established under the provisions of Section 266 of the TULRCA 1992, as amended by the Trade Union Reform and Employment Rights Act 1993. It shares premises and staff with the CRTUM. The Commissioner's role is independent of government and she has the power to grant assistance to any person who is an actual or prospective party to certain High Court or Court of Sessions proceedings, where that individual has been, or is likely to be, deprived of goods and services because of industrial action unlawfully organised by a trade union. The assistance provided can include paying the costs of legal advice and/or representation of the applicant which enable him or her to take proceedings to restrain the unlawful organisation of industrial action by the union. In 1995–96, for example, three formal cases were presented to the Commissioner. In one case the unlawful action had ceased on receipt of the application; in the second case the action was 'unofficial', not unlawful; and in the third case, the application concerned matters 'outside the scope of the Commissioner's powers' (Commissioner for Protection Against Unlawful Industrial Action 1996: page 23).

ASSIGNMENTS

(a) Read Hyman and Brough (1975: especially pages 229–53) and comment on their analysis of the role of social values in employee relations, particularly the concept of 'fairness'. Alternatively read Flanders and Fox (1969: pages 241–76). What did they identify as the sources of 'normative disorder' in British industrial relations at that time and how did these manifest themselves? What relevance does their analysis have for employee relations today?

(b) Interview an employee relations manager and find out the sort of job tasks and activities which he or she does. To whom is this person accountable and what sort of performance targets are set by senior management for this individual?

(c) To what extent is the management style of your employer based on individualism and/or collectivism? Provide illustrations of its employment policies and practices to substantiate your diagnosis.

(d) Read Farnham and Pimlott (1995: pages 44–9) and compare and contrast the unitary (including 'neo-unitary') and pluralist concepts of employee relations.

(e) What are the pros and cons of an employer joining an employers' association:

1. in a labour-intensive industry, where the firm is medium-sized, is one of many operating in a competitive product market, and where there are strong trade unions in the workplace and industry?
2. in a capital-intensive industry, where the firm is a large one operating in a heterogeneous product market, and where the unions are weak in the workplace and industry?
3. in a capital-intensive industry, where the firm is medium-sized and is operating in a homogeneous product market and the unions are strong in the workplace and industry?

(f) Using McIlroy (1988: Chapter 1), how do you account for the absolute and relative decline in trade union organisation during the 1980s?

(g) Interview some trade union members and find out: why they are union members, including the benefits of this; what they see as the purposes of trade unions; and what the main problems facing their union are.

(h) Read Chapter 1 of ACAS's current *Annual Report*. What were the major trends in employee relations for that year? How may these trends be explained? Also read the CRTUM's *Annual Report* and comment on the applications for assistance to the Commissioner during the previous year.

(i) Read Clegg (1976: pages 309–16). What is his defence of pluralism in employee relations?

(j) Comment on the latest annual report of the Commissioner for Protection Against Unlawful Industrial Action.

REFERENCES

ADVISORY, CONCILIATION AND ARBRITRATION SERVICE. 1992. *Annual Report 1992*. London: ACAS.

ADVISORY, CONCILIATION AND ARBITRATION SERVICE. 1996. *Annual Report* 1995. London: ACAS.

ANTHONY, P. 1990. 'The paradox of the management of culture or "he who leads is lost" '. *Personnel Review*. 19(4).

BASSETT, P. 1986. *Strike Free: New industrial relations in Britain*. London: Macmillan.

BROWN, W. 1960. *Exploration in Management*. London: Heinemann.

BROWN, W. *and* WALSH, J. 1991. 'Pay determination in Britain in the 1990s: the anatomy of decentralisation'. *Oxford Review of Economic Policy*. 7(1).

CENTRAL OFFICE OF INDUSTRIAL TRIBUNALS. 1995. *Fact Sheet (for England and Wales)*. London: COIT.

CERTIFICATION OFFICE. 1978. *Annual Report of the Certification Officer 1977*. London: CO.

CERTIFICATION OFFICE. 1981. *Annual Report of the Certification Officer 1980*. London: CO.

CERTIFICATION OFFICE. 1987. *Annual Report of the Certification Officer 1986*. London: CO.

CERTIFICATION OFFICE. 1992. *Annual Report of the Certification Officer 1991*. London: CO.

CERTIFICATION OFFICE. 1997. *Annual Report of the Certification Officer 1997*. London: CO.

CHANDLER, A. *and* DAEMS, H. (eds) 1980. *Managerial Hierarchies*. London: Harvard University Press.

CLAYDON, T. 1989. 'Union derecognition in Britain in the 1980s'. *British Journal of Industrial Relations*. 28(2).

CLEGG, H. 1976. 'Pluralism in industrial relations'. *British Journal of Industrial Relations*. XII(2).

CLEGG, H. 1979. *The Changing System of Industrial Relations in Britain*. Oxford: Blackwell.

COATES, T. *and* TOPHAM, T. 1988. *Trade Unions in Britain*. London: Fontana.

COMMISSIONER FOR PROTECTION AGAINST UNLAWFUL ACTION. 1996. *Annual Report*. Warrington: CPAUIA.

COMMISSIONER FOR THE RIGHTS OF TRADE UNION MEMBERS. 1996. *Annual Report 1995–96*. Warrington: CRTUM.

CONFEDERATION OF BRITISH INDUSTRY. 1991. *Annual Review and Report for 1990*. London: CBI.

CONFEDERATION OF BRITISH INDUSTRY. 1992. *The Voice of British Business*. London: CBI.

CONFEDERATION OF BRITISH INDUSTRY. 1995. *Annual Report for 1995*. London: CBI.

CONFEDERATION OF BRITISH INDUSTRY. 1996a. *Annual Review for 1996.* London: CBI.

CONFEDERATION OF BRITISH INDUSTRY. 1996b. *Prospering in the Global Economy.* London: CBI.

DANIEL, W. *and* MILLWARD, N. 1983. *Workplace Industrial Relations in Britain.* London: Heinemann.

DEPARTMENT OF EMPLOYMENT 1991. *Trade Union Immunities.* London: HMSO.

DICKENS, L. *and* COCKBURN, D. 1986. 'Dispute settlement institutions and the courts'. In Lewis, R. (ed.) 1986. *Labour Law in Britain.* Oxford: Blackwell.

DONOVAN, Lord 1968. *Royal Commission on Trade Unions and Employers' Associations 1965–1968:* Report. London: HMSO.

DUNN, S. 1990. 'Root metaphor in the old and new industrial relations'. *British Journal of Industrial Relations.* 28(1).

EUROPEAN TRADE UNION INSTITUTE. 1987. *European Trade Union Confederation: Profile.* Brussels: ETUI.

EUROPEAN TRADE UNION CONFEDERATION. 1997. *ETUC Info: About the ETUC.* Brussels: ETUL.

FARNHAM, D. 1990. *Personnel in Context.* (3rd edn) London: IPM.

FARNHAM, D. *and* GILES, L. 1995. 'Trade unions in the UK: trends and counter-trends since 1979'. *Employee Relations.* 17(2).

FARNHAM, D. *and* PIMLOTT, J. 1995. *Understanding Industrial Relations.* London: Cassell.

FAYOL, H. 1949. *Industrial and General Administration.* (Translated by G. Storrs.) London: Pitman.

FLANDERS, A. *and* FOX, A. 1969. 'Collective bargaining: from Donovan to Durkheim'. In FLANDERS, A. 1970, *Management and Unions,* London: Faber and Faber.

FOX, A. 1966. *Industrial Relations and Industrial Sociology: Royal Commission on trade unions and employers' associations Research Paper 3.* London: HMSO.

FOX, A. 1974. *Beyond Contract: Work, power and trust relations.* London: Faber and Faber.

FOX, A. 1985. *History and Heritage.* London: Allen and Unwin.

GREGG, P. *and* YATES, A. 1991. 'Changes in wage-setting arrangements and trade union presence in the 1980s'. *British Journal of Industrial Relations.* 29(3).

HUTTON, W. 1996. *The State We're In.* London: Cape.

HYMAN, R. *and* BROUGH, I. 1975. *Social Values and Industrial Relations.* Oxford: Blackwell.

INCOMES DATA SERVICES 1991. *Industrial Relations.* London: IPM.

INSTITUTE OF PERSONNEL MANAGEMENT. 1992. *Occupational Mapping Report.* London: IPM.

INTERNATIONAL CONFEDERATION OF FREE TRADE UNIONS. 1988. *Bread, Peace and Freedom.* Brussels: ICFTU.

KINNIE, N. 1987. 'Bargaining within the enterprise: centralised or decentralised?' *Journal of Management Studies*. 24(5), September.

LIKERT, R. 1961. *New Patterns of Management*. NY: McGraw-Hill.

MCILROY, J. 1988. *Trade Unions in Britain Today*. Manchester: Manchester University Press.

MARGINSON, P., EDWARDS, P., MARTIN, R., SISSON, K. *and* PURCELL, J. 1988. *Beyond the Workplace: Managing industrial relations in multi-establishments*. Oxford: Blackwell.

MILLER, P. 1987. 'Strategic industrial relations and human resource management – distinction, definition and recognition'. *Journal of Management Studies*. 24(2), July.

MILLERSON, G. 1964. *The Qualifying Associations*. London: Routledge.

MILLWARD, N. *and* STEVENS, M. 1986. *British Workplace Industrial Relations 1980–1984*. Aldershot: Gower.

MILLWARD, N., STEVENS, M., SMART, D. *and* HAWES, W. 1992. *Workplace Industrial Relations in Transition*. Aldershot: Dartmouth.

MINISTRY OF LABOUR. 1965. *Royal Commission on Trade Unions and Employers' Associations: Written Evidence of the Ministry of Labour*. London: HMSO.

MINTZBERG, H. 1975. *The Nature of Managerial Work*. NY: Prentice Hall.

PETERS, T. *and* WATERMAN, R. 1982. *In Search of Excellence*. NY: Harper and Row.

PRICE WATERHOUSE CRANFIELD. 1990. *Price Waterhouse Cranfield Survey 1990*. Cranfield.

PURCELL, J. 1987. 'Mapping management styles in employee relations'. *Journal of Management Studies*. 24(5), September.

PURCELL, J. *and* SISSON, K. 1983. 'Strategies and practice in the management of industrial relations'. In BAIN, G. (ed.) 1983, *Industrial Relations in Britain*, Oxford: Blackwell.

SISSONS, K. (ed.) 1989. *Personnel Management in Britain*. Oxford: Blackwell.

STEWART, R. 1982. *Choices for the Manager*. London: McGraw-Hill.

STOREY, J. (ed.) 1989. *New Perspectives on Human Resource Management*. London: Routledge.

STOREY, J. (ed.) 1992. *The Development of the Management of Human Resources*. Oxford: Blackwell.

THOMASON, G. 1991. 'The management of personnel'. *Personnel Review*. 20(2).

TRADES UNION CONGRESS. 1981. *Annual Report*. London: TUC.

TRADES UNION CONGRESS. 1986. *Annual Report*. London: TUC.

TRADES UNION CONGRESS. 1990. *Annual Report*. London: TUC.

TRADES UNION CONGRESS. 1991. *Annual Report*. London: TUC.

TRADES UNION CONGRESS. 1997. *Directory*. London: TUC.

TYSON, S. 1987. 'The management of the personnel function'. *Journal of Management Studies*. 24(5).

UNION OF INDUSTRIAL AND EMPLOYERS' CONFEDERATIONS. 1997. *The Voice of European Business and Industry*. Brussels: UNICE.

Watson, D. 1988. *Managers of Discontent*. London: Routledge.
Wickens, P. 1987. *The Road to Nissan*. Basingstoke: Macmillan.
Winkler, J. 1974. 'The ghost at the bargaining table: directors and industrial relations'. *British Journal of Industrial Relations*. July.

3 Employee relations processes

There are a number of conflict-resolving and decision-making processes in employee relations. Some of these are voluntary, others are legal and can involve either collective or individual methods of conducting employee relations. Employee relations decision-making, in turn, may be unilateral, bilateral or trilateral. This chapter explores these processes in more detail and examines their outcomes, as systems of employee relations rules.

PERSONAL CONTRACTS

With the growth of individualist employee relations policies and patterns of employment since the 1980s (see Chapters 7 and 10), the use of personal contracts of employment, between employers and employees, has been extended within some organisations, especially for managerial and professional staff. A personal contract is the outcome of individual bargaining between an employer and an employee. It normally incorporates an individual salary for the post holder and other specific terms and conditions of employment, pertinent to that individual and his or her job. Personal contracts have always been more common amongst management staff than amongst non-management employees in large organisations, and for all employees in non-union small firms. However, the practice has spread in both the private and public sectors in recent years and has become more common now amongst other groups of employees, such as technical and

Exhibit 1 **Written particulars of the main terms and conditions of employment**

This normally includes:

- the identity of the parties
- commencement of employment
- continuous employment
- hours of work
- holidays
- sickness and injury arrangements
- pensions
- notice period
- job title
- expected length of temporary employment (where appropriate)
- place of work
- collective agreements affecting the contract
- terms relating to abroad
- how grievances and disciplinary matters are to be resolved

professional workers, that have traditionally had their terms and conditions of employment determined collectively rather than individually. Personal contracts are typically linked to staff appraisal and performance review, staff development and performance-related pay.

Like all employees, those on personal contracts are entitled to receive written particulars from their employer setting out the main terms of their employment. This applies to all employees working eight or more hours per week under contracts of one month or more. The information must be provided within two months of commencing employment. Exhibit 1 illustrates the information typically included in such written statements.

In one senior management contract known to the author, most of the items in Exhibit 1 are included but it is stated, regarding hours of work (Portsmouth and South East Hampshire Health Authority 1991), that: 'managers are required to work such hours as are necessary for the full performance of their duties.' It goes on to add that continuation of the appointment is 'subject to satisfactory performance', with the duties of the post being reviewed in 'accordance with the Individual Performance Review arrangements for senior managers.'

> The primary objective of this will be to help . . . achieve the best possible level of performance, but unsatisfactory performance, as assessed under the Individual Performance Review arrangements, may be regarded as grounds for action under the Authority's disciplinary and dismissal procedures.

In this case, this could result from failure to meet agreed objectives after two successive reviews where unsatisfactory performance is identified. Clearly, compared with collectively determined terms and conditions, personal contracts give senior managers much tighter control over the job activities, work performance and pay rewards of the employees covered by such contracts. Personal contracts thus enhance management control of the work process.

COLLECTIVE BARGAINING

Collective bargaining (or joint negotiation) is a voluntary process involving autonomous employers and independent trade unions and remains a common pattern of employee relations in Britain and many other Western countries (see Chapters 8 and 9). Its purpose is to determine:

- the terms and conditions of employment, for particular groups of employees
- the ways in which employment issues such as individual grievances, collective disputes and disciplinary matters are to be resolved at workplace and corporate levels.

Autonomous employers are normally self-governing organisations, operating in the market or public sectors. Independent trade unions are organisations of workers, which are not under the domination or control of an employer, whose activities are not liable to interference from an employer. Unions meeting the criteria for 'independence' set out in Section 5 of the TULRCA 1992 may apply for a certificate of independence from the CO.

Collective bargaining is a power relationship, based on a management policy of union incorporation in the enterprise, and is one of power-sharing, or joint regulation, with management. Its outcomes, resulting from negotiations between management and union representatives, are collective agreements. In Britain, collective agreements are voluntary and non-legally enforceable. In other countries, collective agreements are normally legally binding contracts between employers and unions, with any breaches of such agreements resulting in legal action being taken by the aggrieved party against the other. The relative advantage in collective bargaining is determined by the balance of bargaining power between the two parties in the negotiating process. Where the power balance favours the employer side, this is to the relative disadvantage of the union and its members. Where the power balance favours the union side, this is to the relative disadvantage of the employer and management. The essence of an effective collective bargaining relationship between employers and trade unions is the willingness of both parties to seek negotiated and agreed settlements, by concessions, exchanges and compromises between them, so that each side feels mutually bound, responsible and committed to their joint bargaining outcomes (Clegg 1976).

Any set of collective bargaining arrangements comprises a framework or structure within which the employer and union sides participate. Parker and his colleagues (1971) use the term 'bargaining structure' to describe the permanent features distinguishing the collective bargaining process in any particular industry or organisation. They identify four interrelated features within any collective bargaining structure. These are bargaining levels, bargaining units, bargaining scope and bargaining forms.

Bargaining levels

The bargaining level is where collective bargaining between employer and union representatives takes place. This may be at:

- multi-employer level (otherwise described as industry-wide or national level)
- single employer or company level
- establishment or plant level.

Multi-employer bargaining was common amongst private sector employers in Britain in the 1930s, 1940s and 1950s. For multi-employer bargaining to operate, it is necessary for employers to organise themselves into employers' associations or federations (see Chapter 2), thus providing a collective voice for employer interests in the bargaining process. Unions, in turn, often collaborate at national level through multi-union confederations, consisting of a number of independent trade unions working together. Multi-employer bargaining has also been a common practice in the public services such as local government, the civil service and the National Health Service (NHS). This is changing rapidly, however, with the public services being broken up into a series of executive agencies, NHS trusts and directly managed units in schools, colleges and universities (Farnham and Horton 1996a; 1996b).

Multi-employer bargaining is also common in parts of Europe. In Denmark, for example, industry-wide collective agreements in the private sector are concluded every other year between individual unions and industrial employers' associations. All such agreements, which are legally enforceable, must be ratified by union members in a ballot before they can be signed and implemented by the negotiating parties. In Italy, industry-wide bargaining has traditionally been important because it is the level at which minimum wage rates are set for each industry. These cover the private sector, publicly owned companies and the small business or craft sector. There are around 25 major industries in Italy and about 100 national industry agreements, which are binding on all employers, irrespective of whether they are members of signatory organisations (Incomes Data Services 1991).

Single employer or company bargaining takes place between one employer and the union (or unions) it recognises at corporate level. These arrangements are common either in medium to large, multi-site companies where the employer wants standardised terms, conditions and employment policies across the company, or in single-site companies, which are not involved in multi-employer bargaining arrangements. Company bargaining is becoming more common in Britain, as companies move away from multi-employer bargaining so as to provide themselves with more flexibility, better cost-effectiveness and greater control in the bargaining process. Most collective bargaining in the Republic of Ireland is carried out at company level (Gunnicle and Flood 1990). In the Netherlands, where there used to be a highly centralised collective bargaining system, and where multi-employer bargaining still predominates, company bargaining has increased in importance in recent years, especially in the large corporate sector.

Enterprise or plant bargaining in large multi-site companies takes place between local managers and local union officials. This has been a growing trend in Britain since the 1980s. Patterns vary but, in the private sector, some of the driving forces have been changes in business strategy, decentralised cost and profit centres and management wishes to keep union officials away from strategic decision-making levels. Marginson and his colleagues (1988) show, even where there is plant bargaining, that management freedom to bargain locally may be limited and that guidelines and controls are set at corporate centre. There have also been pressures from government to encourage more decentralised bargaining and pay flexibility in the public services, though not to the extent that has happened in the private sector.

In the USA and Japan, plant bargaining is the norm. In the USA, this is because of its business structures, industrial and commercial regionalisation, immense geographical size and preferred management strategies in employee relations (Kochan *et al* 1986). In Japan, most collective bargaining takes place at enterprise level. Employers favour it because of their paternalist personnel and employment policies. And the unions support it because of their co-operative working arrangements with the employers and their origins as factory and company-based wartime production committees (Shirai 1983).

Bargaining units

A bargaining unit, which is closely related to the bargaining level in an industry or organisation, is the group of employees covered by a particular set of substantive or procedural collective agreements. Separate bargaining units, for example, may cover manual workers, clerical and administrative workers and supervisory workers respectively. A bargaining unit may be narrow or wide in terms of the group of workers it covers. A narrow bargaining unit, by definition, covers a limited group, such as the skilled craft-workers in a manufacturing organisation. A wide bargaining unit covers a much more comprehensive group, such as all the manual workers within an industry, organisation or plant.

There has been a tendency in recent years for bargaining units, especially at company and workplace levels, to become wider. Bargaining units are more likely than in the past to be of a 'single table' type. A single bargaining table covers all the recognised groups of workers at employer or enterprise level including:

- non-manual and manual groups
- workers represented by TUC and non-TUC unions
- skilled, semi-skilled and less skilled workers.

It is an employee relations approach which rationalises and simplifies the bargaining process for employers, harmonises conditions of employment within the employment unit and integrates and focuses collective bargaining for the unions.

Bargaining units are interconnected with bargaining levels. The bargaining unit is particularly concerned with the representative function of the trade unions recognised by the employer, whilst the bargaining level concentrates on the management side of the negotiating table. Within a bargaining unit, it is a joint panel of unions, or a single trade union, that acts as the bargaining agent on behalf of the employees, with the unions normally determining the representative arrangements on behalf of their members. Bargaining levels, in contrast, are predominantly employer-determined and are influenced by a combination of product market, business structure and technological factors (Advisory, Conciliation and Arbitration Service 1983; Palmer 1990).

Bargaining scope

Bargaining scope begins where the right to manage ends. It defines the range of subjects and matters covered within procedural and substantive agreements and may be extensive or limited in content. Again the tendency in Britain in recent years has been for bargaining scope to narrow, as employers and managers become more assertive and confident in the collective bargaining process. This has been helped by relatively high levels of unemployment, falling union membership and better trained management negotiators. Unless changes favourable to unions and their members are made to the balance of power in the labour market, the legal framework of employee relations and personnel policy, bargaining scope is unlikely to be extended in the future.

Bargaining forms

Bargaining forms are the ways in which collective agreements are recorded. They may be formal and written, on the one hand, or unwritten and informal on the other. The tendency in recent years has been towards greater formality in recording collective agreements. This is to avoid arguments about the content and application of collective agreements and to provide stability in collective bargaining arrangements when those who have negotiated procedural or substantive agreements change jobs or roles.

COLLECTIVE AGREEMENTS

Collective agreements are the outcome of collective bargaining and are jointly determined employment rules which may be procedural or substantive in nature. Procedural collective agreements set out:

- the responsibilities and duties of management and unions in employee relations
- the steps or stages through which the parties determine employee relations decisions jointly
- what happens when the parties to employee relations fail to agree.

Substantive collective agreements, in contrast, cover the terms and conditions of employment relating to specific categories of jobs and employment groups.

In Britain, unlike in other western European and North American countries, collective agreements between managements and unions are not legally enforceable. This means that neither party can sue the other where agreements are broken, for example, when either management or unions fail to act in accordance with agreed procedures. Collective agreements become incorporated, however, into the individual contracts of employment of all the employees covered by the bargaining unit, whether they are trade union members or not.

Procedural agreements

There is no such thing as a 'model' procedural agreement. Each employer and the union(s) that they recognise determine their own set of procedural agreements according to a number of contingent factors. These include:

- the size and organisational structure of the company, public service or industry
- the level(s) at which collective bargaining takes place
- the history, location(s) and ownership of the organisation
- the dominant style and philosophy of management
- the union(s) with which the management deal
- union power and organisation.

For the purposes of this analysis, the main types of procedural clauses found in 'traditional' collective agreements between management and unions in the private sector, at employer or enterprise level, are outlined in Exhibits 2–6 below. These clauses typically cover:

- general principles
- union recognition, union representation and facilities
- the rights and duties of the parties
- grievances and the avoidance of disputes
- discipline.

These traditional procedural agreements, which often include multi-union representation, contrast with a less common form of collective agreement, based on single-union representation, called 'new style' or 'single-union' deals. Their procedural clauses incorporate a different approach to the ones outlined below (see Chapter 3).

General principles clauses

These clauses set out the intentions of the various parties to the collective bargaining relationship and the general spirit with which it is to be conducted. The subject matter of these clauses is illustrated in Exhibit 2.

Exhibit 2 **General principles clauses in procedural agreements**

These cover:

- the basis on which discussions and negotiations between the company and the unions take place
- a general statement emphasising the need for good working relations between the company and the unions
- a company statement recognising the right of the unions to represent and negotiate on behalf of their members
- a company statement recognising the right of employees to join and belong to a union
- a union statement recognising the company's responsibility to plan, organise and manage the company efficiently and cost-effectively

- a joint statement reinforcing the common, shared objectives of the company and unions in contributing to its prosperity, increased productivity and operating efficiency
- a joint statement committing the company and the unions to refrain from any form of industrial action, until agreed procedures have been exhausted.

Union recognition, workplace representation and facilities procedure

These clauses set out the unions having recognition rights and how union representatives are to be elected and treated within the procedural arrangements. The subject matter of these procedures is illustrated in Exhibit 3.

Exhibit 3 **Union recognition and facilities procedure**

This covers:

- company recognition of workplace representatives, elected in accordance with union rules
- the appointment of workplace representatives, their numbers, constituencies and co-ordination into a joint panel of unions or joint union committee
- the conditions permitting workplace representatives to undertake union duties and activities and the facilities for these, including time off, pay, administrative support and union training.

The rights and duties of management and unions

These clauses define the roles and responsibilities of the parties in the collective bargaining relationship. The subject matter of these clauses is illustrated in Exhibit 4.

Exhibit 4 **Rights and responsibilities of the parties within procedure**

These cover:

- the importance of the effective use of procedures to all the parties and of mutual confidence and trust amongst them in the conduct of good employee relations
- the right of workplace representatives to take up grievances, disciplinary and other matters on behalf of individuals and workgroups
- the responsibility of workplace representatives to act on behalf of their members where this is justified
- the responsibility of workplace representatives to act fairly, honestly and in a manner befitting their functions
- the responsibilities of management to ensure procedures are used, that workplace representatives are treated fairly, honestly and with the respect due to their positions and that the cases presented to them are given a fair hearing

- the rights of management to object to any breach of procedure through union channels and to expect unions to keep to the principles, spirit and stages of agreed procedures
- the rights of unions to nominate elected workplace representatives to designated areas and to the joint panel of unions or joint union committee
- the responsibility of the unions to see that their workplace representatives adhere to the principles, spirit and stages of agreed procedures.

Procedures for settling grievances and avoiding disputes

These clauses provide means for settling and resolving grievances and disputes between the parties and normally follow a series of stages, with both the employer and the unions undertaking to refrain from taking coercive industrial action against the other, including lockouts or stoppages of work (ie retaining existing arrangements – the status quo), whilst the procedures are being used. Grievance procedures normally cover individual issues (see Chapter 5) and collective 'disputes' procedures normally cover matters of concern to groups of employees. The subject matter of these clauses is illustrated in Exhibits 5 and 6.

Individual issues

Exhibit 5 **Procedure for individual grievances**

These clauses provide for meetings involving:

- Stage 1: the union member and immediate supervisor
  (if the issue is not resolved, it is referred to . . .)
- Stage 2: the union member, workplace representative and supervisor
  (if the issue is not resolved, it is referred to . . .)
- Stage 3: the union member, workplace representative and next level of management
  (if the issue is not resolved, it is referred to . . .)
- Stage 4: the joint panel of unions or joint union committee and appropriate managers, including the personnel manager
  (if the issue is not resolved, and at the request of either management or the union, it is referred to . . .)
- Stage 5: the personnel manager, union full-time official and other invited parties
  (if the issue is not resolved, it is referred to . . .)
- Stage 6: the human resources director, union full-time official and other invited parties
  (if the issue is not resolved, it may be referred to . . .)
- Stage 7: an external party agreed to by management and the union.

Collective issues

Exhibit 6 **Procedure to avoid collective disputes**

- For a group managed by the same supervisor, these clauses provide for meetings involving:
  - Stages 2-7 above
- For a group involving members of one union in more than one department, these clauses provide for meetings involving:
  - the joint panel of unions or the joint union committee and the personnel manager
    (if it is not resolved, it is referred to . . .)
  - Stages 5–7 above
- For a group with members of more than one union in more than one department, these clauses provide for meetings involving:
  - the joint panel of unions or joint union committee and appropriate management representatives, including the personnel manager
    (if it is not resolved, it is referred to . . .)
  - senior management representatives and appropriate full-time union officials.

Disciplinary procedure

The objective of this procedure is to help individuals whose conduct (or performance) gives cause for dissatisfaction, to improve their behaviour (see Chapter 5). Individuals being disciplined have the right to be accompanied by their union representative. The subject matter of these clauses is illustrated in Exhibit 7.

Exhibit 7 **Disciplinary procedure**

The stages typically incorporate interviews involving:

- Stage 1: the individual and the supervisor, which can result in a verbal warning
- Stage 2: unless an improvement in employee conduct (or performance) results, the supervisor reviews the situation with the individual, which, following investigation, can result in a first written warning
- Stage 3: where there is still no improvement in employee conduct (or performance), the supervisor consults his or her manager, which, following investigation, can result in a second written warning
- Stage 4: where there continues to be no improvement in employee conduct (or performance), the manager consults with his or her manager who, if still dissatisfied with the conduct, following investigation, can dismiss the individual.

Where appropriate, Stages 2 or 3 above may be the first steps used in implementing the procedure. Cases of defined and established gross misconduct, for example, may result in instant dismissal, with an individual being suspended on full pay pending a hearing. Appeals systems are normally built into disciplinary procedures, thus allowing individuals to appeal against disciplinary sanctions determined by management.

Other procedures

These clauses include procedures covering:

- recruitment
- induction
- promotion
- redeployment
- training
- redundancy
- retirement.

New-style agreements

New-style collective agreements – sometimes mistakenly described as 'single-union deals' – are typically found in 'hi-tech', foreign-owned, 'greenfield site' companies (Rico 1987). Some new-style procedural clauses are of the same types as those found in traditional procedures, although they incorporate different provisions and emphases, but others are quite distinctive and different from those in normal procedural arrangements between employers and unions. Like traditional procedures, new-style procedures include clauses covering:

- general principles
- union recognition and facilities
- grievances and the avoidance of disputes
- discipline.

Yet they commonly focus on (see also Chapters 1 and 9):

- single-union recognition, not multi-union recognition
- the role of employee representatives in procedure, not union representatives
- single machinery for dealing with negotiation, consultation and information, not multiple machinery
- the need for two procedures for avoiding disputes, not a single procedure – with one for dealing with conflicts of rights (for interpreting existing agreements) and the other for dealing with conflicts of interest (in making new agreements).

Additional procedural clauses typically found in new-style agreements include:

- 'no-strike' arrangements
- 'pendulum' arbitration for disputes of interest, where the arbitrator rules for the final position of one side or the other
- 'labour flexibility' clauses.

The subject matter of typical procedural clauses incorporated in new-style agreements is illustrated in Exhibit 8 (see also Chapter 8).

Exhibit 8 **Procedural clauses in new-style collective agreements**

These cover:

- single-union recognition
- employee representation within the company
- single employment status for all employees
- employee flexibility and multi-skilling, with security of employment and opportunities for training and retraining for employees
- a company council, or forum, incorporating advisory, information, consultative and negotiating functions
- no-strike or peace clauses
- binding pendulum arbitration.

Substantive agreements

These cover how much the various groups of employees are paid for the jobs they do, in terms of either immediate or postponed payments (such as pensions), and the conditions of employment associated with these jobs. Substantive agreements define the market relations between the primary parties to the employment contract and they therefore involve financial costs to the employer and economic rewards for the employees. The main categories are summarised in Figure 4 but the lists are neither exclusive nor exhaustive.

Figure 4 **Main categories of substantive agreement**

Pay	Conditions
Hourly wage rates	Working hours
Annual salaries	Length of working week
Shift work payments	Shift working hours
Unsocial hours payments	Shift working systems
Pay structures	Clocking in arrangements
Payments for performance	Working time arrangements
Pay bonuses	Refreshments facilities
Overtime payments	Overtime arrangements
Holiday pay	Holiday arrangements
Sick pay	Sick pay schemes
Maternity pay	Maternity leave
Redundancy payments	Pensions schemes
'Call-in payments'	Sabbatical leave

JOINT CONSULTATION

In Britain, voluntary collective bargaining and voluntary joint consultation have traditionally been seen as separate and complementary processes, with collective bargaining focusing on the divergent interests of employers and employees and consultation focusing on their common interests. In practice, where bargaining and consultation co-exist, the distinction between them is often institutionalised by having separate negotiating and consultative machinery and separate agendas for their activities. This has meant in many cases that collective bargaining has been concerned with pay determination and conditions of employment and joint consultation with welfare, health and safety, training and efficiency, even where the same representatives are involved in the separate processes in the same organisation.

Although Flanders (1964) argues that this distinction between bargaining and consultation is artificial, McCarthy (1966) accepts the distinction but claims that there is an inverse relationship between trade union power and joint consultation. When union power is strong, joint consultation is neutralised and, when it is weak, joint consultation is reinvigorated. The McCarthy thesis is fairly persuasive, up to a point, since as Millward and Stevens (1986) show, there was a significant growth of joint consultative committees (JCCs) in Britain during the early 1980s which was a period of generally high unemployment, declining union membership and assertive styles of management. By the time of the third Workplace Industrial Relations Survey (WIRS) in 1990, however, the overall proportion of workplaces with JCCs had fallen 'between 1984 and 1990, from 34 per cent to 29 per cent' (Millward *et al.* 1992: page 153). This could be accounted for by the fact that by 1990, there were fewer larger workplaces with recognised unions, where JCCs had previously been common. In the 1960s and 1970s, in contrast, during a period of strong trade union power, successful joint consultation was not widely practised in either private or public industry. Union representatives preferred negotiation because it influenced employment decisions and consultation did not.

One of the problems of analysing joint consultation as an employee relations process is that it has a variety of objectives, subject matter, representative structures and managerial approaches to it. Marchington (1989) identifies four models of joint consultation, in terms of the links between collective bargaining and employee reepresentation. The aims of each of the four models are, respectively:

- to prevent the establishment of independent trade unionism
- to make JCCs a marginal activity within the enterprise
- to upgrade joint consultation, as a substitute for collective bargaining
- to make JCCs a valuable adjunct to collective bargaining.

Clearly, from Marchington's research, management's motives for setting up and participating in joint consultation, and its attitudes towards it, are crucial determinants of its effectiveness, efficacy and impact on employee relations behaviour.

The *non-union* model is established by management to prevent unions organising in the workplace. It is based on information-giving from management, either of a 'hard' business nature or on 'soft' welfare and social matters. Non-union consultative committees are normally chaired by a senior line or personnel manager, and the employee representatives, chosen from amongst the workforce, are encouraged to identify with management and not to challenge management prerogatives or management's decision-making authority. JCCs of this sort are usually at establishment level and are not linked to committees on other sites in multi-plant firms.

The *marginal* model of joint consultation is one in which the JCC has a symbolic role and the JCC's employee representatives are kept busy on non-controversial issues. Fairly trivial information is provided to employee representatives. These JCCs tend to be chaired by the personnel manager and employees are represented by both union and non-union members. Like the non-union model, the marginal model of joint consultation is organised at plant or establishment level with no links to other parts of the organisation.

The *competitive* model aims to reduce union influence, by upgrading joint consultation so as to render collective bargaining less meaningful. Hard, high-level information is provided by management to shop stewards and other employee representatives. Meetings are chaired by senior line managers at establishment level, although in larger organisations there may be departmental JCCs, allowing ideas and information to be passed up and down the organisation to reinforce the line management chain of command. According to Marchington (1988), this sort of consultation may be linked with other types of employee involvement such as quality circles, team briefings and similar direct forms of management-employee communications (see Chapter 10).

The purpose of the *adjunct* model of joint consultation is to provide a problem-solving forum, for management and union representatives, at plant and company levels, in parallel with the collective bargaining machinery. With this approach, collective bargaining tends to deal with matters of conflict between management and unions, such as pay and conditions of employment, whilst joint consultation fills in the gaps left by negotiation. This type of joint consultation therefore deals with issues of common and shared interests between the parties but may also be seen as a process preceding the negotiation of matters of conflict. The adjunct consultative process tends to be based on high trust and mutual collaboration between management and union representatives, with hard, high-level information, covering trading prospects, business plans and customer relations, being provided by management. Adjunct JCCs are likely to be chaired by the most senior line manager in the plant or company and there are normally links between JCCs at workplace and corporate levels in multi-site companies. Managements are also likely to encourage workplace representatives to have their own discussions prior to JCC meetings, to reinforce good working relations amongst management, unions and staff.

CONCILIATION, ARBITRATION AND MEDIATION

Where the secondary parties to employee relations (management/management organisations and unions) are unable to resolve their employee relations differences by agreed negotiating or consultative procedures, or where no procedures exist, then the only means by which they can avoid damaging industrial conflict is by voluntary conciliation, arbitration or mediation. Normally, these are provided through the agency of ACAS (see Chapters 1 and 2).

Conciliation

Where the parties in dispute request or agree to collective conciliation, it is ACAS which provides a conciliator. The task of the conciliator is to help employer and unions settle their differences by agreement. Conciliators work through confidential, informal meetings between the parties, sometimes separately, sometimes jointly. They also work with certain broad assumptions. These include:

- that the parties wish to reach agreement
- that they wish to avoid or end disruptive industrial conflict
- that they will be generally co-operative in the conciliation process.

To be effective, conciliators have to gain the confidence of all parties to the dispute and establish good working relations with them. This depends on the personal qualities, knowledge, experience and, most importantly, the neutrality and impartiality of the conciliator.

According to ACAS (Advisory, Conciliation and Arbitration Service 1979: page 8):

> The process of conciliation is a dynamic one, requiring a continuous assessment of developments as they occur, and the conciliator adapts his conduct of each case accordingly.

The initial stage in collective conciliation is the preliminary briefing meeting. The conciliator's prime objective at this stage is to obtain a clear understanding of the issues in dispute and the attitudes of the parties. This involves collecting information from a variety of sources including oral evidence, documents, press cuttings and informed observers. It is at this stage that the conciliator has to decide whether it is appropriate to proceed with conciliation or not.

Conciliation normally consists of a series of 'side' meetings, with each party separately, and joint meetings chaired by the conciliator. Each party is free to choose its own representatives, though the level of seniority and extent of representation is important. The length of meetings varies and, at an appropriate time, the conciliator tries to direct the discussions into an accommodation between the parties. If successful, this can result in a settlement. If not, the conciliation process fails.

Side meetings enable each set of participants to speak freely, to reduce tensions and to adopt a problem-solving approach. Proposals and counter-proposals are examined, with a view to inducing movements towards a position where a settlement is likely. The conciliator moves between the parties in an attempt to bring their positions closer together. Joint meetings provide an opportunity for negotiations to proceed under an impartial and independent chairperson. They can also be the appropriate place for proposals for resolving the dispute. Joint meetings proceed by each side explaining its position, asking questions of the other and being questioned by the conciliator.

During the various meetings, the conciliator constantly looks for signs that the parties are moving to a settlement. If and when agreement has been reached, or appears to be close in side meetings, the parties can be brought together into a concluding joint meeting. This enables the terms of the settlement to be finalised, with the parties indicating their assent. Since conciliators are not party to any agreements reached, they do not sign the agreed document, except possibly as witnesses.

Conventional arbitration

ACAS is also empowered to appoint external arbitrators in trade disputes, under certain pre-conditions. These are:

- that the specific consent of the parties is obtained
- that the likelihood of the dispute being settled by conciliation is considered
- that generally any agreed procedures have been used and a failure to agree has resulted.

Most arbitrations are conducted by a single arbitrator from a list maintained by ACAS. This is a relatively simple, flexible and quick method of arbitrating. Boards of arbitration are used for major disputes and may be appointed at the request of the parties.

Requests for voluntary arbitration often come in the form of a joint application from the parties, including their names, addresses and agreed terms of reference. ACAS then appoints a suitable arbitrator and this is confirmed as a signed minute of appointment. Each side is allowed time to prepare and exchange statements. Hearings are held on the employer's premises or at an ACAS office. The parties are notified in writing of all the details, with a request to send their written statements to the arbitrator and to exchange them before the hearing, since the submission and exchange of statements is a normal feature of the arbitration process.

Hearings are normally held in private and are conducted informally. The arbitrator usually meets both parties together and asks the claimant party to state its case in the presence of the other, who is then invited to reply. The arbitrator then questions both parties and invites them to make any closing statements. The arbitration award is submitted to ACAS, about two weeks after the hearing, and is binding on both parties. Awards are confidential and are not published, unless the parties agree to this.

Pendulum arbitration

Pendulum arbitration, known as 'final offer arbitration' or 'last offer arbitration' in the USA, is a relatively new process in Britain (Wood 1985). It is an arbitration process particularly associated with new-style collective agreements (see Chapter 9) and normally requires the arbitrator to choose the 'final offer' of the employer or the 'final claim' of the union side in the negotiation process. The rationale for pendulum arbitration derives from the fact that new-style negotiating procedures normally distinguish between conflicts of rights and conflicts of interests. Rights relate to the application or interpretation of agreements, whilst interests relate to matters not covered by agreement (eg new claims on terms and conditions of employment).

In essence, the negotiating procedures and procedures to avoid disputes in new-style agreements are based on the rights of the parties, incorporated in the recognition agreement. The intention is normally to reconcile the few remaining conflicts of interest on substantive issues through in-company negotiation. Where differences of interest persist, pendulum arbitration is used. This is claimed to encourage collective bargaining in the last resort, to keep bargaining claims within reasonable limits and to provide a means for resolving impasses (Burrows 1986).

In pendulum arbitration, the management side states its case and its 'final offer' and the union side states its case and its 'final claim' to the arbitrator. The arbitrator might try by persuasion to bring the two sides closer together but eventually has to settle for one side's case or the other's. There is no 'splitting the difference'. It is argued that one of the benefits of this approach to arbitration is that little face is lost by either side. This is because their original positions are less far apart than in conventional arbitration, with even the losing side ending up not that far from its stated position. Another advantage is claimed to be that, whilst one side is entirely satisfied with the arbitrator's award, the other side does not feel that it has lost so much ground as with conventional arbitration.

Mediation

Voluntary mediation in trade disputes is half-way between conciliation and conventional arbitration. Mediators proceed by way of conciliation but are also prepared to make their own formal proposals or recommendations. These may be accepted as they stand or provide the basis for further negotiations leading to a settlement. Since it provides more positive intervention, mediation tends to constrain the parties more than conciliation does. But it is more flexible and less decisive than arbitration.

As with arbitration, in mediation ACAS may appoint a single mediator or a board of mediation. The three pre-conditions, listed above, need to be observed and the formulation of the terms of reference requires careful drafting. Written statements are exchanged and sent to the mediator but the conduct of meetings differs from arbitration. Sometimes the mediator meets the parties in joint and separate meetings. In other cases, hearings proceed in the style of arbitration. In other cases, the mediator acts as the chair of a working party, making recommendations on any points which the parties themselves cannot agree. Where a settlement is reached by mediation, the mediator's final report records the terms of the agreement and no further action is required. In other cases, it may be necessary for ACAS conciliation officers to assist the parties further, if required.

UNILATERAL ACTION AND INDUSTRIAL SANCTIONS

Having examined the main voluntary, bilateral and trilateral processes of conflict resolution and accommodation in employee relations, we now turn to unilateral action and industrial sanctions. Unilateral action and industrial sanctions in employee relations involve management and unions acting as discrete parties. Unilateral action by management or unions, and any industrial sanctions imposed by one side on the other, are voluntary and collective processes of conducting employee relations which differ from other processes in two main respects:

- they involve the ultimate application, by management or unions, of one-sided power in determining and applying employee relations rules
- because of this power dimension, British law impinges more closely on these employee relations processes than on other voluntarist ones, such as collective bargaining, joint consultation, conciliation, arbitration and mediation.

The right to manage

The right of management to manage in organisations is, in all capitalist countries but in Britain, the USA and Japan especially, at the root of employee relations decision-making and controversy. The right to manage or unilateral management decision-making – otherwise known as managerial prerogative, managerial rights or managerial functions – is where management interfaces with employees, the trade union function, collective bargaining and the law, insofar as this supports and constrains the right to manage in private and public organisations.

The origins of the right to manage can be traced to the emergence of capitalist business organisations in the nineteenth century and the parallel growth of craft trade unionism. The early capitalist entrepreneurs claimed their right to manage on the basis of property ownership. Since they and their families owned the factories, mines, railway companies, shipbuilding yards and shipping lines that they directed, controlled and organised, then it was they alone, they claimed, who should have the right to employ, pay, deploy, discipline and, if necessary, dismiss the hourly paid and salaried 'black coated' workers employed in their enterprises.

The entrepreneurial class's advocacy and defence of the right to manage, moreover, was reinforced by the demands of the craft unions to settle the terms and conditions of employment of their members unilaterally, without reference to the employers, and to enforce pre-entry closed shops on the employers, to control the supply of labour into the labour market (Clegg, Fox and Thompson 1964). This right to manage was embodied in the common law duty requiring workers to obey all reasonable and legitimate instructions given to them by their 'masters' or their supervisory agents. It was also incorporated into statute law by making companies solely accountable to corporate shareholders and stockholders and, unlike in Germany and France after the second world war, by not providing workers with a collective legal status, through, for example, statutory works councils and enterprise committees (Bercusson 1986).

Today, the right to manage is largely based on different claims for managerial authority (Storey 1980 and 1983). In essence, management justifies the right to manage on the grounds of economic efficiency, technical expertise and professional competency. The arguments run along these lines:

- it is management's responsibility to achieve organisational efficiency and success in the interests of those to whom they are accountable
- it is management alone who have the knowledge, skills and abilities to carry out the tasks of effective managing
- it is essential, if the organisation is to remain profitable, viable and cost-effective, that managers have the autonomy and authority to take and implement corporate decisions, including employment ones, without interference from internal or outside parties.

It is these sorts of ideas and interests which have led British employers to resist a statutory minimum wage, the European Community Charter of Fundamental Social Rights for Workers (Commission of the European Communities 1990) and the Social Chapter of the Treaty of Maastricht.

The contemporary justification of the right to manage is both an attractive and a flawed concept. It is attractive because it makes economic sense to argue the necessity of management leadership and know-how in creating, administering and co-ordinating effective organisations. It is flawed, however, because the right to manage can never be absolute in enterprises for four main reasons:

- in practice, managerial authority has to be counterbalanced by the consent of those governed even by unilateral management rules
- where employees are organised into trade unions, the right to make unilateral management decisions is constrained by collective bargaining
- the law provides a floor of legal rights for employees (see Chapter 4)
- the right to manage is not a static concept, either organisationally or societally. What was a managerial right yesterday can become a workers' or a union's right today and what are workers' rights today can regress to managerial rights tomorrow. It depends on the balance of power in the

employment relationship, as affected by market factors, trade union organisation, public policy and the law.

It is clear that the right to manage and to take management decisions unilaterally is a difficult employee relations process to examine definitively. It is also clear that since the early 1980s the right to manage has been strengthened. Even where employers recognise trade unions, 'right-to-manage' clauses are now being put in recognition and procedural agreements and 'status quo' clauses are being omitted. The latter provide that actions proposed by management cannot be implemented, if disputed by workers, until agreement has been reached or the procedure for avoiding disputes exhausted. Recent right-to-manage clauses state, for example, 'that the Union recognises the right of the Company to plan, organise, manage and decide finally upon the operations of the Company'. Another example, in the public sector, states that 'The [employers' federation] and the signatory Unions recognise that it is the right and responsibility of the institutions to manage their domestic affairs in the context of this Agreement' (Polytechnic and Colleges Employers' Forum 1989).

However complex the concept of the right to manage is, unilateral management rules normally take the form of what used to be called 'works rules' but are now normally referred to as 'company rules'. These are usually included in employee handbooks, along with background information about the employer, other employment matters, personnel policies and employee relations procedures, and they become incorporated into individual contracts of employment (Marks 1978). The right to manage is also closely linked with management use of employee involvement processes such as briefing groups, quality circles, total quality management (TQM), profit-related pay and employee share ownership (see Chapter 10).

Union rules

The union equivalents of the right to manage are union rules and custom and practice (C and P). Union rules are subsumed in:

- union rule books
- union policies determined at their national policy-making conferences
- operational policies determined amongst union activists locally.

Unilateral union-made rules are imposed on management where unions are strong and well organised at employer and workplace levels. C and P are unwritten and informal rules regulating employment and work at enterprise level. They are generally unilaterally determined, with management having no say in making them but tacitly accepting them. Some C and P, however, takes the form of 'shared understandings' between management and unions, which management accept but are unwilling to legitimise formally.

Formal union rules affecting employee relations at employer and workplace levels, deriving largely from union rule books, cover a wide range of working arrangements. They are traditionally associated with craft unions, such as those in the printing, skilled engineering and metal trades. With the relative decline of skilled manual occupations and the craft unions in recent years – largely due to technological change, market pressures on employers and new product markets – unilateral union rules are less important now than they were in the past (see Chapter 6). This has resulted in multi-skilling, job flexibility and union mergers. However, examples of such rules cover:

- the training of apprentices
- the closed shop
- job demarcation
- working arrangements
- 'manning' levels
- working with other unions.

C and P rules are established by trade unionists either where such rules have been traditionally accepted by management without challenge, in order to maintain industrial peace, or where management rules – or joint rules – have lapsed and management turns 'a blind eye' to them, because it has lost control of them. Examples include:

- time-keeping
- working practices
- worker behaviour.

Workers may be required to finish at an agreed time on a Friday afternoon, for example, but C and P dictates that, within the last hour of work, workers who have completed their current job tasks may 'job and finish' and leave the employer's premises, before the official finishing time.

C and P are used as precedents by trade unionists either when arguing with management for a solution to conflicts about new employment rules or in applying existing rules to new situations. As such, C and P rules are jealously guarded by workgroups and unions. Management is only likely to challenge them when organisational efficiency is threatened, enterprise effectiveness is at risk and trade union power is weak. This was the case in many organisations in the 1980s and early 1990s.

Industrial action

Both management and unions are prepared, in certain cases, to use industrial sanctions against one another in order to achieve their employee relations goals. These sanctions, known as industrial action, involve disruption of normal working and can take a number of forms. On the employers' side, the lockout is the best known. But other sanctions open to employers include:

- withdrawing union recognition
- withdrawing union facilities
- transferring workers to less pleasant jobs
- tighter workplace discipline
- taking away bonuses
- reducing overtime
- changing working arrangements unilaterally.

On the union side, industrial sanctions include (see also Chapter 11):

- going slow
- working to rule
- banning overtime
- working without enthusiasm
- stoppages of work.

Sanctions are the means of last resort, for both sides, since they involve economic and social costs to both parties. Where employers take industrial action against their workers, the economic and social costs may be lost sales revenue or, in the public sector, withdrawn public services. The cost to workers is lost pay and benefits and possibly lost job security.

In participating in industrial action, unions, union leaders and employees are constrained by the law. In outline, the law seeks to regulate industrial action in a number of ways. This is done through a combination of:

- judge-made law, both criminal and civil
- legislation
- codes of practice, such as for picketing.

First, trade unions and individuals organising and taking part in industrial action may be liable for certain civil wrongs or 'torts' in circumstances which are not protected by statutory 'immunities'. There is no legal 'right to strike' in Britain, as there is in most of western Europe, but immunities provide legal protections for unions and individuals taking part in lawful industrial action, providing the acts are done 'in contemplation or furtherance of a trade dispute'. Second, the law seeks to impose limits on physical manifestations of industrial conflict, such as picketing, occupations and sit-ins (Simpson 1986; see also Chapter 4 below).

Industrial action also affects the legal rights and obligations of employer and employee under the contract of employment. This is because the common law tends to treat all forms of industrial action by employees as breaches of contract, since they violate the employee's central obligation under the contract to work for the employer. This breach of contract is important in two respects. First, it may provide one of the ingredients of the economic torts for which trade unions may be liable. Second, it may entitle the employer to take disciplinary action against individual employees.

In theory at least, employers can respond to industrial action by individual employees in several ways (Mesher and Sutcliffe 1986):

- they may dismiss the employees, though dismissal letters often contain offers of re-engagement provided the workers return to work by a given date
- it is common for employers to claim that the employees have dismissed themselves
- it is possible to sue individual employees for damages, as they have repudiated the employment contract, though this is rare in practice
- with a complete stoppage of work, the employer is entitled to stop the employee's pay, but problems may arise where there is partial stoppage, as in working to rule.

LEGAL ENACTMENT

The traditional ways of conducting employee relations in Britain are voluntary joint regulation, though collective bargaining between employers and unions, or voluntary employer regulation, through individual bargaining between employer and employee. In most other developed countries, the law plays a much more central role in regulating collective bargaining and the individual contract of employment. Until the 1960s, legal enactment or legal regulation played a relatively minor role in employee relations in Britain, with the general thrust of state policy being non-interventionist (see Chapters 4 and 7). It was largely the common law that regulated the contract of employment (Lewis 1997). And it was the so-called emancipatory legislation provided by the Trade Union Act 1871, the Conspiracy and Protection of Property Act 1875 and the Trade Disputes Act 1906 that regulated relations between employers and trade unions, industrial conflict and trade union activity (Lewis 1976). Both employers and unions, unlike in most other industrialised countries, preferred voluntarism and the abstention of the judges and the courts in employee relations to legal interventionism.

The first indications of the growing influence of legal regulation in British employee relations emerged with the Contracts of Employment Act 1963 and the Redundancy Payments Act 1965. The Industrial Relations Act 1971, though repealed in 1974, was followed by further employment legislation enacted by Labour governments in the 1970s and by Conservative governments in the 1980s and early 1990s. The main legislation is largely incorporated in:

- Equal Pay Act 1970
- Equal Pay Amendment Regulations 1983
- Health and Safety at Work etc. Act 1974
- Employment Protection Act 1975
- Sex Discrimination Acts 1975 and 1986
- Race Relations Act 1976
- Transfer of Undertakings (Protection of Employment) Regulations 1981
- Wages Act 1986
- Trade Union and Labour Relations (Consolidation) Act 1992

- Trade Union Reform and Employment Rights Act 1993
- Employment Protection (Part Time) Regulations 1995
- Disability Discrimination Act 1995
- Employment Rights Act 1996.

Some of these legal provisions regulate individual employee relations by providing statutory employment protection rights for employees and statutory union membership rights for trade unionists. Others provide statutory rights for trade unions. And others regulate collective employee relations such as industrial conflict and trade union activities (see Chapters 4, 7 and 11). The main statutory rights are summarised below.

Employment protection rights

Individual employees have over 20 statutory rights, subject to some qualifying conditions, as illustrated in Exhibit 9.

Exhibit 9 **Main employment protection rights**

These include the right to:

- join or not to join a union
- not be refused employment on the grounds of union membership
- not be dismissed, or have action short of dismissal taken, because of trade union membership
- written particulars of the main terms of the contract of employment
- an itemised pay statement
- not have unlawful deductions made from wages
- guarantee payments when not provided with work by an employer on a normal work day
- medical suspension payments
- statutory sick pay
- equal treatment in terms and conditions of employment, irrespective of gender
- time off work for ante-natal care, maternity pay and maternity leave for female employees and, after giving birth, to return to work
- time off work for public duties
- not be discriminated against on the grounds of sex, marital status, disability or race
- not be dismissed in connection with medical suspension
- minimum periods of notice
- a redundancy payment when a job disappears
- time off to look for work in a redundancy situation or to arrange training
- payment from the Secretary of State in the event of employer insolvency;
- not be unfairly dismissed
- a written statement of the reasons for dismissal.

If an employer infringes any of these statutory rights, an employee may make a claim to an industrial tribunal (IT). ITs have the power to make awards, including compensation, and enforce certain rights where an employer has acted unlawfully (Lewis 1990).

Union membership rights

In addition to their statutory rights as employees, trade union members have a number of rights relating to union membership. These are illustrated in Exhibit 10.

Exhibit 10 **Main membership rights of trade unionists**

These include the right to:

- not be unreasonably excluded or expelled from a union
- compensation for being unreasonably excluded or expelled from a union
- elect union executive committees, union presidents and general secretaries by secret ballot
- secret ballots endorsing official industrial action
- secret postal ballots for union political funds
- not be unjustifiably disciplined by a union for failing to take part in official industrial action
- apply to the High Court for an order that a union has taken industrial action without a ballot
- stop deductions of union subscriptions at source.

Where trade union members claim that any of these rights have been infringed by a union, they may take their complaint to one of the following agencies, depending on the nature of the complaint: an industrial tribunal, the Certification Officer, Commissioner for Protection Against Unlawful Industrial Action or the Commissioner for the Rights of Trade Union Members.

Trade union rights

Independent trade unions recognised by employers, the officials of independent recognised unions and members of recognised independent unions all have a series of statutory rights (Farnham 1990). These are illustrated in Exhibit 11.

Exhibit 11 **Rights of independent, recognised trade unions and time-off provisions**

These include the right to:

- appoint safety representatives and to establish safety committees at work
- consultation on pensions in firms contracted out of the state earnings related pension scheme

- consultation on collective redundancies involving 20–99 employees in one establishment, within 90 days, where the consultation must take place at least 30 days before the first redundancy, and those involving 100 or more employees within 90 days or less, where consultation must take place at least 90 days before the first redundancy
- information and consultation in business transfers including their reasons, timing and implications and the measures which the employer proposes taking in relation to employees
- disclosure of information for collective bargaining purposes requested by trade union representatives
- secret ballots on employers' premises for industrial action, union elections and related matters
- time off with pay for officials undertaking trade union duties and training
- time off with pay for safety representatives and training
- time off without pay for union members undertaking trade union activities and representing the union.

WORKER PARTICIPATION IN WESTERN EUROPE

Employee relations in western Europe have two main characteristics distinguishing them from those of Britain. First, there are frequently multiple systems of employee representation. These include collective bargaining, employee representatives on company boards and plant-based works councils. The second feature of European employee relations is their far greater reliance on legal enactment in regulating both collective relations between employers and unions and individual relations between employers and employees than is the case in Britain.

Co-determination at corporate level

Worker participation with management in corporate decision-making at board level takes place, in its most advanced form, in Germany. The form of co-determination in Germany depends upon company size, the legal structure of the company and the industry in which it is located. In essence, board-level worker participation is facilitated through two-tier boards. These consist of a supervisory board (*Aufsichtsrat*) and a management board (*Vorstand*). The supervisory board is legally charged with appointing the management board, or its managing directors, and with overseeing its activities. Employee representatives sitting on the supervisory board have the same rights and duties as shareholder representatives. This, it is assumed, will result in entrepreneurial decisions which serve the joint aspirations of both shareholder and employee interests. Employee representatives may request information from the management board on all aspects of the business, including proposed corporate policies, profitability and sales. The management board is the legal employer, represents the company legally and is responsible for conducting the organisation's business operations.

In companies employing over 1,000 employees in the coal, steel and iron industries, supervisory boards consist of equal numbers of employee and shareholder representatives, though this is a declining sector of employment. Under the Works Constitution Act 1952, companies with over 500 employees but under 2,000 are required to have a supervisory board, a third of whose members are employee representatives.

In organisations with over 2,000 employees (whether joint stock companies, limited liability companies or limited partnerships based on share capital), supervisory boards consist of equal numbers of employee and shareholder representatives. The size of the supervisory board varies according to company size but some seats are reserved for trade unions that have members in the organisation, and for managerial employees. This means that 'workers', as a group, do not have full parity of representation on the supervisory board. In smaller firms, the employee representatives are directly elected by employee groups and in larger companies, with up to 8,000 employees, there are electoral colleges. The most important roles of the supervisory board are to appoint the management board and supervise management (Berghahn and Karsten 1987).

In Sweden, by comparison, the approach to co-determination is based on collective bargaining rights. Its source is the Act of Employee Participation in Decision Making (MBL) 1977. It is an expansion of earlier rights of trade unions to negotiate with employers. Employers are obliged to take the initiative in negotiating with trade unions at company level before decisions on major issues are made. These include closure, reorganisation and expansion of operations. The Act also requires employers to keep local unions informed about how company operations are progressing and about the guidelines for company personnel policy.

The MBL also presumes and encourages the signing of collective agreements on co-determination. The so called 'residual right' to industrial action means that unions are entitled to resort to industrial action if their requests for co-determination agreements, presented in connection with pay negotiations, are not met. The law also gives the unions priority of interpretation in most types of disputes. This is a major strengthening of employee influence, since most disputes of interpretation do not result in negotiations, and the unions have immediate enforcement of their interpretation. It is management which has to request negotiations in these circumstances, with negotiations being referred to national level if necessary or the unions being sued by the employer in the Labour Court (Forsebaick 1980).

Works councils at plant level

Works councils are widespread in Europe. They are prominent in France, Germany and the Netherlands. Basically, a works council is a body, established in law, normally organised at enterprise level, consisting of elected employee representatives with certain rights and responsibilities in their dealings with management and the employer.

In France, there is a multiplicity of representative bodies that have been set up in response to specific social and political pressures, at particular times. Employee delegates (*délégués du personnel*), which were instituted by the Popular Front in 1936, deal with individual employee grievances covering wages, conditions of employment and legal agreements. They are elected by the whole workforce in organisations employing over 10 employees, by a system of proportional representation, though in practice most of them are elected on a union slate. Workplace union branches (*sections syndicales*), established in 1968, can appoint their own stewards, collect dues, use notice boards and organise monthly meetings. In some firms, these branches have offices and other facilities.

Works committees in France (*comités d'entreprise*), set up in 1945 after the Liberation, deal with workplace consultation. They can be established in all firms employing at least 50 employees. They have the legal right to be informed and consulted on issues such as the number and organisation of employees, their hours of work and employment conditions. Managements have to submit an annual written report to the works committee covering the business's activities, profits or losses, allocation of profits, investments and salaries. Agreement by the works committee is required on arrangements for profit-sharing and changes in individual working hours. Works councils may create subcommittees to examine specific problems and, in companies with at least 50 employees, health, safety and improvement of working conditions committees are compulsory. Firms with at least 350 employees have to set up an employment-training committee and those with at least 1,000 have to set up an economic committee (Goetschy and Rojot 1987).

In Germany, works councils are directly elected by the workforce at establishment level, though in multi-plant companies a central works council can be formed by delegation from individual works councils. They may be elected in any establishment with at least five employees and must be recognised by the employer. White-collar workers, blue-collar workers and trainees are eligible for election but executive employees, who have their own employee representative committees, are excluded. The size of the works councils increases with the size of establishment, and representation of employee groups is in proportion to their numbers in the establishment. The members of the works councils are released with pay for their council activities, entitled to relevant training for their roles and protected by law against dismissal by the employer. Works councils in Germany have a wide range of functions (Berghahn and Karsten 1987). Basically, works councils exist to protect the interests of workers in the plant. At the same time, works councils and the employers are expected to work together in a spirit of mutual trust, and in co-operation with the trade unions and employers' associations, for the good of the employees and the plant. Under Article 37 of the Works Constitution Act 1972, works councils have 'to see that effect is given to Acts, ordinances, safety regulations, collective agreements and plant agreements for the benefit of employees' and make 'recommendations to the employer for action benefiting the plant and staff' (Berghahn and Karsten: page 108). Works councils in German companies have the right to co-determination in matters outlined in Exhibit 12.

Exhibit 12 **The rights and responsibilities of works councils in Germany**

These cover:

- the conduct of employees in the plant
- daily working times and distribution of working hours
- the reduction or extension of hours normally worked
- the time, place and form of payment of remuneration
- establishing the general principles of leave arrangements and the preparing of leave schedules
- introducing and using technical devices designed to monitor the behaviour or performance of employees
- preventing workplace accidents and occupational diseases
- the form, structure and administration of social services in the plant, company or combine
- assigning and vacating accommodation rented to employees
- establishing the principles of remuneration and introducing new remuneration methods
- the fixing of job and bonus rates and comparable performance-related remuneration
- the principles for suggestion schemes in the plant.

Where agreement is not reached on these matters, a conciliation panel takes the decision and its award replaces agreement between the works council and the employer. Employers have to gain the consent of works councils for individual measures of personnel policy, such as staff grading or regrading, and vocational training. Works councils also have to be heard where employees are dismissed for the dismissal not to be void in law.

European Works Councils

Since the early 1970s, there have been a series of initiatives within the EU to legislate for more systematic employee participation structures within the corporate sector. The draft European Works Council (EWC) Directive, published by the Commission of the European Communities in January 1991, was one in a line of controversial proposals for employee participation measures in companies operating within European member states over the last 20 years (Commission of the European Communities 1991). Up till then, only those measures requiring information disclosure and consultation on specific issues by employers had been adopted by the Council of Ministers (CoM). These included the directive on collective redundancies 1975, the directive on transfers of undertakings 1977 and the framework directive on health and safety 1989. Proposals for Euro-legislation on a European company statute in the early 1970s, on company law reform from the early 1970s until the early 1980s and on the Vredling measures in the early 1980s have been continually blocked within the EC's decision-making institutions.

The draft 1991 European Works Council Directive was adopted by all member states of the EU, except the UK, together with Iceland, Norway and Liechtenstein, under the Social Policy Agreement of the Treaty of European Union at Maastricht 1991. It provides for a European-level information and consultation system to be set up in all companies with 1,000 or more employees in member states employing more than 150 employees in each of two or more countries. A EWC, or an alternative system, must be agreed with central management and a 'special negotiating body' of employee representatives. If no agreement is reached after three years, a fall-back system applies. This requires the establishment of an EWC of employee representatives under rules defined in the annexe to the Directive. These provide the EWC with the right to meet central management at least once per year for information and consultation about the progress and prospects of the company and to request extra consultation meetings, before certain major decisions are taken affecting more than one member state.

Until the UK 'opt-in' to the Social Protocol, under the Blair government elected in May 1997, the UK and other foreign companies here only had to comply with the Directive if their operations in member states other than the UK met the thresholds. In practice, most large UK and foreign companies covered by the legal requirements in other member states included UK representatives in their EWCs, along with employee representatives from other countries, even though they were not legally required to do so. Companies with agreed trans- European information and consultation systems already in place before the end of September 1996 are exempt from these requirements.

EWCs have the right to meet central management annually and be informed of the undertaking's or group's progress and prospects. They also have the right to be consulted on management proposals likely to have serious consequences for the interests of employees. These matters include mergers, closures, relocations, organisational change and new working or production methods. For these purposes, the EWCs are able to request an additional meeting with management, if necessary.

EWCs have a maximum of 30 members, drawn from existing employee representatives, or specially elected ones where none exist. The operating expenses of the EWCs are met by the undertaking or group concerned. The original directive provides that members of the EWC do not have to reveal any information of a confidential nature and that information can be withheld where it would substantially damage the interests of the undertakings or groups concerned.

Hall (1992) argues, on the issue of the legal compulsion underpinning the establishment of EWCs, that the approach was inconsistent with the then government's emphasis on minimising employers' legal obligations in their dealings with employees and unions. Britain would therefore have been required to fill in the gaps left by the existing reliance on voluntary trade union recognition by employers. A fear of the employers is that mandatory EWCs could potentially be the vehicle for developing European-level collective bargaining within multinational companies. Indeed, it can be expected that collective bargaining strategies in Britain will be influenced by the provision of European-level corporate information.

From the union point of view, the EWC Directive presents, on the one hand, a valuable opportunity for those unions seeking employer recognition. On the other hand, alternative channels of employee representation might have emerged which could inhibit union organisation (Trades Union Congress 1991). It is also likely, since mandatory EWCs are relatively small bodies, that trade unions might have problems agreeing representatives in multi-union situations and where they represent more than one establishment or company.

The social dimension

At a meeting of the European Council in Strasbourg on 8 and 9 December 1989, the heads of state or government of the member states, except that of the UK, adopted the Community Charter of Fundamental Social Rights of Workers, known in short as the 'Social Charter' (SC). The signatories intended the SC to be a statement of the progress already made in the social field in the then Economic Community and a preparation for new advances in it. In the preamble, the heads of state also underlined the priority attached to job creation, social consensus as a factor in economic development and rejection of all forms of discrimination or exclusion. The SC demands a series of initiatives to develop workers' rights, with the responsibility for these initiatives lying with the EU itself, member states and the 'social partners', that is employers and trade unions.

Accordingly, the Commission of the European Communities drew up an action programme for parts of the SC to be implemented at Community level. The programme covered 90 areas whose aims were to develop the social dimension of the single market, thus increasing the economic and social cohesion of the member states. In some areas, falling within the competence of member states or the social partners, but arising in similar terms in all countries of the EU, the Commission initiated non-binding measures encouraging some convergence of efforts, whilst respecting national practices.

The SC identified and defined 12 areas where the fundamental social rights of workers were to be advanced and protected (Commission of the European Communities 1990). The aim of the SC was to set out the principles on which the European pattern of labour law, and the European concept of society and the place of labour within it, are based. They basically cover the social rights illustrated in Exhibit 13 (see also Chapter 4).

After the Treaty of Maastricht 1993, the principle of qualified majority voting was extended to the field of social policy. This meant that decisions within the Council of Ministers could be taken without the unanimous agreement of all member states. These matters included:

- improvements in the working environment
- working conditions
- the provision of information and worker consultation
- equal opportunities
- the integration of persons excluded from the labour market.

Exhibit 13 **The European Community Social Charter**

This set out rights covering:

- the improvement of living and working conditions
- freedom of movement
- employment and fair remuneration
- social protection and appropriate social assistance
- freedom of association and collective bargaining
- vocational training
- equal treatment of men and women
- information, consultation and worker participation
- health protection and safety at work
- the protection of children and adolescents
- pensions and a decent standard of living for elderly people
- the integration in working life of disabled persons.

The UK government was unable to support these Treaty amendments. This meant, when the Treaty came into effect, that the protection offered by the SC did not apply to workers in Britain.

Following their intergovernmental conference in June 1997, the heads of state and governments of the 15 members of the EU agreed a new treaty for Europe, the Treaty of Amsterdam. These new provisions were to be debated in each country and submitted to their electorates for approval, by either referendum or parliamentary decision. The Treaty has four main objectives (Office of the European Communities 1997):

- placing employment and citizens' rights at the heart of the EU
- sweeping away the last remaining obstacles to freedom of movement and strengthening security
- giving Europe a stronger voice in world affairs
- making the EU's institutional structure more efficient, with a view to enlarging the Union through more member states joining.

The Treaty of Amsterdam consolidates the three 'pillars' which have been the foundation of the EU's work since Treaty of Maastricht 1993: the European Communities; the common foreign and security policy; and co-operation in the field of justice and home affairs.

With a view to enlargement, the Treaty extends the area where decisions can be taken by a qualified majority of 71 per cent of the votes to cover new areas. Unanimity remains the rule in respect of constitutional matters and for a hard core of highly sensitive areas, such as taxation. By summer 1997 it was announced that invitations would be extended to Cyprus, Estonia, Hungary, Poland and Slovenia to join the Union by the early twenty-first century.

ASSIGNMENTS

(a) Why has there been a shift to personal contracts of employment in some organisations? Examine the pros and cons of personal contracts for employers and management.
(b) Identify the bargaining level(s), for a named bargaining unit, at which collective bargaining takes place in your organisation. Explain the likely influences on why collective bargaining takes place at the level(s) identified. What other bargaining units, if any, are there in the organisation? Identify the bargaining agents in each case and outline the bargaining scope, in terms of procedural and substantive agreements, for each bargaining group.
(c) Make a presentation describing and analysing the procedural agreements between management and the unions in your organisation.
(d) Read Marchington (1988) and make sure that you fully understand his four models of joint consultation. Using his framework, describe and analyse the joint consultative arrangements in your organisation. How are they linked, if at all, with the collective bargaining machinery in the organisation/industry?
(e) Your organisation's annual pay negotiations with the unions representing manual workers have broken down. Examine the circumstances in which the management side would resort to: (1) conciliation, (2) arbitration, (3) mediation, (4) industrial sanctions. Indicate the pros and cons of using each of these processes.
(f) Read Lewis (1986: pages 3-43). To what extent have British employee relations become juridified in recent years? Give reasons for your conclusion.
(g) Argue the case for introducing a (non-statutory) 'works council' in the establishment where you work. Provide a draft constitution for such a body and indicate the sorts of issues which would have to be addressed if the council was to operate effectively.
(h) Read Hall (1992). (1) Identify and analyse the developments and pressures which have shaped the current Directive on EWCs. (2) Examine the reasons why the British government and some employers are opposed to the Directive. What would have been the consequences for British trans-national companies, operating in Britain, Germany and the Netherlands, if, say, the European Works Council Directive had been adopted, using the 'qualified majority' principle?

REFERENCES

ADVISORY, CONCILIATION and ARBITRATION SERVICE. 1979. *The ACAS Role in Conciliation, Arbitration and Mediation*. London: ACAS.

ADVISORY, CONCILIATION and ARBITRATION SERVICE. 1983. *Collective Bargaining in Britain: Its extent and scope*. London: ACAS.

BERCUSSON, B. 1986. 'Workers, corporate enterprise and the law'. In Lewis, R. (ed.) 1986, *Labour Law in Britain*, Oxford: Blackwell.

BERGHAHN, V. *and* KARSTEN, D. 1987. *Industrial Relations in West Germany.* Oxford: Berg.

BURROWS, G. 1986. *No-Strike Agreements and Pendulum Arbitration.* London: IPM.

CLEGG, H. 1976. 'Pluralism in industrial relations'. *British Journal of Industrial Relations*. XIII (3).

CLEGG, H., FOX, A. *and* THOMPSON, A. 1964. *A History of British Trade Unions since 1889: Volume I 1889-1910*. Oxford: Oxford University Press.

COMMISSION OF THE EUROPEAN COMMUNITIES. 1990. *Community Charter of the Fundamental Social Rights of Workers*. Luxembourg: Office of Official Publications of the European Communities.

COMMISSION OF THE EUROPEAN COMMUNITIES. 1991. *Amended Proposals for a Council Directive on the Establishment of European Works Councils in Community-Scale Undertakings or Groups of Undertakings for the Purposes of Informing and Consulting Employees*. Luxembourg: Council of Ministers.

FARNHAM, D. 1990. *Personnel in Context*. London: IPM.

FARNHAM, D. *and* HORTON, S. (eds) 1996a. *Managing the New Public Services*. Basingstoke: Macmillan.

FARNHAM, D. *and* HORTON, S. (eds) 1996b. *Managing People in the Public Services*. Basingstoke: Macmillan.

FLANDERS, A. 1964. *The Fawley Productivity Agreements*. London: Faber and Faber.

FORSEBAICK, L. 1980. *Industrial Relations and Employment in Sweden*. Uppsala: Swedish Institute.

GOETSCHY, J. *and* ROJOT, J. 1987. 'France'. In Bamber, G. and Lansbury, R. 1987, *International and Comparative Industrial Relations*, London: Allen and Unwin.

GUNNICLE, P. *and* FLOOD, P. 1990. *Personnel Management in Ireland.* Dublin: Gill and Macmillan.

HALL, M. 1992. 'Legislating for employee participation: a case study of the European Works Councils Directive'. *Warwick Papers in Industrial Relations*. Number 39.

INCOMES DATA SERVICES. 1991. *Industrial Relations*. London: IPM.

KOCHAN, T., KATZ, H. and MCKERSIE, R. 1986. *The Transformation of American Industrial Relations*. NY: Basic.

LEWIS, D. 1997. *Essentials of Employment Law*. (5th edn.) London: IPD.

LEWIS, R. 1976. 'The historical development of labour law'. *British Journal of Industrial Relations.* March.

MCCARTHY, W. 1966. *The Role of the Shop Steward in British Industrial Relations. (Royal Commission Research Paper 1)*. London: HMSO.

MARCHINGTON, M. 1988. 'The four faces of consultation'. *Personnel Management*. July.

MARCHINGTON, M. 1989. 'Joint consultation in practice'. In Sisson, K. (ed.) 1989, *Personnel Management in Britain*. Oxford: Blackwell.

MARGINSON, P., EDWARDS, P., MARTIN, R., SISSON, K. *and* PURCELL, J. 1988. *Beyond the Workplace: Managing industrial relations in multi-establishment enterprise*. Oxford: Blackwell.

MARKS, W. 1978. *Preparing an Employee Handbook*. London: IPM.

MESHER, J. *and* SUTCLIFFE, F. 1986. 'Industrial action and the individual'. In Lewis, R. (ed.) 1986, *Labour Law in Britain*, Oxford: Blackwell.

MILLWARD, N. *and* STEVENS, M. 1986, *British Workplace Industrial Relations 1980-84*. Aldershot: Gower.

MILLWARD, N., STEVENS, M., SMART, D. *and* HAWES, W. 1992. *Workplace Industrial Relations in Transition*. Aldershot: Dartmouth.

OFFICE FOR OFFICIAL PUBLICATIONS OF THE EUROPEAN COMMUNITIES. 1997. *A New Treaty for Europe*. Luxembourg: OOPEC.

PALMER, S. 1990. *Determining Pay*. London: IPM.

PARKER, P., HAWES, W. *and* LUMB, A. 1971. *The Reform of Collective Bargaining at Plant and Company Level*. London: HMSO.

POLYTECHNIC AND COLLEGES EMPLOYERS' FORUM. 1989. *Recognition and Procedure Agreement creating the Polytechnics and Colleges National Negotiating Committee*. London: PCEF.

PORTSMOUTH AND SOUTH EAST HAMPSHIRE HEALTH AUTHORITY. 1991. *Contract for Senior Managers*. Portsmouth: PSEHHA.

RICO, L. 1987. 'The new industrial relations: British electricians' new-style agreements'. *Industrial and Labor Relations Review*. 41(1), October.

SHIRAI, T. 1983. *Contemporary Industrial Relations in Japan*. Wisconsin: University of Wisconsin Press.

SIMPSON, B. 1986. 'Trade union immunities'. In Lewis, R. (ed.) 1986, *Labour Law in Britain*, Oxford: Blackwell.

STOREY, J. 1980. *The Challenge to Management Control*. London: Kogan Page.

STOREY, J. 1983. *Management Prerogative and the Question of Control*. London: Routledge and Kegan Paul.

TRADES UNION CONGRESS. 1991. *Unions and Europe in the 1990s*. London: TUC.

WOOD, J. 1985. 'Last offer arbitration'. *British Journal of Industrial Relations*. XXIII (3), November.

4 The contexts of employee relations

The roles of the state, its government agencies and the law are crucial in influencing the structures, patterns and processes of employee relations. The government's economic policies and its legal policies on trade unions, the regulation of industrial conflict and employment protection rights have major implications for employee relations (see Chapters 1 and 7). Where economic policy focuses on creating the economic conditions necessary for full employment (Keynesianism), it strengthens union bargaining power in the labour market and the workplace, whilst weakening that of management. Where economic policy focuses on containing price inflation primarily through the instruments of reducing public expenditure, encouraging free market forces and using changes in interest rates to influence economic activity (monetarism and supply-side economics), this strengthens employers and management in their market relations with trade unions and their managerial relations with employees.

Economic management is the actions taken by government to influence economic performance within the macro- and micro-economy. With the demise of classical *laissez-faire* in the mid-nineteenth century, governments became steadily more interventionist in economic affairs – but not in employee relations, which were dominated by voluntarist values. This was in response to a series of political, social and democratic pressures. Political interventions in economic affairs by the state were also influenced by significant events, such as the First and Second World Wars. These marked a discontinuity with the past in terms of increased levels of government expenditure but also pointed to the future in terms of more government involvement and intervention in the economy. During both of these wars government expenditure rose rapidly, both absolutely and relatively, only to decrease again when hostilities had ceased, but not to pre-war levels (Farnham and Horton 1993 1996). These incremental increases in government intervention in the economy were paralleled by searches for appropriate methods of economic management to accompany them.

Economic management in Britain since the end of the Second World War, in 1945, can be divided broadly into two periods. First, there was the era of Keynesianism which was the dominant economic orthodoxy supported by successive governments between 1945 and the mid-1970s. Second, there is the period of monetarism and supply-side economics which has dominated government economic policy since the mid-1970s. Both approaches to economic management have implications for the parties to employee relations, employee relations processes and their outcomes. To what extent the Blair administration, post-1997, represents a 'new' set of economic policy initiatives, a 'new' approach to economic management and a 'third' way to solving the UK's economic problems is to date an open question.

Similarly, where there is an 'abstentionist' legal policy supportive of trade union organisation, which encourages collectivist approaches to employment policy on the part of employers, the role of trade unions in employee relations is both legitimised and reinforced and limitations are placed on the right to manage. Where legal policy is 'restrictionist' and is aimed at weakening trade unions and encouraging individualism in employee relations, the power of management is strengthened and that of employees, collectively and individually, is weakened.

A further extension to political interventionism in employee relations is the 'social dimension' of the single European market. Ever since the European communities were created, there have been a series of attempts by the European authorities not only to expand the internal European market but also to extend the coverage of its social policies to employees, citizens and their families in the member states. These social initiatives, whilst important to workers and individuals, have not always met with the approval of some British governments or management organisations such as the CBI.

KEYNESIANISM

The economic ideas associated with John Maynard Keynes (1936), most commonly referred to as Keynesianism, emerged out of the experiences of industrial depression, high unemployment and social deprivation during the 1930s. In the years immediately following the Second World War, Keynesian economic policies became the new conventional wisdom of both academic economists and social democratic politicians in Britain and western Europe.

Until Keynes's writings, economic theory was mainly concerned with the determinants of the general price level. Keynes, instead, focused on the determinants of the level of output in the economy, stressing the importance of aggregate demand. It is aggregate demand, he argued, that determines the level of employment, with a given population and existing technology. This contrasted with the prevailing economic orthodoxy of the time – classical economic theory – which attributed high unemployment to excessive real wages and high interest rates. According to classical theory, if money wages were reduced, and interest rates were cut, employment would increase because firms would employ more labour – at lower wage rates – and because increased savings would lead to greater investment spending.

In Keynes's *General Theory*, he argues that far from increasing employment, wage cuts, by depressing aggregate demand, reduce it. This is because the level of employment is determined, not by the level of wages, but by the level of aggregate demand. This, in turn, depends on the level of consumption, investment and government expenditure in the economy. He also argues that full employment occurs at a unique level of investment and unless there is some mechanism to ensure the 'correct' level of investment, full employment does not occur spontaneously. The orthodox view, in contrast, was that investment adjusts to the full employment level automatically, via the interest rate. But in Keynes's analysis, there is no automatic adjustment mechanism through the interest rate, so there is no certainty of creating full employment. In Keynes's system, the equality of savings and investment in the economy is achieved, not by changes in the interest rate, but by changes in the level of aggregate demand. It is government intervention in the economy, largely through its fiscal policy, that results in full employment, if current demand, including investment spending, fails to produce it.

Fiscal policy

The Keynesian emphasis in economic management is on creating the economic conditions necessary for achieving four policy objectives. These are:

- full employment
- price stability
- balance of payments equilibrium
- economic growth.

The aim underpinning all Keynesian policy is that of achieving the level of aggregate demand commensurate with full employment. The policy instruments used by government for this purpose are largely fiscal (Donaldson and Farquhar 1988). This means that when unemployment is rising, due to falls in consumption or in investment spending, fiscal policy is used to inject spending power into the economy by cutting taxes and/or raising public expenditure. The latter is achieved by increasing the public sector borrowing requirement (PSBR), which is the amount by which government revenue falls short of government expenditure in a given expenditure cycle. These 'countercyclical' fiscal measures aim to increase aggregate demand and, in consequence, lead to a higher demand for labour by employers, thus reducing unemployment.

One problem of full employment is that it results in increased collective bargaining power by the trade unions in the labour market (Robinson 1937). In the private sector, unless the unions restrain their wage bargaining claims, or employers resist them, this leads to rising money wages, not necessarily matched by rises in labour productivity or falls in unit labour costs. These wage rises contribute to a wages-prices spiral by inducing: companies which have conceded 'unearned' wage increases to their workforces to raise the prices of their products in 'soft' product markets; other bargaining groups to seek higher wages for themselves in 'soft' labour markets; and these companies, in turn, to pass on the cost of their wage increases to their customers.

In the public sector, wage rises achieved in private industry act as benchmarks for trade union negotiators. This puts pressure on public sector employers to provide comparable wage levels to those in the corporate sector. These can only come out of increases in productivity, taxes or the PSBR. Tax increases are unpopular with government and the electorate;

productivity increases may be resisted by the unions and their members; and the effects of increases in public borrowing are likely to be inflationary, especially where financing the PSBR takes the form of injecting new currency into circulation from the banking sector. Further, public sector borrowing raises interest rates through the increased sales of bonds, thus making borrowing by companies more expensive, with possible adverse effects on private investment.

Governments using Keynesian demand management techniques have two possible policy prescriptions to deal with these economic pressures. One is to deflate the economy through fiscal measures. This is done by cutting back purchasing power through raising taxes and/or cutting public spending. This raises unemployment, strengthens the hands of management negotiators at the wage bargaining table and weakens trade union bargaining power. But it can also result in trade union militancy, slow economic growth and reductions in exports. The result is a 'stop-go' economic cycle, relieved only by the reversal of government economic measures when unemployment and economic recession have brought stabilising pressures to bear on prices and the balance of payments. Reflation, in turn, leads to increases in public spending, renewed growth, falling unemployment, rising wages and rising prices and, eventually, to further attempts at deflation and price stability, thus completing the stop-go economic cycle once more.

Incomes policy

The second policy prescription available to governments pursuing Keynesian economic measures is an 'incomes policy', to complement fiscal policy. An incomes policy is where the government attempts to control wage inflation by intervening in the pay bargaining process between employers and trade unions (Panitch 1976). There are three main types of incomes policy:

- pay freezes
- statutory norms
- voluntary norms.

Pay freezes have been used for short periods in Britain on a number of occasions since the war. They prohibit the implementation of pay settlements during the period of the freeze. They therefore disrupt established internal pay differentials, and external pay relativities, between those who have implemented a settlement immediately before the freeze and those who have been constrained by it.

A *statutory pay norm* traditionally follows a pay freeze. This further defers the re-establishing of traditional wage differentials and relativities, as well as contributing its own distortions to the wages structure. A statutory pay norm imposes a zero increase, or a small ceiling, on all wage settlements. Settlements in excess of the statutory norm are usually permitted only where one of a number of criteria for exceptional treatment is satisfied. These may include:

- to reward work groups for rises in productivity
- to help employers respond to labour shortages
- to help the low paid
- to restructure distorted pay differentials.

Statutory pay norms are also accompanied by a restriction on the number of pay settlements that any single negotiating group can achieve in a year, normally only one every 12 months. Statutory norms may be specified in terms of either a percentage pay increase or some absolute money sum to be added to existing pay levels. In practice, pay norms come to be regarded as the 'going rate' or target rate of increase for most negotiating groups. Where the sum specified is an absolute money sum, this results in a narrowing of percentage wage differentials. The specification of the norm in absolute terms in a succession of incomes policies in Britain in the early 1970s was a main reason for the substantial erosion of occupational wage relativities at that time.

Voluntary pay norms usually involve specifying a maximum permissible level of wage settlements but, unlike statutory policies, they do not have legal force. For this reason, there is normally less compliance with them. And such policies are effective only where government can exert its own direct control over wage levels, as amongst public sector employees.

Incomes policies have suffered from a number of shortcomings. First, it is suggested that they merely defer rather than cancel large wage increases, because once the policy is off, employee groups try to catch up lost ground. Second, where the norm relates to basic wage rates, earnings drift (or rises in weekly earnings in excess of negotiated wage increases) emerges to compensate for this, causing resentment among those who remain constrained by wage policy norms. Third, incomes policies tend to ossify the wages structure, preventing differential rates of change in money wages amongst competing job sectors. Fourth, there is the issue of policing incomes policies. In Sweden, in the 1960s and 1970s, both management and unions policed incomes policy voluntarily, without government intervention. In Britain, in contrast, state agencies such as the National Board for Prices and Incomes and the Pay Board were used in the late 1960s and early 1970s, but with varying degrees of success.

The new Keynesianism

After the election of the first Thatcher government in Britain in June 1979, and the first Reagan administration in the USA in November 1980, Keynesian approaches to economic management were largely rejected by both British and American governments in favour of market liberal policies, associated with monetarism and supply-side economics (see below). The market liberal emphasis in economic policy is on rational individuals pursuing their own self-interest in the market place, with the minimum of government intervention, supported by sound monetary policy to control inflation and by economic measures aimed at improving the ability of producers to supply goods and services to the market, efficiently and cost-effectively. The market liberal critiques of Keynesianism in Britain were fuelled by the onset of 'stagflation', that is rising inflation and rising unemployment, and by the failures of successive incomes policies in the 1960s and 1970s.

The economic experiences of the 1970s and 1980s have modified Keynesian thinking (Shaw 1988). First, few Keynesians would still argue that unemployment always represents a problem solely of effective demand without taking account of the supply side of the economy. Second, few Keynesians would argue today that an overall increase in public spending would continue to reduce the level of unemployment, without conceding that the problem is not just one of demand but also of training in human capital. Keynesians are now aware of the need to target public expenditure, by using it, for example, to produce a better-trained workforce, able to produce goods and services to meet consumer demand in the market place. Third, Keynesians are also aware of regional variations in unemployment, of unemployment in the inner cities and of the long-term unemployed. Structural unemployment, for example, is due to declining industries, economic change, new technology and global competition. All these problems require different solutions.

Keynesians now also accept that increasing aggregate demand in the classical Keynesian way will not deal with the problems of unemployed ethnic minorities, of women entering the labour market when there are no childcare facilities or of the unskilled, lacking training, qualifications and work experience. Unlike some of the market liberals who see these problems in micro-economic terms, Keynesians still see them as of macro concern, justifying a more interventionist approach by government in economic management.

MONETARISM AND SUPPLY-SIDE ECONOMICS

The mid-1970s marked a watershed in economic policy in Britain, as the decade ended in a break with the postwar settlement of full employment, Keynesianism and the welfare state. The wider economic contexts of the 1970s also provided new challenges for government policy-makers. First, there was the replacement of fixed exchange rates, agreed at Bretton Woods in 1944, by countries floating their own domestic currencies in 1973. Second, the spirit of policy co-operation internationally was replaced by foreign competition and freer markets as countries used the mechanism of interest rates to deal with the dual problems of inflation and balance of payments deficits. Third, rises in oil prices in the early 1970s and late 1970s produced very difficult challenges in economic management for governments of the major industrial countries (Keegan 1984).

Keynesian economics had become associated with interventionism and big government, whilst monetarism and supply-side economics were becoming associated with rational individualism, the market and less government. Mullard (1992: page 248) relates the demise of Keynesianism in

Britain 'to the failure of UK governments to establish both a Keynesian economic and political agenda similar to that established elsewhere in Europe.' It is monetarism and supply-side economics that have dominated British and American economic management since the mid-1970s.

Monetarism

Monetary policy is concerned with the measures taken by government to influence the price and supply of money in the economy, through changes in the rate of interest. Clearly, in a free, deregulated money market, government can attempt to control either the supply (quantity) of money in circulation or its price, but not both. The growth in importance of monetary policy as an instrument of macro-economic management in recent years is explained to a large extent by the apparent failure of fiscal policy in the 1970s to resolve the problem of stagflation. Monetarist economists explain this failure in terms of excessive government spending, financed by spiralling budget deficits, not only through borrowing – from the banking and non-banking sectors – but also increasingly as a result of printing new money (Friedman and Schwarz 1963; Friedman 1991). Both of these lead to increases in the money supply in excess of the amount needed to finance the transactions that arise from growth in the physical output of the economy.

Monetarists argue that if the money supply is allowed to grow faster than the economy's output, then firms and households find themselves holding larger money balances than they want. This surplus of money balances is then spent on goods and services, leading to an increase in aggregate demand which it is beyond the capacity of the economy to supply. According to monetarists, this results in a general rise in prices. Additionally, any upward pressure on prices also fuels expectations of future inflation. This results in higher wage demands from trade union negotiators and an ensuing wages-prices inflationary spiral. A related consequence of excessive monetary growth, it is argued, is unemployment, as the competitiveness of firms declines and workers 'price themselves out of jobs'. In monetarist analysis, unemployment will fall, in the longer term, only if the productive efficiency of the economy is increased and inflationary expectations are reduced.

The monetarist analysis of the role of money in the economy is based on the quantity theory of money. This relates monetary growth to the rate of inflation. The monetarist prescription is to allow the money supply to grow at a constant rate approximately equal to the growth in national output (the money supply rule). Money supply in excess of this, it is believed, is likely to result in inflation. Monetarists also believe that there are strong links between changes in the money supply and changes in interest rates, when interest rates (or the price of money) are determined in a free market. This is based on the assumption that people's willingness to hold assets in the form of money balances is relatively sensitive to the rate of interest.

Monetarists also argue that the rate of interest is a main determinant of investment decisions. The reasoning is that a fall in interest rates makes some investments profitable, which were previously unprofitable, and therefore aggregate investment should increase. Conversely, when interest rates rise, aggregate investment should fall. Aggregate investment, therefore, is inversely related to the rate of interest.

In the 1980s, monetary policy in Britain reflected the predominance given by governments to the importance of money in determining economic performance. In March 1980, the newly elected government unveiled its anti-inflation policy, with the announcement of its first medium-term financial strategy. Sterling M3 (broadly defined as notes, coins, current and deposit accounts in UK banks, and private sector holdings of sterling bank certificates of deposit) was the targeted money supply. However, achieving the desired growth in M3 in the following years proved problematic (Smith 1987). And in 1987, the Chancellor of the Exchequer quietly announced the end of targeting broad money in the Budget that year. This decision came after more than a decade of unsuccessful targeting. The main reason for this policy failure was the dramatic deregulation of the financial services sector in the 1980s, with the consequent acceleration in the rate of financial innovation in money markets.

With the abolition of exchange controls and with financial deregulation in Britain, governments felt it necessary to fall back on interest rate policy to restrain the rise of credit in the economy. But high interest rates, in turn, proved difficult to sustain over long periods for economic and political reasons. Moreover, from the mid-1980s, interest rates appeared to be set more with a view to influencing the level of the exchange rate rather than with a view to constraining growth in the money stock. Interest rates alone seem to be inadequate in restricting monetary growth sufficiently to squeeze out inflation. As such, their use is viewed as a blunt policy instrument.

It is further argued that monetarist measures to reduce inflationary pressures are likely to have a number of negative consequences for businesses (Ellis and Parker 1990). First, high interest rates, since they attract foreign currency into the economy, and cause the external value of the currency to rise, tend to hit exporters. Similarly, as the value of the domestic currency rises, domestic producers suffer as imported goods gain a price competitive advantage over home produced ones. Second, high interest rates, coupled with a high exchange rate, tend to decrease aggregate demand for domestically produced goods. This is likely to squeeze profits, to increase stocks of unsold goods and to result in more borrowing to finance this. Third, firms may not be able to survive a combination of high interest rates and a high exchange rate, since these have implications for employment, investment and the productive capacity of the economy.

Supply-side economics

Keynesian and monetarist macro-economic policies are both concerned with influencing the level of aggregate demand in the economy. Keynesian economics operates primarily through fiscal measures, whilst monetarist economic policy seeks to control growth in the supply of money and interest rates. The branch of economics which focuses on the micro-economic factors determining aggregate supply is referred to as 'supply-side' economics. The aggregate supply of an economy consists of the amount of total real output that producers are willing and able to produce at various prices in the short term.

Supply-side economists argue that the key to reducing unemployment and inflation lies in improving the ability of the economy to supply goods and services to the market efficiently and cost-effectively. In practice, most supply-siders also favour a sound monetary policy to keep down inflation so as to provide a favourable economic climate for employment and production. Recent supply-side economics differs from earlier attempts at dirigiste industrial policy in its emphasis on creating an economic environment conducive to private enterprise and free markets, rather than state planning, government intervention and investment subsidies. Supply-side measures are therefore aimed at creating an economic environment in which there are incentives for individuals to work and for firms to invest, produce goods or services and employ workers. The role of government is not to plan industry and manage demand but to liberalise markets, reduce taxes and public spending and deregulate the labour market.

The primary objective of supply-side policies is to create the economic conditions necessary for fast growth, low inflation and full employment. In essence, supply-side economics is concerned with increasing aggregate supply so that more demand can be accommodated, without inflation. The supply-side measures pursued by Conservative governments in Britain between 1979 and 1997 involved:

- reducing direct taxation and creating incentives to work and invest
- privatising public industries
- using the law to restrict union power in the labour market.

Improving economic incentives

Exhibit 14 **Major tax incentives 1979–97**

These included:

- reductions in the marginal rate of income tax on high earned incomes and the introduction of a uniform rate of tax on earned and unearned incomes
- reductions in the basic rate of income tax
- reductions in the rates of corporation tax on profits
- increases in income tax thresholds, taking more people out of paying tax
- introduction of technical changes to taxation legislation, to alleviate the impact of capital gains tax
- introduction of tax exemptions and other incentives for investment in plant, buildings, enterprise zones, share options and personal equity plans.

After 1979, a number of major tax changes were introduced by successive Conservative governments to act as incentives to work, invest and encourage private enterprise. These are illustrated in Exhibit 14.

The unanswered questions which remain are whether pre-1979 taxes damaged the British economy and whether the changes introduced since then have improved incentives to work, invest and save and encouraged economic growth or not.

Privatisation and deregulation

These measures involved:

- selling off state monopolies to private shareholders
- introducing market competition into the remaining public services
- introducing more competition into the private sector.

Underpinning them was the assumption that market competition is the key to higher productivity, wider consumer choice and lower prices. First, a wide range of public industries was sold off and denationalised by government after 1979, starting with Associated British Ports, British Aerospace, Enterprise Oil and Jaguar Cars (Farnham and Horton 1996). Second, more competition was introduced into the Civil Service, local government and the National Health Service (NHS), through compulsory competitive tendering. This required these sectors to compete with external contractors for the provision of certain services such as cleaning, catering and some professional services. Third, more competition was introduced into the private sector through reforming some monopolies and removing restrictive practices, such as in the Stock Market, legal services and the supply of spectacles.

Improving labour market flexibility

Another supply-side policy goal of Conservative governments in the 1980s and 1990s was to make the labour market more competitive to enable wages to find their free market levels. The Thatcher and Major governments believed that real wages were not responsive enough to labour market factors and saw the unions as a prime cause of this. They were convinced that unions destroy jobs by raising wages above levels that employers can afford. They therefore enacted measures attempting to curb trade unions and their bargaining power through a series of trade union laws: the Employment Acts of 1980, 1982, 1988, 1989, 1990 and the Trade Union Act 1984. This legislation was subsequently consolidated, with other trade union legislation, as outlined in Figure 5, into the Trade Union and Labour Relations (Consolidation) Act 1992.

Figure 5 **Principal legal sources of the TULRCA 1992**

Conspiracy and Protection of Property Act 1875
Trade Union Act 1913
Industrial Courts Act 1919
Trade Union (Amalgamations, etc) Act 1964
Industrial Relations Act 1971
Trade Union and Labour Relations Act 1974
Employment Protection Act 1975
Trade Union and Labour Relations (Amendment) Act 1976
Employment Protection (Consolidation) Act 1978
Employment Act 1980
Employment Act 1982
Trade Union Act 1984
Employment Act 1988
Employment Act 1989
Employment Act 1990

Another of the Conservative governments' aims was to reduce 'involuntary' unemployment, by making the labour market more flexible and thus enable all those seeking employment to be in work. It was also felt that the structure of employment and levels of social security benefits distorted the labour market. Governments therefore attempted to make the trade-off between receiving social security payments and working less favourable to remaining unemployed. These measures included:

- indexing benefits to retail prices, rather than to earnings
- reforming social security payments
- making the obtaining of benefits more difficult for school-leavers
- abolishing earnings-related supplements, based on the previous level of earnings at work.

NEW LABOUR'S APPROACH: A THIRD WAY?

With the election to political power of a 'New Labour' government, led by Tony Blair, in May 1997, there was much speculation about the possible implications for the UK having its first Labour administration for 18 years and the impact which this would have on economic and employment policy. In economic terms, Labour is likely to be fiscally cautious. It had no plans for increasing public spending during its first two years of office, and one of the Chancellor of the Exchequer's first actions was to give the Bank of England full independence in monetary matters and freedom to raise interest rates independently of government and the Treasury. This subsequently resulted in four rises in interest rates in the first 100 days of New Labour's administration. Similarly, the Chancellor's first post-election budget contained few surprises: a windfall tax on the public utilities to fund training for the young unemployed; rises in duties on alcohol, tobacco and petrol; and no income tax rises. The new government's overall objective was to provide the conditions for continuing the steady growth of the economy, already apparent under the previous Conservative administration, promote long-term investment, keep a tight target for inflation and not undermine business confidence.

The overriding economic goals of the New Labour government were stated in its election manifesto (Labour Party 1997: page 11): 'low inflation, rising living standards and high and stable levels of employment.' With economic stability seen to be the essential platform for sustained growth within a global economy, Labour's economic priority was stable, low inflation conditions for long-term growth. To these purposes, Labour claimed, by spending wisely and taxing fairly, government could help tackle the country's central economic problems. Its main policy proposals included:

- ensuring that public money was used better, underpinned by a partnership with the private sector
- promoting fair taxes to encourage work and reward effort
- making monetary policy more effective, open, accountable and free from short-term political manipulation
- maintaining strict rules for government borrowing by enforcing the 'golden rule' of public spending – borrowing only for investment, not to fund current public expenditure
- sticking to planned public spending for the government's first two years' of office
- switching public spending to investment by using resources better and eliminating public-sector waste
- promoting saving and investment
- reforming competition law to facilitate competition wherever possible
- reinvigorating the private finance initiative
- promoting local economic growth and small businesses
- strengthening the UK's capability in science, technology and design
- taking action on long-term unemployment, through initiatives involving government, businesses and local authorities
- promoting new 'green' technologies.

It was also Labour's stated objective 'for Britain to be a high-quality, high-added-value economy, supported by sustained long-term investment, social cohesion and an ethos of democratic participation and citizenship' (Labour Party 1997: page 1). To these ends, Labour believes that to sustain economic opportunity and prosperity in a global economy, government needs, as outlined above, to provide a supportive environment for the business sector, including a stable currency, adequate level of public investment, a fair tax regime and promotion of fair competition amongst businesses in the market place. In parallel with its concern for promoting the conditions necessary for steady economic expansion and business confidence, New Labour also believes – unlike Conservative governments in the 1980s and 1990s –

that, to be economically successful, the UK needs to use the talents of its workforce fully, rather than exploitively. It recognises that competitive success is best achieved through partnership between employers and employees, rather than confrontation. This requires, in its view, leading-edge companies' recognising that high business performance is directly associated with maximising the potential of all of its employees in the workplace. In Labour's view, 'the way to achieve this is through trust, consultation, teamworking and offering people real security.'

The challenge for the Labour government is, in its opinion, how to create both opportunity for businesses in the modern, rapidly changing, globalised economy – especially in terms of market opportunities, technology and patterns of working – and security for workers. Its prognosis is that companies and individuals need both the capability and flexibility to succeed in this 'new world' of fierce competition, constant innovation and continuous change. Accordingly, there are three principles underlying Labour's approach in trying to balance the creative tensions between economic efficiency, employment flexibility and fairness at work:

- every person at work should be entitled to a basic minimum of standards of fairness, properly enforced
- rigidity should be avoided in labour market regulation to promote the flexibility required
- the best route to job security in the long term is a highly educated and skilled workforce able to succeed in the labour market.

Whilst these standards are based on the notion of individual rights, New Labour accepts that some of them may be best realised through membership of a union. However, Labour's overall purpose is to provide a 'new deal' for people at work, by giving them a decent minimum threshold of fair treatment, whilst recognising that social partnership is at the heart of successful businesses.

Its starting point in terms of its employment policy is that the modern labour market is changing:

- jobs are changing, with around a third of them classified as professional, managerial and technical
- firms are changing, with a growing proportion of the workforce employed in small to medium-sized businesses
- there are more atypical workers, not employed on full-time, permanent contracts
- more women are working, making up some half of the total workforce
- there is less job security and more individuals are experiencing periods of unemployment
- there is growing inequality and widening pay relativities
- only about 50 per cent of the workforce are covered by collective agreements, compared with 75 per cent in the mid-1970s
- only one in three workers is unionised, compared with more than one in two in the mid-1970s.

Whilst Labour accepts that this new labour market can bring new opportunities for people, it can also bring abuses and unfairness (Farnham 1996). And, since the UK has amongst the fewest basic legal standards to protect working conditions in the developed world, government's objective is to establish a framework of minimum standards in both the labour market and workplace. This is aimed to support flexibility, on the one hand, and provide protection against unfair treatment by less scrupulous employers on the other.

New Labour's proposals for setting basic standards at work should, in its view, be regarded as being part of an individual's citizenship rights. 'They should be regarded as natural as the rule of law and the protection against the abuse of power', at whatever level (Labour Party 1997: page 3). Yet to what extent New Labour's economic, employment and labour market policy initiatives represent a break with the harsher New Right approach to economic management and supply side economics – and represents a 'third way' in managing the economy, combining economic efficiency with social fairness – has yet to be effectively demonstrated.

LEGAL POLICY

The state and the law are never neutral in employee relations. The state, through the application of the law, is the ultimate source of authority and power in society and employee relations are not excluded from its influence. Figure 6 illustrates how the law regulates relations between the primary parties to the wage–work bargain (through the contract of employment and employment protection rights), between unions and their members (through the contract of membership and union membership rights) and between the secondary parties (through voluntary collective agreements, trade union rights and the law on trade disputes).

Figure 6 **The law and employee relations**

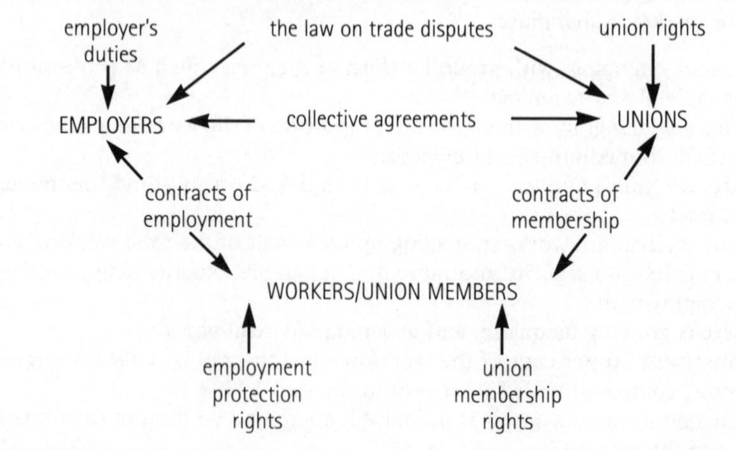

The key to understanding the role of the law in employee relations is identifying its emphasis and impact at particular times. These include:

- whether the law focuses on legal rights or legal freedoms for the parties to employee relations
- whether it is abstentionist or interventionist in employee relations processes
- whether it prioritises individual or collective patterns of employee relations
- whether it affects the balance of bargaining power between employers and employees and between management and unions in the labour market
- whether it seeks to regulate intra- and inter-union affairs
- whether the law counterbalances management power by supporting union and employee interests or reinforces this power.

The law is a dynamic and iterative process and its outcomes depend on the legal sources regulating employee relations, the decisions of the courts and whether Parliament enacts Conservative or Labour government policies.

The sources of English employment or labour law are:

- legislation
- codes of practice
- the common law.

Legislation or statute law is determined by Parliament, whilst delegated legislation is actioned through statutory instruments, which are normally subject to approval from Parliament or from the European Commission and Council of Ministers. Codes of practice, such as those from ACAS, the Health and Safety Commission and the Equal Opportunities Commission, are guidelines to good employment practice, similar to those of the Highway Code for road users. The common law or case law is based on judicial decisions in the courts, which form binding precedents on lower courts. These legal decisions are based on certain legal principles identified by the judges.

THE EMPLOYMENT CONTRACT AND STATUTORY EMPLOYMENT PROTECTION RIGHTS

The individual legal relationship between employer and employee, embodied in the contract of employment, is the cornerstone of British employee relations. The contract of employment originated in the common law and the law of 'master' and 'servant' in early capitalism. Today, the contract of employment is still largely regulated by the common law and the rules of contract built up by the judges. In theory, the contract of employment, made orally or in writing, is determined between two equal parties, employer and employee. As a legal relationship, it is one whereby the employer agrees to provide employment, wages and conditions to the individual employee who, in return, provides effort and skills in carrying out the job's tasks, is expected to take reasonable care in fulfilling the duties of employment and accepts the legal constraints of employment, such as not acting in conflict with the commercial interests of the employer.

In practice, the legal equality between an employer, normally a corporate body, and an employee, who is an individual, is a fiction. This is because once employed, employees put themselves under a common law obligation to obey all reasonable and lawful instructions given to them by the employer in carrying out their work tasks. This in reality is an act of subordination. As Kahn-Freund (1977: page 7) comments:

> There can be no employment relationship without a power to command and a duty to obey, that is without this element of subordination in which lawyers rightly see the hallmark of the 'contract of employment'.

An element of co-operation can be built into the employment relationship, and the power to command and the duty to obey can be ameliorated, but the ultimate power of command by management remains. A crucial legal issue is how far the courts interpret the contract in order to preserve the employer's power to command and management's right to manage.

A complementary legal issue is how far statute law, enacted by Parliament, offsets employer and managerial power under common law, by providing a series of workers' or employment protection rights for employees, thus redressing, to some degree at least, the inherent economic, social and common law imbalances in the relationship between individuals and their employer. The majority of these statutory rights are not incorporated into the contract of employment itself. The statutory right not to be unfairly dismissed, for example, is separate from the employee's common law contractual rights to wages, work and co-operation from the employer. And the right not to be unfairly dismissed, along with other statutory employment rights, does not become part of the contract. As Wedderburn (1986: page 5) points out, there are certain common law rights enshrined in the employment contract and enforceable by civil actions in the ordinary courts and, on the other hand, 'a separate, minimum "floor of rights" for individual workers gradually added to over recent years by statutes and enforced largely by civil claims in the industrial tribunals.' Claims for 'wrongful' dismissal – sacking without notice or payment in lieu of notice – used to go to the ordinary courts, whilst claims for 'unfair' dismissal, for unfair reasons and carried out in an unreasonable way, which are based on employment protection legislation, were settled in ITs. Now both types of claim are determined by ITs.

The statutory floor of employment protection rights extends into many areas of employment law, including:

- unfair dismissal
- redundancy payments
- discrimination on the grounds of gender, ethnic origin, nationality and disability

- union membership
- maternity pay and maternity leave
- minimum periods of notice
- security of earnings.

This floor of legal rights was created in Parliament by governments sympathetic to the view that there should be a basic level of employment protection, below which no employee should fall. It was a level, moreover, over and above which trade unions could negotiate superior conditions through collective bargaining.

In the 1960s and 1970s, statute law sought to weaken employer power and strengthen that of employees by extending the floor of employment protection rights, underpinned by a system of ITs with legal remedies for those claiming that their rights had been infringed by law-breaking employers. Since the 1980s, although the case must not be overstated, the law has tended to strengthen employer power and to weaken the legal position of employees by making adjustments to the statutory floor of employment protection rights. Both unfair dismissal and maternity rights were restricted, especially for workers in small businesses. In 1980, the qualifying period for unfair dismissal claims by employees was increased from six months' continuous service to one year. In 1985, it was further extended to two years for newly appointed employees. Guarantee payments in cases of short-time working were reduced, limitations were placed on social security payments – by phasing out earnings-related benefits – and deductions were made from the supplementary benefit payments to families of striking workers. This is because governments since 1979 have believed in using market forces and competition to contain inflation and achieve prosperity, with changes in employment law mirroring these economic policy changes.

It may be inferred, therefore, that the content of the contract of employment has changed significantly since the 1970s, largely because of the new framework of statutory rights provided for employees by Parliament. These rights complement rather than replace the common law of the contract. As Napier (1986) argues, the role of the common law is two-fold. First, it acts as a legal backcloth and provides a set of rules in those situations unregulated by specific statutory measures or where the legal remedies which exist are inadequate or restricted in their application. Second, it plays a crucial role in the operation of the statutory floor of employment rights themselves. This is because Parliament has used certain contractual terms and concepts in defining the statutory rights of employees in the workplace.

STATUTORY UNION MEMBERSHIP RIGHTS

A statutory floor of rights for trade union members has been enacted and extended in recent years. Some of these statutory rights, enacted under Labour governments, provide a set of positive rights for individuals to associate into unions, to be active within them and not to be dismissed on the grounds of union membership or for taking part in trade union activities. Others, enacted by Conservative governments since the 1980s, provide negative rights to abstain from union membership, or the right to dissociate. And a third set, also enacted since the 1980s, provides positive rights for union members to participate in or restrain union decision-making on specific issues (see Chapter 3).

The right to associate

Traditionally, there was no legal right for individuals to join trade unions in Britain, unlike in most other countries in western Europe. This was because of the philosophy of legal abstentionism or voluntarism in British employee relations. This specifically excluded the law from intervening in relations between employers and unions, in trade disputes and in supporting or preventing individuals joining trade unions.

The case for legal protection of the positive right to associate was put by the Donovan Commission (1968), largely in terms of the reform and extension of collective bargaining. If, as Donovan concluded, voluntary collective bargaining was the best method of conducting employee relations, then a necessary condition for this was effective trade union organisation amongst the workforce. The Commission therefore recommended that any condition in a contract of employment prohibiting union membership should be void in law and that dismissal for union membership should be deemed to be unfair. After the repeal of the Industrial Relations Act 1971, by the Trade Union and Labour Relations Act 1974, statutory rights to time off work for trade union lay officers and safety representatives were established, as well as the rights not to be dismissed, or subject to action short of dismissal, because of union membership or union activity.

The right to dissociate

The right to dissociate from union membership is related in part to opposition to the practice of the closed shop. A closed shop is any agreement or arrangement between an employer and union(s) which requires employees to be a union member as a condition of employment. Pre-entry closed shops limit jobs to those who are members of a specified trade union, whilst post-entry closed shops require those recruited by an employer to join an approved, recognised union within a set period after starting employment.

In the Employment Act (EA) 1980, protections were given for the first time to individuals against dismissal for non-union membership in a closed shop in the case of strongly held personal convictions. This derived from the government's objections to the closed shop in principle. As the Department of Employment (1981: page 66) stated:

> The Government's view of the closed shop is clear: it is opposed to the principles underlying it. That people should be required to join a union as a condition of getting or holding a job runs contrary to the general traditions of personal liberty in this country. It is acceptable for a union to seek to increase

its membership by voluntary means. What is objectionable, however, is to enforce membership by means of a closed shop as a condition of employment.

Subsequent legislation first increased the protection and compensation of employees if they were dismissed because of a closed shop, under the EA 1982. The EA 1988 then made post-entry closed shops unenforceable, removed trade union immunity from any industrial action taken to enforce a closed shop and provided legal protection against dismissal for non-union membership, by making dismissal or discrimination against employees refusing to join a union automatically unfair. Under the EA 1990, pre-entry closed shops became void in law, thus effectively making all forms of closed shop arrangement unlawful.

Another example of the right to dissociate was incorporated in the EA 1988. The TULRCA 1992 now provides protection for union members against what the law describes as 'unjustifiable discipline' by their unions. This upholds the right of individual trade members not to participate in lawful trade dispute, even where the action has previously been legitimised in a properly conducted industrial action ballot, and not to be disciplined by their union for failing to take part in the industrial action with which they disagree.

Intra-union rights

Membership participation in the internal affairs of trade unions has traditionally been provided under the union rule book and, where the rule book was infringed, there was the right to seek its enforcement through the courts. In the 1980s, governments increasingly held the view that the law needed to be changed in order to democratise the trade unions and make them more accountable to their members. A government green paper (Department of Employment 1983: page 37) stated that there was much public concern about the need for trade unions to become more democratic and more responsive to the wishes of their members and that 'society, including individual trade unionists themselves, is entitled to ensure that union power is exercised more responsibly, more accountably and more in accordance with the views of their members.'

It was this analysis which led to the passing of the TUA 1984. Its provisions, now incorporated in the TULRCA 1992, are:

- the right for union members to have the opportunity to participate in regular ballots to decide whether or not their union should undertake political activity, through union political funds and the political levy, at least once every 10 years
- the right for trade union members to elect all voting members of their union's executive by secret ballot, at least once every five years
- the right to participate in secret ballots before a union takes organised industrial action against an employer.

A further green paper (Department of Employment 1987: page 2) went on to argue that there was more to be done, stating:

> It is the view of the Government that, having embarked on the process of giving proper and effective rights to union members, it should ensure that those rights are fully developed so that they provide the ordinary member with the effective protection that he or she is entitled to enjoy in a free society.

Accordingly, the EA 1988, also now incorporated in the TULRCA 1992, extended the rights of union members:

- to elect all the principal union officers by secret postal ballot
- to take part in political fund review ballots by secret postal ballot
- to restrain their union from calling on them to take part in industrial action not supported by a properly conducted secret ballot
- not to be unjustifiably disciplined by their union
- to inspect their union's accounting records.

The office of the CRTUM, created by the 1988 Act, and that of the Commissioner for Protection Against Unlawful Industrial Action, have the power to support individual union members, by giving them advice and paying their costs, when making complaints against their union.

THE LAW AND TRADE DISPUTES

Whether the issues are substantive or procedural in nature, employees who are organised into trade unions are likely to take collective industrial action or industrial sanctions against their employer when alternative forms of conflict resolution, such as collective bargaining, conciliation or arbitration, have failed to resolve the differences between the parties. Employee industrial action involves a range of possible activities taken unilaterally by unions and their members against an employer. These include working to rule, banning overtime and stoppages of work, with concomitant legal implications (see Chapters 1, 3 and 7).

Breach of contract

A central legal issue arising from most forms of industrial action taken by employees is that they commonly breach their contracts of employment, by violating the employee's common law obligation to work for the employer under the terms of the contract. But the law is complex in this respect and there are areas of legal uncertainty. Where, for example, working to rule focuses on working strictly in accordance with the terms of the contract of employment, this is not normally taken to be a breach of the contract. Where working to rule refers to the employer's works rules, this too is unlikely to involve a breach of contract in the first instance, since this is within the implied terms of individual contracts of employment. Where overtime is not normally a contractual requirement, a union ban on overtime would also not normally be taken to be a breach of contract by individual employees.

Where, however, an employer unilaterally changes the works rules, employees would normally be expected to conform with them, in all circumstances, since they become incorporated into individual contracts of employment as implied terms. Where working to rule refers to the union rule book, this too is likely to be in breach of contract, since the terms of the contract are likely to be ignored by employees 'working to rule' in this manner. Similarly, where overtime is contractually required, an overtime ban would be in breach of contract. It is in the cases of stoppages of work that the law is most clear-cut, since such actions are obviously in breach of the employee's common law obligation to work for the employer and not to impede the employer's business.

All forms of industrial action have profound legal implications for individual employees, since the judges tend to see any industrial action as a challenge to the legitimate authority of the employer to employ labour and to deploy it, as embodied in the contract of employment. The employer's capacity to coerce through its economic power is not seen as problematic by the courts but as a legitimate property right. As outlined above, under common law, all forms of industrial action are treated in essentially the same way, as breaches of contract by the employee.

This means, first, that breach of contract may provide one of the ingredients of the economic torts (see below) for which trade unions may be liable. Second, it may entitle the employer to take disciplinary action against individual employees. Third, although continuity of employment is not broken by employees taking strike action, any such period does not count towards continuous service for the purposes of claiming employment protection rights.

Economic torts

A second legal issue arising from industrial sanctions taken by unions and their members against employers is that of 'economic torts'. Because the economic interests of employers and other organisations are damaged by collective industrial action, certain torts (civil law 'wrongs') may be committed in the process of conducting strikes, overtime bans and work to rules. The most common economic tort is that of inducing breach of contract.

The inducement may be direct or indirect. Direct inducement takes place when an outsider to the contract persuades one of the contracting parties to break the contract. The necessary elements of the tort are that the inducer must act intentionally, there must be evidence of inducement and the inducer must know or have the means of knowing of the existence of the contract, although that party need not know its actual terms. An example of direct inducement would be if a union official were to persuade union members to go slow or to refuse to work mandatory overtime. The official would then have induced a breach of the employment contract. The employer could obtain an injunction to end or prevent the inducement and/or obtain damages relating to any commercial loss it has suffered as a result of the breach of contract. The employer could sue both the official and the union itself.

Indirect inducement is more complicated. This occurs whenever a person (A) persuades a second person (B) to act unlawfully, with the intention of inducing a third person (C) to break a contract entered into with a fourth person (D). Because the inducement is indirect there is a further key requirement that the inducement must be obtained by unlawful means. For example, a union official (A) may persuade members (B) to break their employment contract with their employer (C), to prevent it supplying goods under a commercial contract with (D). The means of achieving the intended breach between (C) and (D) involves inducing a breach of the employment contract between (B) and (C) – in other words, the commission of an unlawful act. All the key requirements are present, and the fourth party (D) may bring an action for damages and/or seek an injunction against both the official and the union.

The tort of intimidation differs from inducing breach of contract in that it is concerned with threats rather than action itself. Intimidation occurs whenever there is a threat to commit unlawful action. Unlawful has been widely defined and includes, as well as criminal acts, tortious acts and breaches of contract. So a threat by a union official that members will strike in breach of contract unless wages are increased would amount to intimidation. As with inducing breach, there may be direct or indirect intimidation. Both intimidation and inducement can occur in the same dispute. First there may be a threat of unlawful action such as strike (intimidation) followed by the strike action itself (inducement).

Legal immunities

A third legal issue arising from industrial action is the common law liabilities of those organising or participating in industrial action and the statutory protections, or legal immunities, provided during stoppages of work and other sanctions. Unlike in other Western European countries, there is no legal right for workers or their unions to take industrial action in Britain. The situation differs in countries like France, for example, where the Constitution guarantees the individual worker the right to strike, and in Germany, where strikes are lawful, provided that they are in furtherance of improvements in working conditions and do not break a collective agreement (Department of Employment 1981). This means that in these countries workers and their unions are legally authorised, through systems of positive legal rights, to take industrial action against employers, subject to certain statutory conditions and qualifications.

In Britain, the law has taken a quite different path from that in other countries (Wedderburn 1986). Here the law governing industrial action and trade disputes starts with the common law. It is this which provides the basic legal principles which underlie subsequent statute law. The statutes governing strikes and other forms of industrial action have defined a system of 'legal immunities'. These protect those organising and taking part in industrial action from the civil (and possible criminal) liability arising from the imposition of industrial sanctions on employers. Without legal immunities, most industrial action would be illegal and trade unions, their officials and their members would be liable to civil actions for damages, and even criminal prosecution, every time they were involved in a strike, unless due notice, under the terms of the contract of employment, were given by the employees to the employer.

Legal immunities do not abolish civil wrongs (or 'torts'), or criminal liability, but they suspend liability in the circumstances of a trade dispute. Where these immunities are reduced, the common law liabilities are restored. Where they are extended, the common law liabilities relapse. If there were no immunities, then unions and individuals would be at risk of legal action by employers every time they organised a strike. The history of trade union law in Britain over the past 20 years reflects the differing views of Labour and Conservative governments about the role and scope of immunities in regulating industrial conflict. In general, Labour governments have strengthened immunities and Conservative ones reduced them.

To be protected in law, industrial action by unions and their members must: (1) fall within the legal definition of a 'trade dispute'; and (2) take place 'in contemplation of furtherance of a trade dispute' – the so-called 'golden formula'. It is the golden formula which provides the basis for legal immunities. A trade dispute is now defined in law by Section 218 of the TULRCA 1992 as any dispute between 'workers and their employer' which relates 'wholly or mainly to':

- terms and conditions of employment
- engagement or non-engagement of workers or termination or suspension of employment
- allocation of work or the duties of employment
- matters of discipline
- membership or non-membership of a trade union
- facilities for trade union officials
- machinery for negotiation, consultation or other procedures, including trade union recognition.

In contrast to earlier legislation, secondary disputes (between workers and employers other than their own), inter-union disputes and political disputes are no longer incorporated within the statutory definition outlined above.

Legal immunities, as provided by Section 219 of the TULRCA 1992, were incrementally limited during the 1980s by amendments to the law through the Employment Act 1980, 1982, 1988, 1990 and the Trade Union Act 1984. In outline, immunity in law is now provided only where:

- the industrial action is between an employer and their direct employees, with all secondary or sympathy action being unlawful

- a properly conducted industrial action ballot has been conducted by the union, authorising or endorsing the action
- peaceful picketing is limited to the workers' own place of work.

Immunity is specifically removed where industrial action is taken to impose or enforce a closed shop or where the action is unofficial and not repudiated, in writing, by the union. Where the 'golden formula' does not apply, it is relatively easy for an employer to show that one of the economic torts is being committed and to obtain an interlocutory injunction on that basis. Moreover, since the EA 1982, trade unions are now treated as ordinary persons. This means that they can be sued if responsible for unlawful industrial action (see Chapters 7 and 11).

THE SOCIAL DIMENSION OF THE SINGLE EUROPEAN MARKET

In recent years, the single market programme of the EU has led to the expansion of a social dimension within the Union. This includes employment-related policies and objectives relating to improved living conditions in general. This commitment to social progress is not new in Western European politics. It has been a feature of national and supra-national politics in EU member states for many years. Issues such as comprehensive social security schemes, employee protection, job security and paid leave from work have been a much more important feature of western European states than in the USA and Japan.

Another feature of western Europe is the protection given to individual employees' rights to organise and take part in industrial action and the legal regulation of employee relations. In addition, politics in western Europe has had a strong corporatist dimension, with the 'social partners' – employers and unions – having a formalised consultative role in national policy-making. According to one student of Europe, 'social policy in the widest sense is very much a hallmark of politics in Western Europe, regardless of country or government. Social policy is indeed a European invention' (Holmstedt 1991: page 39).

Employment and social policy

EU policies on employment and social issues do not form a coherent or comprehensive programme but a patchwork of different policy areas. They include legislation, action programmes and funding and cover such diverse subjects as health and safety, equal opportunities and training. The rationale for EU legislation in the field of employment is three-fold. The first is to harmonise provisions in member states to produce a 'level playing-field' for enterprise. The second is to facilitate freedom of movement of people within the EU and this requires some regulation and protection of workers' rights. A third reason is the need to create a community that is relevant to the people of Europe as well as to its entrepreneurs and business sector.

In the area of health and safety, for example, which is already covered by extensive legislation, the European Commission is proposing a long list of future legislation. In other areas, in contrast, such as trade union rights and collective agreements, recommendations rather than legislation are proposed and the European Commission is taking no co-ordinated action but leaving matters to governments, without seeking to enforce minimum safeguards.

This lack of cohesion in EU policies on employment and social policy is a consequence of the EU political institutions not being the machinery of an integrated, nation state, nor even of a federal one, but having very circumscribed political powers. The EU institutions are limited to framework legislation and pilot projects, without the powers of command that national, regional or local administrations have. Political power is still largely the prerogative of national governments. Despite the political difficulties attached to harmonising provisions in the area of labour law and employee relations, however, the European Commission has been active in developing draft legislation in this field for many years.

The roots of the social dimension of the EU run deep. The Treaty of Rome stated a commitment to common action on economic and social progress, as did the European Coal and Steel Community, which had extensive powers to fund and promote improvements in the working and living conditions of coal and steel workers. The European Economic Treaty contains a number of Articles authorising Community institutions to take action in various areas of social policy. The European Social Fund provides funding for retraining or settlement allowances for workers threatened by loss of employment. The Social Action Programme of 1974 laid the foundation for all future action in the social sphere for two decades. Many of the new proposals for legislation and action in this area which are being launched, as part of the single market programme, have their roots in the 1974 Action Programme.

The single market programme has brought a new momentum to the development of the EU's social policy. Its roots lie in the belief that achieving support for a single market from both sides of industry, and all major political parties, requires parallel efforts in the social field. The single market programme includes measures to complete the traditional aims of Community legislation, such as full freedom of movement for people. It also commits member states to encourage improvements in social policy. And there is a general commitment to strengthen the EU's economic and social cohesion, especially by reducing disparities between the various regions and the backwardness of the least favoured regions. Freedom of movement, health and safety, and reform of the structural funds are included in the Single European Act 1987, as are various programmes to combat unemployment and to emphasise the need for social progress towards a 'people's Europe'.

The European Community Charter of Fundamental Social Rights of Workers

Discussion about the social dimension of the single European market has led to the adoption of the Social Charter by the various member states, except the UK (see Chapter 3). The Charter was intended as a bill of rights for European citizens in the social sphere, although it is no more than a series of recommendations on minimum standards. What it provides, in effect, is a collection of targets for European action and minimum standards for member states to achieve.

The European Commission's action programme on the Social Charter provides the framework for action in the employment and social fields for many years ahead. The Commission is, for example, proposing to make the European labour market operate more smoothly and is proposing legislative action on a number of issues including:

- revision of the 1976 Directive on Equal Treatment
- revision of the 1986 Directive on Equal Treatment in Occupational Social Security Schemes
- protection of employees' supplementary occupational rights as they move between member states
- rights of establishment of foreign lawyers
- extension of recognition of professional qualifications.

Although the Commission is not proposing any fresh initiatives under the controversial chapter on freedom of association and collective bargaining, it does intend taking initiatives on employee consultation and participation.

The Social Charter proclaims the major principles underlying the following declared rights of individuals in the EU. In outline, these rights can be summarised as follows (Commission of the European Communities 1990):

- *Freedom of movement.* Every worker shall have the right to freedom of movement throughout the EU and to engage in any occupation or profession in accordance with the principles of equal treatment and access.
- *Employment and remuneration.* Every worker shall be free to choose their occupation and all employment shall be fairly remunerated, with workers having a wage sufficient to enable them and their families to have a decent standard of living.
- *Improvement of living and working conditions.* This principle states that the completion of the internal market must lead to an improvement in the living and working conditions of workers in the EU. Workers shall have a right to a weekly rest period and to paid annual leave. The conditions of employment of every worker shall be stipulated in laws, a collective agreement or a contract of employment, according to the arrangements applying in each country.

- *Social protection.* Every worker shall have a right to adequate social protection and shall enjoy an adequate level of social security benefits. Persons unable to enter the labour market must be able to receive sufficient resources in keeping with their circumstances.
- *Freedom of association and collective bargaining.* Employers and workers shall have the right to associate and their organisations shall have the right to negotiate and conclude collective agreements together. The dialogue between the two sides at European level must be developed. There shall be a right to strike and the utilisation of conciliation, mediation and arbitration machinery should be encouraged.
- *Vocational training.* All workers must be able to have access to vocational training and to benefit from it throughout their working lives. There should be leave for training purposes to improve skills or to acquire new skills.
- *Equal treatment for women and men.* Equal treatment must be assured and equal treatment for women and men must be developed. Equality of access should be provided to employment, remuneration, working conditions, social protection, education, vocational training and career development.
- *Information, consultation and participation of workers.* These principles must be developed along appropriate lines and shall apply especially in companies operating in two or more member states. These processes should be implemented particularly during: technological change; corporate restructuring; collective redundancies; and when transfrontier workers are affected.
- *Health protection and safety at the workplace.* Every worker must enjoy satisfactory health and safety conditions in the working environment. The need for training, information, consultation and the participation of workers in this area is stressed.
- *Protection of children and adolescents.* The minimum age of employment must be no lower than the minimum school leaving age. The duration of work must be limited, night work must be prohibited and initial vocational training must be an entitlement.
- *Elderly persons.* All retired workers must be able to enjoy resources affording them a decent standard of living. They must also be entitled to sufficient medical and social assistance.
- *Disabled persons.* The disabled must be entitled to additional concrete measures aimed at improving their social and professional integration.

The Social Action Programme

The Social Action Programme is a set of legal proposals from the European Commission to provide ways of enforcing the Social Charter's principles. Most of the major proposals are for legal instruments which, once adopted, are applicable to all member states. Other proposals are for studies or communications which may then lead to legislative proposals. The third

Social Action Programme of the European Commission, published in 1995, aims to consolidate existing legislation and strike a balance between employers' demands for a social policy which provides for increase competitiveness, and creation of new jobs, and the Commission's commitment to protecting minimum social standards. Proposals include completion of outstanding measures on (Institute of Personnel and Development 1996):

- part-time work
- reversal of the burden of proof in sex discrimination cases
- posted workers
- transport for disabled workers
- health and safety issues
- transfer of undertakings
- information and consultation of employees.

This Social Action Plan also provides a raft of non-legislative proposals, including discussions with the EU social partners on measures such as:

- dismissal and paid leave
- working time in sectors and activities outside the Working Time Directive
- home working
- health and safety.

ASSIGNMENTS

(a) Consider the situation where unemployment has risen to three million and inflation to 4 per cent. What would be a Keynesian economic response to this and how would this affect wage bargaining in your organisation? What would be a supply-side economic response to this situation and how would this affect wage bargaining in your organisation?

(b) Examine the reasons for introducing incomes policies, the forms they take and the conditions necessary for them to be effective. Compare and contrast how (1) a named public sector organisation might respond to a wages freeze; (2) a multi-plant manufacturing company negotiating with trade unions might respond; and (3) a small non-union company with 25 employees might respond. Provide a rationale for your answer in each case.

(c) Present a report summarising what 'unfair dismissal' is and the legal remedies available to those whose claim for unfair dismissal is upheld by an industrial tribunal.

(d) Union membership agreements are now unlawful. What action would you take, as a newly recruited personnel manager, if the chief executive of your company asked you to continue enforcing, on behalf of the company, an informal, closed shop arrangement with the unions?

(e) Read Simpson (1986: pages 161-92) and outline the development of trade union immunities in Britain and how the law on immunities has changed since 1980.
(f) What are the cases for and against employers supporting the Social Charter?

REFERENCES

COMMISSION OF THE EUROPEAN COMMUNITIES. 1990. *The Community Charter of Fundamental Social Rights for Workers*. Brussels: European Commission.

DEPARTMENT OF EMPLOYMENT. 1981. *Trade Union Immunities*. London: HMSO.

DEPARTMENT OF EMPLOYMENT. 1983. *Democracy in Trade Unions*. London: HMSO.

DEPARTMENT OF EMPLOYMENT. 1987. *Trade Unions and Their Members*. London: HMSO.

DONALDSON, P. *and* FARQUHAR, J. 1988. *Understanding the British Economy*. Harmondsworth: Penguin.

DONOVAN, Lord 1986. *Royal Commission on Trade Unions and Employers' Associations 1965-1968*: Report. London: HMSO.

ELLIS, J. *and* PARKER, D. 1990. *The Essence of the Economy*. Hemel Hempstead: Prentice Hall.

FARNHAM, D. 1996. 'New Labour, the new unions and the new labour market'. *Parliamentary Affairs*. 49(4), October.

FARNHAM, D. *and* HORTON, S. (eds) 1996. *Managing the New Public Services*. Basingstoke: Macmillan.

FRIEDMAN, M. 1991. *Monetarist Economics*. Oxford: Blackwell.

FRIEDMAN, M. *and* SCHWARZ, A . 1963. *A Monetary History of the United States*. Princeton: Princeton University Press.

HOLMSTEDT, M. 1991. *Employment Policy*. London: Routledge in association with the University of Bradford.

INSTITUTE OF PERSONNEL AND DEVELOPMENT. 1996. *Europe: Personnel and Development*. October. London: IPD.

KAHN-FREUND, O. 1977. *Labour and the Law*. London: Stevens.

KEEGAN, W. 1984. *Mrs Thatcher's Economic Experiment*. Harmondsworth: Penguin.

KEYNES, J. M. 1936. *The General Theory of Employment, Interest and Money*. London: Macmillan.

LABOUR PARTY. 1997. *Road to the Manifesto*. London.

MULLARD, M. 1992. *Understanding Economic Policy*. London: Routledge.

NAPIER, B. 1986. 'The contract of employment'. In Lewis, R. (ed.), *Labour Law in Britain*, Oxford: Blackwell.

PANITCH, L. 1976. *Social Democracy and Industrial Militancy: The Labour Party, the Trades Union and Incomes Policy 1945-74*. Cambridge: Cambridge University Press.

ROBINSON, J. 1937. *Essays in the Theory of Employment.* London: Macmillan.

SHAW, G. 1988. *Keynesian Economics: The permanent revolution*. Aldershot: Elgar.

SMITH, D. 1987. *The Rise and Fall of Monetarism*. Harmondsworth: Penguin.

WEDDERBURN, Lord. 1986. *The Worker and the Law.* Harmondsworth: Penguin.

5 Employee relations skills

Stephen Pilbeam and Marjorie Corbridge

There are several personnel management activities that everyone managing employee relations becomes involved in at some time or other. Employees raise dissatisfactions and grievances with managers, arising from their jobs, terms and conditions or the management decisions affecting them, and this potential for conflict needs to be resolved. This necessitates managers using relevant grievance procedures, interview skills and appropriate judgement to ensure that such issues are dealt with fairly, consistently and efficiently. Similarly, managers who are concerned about the job performance, conduct or effectiveness of employees may need to take disciplinary action against them and this might ultimately result in terminating their employment contract. Disciplinary action by managers has ethical, legal and procedural implications and it also requires appropriate interpersonal and professional skills. Procedures need to be applied, legal requirements to be adhered to and management competency to be demonstrated. Where organisations are being restructured, skill mixes changed or market demand for a product – or citizen need for a service – falls, job losses can occur and a redundancy programme has to be implemented and managed.

It is the employee relations issues and activities associated with the handling of grievances, dealing with discipline and managing of redundancy that are addressed in this chapter. The essential principles underpinning negotiating activity are also examined briefly, because negotiating is something that all managers are involved in, not just personnel practitioners. A more detailed analysis and examination of formal collective bargaining is provided in Chapter 9.

NEGOTIATION BASICS

Negotiation is a process whereby two or more interested groups seek to reconcile their differences through attempts to persuade the other group to move from their initial position, with the overall aim of reaching an agreement. Implicit in this process is an intention and a willingness to compromise in pursuit of an agreement which, although it may be less than ideal, is acceptable to all the groups involved. The precise definition of acceptability is subject to many influences and the contingencies of the negotiating situation, not least of which is the balance of bargaining power between the negotiating groups. It could be argued that the relative power between the negotiating groups influences the outcome of the process to a much larger extent than the skills and abilities of the negotiators. Negotiation is therefore a conflict-resolving activity involving compromise but will often incorporate collaboration, confrontation, accommodation and avoidance (Thomas 1979).

Negotiations pervade organisational life and essential negotiating skills developed within an employee relations framework are transferable to many other areas of management. More flexible organisational structures, with reduced emphasis on hierarchical relationships, necessitate effective intra-organisational negotiation between teams, groups, and individuals. In the public sector the development of purchaser and provider relationships, both internal and external, heightens demand for effective negotiation skills. The aim of any negotiating cycle therefore, whether formal or informal, is to reconcile conflicting viewpoints through concessions, compromise and exchanges between the parties involved. To analyse the negotiation process three distinctive and sequential elements can be identified: preparation, negotiation and implementation. Negotiation also incorporates certain skills such as tactical adjustment, listening skills and some basic competences.

Preparing for negotiation

Preparation includes:

- defining negotiation objectives
- the development of group cohesiveness
- information gathering
- the allocation of roles
- achieving intra-group consensus
- considering the abilities and skills of the other negotiating team
- determining the relative power balance
- determining tactics and strategy
- defining negotiating parameters in terms of optimum and minimum outcomes
- predicting the expectations, arguments, counter-arguments and strategies of the other side.

Thorough and careful preparation is arguably the key to successful and effective negotiation. The definition of clear objectives is essential because it enables each team to distinguish between the important and the less significant issues it wishes to address and it serves to clarify and synchronise the expectations of negotiators. A by-product of good planning can be the development of effective working relationships and cohesiveness within the negotiation team.

A starting point in negotiation is the identification, clarification and consideration of the issues involved. Until a common understanding is achieved, it is inappropriate to make any strategic or tactical decisions. This exploration of the issues needs to be accompanied by information-gathering activity. This activity is largely self-explanatory but involves accessing appropriate information sources, including any facts surrounding the issue, employer information relevant to the negotiation, statistical material, and company rules and agreements. It also includes external information, for example, market rates in the case of pay negotiations and any relevant legislation. There needs to be an assessment of who should be involved in the negotiations and consideration given to the size of the negotiating team. The need for particular skills, knowledge and expertise in relation to the particular negotiation also influences the composition of the negotiating team.

The allocation of roles within the negotiating team is of critical importance and can be addressed by answering the following questions. Who will take a lead role? Where will the locus of decision-making lie? What control mechanisms are necessary to ensure a co-ordinated approach? Should a lead negotiator, observer and note-takers be allocated in advance? Who will have the authority to call adjournments? In essence, the decisions revolve around creating a cohesive team with members who are able to present a united front, or at least avoid overt disagreement in dealing with the other side. The negotiation process starts in the preparation stage because it enables intra-group negotiation to take place prior to the actual negotiations with the other interest group or party. The achievement of intra-group consensus gives confidence to the negotiating team. It also reduces the possibility of exposing weaknesses, or any apparent dissonance within the team, which might have a negative impact on the negotiating position, during the negotiations.

In assessing the strength of the other side, negotiators need to take account of the skills, experience and expertise of the other team. In parallel with this, an important judgement to make is the level of commitment to the issue likely to be exhibited by the other side and its significance for them. The validity and logic of their arguments needs to be assessed and the power balance, as defined by the ability to impose unilateral action or take sanctions against the other side, is a crucial factor. Identifying the comparative strengths of negotiating positions are prerequisites to the determination of strategy and tactics. The negotiating team also needs to focus upon the outcomes it seeks in relation to its pre-determined objectives. This process is facilitated by identifying the team's optimum and minimum acceptable outcomes. These polar points can be refined by considering what the team *would like* to achieve, what it *intends* to achieve, and what it *must* achieve – 'likes', 'intends', 'musts' or LIMs (Kennedy *et al* 1984). Some writers describe these as the ideal settlement point, realistic settlement point and fall back position (Atkinson 1980). Whatever analytical tool is used, the principle remains the same: defining the negotiating parameters as a focal point for the negotiating team. These parameters allow some flexibility, provide a framework for negotiating and give direction to the negotiation activity. Such decisions, or more accurately expectations, are not, of course, disclosed to the other side. But they are the subject of probing and speculation by the other party during the negotiation process.

It is useful to try to perceive and evaluate your own expectations from the standpoint of the other side. Thus an associated aspect of preparation is to predict the parameters and expectations of the other group and the responses and arguments likely to occur in order to plan appropriate counter-responses and counter-arguments. This predictive process can include an assessment of the potential strategies available of the other side.

Decisions have to be made about the nature of the negotiations. Some are problem-centred or integrative. Others are competitive or distributive. Which predominates, however, is determined largely by the negotiation issue (Walton and McKersie 1965). Integrative negotiation exists where the parties believe that co-operation and a problem-solving approach will produce a mutually acceptable outcome. The negotiations are more likely to be characterised by openness and a degree of trust between the parties. It is potentially a 'win/win' situation. In contrast, distributive negotiation is more likely to be perceived as a 'win/lose' situation because of the incompatibility of negotiation objectives between the parties and the behaviour within the negotiations is likely to be influenced by this conflict perspective. There are rarely pure forms of either integrative or distributive negotiations. A more realistic strategy is to attempt to define the likely mix and develop an awareness of oscillation and fluctuation during the negotiation process. Within these limits, there is advantage in appreciating that the purpose of negotiating is the pursuit of mutual benefit rather than just the scoring of points by one side at the expense of the other. Also within the preparation it is useful to consider the implications of a failure to agree within the negotiation process and what action may become necessary if this happens.

Whilst detailed preparation is vital, this should not predispose the negotiating team to developing a rigid position. Flexibility and the ability to manoeuvre within the negotiating process are essential and desirable characteristics. A further caveat is that the attitudes, personalities and relationships of the negotiators are likely to influence the negotiations independently of the strength of argument because negotiations are a psychological encounter. Additionally, within each negotiating team the power, influence and accountability of the participants in relation to each other create an internal dynamic which should not be discounted. These factors suggest that the negotiation process and the negotiation cycle should be viewed through an interactive and behavioural, rather than a purely mechanical, frame of reference.

Negotiating

An awareness of the negotiating cycle offers valuable insights to the manager. This cycle involves a number of phases which, although initially sequential, often oscillate in order to reflect the ebb and flow of the negotiations, which are also likely to be punctuated by adjournments and side meetings. The three phases can be described as arguing, proposing, and exchanging and agreeing (see Chapter 9).

Arguing

This formative phase begins with the opening statements and supporting arguments from the negotiating parties. The party presenting first has considerable influence in setting the tone of the negotiations. Initial negotiating positions are established by the rejection of demands and demonstrations of inflexibility. This phase is highly ritualistic and challenging, but affords an opportunity to test commitment, to identify tactics and to assess strengths. The arguing phase reasserts itself throughout the negotiations. It is manifest each time one side seeks to convince or persuade the other side of its strength of argument. Arguing is an inevitable precursor to compromise and agreement.

Proposing

Having established their relative positions, the negotiators enter an exploratory phase in which each side seeks to discover some potential for flexibility and movement away from initial statements of position. This incorporates tentative offers and concessions of a highly conditional nature. The proposing stage is characterised by probing and encouraging the other side to reveal their real expectations whilst to some extent concealing your own. Positions are summarised and attempts are made to move forward by finding common ground. It is a delicate phase with progress often dependent upon allowing the other side to concede certain points without necessarily losing face. Concession may be implicit and disguised by the appearance of not having given way and this should be respected. Triumphalism is to be avoided as it may set back the negotiations to the arguing phase. A patronising approach is also likely to have negative consequences.

Emotional language can undo a fragile, emerging or embryonic agreement. As well as avoiding emotionally charged words, personal attacks and put-downs, negotiators need to focus upon the positive and constructive rather than the negative and destructive, in terms of language and approach. It is also important during this phase to listen actively, observe behaviour and make appropriate judgements to enable progression to the next phase of the negotiations.

Exchanging and agreeing

This phase is about exchanging concessions, giving and receiving, and consequently it moves the negotiations towards agreement. It is dependent on an overlap in the predetermined expectations of the parties involved. Clearly, if there is too wide a gap between negotiating positions, exchange is unlikely to occur. However, if concessions are made, a degree of convergence characterises the negotiations as the parties seek areas of agreement. The exchange process can generate a momentum of its own. The optimism and expectation of concluding the negotiation can result in concessions which may have been unthinkable earlier in the negotiations. Experienced negotiators may seek to exploit this situation, although they may pay a price for this if any exploitation becomes apparent to the other side.

As it becomes evident that compromise is possible, the negotiations move quickly to the agreement phase. The exchange process is checked, precise statements are made and potential misunderstandings are addressed. A written record serves the purpose of promoting common understanding of the outcomes to the parties – an agreement is not an agreement until it is agreed in writing.

Implementation

Ultimately negotiation has little benefit or value to those involved unless the negotiated outcomes are converted to action. This action has two aspects. The first is the effective communication with and dissemination of information to those affected by the agreement. The second is the devising of a programme of implementation which includes allocating responsibility, determining resources required and setting time-scales. A part of the implementation strategy is to evaluate the outcomes of the negotiations in relation to the agreed objectives and to make an assessment of negotiating performance. This evaluation may include learning points for future negotiations.

Sometimes there is a failure to agree in negotiations. This largely unsatisfactory outcome prompts a reassessment of the options available and an evaluation of whether or not agreement remains a viable proposition. If agreement appears unlikely, an examination of the alternatives becomes necessary. These may include an imposition of terms by one party, should it have the unilateral power to do so – although there are clearly implications for the relationship between the parties if this course of action is pursued. Alternatively, the parties can consider the value and practicability of third-party intervention, either internal or external to the organisation, in order to conciliate, mediate or arbitrate according to the situation (see Chapter 3).

Tactics and skills

As a general principle the making of concessions in negotiation without gaining something in return is to be avoided – if negotiation is about giving and receiving, why give something for nothing? Where a concession is unavoidable some conditions for acceptance can be attached. These conditions should be injected into the negotiations prior to indicating a willingness to concede because they are then likely to stand more chance of being accepted. Once given, concessions cannot be withdrawn without inflicting some damage on the negotiation process and losing good faith. On the same basis, final offers must be final offers or credibility is affected.

Whilst it is potentially attractive to separate out the negotiating items within a set of negotiations and deal with each in turn, this imposes a constraint on exchanges and concessions. A holistic approach incorporating all the negotiating items, whilst not necessarily as easy to manage as a segmented approach, is ultimately likely to be more balanced and fruitful. Threats and posturing are not illegitimate tactics within the ritualism of negotiation. 'Trickery', however, may be destructive, and can affect not only the immediate negotiations, but also any future negotiations by eroding mutual trust and confidence.

Adjournments are a valuable tactic for negotiators but their value and scope goes beyond the tactical level. The skilled use of adjournments can have a significant impact upon the progress of the negotiations. Some potential uses of adjournment are shown in Exhibit 15.

Exhibit 15 **The uses of adjournment during negotiation**

These include:

- to consult privately when it is apparent that there is divergence or disagreement within the negotiating team
- to discuss privately when a new argument becomes evident
- to evaluate progress or lack of it
- to allow an opportunity to consult with others
- to consider whether or not to reject an offer
- to take a break in order to regroup or relieve fatigue
- to allow a cooling-off period if breakdown appears to be a probability
- to consider the breaking-off of negotiations, or unilaterally withdrawing, when the negotiations have turned sour
- to afford an opportunity for off-the-record communication between negotiation teams.

Frequent adjournments can be disruptive and may suggest a weakness of argument or lack of cohesion or co-ordination on the part of the side asking for them. They can also be an undesirable irritant to the other party if they are too frequent, unless of course the aim is to cause irritation. It is advisable to set a time limit for reconvening the negotiations in order to focus effort and ensure that the negotiations are not unnecessarily protracted. This time-scale must be realistic, as failure to adhere to an agreed resumption time can be a source of considerable antagonism, with negative implications for the tenor of the negotiations when resumed. This latter point is more likely to apply in the case of adjournments during negotiations in process. It is less likely where a formal adjournment until another day is agreed.

The importance of listening skills in negotiation warrants special attention. It is self-evident, although not always appreciated, that most information can be gathered and obtained through listening actively.

There is a good argument for allocating some team members to exclusively listening roles or even allocating observers to listen to specific members of the other side. Examples of active listening skills are indicated in Exhibit 16 overleaf.

Clearly natural ability features as a variable in determining negotiation competence. However, there are elements of competence that can be developed through exposure to negotiations, training and experience. Some of the necessary interpersonal and analytical skills are indicated in Exhibit 17.

Exhibit 16 **Active listening skills**

These include:

- concentrating on what is being said
- observing and interpreting associated body language
- encouraging through appropriate verbal and non-verbal responses
- seeking clarification of understanding
- using pauses and silences through conscious attempts to avoid jumping in
- using appropriate questioning techniques and valuing the importance of open questions
- drawing appropriate and accurate inferences from what may be coded language.

Exhibit 17 **Interpersonal and analytical skills in negotiation**

These include:

- effective oral communication skills
- interpreting non-verbal cues
- awareness and control of body language
- active listening
- sensitivity to people and situations
- ability to think on one's feet (or seat) and articulate appropriately
- creative thinking and problem-solving
- persuasiveness
- awareness of power relationships
- judgement
- assertiveness
- quality of presentation
- information processing and evaluation
- teamwork and group dynamics
- recognition of the ritualistic nature of the negotiation encounter.

Effectiveness as a negotiator is founded on these competences, which include not only skill but also a firm knowledge base.

Stress in negotiation

Linked with the idea of negotiation competences is the concept of negotiation stress. The degree of stress is likely to influence the degree of competence exhibited in negotiations. Pressure, or stress, is a natural facet of negotiation, but it is useful to identify the potential sources of stress. First, there is the pressure associated with the need and desire to achieve the predetermined negotiation objectives in the face of opposition. Additionally, in the case of team negotiations, there is the desire to be seen to be making an effective contribution to the team effort. Second, personal credibility is at risk in negotiation. Personal performance may enhance or diminish this and has implications not only for the next negotiation but also for the negotiator's general organisational reputation. The stress derives from wanting to preserve individual credibility and reputation. Third, the negotiating process itself is fertile ground for stress. This may be produced by the environment, the disparity in objectives, the emotional context, general fatigue or being the object of personal inference or attack. The skill for the negotiator is to recognise this possibility and to adopt appropriate compensating and personal adaptation strategies. To the list of general competences can be added the ability to manage stress.

GRIEVANCES

A grievance is an expression of perceived dissatisfaction or injustice that an employee feels towards the employer. It is based on the procedural right of individuals at work to express their dissatisfaction with any aspect of their work situation and the employer's legal obligation under the Employment Rights Act 1996. This legislation requires the employer to notify the employee, within the statement of terms and conditions of the person to whom the employee can address a grievance, how it may be done, and any further steps that should be taken. However, employees have only limited legal remedy if the employer denies them access to a grievance procedure. There are positive benefits to the employer in encouraging the appropriate use of an agreed grievance procedure. It may be possible to assess the attitude and morale of the workforce from the extent of use of the grievance procedure and the nature of the issues that are raised. It may also be the case that time spent on identifying and resolving issues may reduce the possibility of major disputes.

Whilst disciplinary procedures allow the employer to express and try to resolve dissatisfactions it may have identified with the employee, in a grievance the employee is highlighting an issue of dissatisfaction with the employer. Many work situations have the potential to cause dissatisfaction and often the expression of a formal grievance is triggered by a particular event.

Salamon (1992) points out that the terms dissatisfaction, complaint, grievance and dispute may be regarded as overlapping segments of a continuum based primarily on the manner and formality of the presentation of employee dissatisfaction. These range from personal dissatisfaction to informal complaints, to formal grievances, to collective disputes. Not every employee dissatisfaction or complaint results in a grievance or a dispute. Whether it does or not depends on the employee's presentation of it and the employer's response to it and whether it is resolved to the satisfaction of the employee. The way in which the dissatisfaction is presented to management can range from an informal discussion to the formal presentation of the issue using the grievance procedure. The progression from the informal to the formal machinery may be seen as a failure to resolve the situation at the informal level or to deal with it or explain it to the satisfaction of the aggrieved individual.

The culture of an organisation has a major effect on the way in which grievances are received and handled. In a unitary or neo-unitary organisation there are assumptions that there are common values and common objectives and that management's right to manage is accepted by all (Farnham and Pimlott 1995). Therefore conflict within the organisation is seen as dysfunctional. Individuals may feel inhibited from raising a formal grievance because of the effect it may have on their career prospects and for fear of being labelled 'a trouble maker' or a 'deviant'. In a pluralist organisation, conflict is seen as inevitable and it is assumed that employees have a right to question management decisions and management's application of policies and procedures. Employees therefore normally accept that they have a right to raise grievances where they feel that this is necessary and the formal grievance procedure is likely to be more commonly used.

The need for formal mechanisms for resolving conflict is taken for granted, certainly in pluralist employee relations. Indeed, the requirement in law on the part of the employer to have a grievance procedure was first included in the Industrial Relations Act 1971 and it is now incorporated in the Employment Rights Act 1996. The subjects of grievances vary. They can range from issues affecting one individual with no organisational implications, to issues affecting a group of workers which challenges management decisions and with the potential to escalate to a dispute before being finally settled.

Grievance procedures

Grievance procedures provide the formal means for the presentation and resolution of employee dissatisfaction. Exhibit 18 indicates the basic elements to be incorporated within grievance procedures.

Exhibit 18 The basic elements of a grievance procedure

These are:

- management should agree with the recognised trade unions the procedure for raising grievances and for settling them promptly and effectively
- there should be a formal procedure
- if there are separate procedures for grievances and disputes these should be linked
- an individual grievance should be settled as near to the point of origin and as quickly as possible
- the procedure should be in writing.

Grievance procedures should set out the stages through which a grievance is heard within the organisational hierarchy. This recognises the authority and responsibility of the parties at the different levels within the organisation and allows for a structured approach to the situation. The stages also define the time-scale for the resolution of the problem. This, in theory, allows for a review of the decision at each stage. Larger organisations are more likely than smaller organisations to include additional stages. The number of stages in a procedure is, to some extent, determined by the structure of the organisation, but in practical terms three to four stages are most appropriate. Any more than this can lead to a procedure that is unwieldy, slow and potentially confusing in the way it operates.

There are usually three levels for hearing grievances: departmental, functional and senior level. The departmental level provides the first hearing of the grievance through the line manager of the aggrieved person. The functional level – the next hearing of an unresolved grievance – involves the line manager's manager or the functional manager. And the senior level – the third (usually final) hearing of an unresolved grievance – is with a member of the senior management team or the managing director or chief executive. There may also be provision for an external review of the grievance or dispute, although this is more common in the disputes procedure, with many organisations providing for third-party intervention such as through ACAS or an employers' association. An example of a grievance hearing structure is provided in Figure 7.

Figure 7 **Grievance-hearing structure**

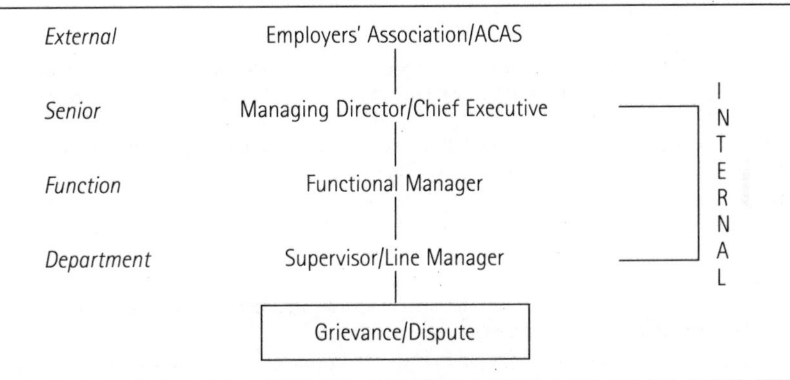

The time-scale for the resolution of a grievance from receipt of the written grievance to its settlement must be clearly defined and the aim should be to settle the grievance in the shortest possible time. The outcome of the grievance must be notified to the aggrieved employee in writing, with a statement of their right to take the grievance to the next stage of the procedure if they are dissatisfied with the reviewing manager's decision. The grievance procedure should identify, if possible, the type of issues that can be raised within it. This should not be used as a means of restricting the use of the procedure. There are problems, such as personality clashes, that really cannot be resolved using a grievance procedure but only through effective communication and management. The procedure is used for such issues as implementation of national or local agreements, terms and conditions of employment, allocation of pay, overtime and so on. An example of a grievance procedure is shown in Figure 8.

There is one area of potential grievance that needs careful handling and may be best dealt with within a different procedure. Discrimination and harassment are highly sensitive and may in fact be perpetrated by the immediate line manager. The normal procedure for grievances is through the line manager, therefore there must be a facility for the resolution of these problems outside the usual reporting structure. It may be possible to have named people for the reporting of this type of incident or they can be dealt with through a separate harassment procedure.

Figure 8 **Example of a grievance procedure**

Grievance procedure

Management respects the right of employees individually or collectively to present grievances to management. It is in the interests of all that there are established formal procedures for handling these complaints.

a) Stage 1 – If you are unhappy about any aspect of your employment* you should raise the issue with your immediate supervisor or line manager. You will receive a response to your grievance within three working days.

b) Stage 2 – If the issue is not resolved to your satisfaction you may progress the matter in writing to your functional manager who will respond to you within five working days.

c) Stage 3 – If the matter is still unresolved you may take your complaint to a Senior Manager who will arrange a meeting within a further ten working days.

You have the right to be accompanied at any or all of these meetings by a representative or work colleague.

*Health and safety matters and incidents of racial or sexual harassment may be raised if you wish with the Safety Officer/Personnel Manager respectively.

Grievance interviews

The importance of management taking any grievance seriously must be emphasised. If any employee feels strongly enough to use the formal grievance procedure to raise a complaint then that person has the right to a fair and respectful hearing. However, as was discussed earlier, there are dissatisfactions and complaints that are raised outside the formal process. Again, it is important that issues raised outside the formal procedure are treated with care as that will reduce the likelihood of the formal procedure being needed. Indicators of problems are high levels of labour turnover, absenteeism and problems with morale. Although these may indicate different problems, they should never be ignored.

The grievance interview requires the skills of any interview situation. This includes the need to:

- *Provide an appropriate physical environment free from interruptions.* It is important that the employee feels that the situation is being taken seriously, therefore a room where the complaint can be heard, in private, free from telephone and personal interruptions, must be made available. The employee must be given prior notice of the date, time and venue of the interview and of their right to be accompanied by a union representative or a colleague if that is within the procedure.
- *Listen to, and hear, what is being said by the aggrieved individual.* Any interview requires good active listening skills, and appropriate body language and eye contact are important if the aggrieved individuals are to feel that they are being listened to.
- *Ask appropriate questions in a non-threatening way.* In order that the manager understands the nature of the grievance and how the aggrieved feels, the situation causing the complaint must be presented in full by the employee. This may need careful probing and questioning so that all of the facts can be identified or clarified. It should be done in a calm and non-threatening way so that the employee feels that speaking openly will not disadvantage the case. It is often worth identifying what outcome the aggrieved is looking for, because it is not uncommon for the situation to require negotiation. Compromise may be the only way forward.
- *Prepare.* The nature of any grievance is that it is initiated by the employee. There may therefore be little that the manager can do to prepare for the first interview. The facts of the case need to be identified and it is at the second and subsequent stages that management's preparation is mainly undertaken. However, the written grievance should be read carefully and any information that the manager feels may be relevant should be gathered.
- *Analyse the facts and take a decision.* Having heard all the facts of the case, consulted the relevant policy and looked at any possible situation that may have set a precedent, the manager is then able to take a decision on the outcome of the grievance. Whilst there may be a need to discuss the case with a personnel manager or another manager, for advice, care must be taken that this does not jeopardise the fairness of treatment of the employee. The manager is taking the decision in the framework of the policies and procedures of the organisation and therefore contributing to its 'case-law'. The decision may set a precedent that others will have to follow, therefore any management interpretation must be one that the employer can live with. The decision should be communicated in writing to the employee within the procedural time-scale. If further time is needed to allow for a full investigation of the situation then agreement

should be sought with the employee for the time-scale to be extended. This ensures that the employer does not attract further complaint of not adhering to the agreed procedure.

Any individual grievance ends with an outcome that is ultimately accepted by the individual or the procedure is exhausted. However, the situation should not end there. It is important, as stated previously, that the decision is communicated clearly to the employee and that both parties understand exactly what has been agreed. There is also benefit to the employer in monitoring grievances both in terms of issues that are raised and outcomes that are agreed. It may be that some of the employer's terms and conditions of employment need to be re-written in a more easily understood form or that training needs to be given to explain the implementation of policies. Issues that are constantly giving rise to grievances may highlight a communication problem.

DISCIPLINE AT WORK

Discipline at work incorporates concepts of self-discipline, peer discipline and managerial discipline. It is managerial discipline which is the focus of this section as a disciplinary procedure emphasises managerial values and standards. Discipline can be defined as action instigated by management against an employee who fails to meet reasonable and legitimate expectations in terms of performance, conduct or adherence to rules. Ethics and professionalism argue for an emphasis on problem-solving, prevention and constructive approaches to discipline issues as these are more likely to encourage a positive response from the employee. It also maximises the opportunity for acceptance of the problem, correction of the behaviour or performance, and reconciliation of the parties. A disciplinary process can therefore be viewed as an individual conflict-resolving mechanism within the employment relationship, with an emphasis on improvement and remedy rather than on punitive measures. Where encouragement, guidance, support or training do not result in employee improvement to an acceptable managerial standard, punishment may however be necessary. Sanctions against the employee can act as a deterrent to the individual behaviour or conduct and, by example, for the workforce as a whole. Fairness, equity and consistency in the management approach to discipline will minimise disagreements and benefit employee relations within the organisation. As the ACAS code of practice states (ACAS 1987, page 3): 'disciplinary procedures should not be viewed primarily as a means of imposing sanctions. They should also be designed to emphasise and encourage improvements in individual conduct.'

Disciplinary rules and procedures

Disciplinary rules are necessary for promoting order and avoiding ambiguity and inconsistency in employee relations. By setting standards, rules determine acceptable and unacceptable employee behaviour and importantly let employees know where they stand. Disciplinary rules are normally formulated by management but need to be perceived as reasonable by employees and employee representatives, and accepted as workable by managers who have to enforce them, if they are to be effective. Rules reflect legitimate management authority, based on the common law duty of employees to obey reasonable and legitimate instructions given by the employer, and enable management to obtain compliance to instructions in the pursuit of organisational effectiveness. Whilst rules are determined by management, they encompass obligations incurred under statute, for example health and safety at work and non-discrimination in employment, and also reflect 'acceptable behaviour' within a wider societal sense, for example, values associated with honesty, propriety and non-violence. Management has the responsibility for ensuring that disciplinary rules are clear, accessible and understood. This has implications for the appropriate use of language and the means of communication. This may include prominent display, word of mouth and incorporation into an employee handbook and other documents. Above all, rules should be designed on the principle of voluntary compliance rather than on the imposition of sanctions for breaking the rules.

Rules set standards and disciplinary procedures provide a means of ensuring that these standards are met and a method for dealing with a failure to meet them. The Employment Rights Act (ERA), 1996 creates an obligation to ensure that the principal statement of employment conditions makes reference to rules, disciplinary procedures and appeals procedures. A disciplinary procedure should include a general statement regarding the employer's attitude towards discipline and this should indicate that a precursor to formal disciplinary action will be counselling or informal management intervention with the aim of resolving disciplinary problems at the lowest possible level. Only when this informal approach fails will it be necessary to

Exhibit 19 **The principles of natural justice in employment**

These incorporate:

- a knowledge of the standards or behaviour expected
- a knowledge of the alleged failure and the nature of the allegation
- an investigation to establish a prima facie case should normally precede any allegation
- the opportunity to offer an explanation and for this explanation to be heard and considered fairly
- the opportunity to be accompanied or represented
- any penalty should be appropriate to the offence and take account of any mitigating factors
- the opportunity and support to improve behaviour except when misconduct goes to the root of the contract, should normally be provided
- a right of appeal to a higher authority.

escalate the matter and enter a formal disciplinary procedure.

Disciplinary procedures should conform to the principles of 'natural justice'. These principles have emerged from ideas of equity, due process and model legal practice. An illustration of these principles in an employment context is provided in Exhibit 19. The incorporation of these principles into disciplinary procedures is likely to enhance the perceived equity of procedures and foster voluntary compliance with the rules. Any perceived unfairness may create resentment and militate against compliance. In order to command respect and support, and to operate effectively, disciplinary procedures must also be accepted as fair and equitable by managers and facilitate consistent managerial action.

According to ACAS (1987: page 55) disciplinary procedures should:

(a) be in writing
(b) specify to whom they apply
(c) provide for matters to be dealt with quickly
(d) indicate the disciplinary actions which may be taken
(e) specify the levels of management which have the authority to take the various forms of disciplinary action, ensuring that immediate superiors do not normally have the power to dismiss without reference to senior management
(f) provide for individuals to be informed of the complaints against them and to be given an opportunity to state their case before decisions are reached
(g) give individuals the right to be accompanied by a trade union representative or by a fellow employee of their choice
(h) ensure that, except for gross misconduct, no employees are dismissed for a first breach of discipline
(i) ensure that disciplinary action is not taken until the case has been carefully investigated
(j) ensure that the individuals are given an explanation for any penalty imposed
(k) provide a right of appeal and specify the procedure to be followed.

The ACAS Code of Practice on disciplinary practice and procedures is not legally binding upon employers, but it can be taken into account by an industrial tribunal if it is relevant to the case. If disciplinary rules are formulated principally by management and require compliance by employees there is a case for disciplinary procedures being agreed through consultation or negotiation with employees or their representatives in order to enhance moral authority, command respect and ultimately to work effectively.

A disciplinary procedure should be incremental and should provide for a range of progressive actions against employees. If a disciplinary issue is not resolved at an informal level it may be necessary to enter the formal disciplinary procedure. The first stage of the formal procedure may be a recorded oral warning. Warnings should always make clear the consequences of a failure to improve or a repetition of the offence. The next stage of the procedure should be a written warning which, depending upon the severity of the case, may or may not be a final written warning. The final stage may be either action short of dismissal, including disciplinary transfer, or reduction in status and responsibility, or termination of employment. An indicative outline of the stages in a disciplinary procedure is provided in Exhibit 20 but the stages should not be viewed as a strict sequence, as managerial flexibility to enter at an appropriate stage is both legitimate and necessary. The importance of having and following a proper procedure was highlighted by *Polkey* v. *A E Dayton Services* (1987 IRLR 503) where a dismissal was found to be unfair because of a procedural failure. Failure to follow a fair procedure is, therefore, not only bad practice but may also affect the legitimacy of the dismissal itself.

Exhibit 20 **Principal stages of a disciplinary procedure**

Disciplinary matter and the procedural stage	**Management response**	**Management level, with advice from personnel**
1 *Misconduct* which is not serious	Oral warning	Team leader or Supervisor
2 *More serious misconduct* or repeated misconduct	Written warning	Supervisor or Line manager
3 *Serious misconduct* or repeated misconduct	Final written warning and/or Action short of dismissal	Line manager and/or Senior manager
4 *Gross misconduct* or further misconduct	Dismissal or Action short of dismissal	Senior manager

Disciplinary interviews

The importance of thorough investigation in disciplinary matters cannot be over-emphasised. Before disciplinary action is taken there needs to be a prima facie case of misconduct or breach of rules or unacceptable standards of work. It may be appropriate to suspend the employee during the investigation, particularly in cases of apparent gross misconduct. However, an unwarranted suspension will be to the detriment of the problem-solving approach and to the perception of equity referred to earlier. The investigation should include the objective collection of both oral and written evidence. Checking the employee's record is also essential and may contribute to the decision whether or not to proceed. If the evidence suggests that an allegation is justified, the employee should be informed and a suitable time and place arranged. The right to be accompanied or to be represented should be pointed out to the employee.

The disciplinary hearing or interview is potentially an emotional encounter and requires sensitive handling. Professionalism and good interpersonal skills are crucial. An introduction of those present and the reasons for attendance should precede the hearing. The employer should explain the purpose of the interview and where it fits into the formal disciplinary procedure. The allegation should be clearly stated, going through the evidence and concentrating on the facts. The employee should be given the opportunity to respond to the allegation and explain any actions. If it is apparent that there is no case to answer the interview should be terminated and no further action taken. If the employee does not offer an acceptable explanation or justification, a discussion should follow during which the problem is clarified and an acceptance of employee responsibility for resolving or improving the situation is encouraged.

If disciplinary action seems necessary, due consideration of all the circumstances is normally achieved by adjourning the hearing. During the adjournment, proper weight should be given to the employee's explanation and also to any special factors that have emerged or are known. Employers are able to act upon the establishment of a reasonable belief based on the available facts; there is no obligation to prove an allegation beyond reasonable doubt. The decision or outcome of the disciplinary interview should be clearly and unambiguously communicated to the employee, as should the right to appeal against the decision if there is dissatisfaction with the outcome.

This simple description of the interview process belies the managerial skills required. The existence of conflict militates against a smooth process despite the emphasis on thorough preparation and professionalism. The interviewer can be confronted with a range of responses from aggression or distress, on the one hand, to passiveness and disinterest on the other. The employee may reject the allegation outright or engage in self-denial behaviour. It is important in these circumstances to be able to remain calm and rational and demonstrate a professional and objective approach. The information-gathering nature of the interview requires good questioning skills and active listening. The ability to weigh the balance of probabilities, make an objective judgement and decide on appropriate action are skills that will determine the success or otherwise of the disciplinary process. The process should not be treated merely as a means for confirming managerial concerns, but as an opportunity for resolving conflict in the employment relationship through corrective action.

The result of the interview needs to be formally communicated to the employee, with copies to the employee's representative, if appropriate. Clearly this requires effective writing skills, not only because of the need to have an accurate record for the personal file and to demonstrate procedural fairness but also to ensure that the employee understands the decision. Any communication should be constructed in a language that the employee understands. Performance or conduct should be monitored and reviewed, and the employee either told of a satisfactory outcome or failing this the next stage of the procedure may need to be invoked. Warnings, except in extreme cases, should expire and be 'spent' after a predetermined period. This is in the interests of natural justice so that the employee has the opportunity to 'wipe the slate clean' in due course. Fairness and consistency in individual matters of discipline will contribute to good employment relations. Perhaps corrective action procedures is a more appropriate description than disciplinary procedures.

The law and dismissal

Protection against unfair dismissal originated in the Industrial Relations Act 1971 and was consolidated most recently in the Employment Rights Act (ERA) 1996, sections 94 to 134 in Part X. The law provides an employee with a limited job property right and affords some protection against unreasonable behaviour by the employer ending in loss of employment. The employer is in no way denied the freedom to dismiss individuals, in fact the legislation ensures that employers can legitimately dismiss employees for 'fair' reasons in 'reasonable' circumstances (Employment Department 1991). However, employment protection legislation serves to encourage good employment practice and is in reality aimed at persuading employers to act reasonably and fairly in the circumstances. The legislation enhances the role of ACAS as a conciliator and ACAS has a statutory obligation to intervene at the request of either party or on its own initiative when a claim of unfair dismissal is lodged. This has a significant impact upon the number of cases which are settled or withdrawn before reaching an industrial tribunal, with only 30 per cent of claims actually being heard (ACAS Annual Reports). The legal remedies for employees are best viewed as a back stop (see Chapter 2).

Employees are protected against unfair dismissal after two years' continuous service unless they have reached retirement age or the normal retirement age for the organisation. This two-year qualification may be subject to reduction either through precedent created by particular cases, through the interpretation of European Directives or a change in government policy. Employees with fixed-term contracts are not protected against non-renewal of their contract if they have waived their rights in writing following independent legal advice. A succession of fixed-term contracts may constitute continuous employment if breaks in service are interpreted merely as cessations of work. There is normally no service requirement in cases of inadmissible reasons for dismissal. Potential inadmissible reasons for dismissal include dismissal on the grounds of:

- pregnancy, maternity, sex, race or disability
- spent convictions
- refusal to work on a Sunday

- asserting a statutory employment right
- trade union membership, activity or non-membership
- the relevant transfer of an undertaking.

Dismissal takes place when either the employer terminates the contract, with or without notice, or the employee resigns by reason of the employer's behaviour and the employee considers the employer to have repudiated the contract by its actions or behaviour. Constructive dismissal, as this is known, may consist of a serious single act which is deemed to have destroyed the contract or alternatively it may constitute a series of smaller incidents which cumulatively add up to repudiation of the contract. In law, dismissals must be fair and reasonable in the circumstances. Dismissal may be fair for reasons related to:

- the conduct of the employee
- the employee's capability or qualification
- redundancy
- a statutory duty which prevents employment being continued
- some other substantial reason of a kind that justifies dismissal.

Whilst these reasons provide convenient categories, it is the substantial merits of each incident or case that determine whether or not the dismissal is for a fair reason. The reasonableness of each decision relates to whether the dismissal is based upon sufficient factual evidence, whether the correct procedures have been followed, whether dismissal as a penalty is justified, and importantly whether dismissal fell within the range of responses of a reasonable employer. Reasonableness is not an objective standard and takes account also of the employer's size and resources.

An employer does not have to prove employee fault beyond reasonable doubt. The burden of proof is one of establishing a genuine and reasonable belief based on the information available at the time following proper investigation. As part of any investigation, the employer is expected to talk to the employee as well as listen to and consider any explanations. This procedural importance makes it essential that dismissals are well documented. Fair reasons for dismissal require that a distinction is drawn between general misconduct, which is dealt with within the incremental framework of a disciplinary procedure, and gross misconduct, which may justify summary dismissal for one occurrence. Gross misconduct may include acts of drunkenness, theft, violence, breach of confidence, serious and wilful refusal to conform to the legitimate managerial instructions or serious misconduct outside the workplace. Alleged or suspected gross misconduct does not obviate the need for thorough investigation or the opportunity for employees to offer an explanation for their behaviour, but the serious nature of these offences often goes to the root of the contract and effectively destroys it. There is a duty on the part of the employer to ensure that what may constitute gross misconduct, and its potential consequences, are clearly and unequivocally communicated to all employees.

The capability of the employee may be in question if there is a failure to achieve a satisfactory standard of work or of job performance. If this is a failure to exercise competence, this may constitute misconduct. However, if the issue is one of incompetence or relative incompetence, the employer needs to point out the performance shortfall, specify the standard expected, indicate the consequences of a failure to meet the standard and give the employee reasonable time to improve. Within this process, there is an implicit obligation for the employer to provide reasonable and necessary support, training and guidance to the employee.

Incapability through ill health requires particularly sensitive handling and a distinction needs to be drawn between frequent short-term absences and long-term ill health. The issue is ultimately whether the employee is able to give continuous and effective service and each situation requires consultation with the employee and medical practitioners before deciding upon a course of action. The availability of alternative work needs to be considered, although there is no obligation upon the employer to create an alternative job. The age of the employee, the length of service, the likelihood of a return to health and the impact of the absence upon the organisation are all factors to be taken into account. When the employer has exhausted alternatives and can no longer be reasonably expected to accommodate health limitations or hold a job open then the 'enough is enough' point is reached and dismissal may be fair and reasonable. Reasonable adjustments may need to be made for disabled employees (Disability Discrimination Act 1995).

Redundancy occurs when the requirements for a particular type of work cease or diminish. Selection for redundancy requires employers to act reasonably and from genuine motives. There is a legal requirement to consult employees and their representatives (see below).

Dismissal for the reason that a statutory duty prevents employment continuing relates to a situation where it would be unlawful for an employee to continue working in the position for which they were contractually employed. Although this appears straightforward, the experience is that dismissal on these grounds is rarely justified. Examples include loss of a driving licence in certain circumstances or failure to renew a work permit.

Some other substantial reason is included as a fair reason for dismissal to give ITs some scope to accept a dismissal that is for reasons which do not conveniently fall into one of the other four categories discussed above. The reason for dismissal must be substantial, and not trivial, and it must justify dismissal. Described by some as an 'employer's charter', it has been used for dismissals relating to third-party pressure to dismiss, personality conflicts, relationships between employees and business reorganisation requiring variation to contractual terms. In the latter category, decisions by ITs are generally supportive of business needs overriding the interests of the individual employee, where this is justified on commercial or efficiency grounds. This entails an assessment of the balance of advantage to the employer through reorganisation against the disadvantage to the employee. There remains a requirement for employers to achieve change through consultation, persuasion and agreement.

Remedies for unfair dismissal

Where an industrial tribunal finds that there has been no unfair dismissal the matter ends, subject to any appeal by the applicant on a point of law. In cases where a tribunal is satisfied that dismissal is unfair, it has powers to order reinstatement or re-engagement of the employee. Reinstatement involves a return to the employee's previous job and acting as if dismissal had not taken place. Re-engagement involves a return to a comparable or otherwise suitable position. In considering the alternatives of reinstatement and re-engagement, ITs consider the applicant's wishes and any representation made by the employer relating to practicability. An employer cannot be compelled to take back an employee, but refusal to do so may result in an award of additional compensation to the employee. In reality fewer than 1 per cent of successful unfair dismissal claims result in re-engagement or reinstatement, principally because the adversarial nature of the legal process, and the time taken to reach a decision, condemn the employment relationship to irretrievable breakdown.

An alternative to reinstatement or re-engagement, and the most commonly exercised power of ITs, is the award of compensation to the unfairly dismissed employee. This consists of a basic award which is based upon length of service and calculated on the same basis as redundancy payments. The tribunal may also make a compensatory award to take account of the employee's current and future financial losses arising from the dismissal, although the employee has an obligation to mitigate this loss by actively seeking other work. The compensation awarded by ITs takes account of the contribution by the employee to the dismissal and the award may be reduced in proportion to that contribution. An additional award may be made where an employer rejects an order to reinstatement or re-engagement and a special award is available in dismissal which relates to health and safety or trade union matters. Awards are capped except in dismissal relating to unlawful discrimination. The median award is of the order of £2,500 (ACAS Annual Reports).

Preparing for industrial tribunals

An employee, the applicant, with a complaint, normally completes form IT1 identifying the employer, indicating the grounds for the claim and the remedy being sought. The application must be made within three months of the effective date of dismissal. After an assessment of the entitlement to claim by the Central Office of Industrial Tribunals, it is sent to the employer, the respondent, and to ACAS, via the regional office. The employer is obliged to respond on form IT3, normally within 14 days. Clearly the response by the employer has to be preceded by several considerations and points of decision, the first of which is to decide whether to concede or to contest the claim. This decision should take account of:

- an appreciation of the legislation which may be relevant to the case

- the skills required to defend the case and whether legal representation is necessary
- a judgement on how well the case has been handled within the organisation in relation to documentation and the conduct of those involved
- the likely consequences and cost of the decision to proceed; importantly, what is the applicant likely to achieve if successful, and would it be better to seek an out-of-court settlement?

If it is decided to contest the claim, it is necessary for the employer to gather the relevant documentation for consideration and also identify and consult the relevant witnesses and parties to the dismissal. This leads to a review of the situation, with consideration being given to the role of an ACAS conciliation officer who may contact the applicant, or the applicant's representative, with a view to reducing the difference between the employer and employee and seeking to identify areas of consensus as a way of progressing towards an acceptable resolution. A pre-hearing assessment may be appropriate as a means of testing commitment and providing guidance on the merits of the case of both parties (Employment Department 1990).

If, despite these efforts, the case goes to a tribunal the preparation required relates to proper and accurate presentation of the evidence. In addition, a co-ordinated and cohesive approach by those involved is essential, together with the determination of a strategy appropriate to the case. The principles relating to negotiation preparation and negotiation activity (see above) are transferable to defending unfair dismissal claims. Tribunal chairs are not generally sympathetic to surprises or court room antics and these should be avoided. Employers have no grounds for concern if they have acted reasonably, have followed the principles of natural justice, have ensured that disciplinary action is taken according to agreed procedure by skilled interviewers, have documented the case appropriately, and have prepared thoroughly for the tribunal.

REDUNDANCY

Prior to the 1960s, the concept of a right of ownership in a job would have seemed incredible to the average British worker. The right of the employer to decide who to 'hire and fire' was seen as absolute and embodied in the right to manage. The need to shed labour in an economic downturn was seen as inevitable and the worker had no power or legal protection in this situation. The first legislation directed at redundancy was the Redundancy Payments Act 1965 which set out the definition of redundancy and the compensation payment that the redundant workers were entitled to when their job disappeared. Payments were made from a now-defunct state redundancy fund. In the context of the political and economic situation of the time, it can be seen as a way of encouraging more mobility of labour in a situation of relatively low unemployment by discouraging employers from hoarding labour during periods of economic downturn.

The law and redundancy

Redundancy is one of the potentially fair reasons for dismissal, referred to above, and occurs when employees are dismissed because the need for employees of a particular type has ceased or diminished or is expected to cease or diminish.

The law provides for redundancy payments for the loss of employment which is 'wholly or mainly' attributable to redundancy. There are, however, some employees who are excluded from this legislation. These are:

- employees with less than two years' service after the age of 18
- employees who have reached retirement age
- employees on fixed-term contracts of two years or more who have waived their right to claim redundancy payment.

The legislation allows for payment of compensation based on age and length of continuous service. This is illustrated in Table 1.

Table 1 Statutory redundancy payments provisions

Age	Payment
18–21	$^1/_2$ week's pay
22–40	1 week's pay
40–64	$1^1/_2$ weeks' pay
64–65	reduced by $^1/_{12}$ per month

Entitlement is calculated on completed years of service subject to a maximum of 20 years and subject to a maximum weekly 'pay' which in 1997 was £210. From the age of 64, entitlement, calculated using the above formula, is reduced by $^1/_{12}$ for each month of service beyond that age. The redundant employee has a right to a written statement of how the payment has been calculated. Any employee disputing the calculation of a redundancy payment may take their case to a tribunal up to six months after the employment has been terminated.

The Collective Redundancies and Transfer of Employment (Protection of Employees) Regulations 1995 places a duty on employers to consult with elected employee representatives or with recognised trade unions. There is little guidance in law as to what constitutes fair election of representatives or what constitutes an appropriate number of representatives but the law requires that representatives are elected from all affected employees and employers are well advised to document this process to provide a defence if necessary. The employer must notify the Department of Trade and Industry of the numbers of workers to be made redundant. The minimum statutory periods for consultation are as follows:

- where 20-99 employees are to be made redundant in one establishment within a 30-day period, the consultation must take place at least 30 days before the first redundancy
- where more than 100 employees are to be made redundant in one establishment within a 90-day period or less, consultation must take place at least 90 days before the first redundancy
- where there are fewer than 20 employees, or the redundancy is spread over a longer period, management is still required to consult even if there is only one person to be made redundant.

Specific information to be provided prior to the consultation includes:

- the reason for the proposed redundancy
- the numbers and types of employees to be made redundant
- the total number of employees of this type employed
- the selection criteria to be used
- the implementation plan and the period of redundancy.

Management are required to consult and to listen to any representations made to the employer by the representatives. However, there is no legal obligation to come to any agreement with the employees' representatives. Failure to consult can lead to the imposition of a protective award which requires employers to pay employees their normal pay for the period called 'the protected period'.

Redundancy policy

Management must plan ahead for redundancy, in terms not only of numbers to be made redundant but also by having an agreed redundancy policy prior to a redundancy situation arising. If a policy is in place, then the employer and the employees are not dealing with the details under stress or in emotive situations. The agreed policy should be supplemented by a procedure or implementation plan that identifies the process of handling the collective redundancies.

The redundancy policy should be a part of the package of employment policies that any 'good' employer has at its disposal. Any employer that is fearful of having a policy for redundancy because of its possible adverse effects on staff and the concern of employees that it may become a self-fulfilling prophecy is doing both itself and its workers a disservice. The policy should include:

- an opening statement about the maintenance of employment levels and the need for job security together with a recognition that the requirements for labour are not static and therefore change will take place over time
- consultation arrangements
- steps that the company will take to reduce the need for redundancy
- the selection criteria

- details of redundancy payments
- details of redeployment procedures and related payments
- a statement of the appeals procedure
- redundancy support systems such as outplacement, counselling, and training.

Selecting for redundancy

The area most likely to give rise to claims for unfair dismissal is the criteria used for deciding who goes and who stays in a redundancy situation. Selection criteria must be stated in the redundancy policy and management must ensure that they are applied in an even-handed way. Any employees claiming unfair selection for redundancy can claim unfair dismissal at a tribunal provided that they are covered by the legislation. Care must be taken in the determination of selection criteria that discrimination does not take place. Selection based on part-time working will almost certainly be seen as infringing the Sex Discrimination Act 1975, as part-time staff are more likely to be women. The employer must also show that the new work patterns are needed to fit in with the organisation's requirements. Selection based on pregnancy or on trade union membership is automatically unfair.

Non-compulsory redundancy

Voluntary redundancy. An increasingly acceptable method of selection in redundancy is voluntary redundancy. This requires employees to volunteer to be made redundant and for the employer to select individuals from that list. Problems can arise, however, if there are more volunteers than the employer wants to lose, as any subsequent selection the employer makes must be fair. Also voluntary redundancy can be an expensive option for the employer, as commonly the longer-serving members of the workforce come forward and they attract higher redundancy payments. A further problem that can arise is that an imbalance of skills and experience develops in the organisation. This means that the employer must carefully work out the profile of the workforce that it needs to maintain its work activity, efficiently and effectively.

Early retirement. Early retirement can be redundancy. This may also be an expensive option as it requires a long-term financial commitment on the part of the employer. However, it can help in terms of workplace morale. Unfortunately, it can leave a skewed age structure, with little natural retirement for a few years, and this can lead to difficulties in career progression.

Compulsory redundancy

Last-in first-out (LIFO) can provide organisational problems in deciding whether, for example, it is to be applied on a company-wide basis or a departmental basis. In the former case, it can give rise to skill mix difficulties, if the latter, then the employer must make sure that internal transferees are excluded. The fairness of selecting long-service employees on LIFO, simply because they have been recently transferred to a new department, may well be open to question.

Skills or qualifications. The employer is likely to see the retention of a balanced workforce as the main priority in a redundancy situation. Here selection on the basis of skills or qualifications is appropriate. Again the importance of objectivity must be stressed and the profile of the required workforce should be decided before any individual decisions are made.

Efficiency or work performance. Management may decide to select employees on the basis of efficiency, which may include attendance and timekeeping. There are potential problems with this approach as it requires records that are absolutely accurate. Poor application of this criterion can lead to claims that the reason for dismissal is not redundancy but other factors.

Multiple criteria. There is an increasing tendency for employers to use a combination of criteria for selection based on length of service, performance, attendance and skills or competence. This is clearly a more complex method and means that the employer must have up-to-date and accurate data from which the total score is derived. The process requires points to be allocated, decided against the individual criteria according to agreed and defined categories, these points to be aggregated and an objective points score to be calculated. This in theory provides an objective method but if any individual score is based on subjective judgement then the system may be flawed. All of the data required for this type of system should be available and agreed, and the employees should know the criteria and also what they scored. Failure to notify any individual employee of the score may be seen by an industrial tribunal to be unfair (*John Brown Engineering* v *Brown and others 1997*).

Providing support

The announcement of redundancy in any organisation gives rise to feelings of anxiety and insecurity amongst the workforce. There is a need to communicate the issues, procedures and criteria with employees in general. There is no right time to communicate a redundancy situation and some may argue that it is best delayed as long as possible. This is fine if it does not give rise to rumour, as this will lead to a loss of trust and confidence in management and may well lead to greater problems in the long term. When the general announcement is made, the individual employees who are affected by the redundancy should then be seen by their manager. Managers need to have the skills to handle what may be one of the most difficult interviews they ever have to conduct. They must be prepared for the 'who', 'what', 'why' and 'how' questions and be given the information to answer them accurately and confidently. The interviews need to be handled in a confident and assertive way but also with empathy. Not all managers feel able to do this. Alternatives available to the employer in a redundancy situation are:

- to handle the whole process within current resources
- to handle the redundancies using permanent managers (usually personnel

managers) and appoint temporary staff to free up those managers
- to use the services of outplacement consultants.

Outplacement

The term 'outplacement' is defined by Eggert (1991: page 3) as 'the process whereby an individual or individuals compelled to leave their employer are given support and counselling to assist them in achieving the next stage of their career'. The aim is to facilitate the transition from the redundant job to the next employment. It usually consists of practical support such as job search, individual assessment programmes and employee counselling. Internal skills may be enough to handle small numbers of redundancies. Large-scale redundancies, however, often require additional support, either in the form of outplacement consultants, which are increasing in number, or through the Job Centres. This depends on the numbers involved and arrangements can be made at the place of employment to provide assistance to redundant workers. Outplacement specialists have the knowledge and skills to assist in a variety of situations. Senior and middle managers being made redundant need a different approach from manual workers, but all need careful handling, financial advice, possibly retirement programmes and skill development programmes. The use of psychometric tests to assist in identifying the skills and aptitudes of individuals can be of positive value. Many long-term employees may never have stood back and assessed their work and individual abilities. Sometimes the 'opportunities' which redundancy provides can be very fulfilling for the outplacement staff when they see the redundant worker move through the stages of disbelief and shock to success and hope in a new job role.

Counselling

Counselling redundant workers is increasingly recognised as a positive benefit by employers. In a redundancy situation, it is not only the employees under notice of redundancy who feel under stress and suffer anxiety. The provision of counselling services is obviously needed and may be required for both those going and those staying. However, individuals respond differently to redundancy depending on several factors such as age, financial situation, personality, gender and length of service. Counsellors should be able to assess individuals and identify their different responses on a personal basis.

Rebalancing the organisation

A redundancy situation is distressing in any organization, not just for the individual or individuals who are to be made redundant, but for all employees. The concept of the 'survivor syndrome' needs to be recognised and addressed if the business is to progress. Whilst redundancy affects those being made redundant it also affects those remaining. There may be relief that 'my name is not on the list' but feelings of insecurity amongst those remaining become more pronounced and concerns about 'will I be next?' are difficult to ignore. However, in order to move forward following redundancies, the employer has to manage the redundancy in a fair way, recognise the feelings of the remaining workforce and turn these feelings around. A very important consideration often not given sufficient thought is the restructuring and rebalancing of the organisation following a redundancy situation, and the role of staff in achieving a successful outcome.

Communication is important, particularly about the shape of the new organisation and the effect on jobs. Staff who are required to cover for others who have been made redundant, without support, or with little information about the future, are unlikely to perform well or be committed to the organisation. Consideration needs to be given to:

- communication strategies
- workforce planning
- job redesign and work restructuring
- skills audit and training needs analysis
- investment in training and development.

A positive response by management indicating that a planned and considered approach is being taken will add to the confidence of the remaining staff and help to build commitment and, hopefully, a return to a successful enterprise.

ASSIGNMENTS

(a) Observe or participate in a negotiation in your organisation.
- (i) Analyse the negotiation process in terms of the skills required. To what extent were these skills evident and how effectively were they utilised?
- (ii) Did adequate planning take place?
- (iii) Was it possible to detect movement through the negotiation cycle?

(b) Identify a situation where you have been required to negotiate on a one-to-one basis.
- (i) Describe the situation.
- (ii) Was there a successful outcome?
- (iii) What contributed to the success or otherwise of the outcome?

(c) Identify a situation at work where you will have to negotiate on a particular issue.
- (i) Decide upon your ideal settlement, realistic settlement and fall-back position.
- (ii) After the negotiation review the outcome in relation to your expectations.

(d) Body language or non-verbal cues make a vital contribution to the communication process. Keep a confidential log of body language which you observe in your organisation.
  (i) How does body language manifest itself?
  (ii) What do you interpret from the signs?
  (iii) How does it help or hinder the communication process?

(e) Attend an industrial tribunal and observe an unfair dismissal case.
  (i) Write a brief report on the proceedings and the outcome.
  (ii) Was a proper procedure followed by the employer?
  (iii) Comment upon whether the employer acted 'reasonably in the circumstances'.
  (iv) Discuss whether and to what extent the employee contributed to the dismissal.
  (v) Using the laws of natural justice outlined earlier in this chapter, examine each one in relation to the case and comment upon whether they have been adhered to.

(f) Obtain a copy of disciplinary procedures from two or more organisations.
  (i) Discuss to what extent they include the features recommended by the ACAS Code of Practice.
  (ii) Compare and contrast the disciplinary procedures, identifying strengths and weaknesses.

(g) Interview a manager who is experienced in disciplinary interviews.
  (i) Using open questions identify the skills required for effective disciplinary interviews.
  (ii) Write a brief report on your findings.

(h) Interview a number of managers in your organisation who may have some potential for involvement in grievance matters.
  (i) Question them about their understanding of the grievance procedure.
  (ii) Comment upon whether any training is warranted.

(i) Investigate the number of grievances you have had in your organisation over a specific period.
  (i) Analyse the subjects of the grievances and the outcomes of the hearings.
  (ii) Write a brief report on your findings paying particular attention to any organisational implications.

(j) Critically evaluate your organisation's redundancy policy. Comment on the effectiveness of the selection criteria identified in the policy.

(k) What support does your organisation offer to employees who are being made redundant. Evaluate the effectiveness of this and make recommendations for support for remaining staff.

REFERENCES

ADVISORY, CONCILIATION and ARBITRATION SERVICE. 1987. *Discipline at Work – advisory handbook*. London: ACAS (periodically revised).

ADVISORY, CONCILIATION and ARBITRATION SERVICE. 1988. *Redundancy Handling – advisory handbook*. London: ACAS (periodically revised).

ATKINSON, G. 1980. *The Effective Negotiator*. Newbury: Negotiating Systems Publications.

CORBRIDGE, M *and* PILBEAM, S. 1998. *Employment Resourcing*. London: Pitman.

DEPARTMENT OF EMPLOYMENT. 1987. *Redundancy Consultation and Notification.* London: ACAS.

DOHERTY, N. 1995. 'Helping survivors to stay on board'. *People Management*. January 1995

EGGERT, M. 1991. *Outplacement.* London: IPM.

EMPLOYMENT DEPARTMENT. 1990. *Individual Rights of Employees: A guide for employers*. London: ED.

EMPLOYMENT DEPARTMENT. 1993. *Fair and Unfair Dismissal: A guide for employers*. London: ED.

FARNHAM, D. *and* PIMLOTT, J. 1995. *Understanding Industrial Relations.* London: Cassell.

FOWLER, A. 1990. *Negotiation Skills and Strategies*. London: IPD.

FOWLER, A. 1996. 'How to conduct a disciplinary interview'. *People Management.* November.

INDUSTRIAL RELATIONS REVIEW AND REPORT 570. 1994. *Inconsistent Treatment Not Decisive in Itself.* October.

INDUSTRIAL RELATIONS REVIEW AND REPORT 566. 1994. *Sunday Trading Act 1994: Employment protection rights*. August.

INDUSTRIAL RELATIONS REVIEW AND REPORT 556. 1994. *EC Equality Law Secures Rights for Part-timers*. March.

INDUSTRIAL RELATIONS REVIEW AND REPORT 555. 1994. *Guidance on Identifying Reasons for Dismissal.* March.

INDUSTRIAL TRIBUNALS 1995. *Industrial Tribunals Procedures – England and Wales*. ITL 1.

INSTITUTE OF PERSONNEL MANAGEMENT 1993. *TURERA 1993 – Personnel Practitioners' Checklist*. July.

IRS EMPLOYMENT REVIEW 575. 1995. *EAT Addresses Limits of 'Polkey' reductions*. January.

KENNEDY, G., BENSON, J. *and* MCMILLAN, J. 1984. *Managing Negotiations.* London: Business Books.

SALAMON, M. 1992. *Industrial Relations: Theory and practice*. London: Prentice Hall.

SUMMERFIELD, J. 1996. 'Lean firms cannot afford to be mean'. *People Management*. January.

THOMAS, K.W. 1979. *Organisational Conflict in Organisational Behaviour.* Ohio: Columbus.

TRADE UNION REFORM AND EMPLOYMENT RIGHTS ACT (TURERA) 1993. London: HMSO.

WALTON, R. E. *and* MCKERSIE 1965. *A Behavioural Theory of Labour Negotiations*. New York: McGraw-Hill.

Part 2

MANAGING EMPLOYEE RELATIONS

6 The employee relations environment

Sylvia Horton

Employee relations management takes place within both an internal and external context, and these affect the employee relations strategies, policies and practices of employers. The internal context is one over which managements have some control and is determined by the size, functions, structure, social composition and managerial philosophy of the organisations they manage. The external context is beyond the control of management, at least in the short to medium term, and is therefore a given. The concept of the external environment is an abstraction but it refers to the complex world within which organisations have to operate. Further abstractions enable us to analytically separate the external environment into zones or sub-systems such as the economic, technological, social and political. Empirically, they are interrelated and overlapping but, by conceptualising them separately, we can examine how each dimension of the external environment affects the ways in which organisations are managed, particularly in the area of employee relations.

THE ECONOMIC CONTEXT

Britain is an advanced industrial society located in what is classed as the 'First World'. It had a Gross National Product (GNP), at market prices, of £748 billion in 1996 and, in terms of GNP per capita, it ranked twelfth in the 15 member states of the EU and eighteenth in the world league of the top 25 high-income economies in the OECD. These positions are lower rankings than in the past and reflect a declining relative world economic position. During the last three decades, dramatic changes have occurred in both the international and domestic economies. First, there has been a major restructuring of international markets, with Third World countries developing their own manufacturing industries and becoming important exporters of manufactured and semi-manufactured products to the economies of Europe, North America and Australasia. Second, the First World economies have been de-industrialising and developing service and non-manufacturing industries. Thus the international flow of goods, patterns of trade and capital movements are in a state of flux. Third, the collapse of the former communist regimes in eastern Europe and Russia between 1989 and 1991 and their movement towards open market economies have extended the scope of the international economy by opening up new opportunities for trade. But they have also destabilised the world political order. Britain's economy has been affected by these international trends and by changes in its national patterns of production and consumption.

Table 2 **Changing sector distribution of employment in the UK for selected years, 1971-96**

	1971	%	1979	%	1981	%	1986	%	1991	%	1992	%	1996	%
Manufacturing	8,065	(36.43)	7,253	(31.30)	6,222	(28.42)	5,227	(24.44)	4,793	(21.56)	4,589	(21.09)	3,913	(18.00)
Services	11,627	(52.52)	13,580	(58.60)	13,468	(61.52)	14,297	(66.85)	15,744	(70.83)	15,644	(71.91)	16,490	(76.00)
Other	2,447	(11.05)	2,340	(10.10)	2,203	(10.06)	1,863	(08.71)	1,692	(07.61)	1,524	(07.00)	1,239	(5.700)
All Industries	22,139		23,173		21,893		21,387		22,229		21,757		21,645	

Source: *Social Trends 22, 1992. Annual Abstract of Statistics 1997*

Although Britain's annual rate of economic growth has been on average around 2.5 per cent over this century, it has had periods of cyclical variation associated with booms and slumps. More significantly, its rate of growth has been slower than that of its major competitors. Domestically, the British economy has been characterised by changes in its structure, in the geographical location of industry and in the methods and patterns of work There has been a long-term shift from primary to service industries as traditional industries like coal and textiles have contracted and new ones have emerged. The decline in agriculture throughout the century has resulted in under 2 per cent of the working population being employed in farming. The most significant change, in more recent years, has been the decline in the proportion of the labour force employed in manufacturing industries and the increase in the service sector. As Table 2 shows, between 1979 and 1996 the numbers employed in manufacturing fell from 7.2 million to 3.9 million – a fall of some 45 per cent – whilst those in service industries rose from 13.6 to 16.5 million – an increase of 21 per cent. The service sector now accounts for 76 per cent of the labour force.

Figure 9 **Unemployment in the UK 1971-97**

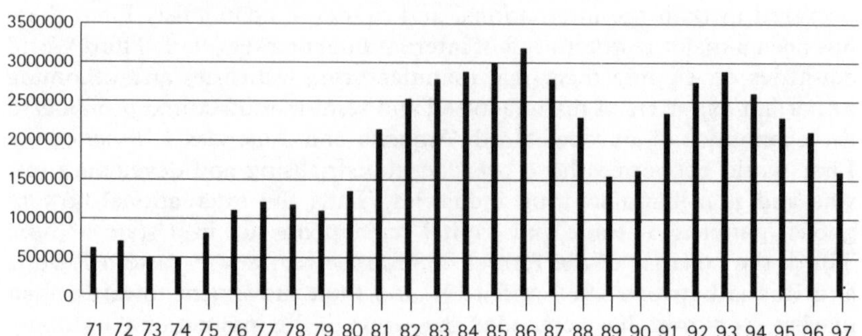

Source: Labour Market Statistics; Annual Abstract Statistics

The changes in employment have not been smooth, however, and throughout the last three decades there have been fluctuating and relatively high levels of unemployment as shown in Figure 9. The numbers unemployed rose above 1 million in 1976, above 2 million in 1981 and passed 3 million in July 1985, peaking at 3.2 million in July 1986. After falling sharply to 1.5 million in early 1990 they rose again to over 3 million at the beginning of 1993. In May 1997 they were back to the lowest level since 1979, with official unemployment at 1.8 million. In the mid-1990s the unemployment rate in the UK was one of the lowest in the EU – in contrast to the early 1980s, when it was the highest. The official unemployment rate is always disputed, as it is based on the numbers of claimants rather than of those looking for work. The independent Unemployment Unit estimated that in early 1997 around 5.4 million people were in fact looking for work.

A significant trend throughout the 1980s and 1990s has been the numbers of long-term unemployed – that is, those out of work for more than one year. The composition of the long-term unemployed consists of unskilled manual and skilled craft workers, older workers, the young between 16 and 25, and blacks. Unemployment is highest amongst the young. The Labour government, elected in May 1997, is committed to tackling that problem with its Welfare to Work programme.

Changes in the structure of industry have been accompanied by changes in the spatial distribution of economic activity within Britain. As extractive and manufacturing industries have contracted, the traditional industrial regions of Wales, the north-east, Lancashire and the Midlands have lost jobs. A census published in 1987 showed that 94 per cent of the jobs lost in manufacturing between 1979 and 1984 had been lost in the north. The Midlands was particularly badly hit by the collapse of the car industry in the late 1980s.

Although the expansion of the new service industries is not confined to the south, the latter has gained most from the rise of new industrial sectors and the growth in the service industries. There is, therefore, an inverse relationship between de-industrialisation and tertiarisation and, as a result, inequalities between British regions have tended to increase. The highest levels of unemployment in 1996 were in Merseyside (13 per cent), Tyneside (11 per cent) and South Yorkshire (9 per cent), whilst the lowest were in the south.

The changing structure of the economy has also been reflected in the occupational distribution of the labour force. The working population grew from 25 million in 1971 to a peak of 28.2 million in spring 1990 and then fell slightly to just below 28 million in 1996. The increase in the labour force was accounted for mainly by the entry of over 3.0 million women workers. In 1996, there were 12.0 million economically active women, representing 45 per cent of the workforce, compared with 15.7 million men (55 per cent). There is an increasing convergence in the economic activity rates of men and women, which now stand at 85 and 71 per cent respectively.

Between 1971 and 1996, there was an expansion of white-collar and professional jobs and a decline in blue-collar ones. Over half of men and more than two-thirds of women are now in non-manual occupations. The fastest-growing area has been managerial and professional occupations, which accounted for 39 per cent of men's and 20 per cent of women's jobs in 1996. Gender segregation continues to be a major feature of employment, with women concentrated in clerical and administration; public services such as teaching, nursing and social work, and the retail and sales sector. In contrast, men dominate in construction, engineering, transport, craft industries and as plant and machine operatives. There is also horizontal gender segregation within organisations, even those occupied mainly by women workers, in that most senior posts are held by men.

De-industrialisation has resulted in many job losses but it has also been accompanied by increases in productivity and output. Between 1980 and 1996, manufacturing productivity grew at an annual average rate of 5 per cent owing to increased investment, the introduction of new technology, and changes in the patterns and structure of the work process. The process of deskilling, reskilling and multiskilling is widespread. Furthermore, employers have sought to increase the flexibility of their workforces by adopting a range of employment modes from full-time 'core' employees to 'peripheral', part-time and temporary workers, so as to control labour costs.

Although part-time employment has increased significantly since the 1980s, most of the jobs (86 per cent) are filled by women. Only 1 million out of 13 million men were in part-time work in 1996. Amongst both men and women it is the youngest and the oldest workers who are most likely to be in part-time work. The high rate amongst the young is because of the number of students who take part-time work, and amongst older age groups there is a disproportionate number of men who have taken early retirement. In the 25 to 45 age range almost all part-time jobs are held by women with children under 16. Part-time working is more common in public administration and the distribution industries, where 34 and 44 per cent respectively are part-time positions. Most people who work part-time do not want to work full-time, and this is particularly true of women, because of their dual role – at work and in the home. Another feature of the labour market in recent years has been the increase in temporary employment. Some 7 per cent of people in work are in temporary posts and most of these again are women. This figure is low compared with most other EU countries: only Austria and Belgium have lower rates, whilst Spain peaks at 35 per cent (Social Trends 1997).

THEORIES OF ECONOMIC CHANGE

There is widespread agreement amongst academics and practitioners about the changes in the international and British economies in the last quarter of the twentieth century including:

- rapid and radical changes in production technology and industrial organisation
- major restructuring of world markets
- changes in the policies of economic management at the international, national and regional levels.

There is disagreement and debate, however, about how to explain what is happening, as Britain passes from an industrial into a post-industrial society. The main competing theories can be grouped under a number of headings including 'neo- and post-Fordism', 'the information society', 'post-modernism' and 'globalisation'. They all overlap, and many themes are common to all or some of the theories, but what distinguishes them is the framework they use within which to examine these common themes and ideas.

Fordism

Fordism is a term used to describe both an epoch and a form of production which dominated that epoch. During the early twentieth century a series of innovations in manufacturing led to large-scale mass production of commodities, using highly specialised machinery, extensive division of labour and assembly-line processes. Labour was highly fragmented, generally semi-skilled or unskilled, and located primarily in factories. Factories produced long runs of standardised products, at relatively low unit cost.

Fordism is also associated with scientific management. Frederick Winslow Taylor (1947), the father of scientific management, demonstrated that where employers adopted a rational scientific approach to production, they could maximise productivity, output and efficiency. This entailed the separation of planning, organising and controlling from the activities of executing and producing. In other words, it was the job of management to plan production scientifically, including the work process, and the job of workers to execute and carry out the work assigned to them. Through time and motion studies, and a careful analysis of the tasks involved in completing an activity, the 'one best way' of doing it could be identified. These ideas were extended to labour and led to scientific approaches to recruitment and training to ensure that management had the right quantity and quality of labour to do the job. The result was not only standardisation and bureaucratisation within organisations but also the emergence of an 'expert' managerial cadre claiming managerial prerogative and the right to manage within the workplace (Rose 1988).

Fordism is also linked to a particular pattern of consumption. Mass production requires mass consumption if it is to be sustained. It also requires market stability. This can be achieved only if purchasing power is sufficient to consume all that is produced. Mature Fordism came to be identified with a period of government regulation known as Keynesianism (see Chapter 4), where governments sought, through macro-economic policies, to manage the level of aggregate demand and maintain high levels of employment.

Finally, the Fordist system of work was reflected in particular social and economic patterns of employment. Full-time male employment was the norm, with workers' families dependent on a single income and a 'social wage' provided by the state. The nuclear family consumed standardised commodities and standardised collective goods and services provided by a bureaucratic state (Jessop 1989a). Conflicts over the industrial and social wage were resolved by political processes within industry and at a national political level. Trade unions sought to increase their members' wages and improve employee relations through collective bargaining, whilst in Britain the two main political parties used parliamentary democracy to resolve conflicts over the size and distribution of the social wage.

Challenges to Fordism

Fordism did not characterise the whole of industry, but in Britain between 1945 and the mid-1970s it was the dominant mode of production. Fordism provided the basis for the full employment, economic growth and rising living standards of the postwar era, as well as the expansion of the welfare state. Several writers (Hobsbawn 1968; Weiner 1981; Jessop 1989a) point out, however, that the prosperity of the period concealed underlying weaknesses of the British economy and its relative decline internationally.

The changes that are occurring in Britain today are seen, by Fordist writers, as a movement from traditional or classic Fordism to 'neo- (new) Fordism' or 'post-Fordism'. This transformation is the consequence of a structural crisis of Fordism. First, there is the inability of Fordism to constantly deliver rising productivity, economic growth and prosperity. Fordism appears to have reached its economic and productive limits. Constantly rising returns to scale have been frustrated by the failure of demand to keep pace with supply, whilst saturated markets, changes in tastes and fluctuating purchasing power have all contributed to a decline in production. Latter-day Fordism was also plagued by employee relation problems, absenteeism and alienated workforces which stemmed from the mass production labour process, the highly bureaucratised method of control and centralised monitoring systems.

Second, allied to these domestic factors, was the instability of world markets and the increase in global competition. The latter has also contributed to the breakdown of international price-fixing and the emergence of globalised free markets for products, raw materials and finance. Political instability in the Middle East, which led to the oil crisis in 1974, seems to have been a turning-point in the fortunes of classical Fordism. There are those who argue that the response has been pragmatic and reformist and that Fordism has been 'modernised' and transformed into 'neo-Fordism'. Others argue there has been a fundamental break with Fordism and a move to a post-Fordist period.

Neo-Fordism

Neo-Fordism focuses on changes in the labour process, including the introduction of new technologies, increased automation and new modes of employment and working practices. Technological innovations, such as computer-integrated manufacturing systems and electronic offices, have led to reductions in the labour force, employment of more multi-skilled technicians, greater flexibility in production methods and diversification in types of product. At the same time, new working practices and the introduction of participative working groups, such as quality circles, have introduced flexibility into socio-technical systems in the workplace (see Chapter 10).

These new technologies and working practices have not only increased flexibility in production but have also led to both domestic and international geographical decentralisation. As Allen *et al* (1992) point out, the neo-Fordist scenario is one in which traditional Fordism is being exported to third-world countries with cheap labour supplies and new potential markets, whilst at home the use of new technologies and increased automation have led to a new, highly skilled technical élite and to a de-skilled, peripheral workforce. But mass production is still widespread, employee relations are still rooted in the capitalist dynamics of class conflict and scientific management has had a revival.

Post-Fordists

In contrast, post-Fordists argue there is a qualitative shift taking place in the economic system which is transforming a mass production, mass consumption system into one of flexible specialisation and fragmented consumption. Murray (1989) argues that across sectors of the economy there have been changes in product life and product innovation, with shorter flexible runs and a wider range of products on offer; in stock control, using 'just-in-time' management processes; and in design and marketing, in response to increasingly diverse patterns of demand. Whilst neo-Fordists stress job de-skilling and increased centralisation of management control, post-Fordists highlight re-skilling and multi-skilling, and less hierarchical work environments that extend employee involvement and employee control of the work process.

Both neo- and post-Fordists share a common emphasis on the role of flexible manufacturing systems to provide for speedy responses to market demand and to ensure high-quality products. They also both emphasise the demise of Keynesianism and the emergence of neo-liberal economic strategies designed to deregulate markets, encourage free enterprise and free trade (Jessop 1989b; Sabel 1982). Both emphasise the globalisation of supply and demand and markets. The differences between them lie mainly in how they perceive technology. Neo-Fordists see technology as being used primarily to save labour and improve productivity, and argue that although task structures and modes of management may deviate from conventional Taylorism, they are not significantly different. Neo-Fordism is capitalism's response to the effects of overproduction and saturated domestic markets and the falling rate of profit. It is exploiting new product and labour markets and reconstructing itself, but the classic characteristics of Fordism are still in evidence.

Post-Fordists, in contrast, perceive technology as the trigger not only for the production of new products but also the basis for the transformation of the production process itself (Coombes and Jones 1988). At the heart of post-Fordism is the theory of flexible specialisation which focuses on the movement away from mass production to batch production and the manufacture of a wide and changing array of customised products, using flexible, general-purpose machinery and skilled, adaptable workers (Hirst and Zeitlin

1991). Changes in taste (which break up mass market demand) and competition from third-world producers force manufacturers to look for new and diverse products, and new technology facilitates a reactive response to complex and niche markets in organising production. The advent of flexible specialisation sees not only the re-emergence of the small firm and craft production but also greater involvement and enhanced work satisfaction of the workers, as it depends on the collaboration between all grades of workers (Piore and Sable 1984).

Hirst and Zeitlin (1991) draw attention to two other features of flexible specialisation. First, it is a system of network production in which firms are aware that they do not know precisely what they have to produce and that they must count on the collaboration of workers and sub-contractors in meeting the market's eventual demand. Second, and linked to this, it creates a complex set of practices at company level, involving relationships with sub-contractors, other firms and the sectoral and district institutions supporting and sustaining the system of production.

Flexible specialisation can take a number of forms including numerical flexibility, functional or internal flexibility and pay flexibility (Atkinson 1985; Wood 1989; Thompson, 1989) which tend to result in a dual labour market in which a core group of workers benefits from flexible specialisation, with its multi-skilling and employee involvement practices (see Chapter 10), whilst a peripheral group of part-time, sub-contract labour is de-skilled and without secure employment.

Another theory, which has much in common with flexible specialisation and is encompassed within the neo-Fordist camp, is regulation theory. Regulation theorists (Aglietta 1979; Boyer 1990; Lipietz 1985, 1988, 1992) are mainly French sociologists who adopt a very broad concept of Fordism and offer a more radical analysis of contemporary economic change than other Fordist writers. For them, Fordism is more than a production system and a particular labour process: it is a specific regime of capital accumulation, or a paradigm of production and consumption in which the economy is regulated in a particular way. It is the form of regulation which is the key to understanding economic activity, stability and change. The mode of regulation acts as a support system for the economy and pulls together and directs the wide variety of actions taken by firms, banks, retailers, workers and state employees. It takes place at two levels – the national and international. The mechanisms within each national economy regulate labour and capital, on the one hand, and different types of capital on the other. These controls include the system of management, the labour process, the system of wage payments, the role of market forces in determining prices and wages and the policies of the state towards incomes control and welfare provision (Harris 1988). At the international level, it is the international monetary system which is the key regulator.

Regulationists see the breakdown of both internal and international regulators in the 1970s as the turning-point for the economies of the West generally and for Britain in particular. Keynesianism, the mode of regulation compatible with Fordism, failed to cope with the crisis of capitalism in the

1970s. Regulationists trace the structural crisis of Fordism, first, to the Fordist labour process and the inability of mass production methods, for both technical and social reasons, to realise further productivity gains. In addition, insufficient demand for everything that was or could be produced resulted in a fall in profits. The second cause was a change in the global level of demand and an increase in world competition. Capital had to search for new sources of profit and so structural reorganisation became necessary. The regulationist school sees the explanation for the changes in the economy in the inherent contradictions of capitalism and its tendency towards a falling rate of profit. At the present time, capitalism is in the process of being reconstructed and there are elements of the old and the new in evidence. For this reason, they argue, both neo- and post-Fordist theories co-exist and have explanatory power and plausibility. Capitalism's response to the current crisis is to establish a global system on the one hand, which bears the hallmark of classic Fordism with its mass production and mass consumption patterns, along with flexible forms of small batch production in flexible smaller units of production responding to changing tastes and markets mainly in the first post-industrial societies (Kumar 1995).

Post-industrialism and the information society

It was Daniel Bell (1973) who first identified what he thought were the characteristics of a new emergent economic system which he called the 'post-industrial society'. These were:

- the change from a goods-producing to a service economy
- the emergence of a new professional and technical class
- the central role of theoretical knowledge as the source of innovation
- the creation of new information-based technologies.

Bell described post-industrial society as one in which most people would be employed in service industries and white-collar and professional workers would become a new occupational élite. It would be dominated by information and information technologies, which would transform organisational structures and processes as well as the location and content of work. In post-industrial society, information would become the key commodity and it would be an 'information society'. The generation of knowledge and information and new information technologies would be the motors of economic growth rather than profit and production which had been the motivating force – the 'axial principle' – underlying the dynamics of change for the industrial society. Bell was optimistic about the liberating effects of information technologies that would lead to the increasing automation of work processes and to high productivity. He predicted that people would work less and enjoy more leisure. The information society would guarantee sufficient wealth to raise standards of living for all and reduce the class conflicts endemic in the industrial era. There would be an 'end of ideology' as all societies moved to the post-industrial stage of development. He did not envisage the end of ideology as coinciding with the end of the cold war.

Alvin Toffler's (1980) analysis is more wide ranging than that of Bell's. He describes the post-industrial society as a 'third wave' after the 'first wave' agricultural and the 'second wave' industrial societies. New sciences and knowledge and new technologies transform the economy structurally, geographically and socially. The new 'information society' is characterised by desynchronisation, decentralisation, matrix structures, multiple command structures, networking, new lifestyles and prosumers. Whilst second wave industrial societies sought out predictability and principles compatible with mechanical causality, third-wave societies would be governed by a perception of things as inherently and unavoidably unpredictable. In this type of society, order emerges out of chaos and chance dominates change. Toffler, like Bell, was optimistic about this post-industrial society and predicted that information and communication would be the main means of integrating society and societies and empowering the individual. He also saw the information society as one in which knowledge would replace labour as the main source of value. However, he went further than Bell in predicting changes not only in the 'techno-sphere' and the 'info-sphere' but also in the 'socio-sphere',the 'bio-sphere' and the 'psycho-sphere'.

A less optimistic view of post-industrial, information society is presented by the French theorist Alain Touraine (1974), who describes the emerging society as a programmed society in which knowledge and information and 'technocracy' dominate. Unlike Bell, Touraine does not envisage an end of ideology and social conflict but a new class conflict between those who control information and its uses and those who do not. The root of conflict between social classes will no longer be ownership and control of property but access to information and its uses.

Two further writers, Castells (1989) and Gorz (1982), both in the Marxist tradition, are often grouped together in the same school as Bell and Toffler, although they tend to distance themselves from the post-industrial emphasis. Castells states that the new information-based society is no more post-industrial than the industrial society was post-agrarian. It represents a further stage in the evolution of capitalism in which new technologies have enabled companies to operate in new ways. In particular, new information technologies now traverse continents, space and time, shrinking the world and markets and enabling flexible and fragmented multinational corporations to emerge. Similarly, within organisations, core 'information workers' now function alongside a peripheral workforce of low-skilled workers, thus segmenting the organisation and polarising the 'knowledge élite' and the supportive mass.

Gorz agrees with Castells that the new information technologies are altering the structure of work and producing a core of secure, well-paid workers, on the one hand, and a peripheral workforce which is poorly paid and lacking any job security, on the other. In addition, increased automation is creating 'jobless growth' and a rising pool of unemployed. Gorz describes the new class structure as consisting of a securely employed professional class, a 'servile' working class, increasingly alienated and totally instrumental in their attitude to work, and a swelling underclass of unemployed. For Gorz and Castells, the 'new information society' is characterised by growing inequalities.

The common theme amongst the post-industrial theorists is that knowledge, information and communication technologies are both enabling and driving socio-economic transformation. The result is a changing social and power élite, with old class structures giving way to new social formations. Bell and Toffler are optimistic about the outcomes of change, whilst Castells, Gorz and Touraine point to the differential benefits within a new class formation.

Post-modernism

As Kumar states (1995; page 66): 'like post-industrialism and post-Fordism, post-modernism is a "contrast-concept" . . . . the initial meaning of post modernism is that it is not modernism.' But this begs the question what is modernism? Modernism, like most sociological concepts, is a disputed one, and even the point in time which divides modernism from pre-modernism is not agreed. There is some consensus, however, that modernity refers to a variety of social, political, economic and cultural transformations which separated the Middle Ages from the modern period and that modernism is rooted in several key ideas associated with the enlightenment. The first is that history is a record of humankind's achievements as well as its failures and that it is not predetermined or pre-destined. Second, reason is the source of all knowledge and understanding of the world, and reason, therefore, is the source of human progress and the mastering of nature. Third, social problems can be resolved through the application of reason, whilst science and empiricism are the means to human understanding. Laws of nature and the order of things can be exposed through scientific endeavour. Out of this paradigm emerged the dominant characteristics of modernism, namely capitalism, scientism, bureaucracy, technocracy, liberalism, democracy and socialism, along with social scientific theories of society, economy and psychology. As Kumar observes (1995: page 84): 'History and progress, truth and freedom, reason and revolution, science and industrialism . . . are all the main terms of the "grand narratives" of modernity that post-modernists wish to consign to the dustbin of history.'

Post-modernism and post-modernity arouse highly-charged reactions. As Smart (1993) points out, some writers refer to it as a period extending from the 1970s to the late 1980s when the impact of new-right ideas and neo-liberal economic policies took hold. Others see it as a contemporary phenomenon in which continuous reflection on current social conditions seeks to extend our understanding of the limitations of modernity. A third more radical view is that post-modernity is a form of life beyond modernity and represents a reconstruction of Utopian thought (Giddens 1996).

In the latter sense, post-modernism represents a radical assault on all those traditions of modernism. It rejects the belief that reason and the scientific method can 'discover' the reality of the physical and social worlds. It rejects objectivism and claims there are no facts, only interpretations, and no objective truths, only the constructs of various individuals and groups. In other words, our perception of the world is relative to time and space and experience. One person's reality is as 'real' as any other and should give way to intuition, sentiment and the free play of the imagination. Post-modern culture rejects the Protestant ethic, order and discipline for nihilism, hedonism and experientialism.

A key exponent of post-modernist thought, Foucault (1970, 1980) illustrates, in particular, the rejection of the equation of reason, emancipation and progress, arguing that an interface between modern forms of knowledge and power have created types of domination as irrational as those of the earlier pre-modern age. Foucault, like many other post-modernists, believes that modern rationality is a coercive force rather than a liberating or emancipatory one, and that modernism entails its own systems of subordination and domination. Foucault proclaims difference, fragmentation, relativism and chaos as the antidotes to the repressive features of modernism. He also insists that no single analytic framework can encompass the complexity of the modern world and advocates eclecticism. It is the irreducible plurality and diversity of contemporary society and the impossibility of controlling and directing its shape and meaning which is the key feature of post-modernity.

There are many schools of post-modernist writers which are identified by Best and Kellner (1991), Kumar (1995) and Turner (1990). There are also many overlaps between theories of post-modernism, post-industrialism and post-Fordism – with some writers, such as Bell (1980, 1987) and Jameson (1992), featuring in more than one. Along a continuum there are those at one end who see the present period as representing a post-modern rupture in history (Baudrillard 1988; Foucault, 1970) and at the other end writers who see elements of continuity between the present age and the period of modernity (Jameson, 1992; Laclau, 1990). Jameson, for example, adopting a Marxist perspective, links post-modernism to late capitalism. For him the cultural shifts associated with post-modernism are resulting in a cultural style congruent with the latest stage of capitalist development. Each stage of capitalism has its own cultural style and realism – modernism and post-modernism are corresponding cultures to market capitalism, monopoly capitalism and multinational capitalism. For Jameson, post-modernism is simply a stage in the development of capitalism.

Globalisation

In the mid-1980s ideas about globalisation came to the fore, and it is now the dominant concept of the 1990s having superseded post-modernism. It is a far less controversial concept than Fordism or post-modernism, because most observers agree about the changes that are taking place throughout the world. Although the spread of capitalism and Western culture has been going on for hundreds of years, it is the rate of acceleration of this process and the popular awareness of its happening that distinguishes this era from the past. Globalisation is described by Water (1995: page 2): as 'a social process in which the constraints of geography on social and cultural arrangements recede and in which people become increasingly aware that they are receding'. Globalisation is occurring in the three spheres of social activity: the economy, the polity and culture and, together with a revolution in global communications, is creating a 'global village'.

Again there are a number of theories which attempt to explain this phenomenon. The first is modernisation theory. Sociologists such as Parsons (1966) argue that as societies become industrialised they evolve very similar economic, political and social structures. A pattern of social differentiation emerges in which production and consumption are separated, specialist organisations emerge to provide for the educational, health and support needs of society, and mass media become the means of enculturating people into a new set of values, beliefs and symbols. Those values are ones of rationalism, individualism, universalism and secularism. This transformation amounts to modernisation. Paradoxically, the process of differentiation is also paralleled by processes of integration so that modernisation also leads to greater interdependence and to greater centralisation of decision-making because of the need to co-ordinate and control diversity and specialisation. Modernisation results in economic growth and brings material benefits. Therefore it becomes attractive to non-modernised societies, which seek to emulate wealthier, stronger ones. Societies converge through the process of modernisation because the means to modernisation is the adoption of technologies which are universal and common socio-technical systems are thus globalised.

A second theory that explains the phenomenon of globalisation is 'world capitalism'. Here capitalism is the major globalising dynamic, because it is driven towards constantly increasing the scale of production and consumption. This is resulting in the emergence of world markets and multinational and international corporations which come to control the economy and divide the world between them. This also explains the inter-societal stratification found in the global economy and the existence of First, Second and Third World societies, which refer both to stages of development and power relationships.

The economic changes identified with advanced capitalism are also the driving forces leading to the transformation of both the political and cultural spheres. The nation state, once the appropriate regulatory system within which industrial capitalism thrived, is being supplanted by regional political organisations, such as the European Union, to support the developments of monopoly capitalism, and all parts of the world are being incorporated into a new global system based upon international bodies such as the United Nations, the World Bank, GATT and the IMF. Furthermore, integration is taking place at the transnational level as non-governmental relationships are cementing the global economy and as mass communication systems promote modern consumerist and materialist cultures. Popular culture, 'macdonaldisation' and world-wide webs are compressing time and space, as well as creating similar social formations and social relationships across geographical boundaries.

A third school of globalisation theorists who challenge the capitalist view as too simplistic include Giddens (1985) and Robertson (1992). Both place great emphasis on the importance of international relations and see globalisation as occurring independently of the internal dynamics of individual societies. Globalisation has its roots in the emergence of the culturally homogeneous nation-state. Nation states, competing for resources, markets and territory develop political, economic, military, administrative and diplomatic systems for exchanges with other states which are both co-operative and conflictual. As nation states multiply and the nation state becomes universal, so international relations have to accommodate this. The world comes to be conceptualised as a whole and new systems evolve to make it more unified – but this does not mean it becomes more integrated or less conflictual, only more conscious of its oneness.

Giddens (1985) explains the process as one in which the first European nation states successfully married industrial production to military action and succeeded in colonising tribal societies and dismembering earlier empires. Their rational-bureaucratic systems enabled them to harness resources to industrial development and modernisation and to managing relations with other states. The destabilisation of international relations caused by the total wars of the twentieth century led to the burgeoning of international organisations which offer more security, institutionalise the sovereignty of the nation state and provide an environment within which new nation states can emerge.

Giddens (1990) argues that it is the four dimensions of modernity – namely capitalism, surveillance, military order and industrialism – that are driving globalisation. First, the world is emerging as a universal capitalist system, with the nation state providing the institutional framework for internal surveillance and control. Second, this is enhanced by the development of international information systems and the sharing of knowledge and information across national boundaries. Third, war has been globalised and a system of alliances, revolving around the military dominance of the USA since the end of the cold war, means that only local and peripheral conflicts occur, although that depends on the stability of international alliances. Finally, the industrialisation of the world has eroded Western economic dominance but it has resulted in the commodification of services and information and the globalisation of culture which Giddens describes as the axial determinant of the whole process. For both Giddens and Robertson, and other writers such as Lash and Urry (1987), globalisation is multi-faceted and multi-causal, but all agree that whilst it appears to be inexorable it is an uneven process of development. Taken together these theories and others, which can be found in Water (1995), assert that globalisation

- is a process of economic systematisation, of international relations between nation states and an emerging global culture and consciousness
- unifies and is inclusive and results in the phenomenological elimination of space and the generalisation of time

- is an inexorable process towards a global economy, a world political system and a cosmopolitan culture of great diversity.

Overview

This brief summary of the main theories describing and explaining economic and industrial change over the last two decades points to important environmental factors which are influencing organisations and their production, marketing and employee relations strategies. These are:

- changing industrial structures, modes of production and movement to flexible specialisation
- the globalisation of markets, spread of multinational corporations and geographical relocation
- the emergence of new occupations, the dual labour market and changes in the class structure
- the demise of Keynesianism and its associated patterns of internal and external regulation, and the emergence of new neo-liberal economic policies and state regulation
- the transition from mechanical and electronic technologies to new information technologies
- the challenge to generalised rational, scientific-rooted world views by relativist, intuitive forms of expressionism
- the phenomenon of the global village in which space and time are dissolved in common simultaneous experiences, common cultural symbols and common values, ideas and beliefs.

It is impossible to separate out the interacting forces and to identify a single causal factor, but a necessary condition of the rapid changes occurring in the late twentieth century would appear to be information technology.

INFORMATION TECHNOLOGY

Technology is the application of knowledge to aid human production. There are many types of technology and it is advances in technology that have generally accompanied major waves of economic change. Toffler (1980) points to the fact that in all societies the energy system, the production system and the distribution system are interrelated parts of a 'techno-sphere' which has its characteristic form at each stage of social development. Fossil fuels provided the energy for industrial societies and a new technology spawned, first, steam-driven and, later, electromechanically-driven machines. These were then brought together into interconnected systems to create factories, mass production and Fordist structures.

The new technologies are rooted in 'information technology' (IT). IT in its strictest sense is the science of collecting, storing, processing and transmitting information (Forester 1985). It is the result of a convergence of the three separate technologies of electronics, computing and communications, and the invention of the silicon chip. Naisbitt (1982) points to the launching of the Russian satellite Sputnik I in 1957 as the trigger for a technological and communications revolution which has transformed the world. From the late 1960s, a series of scientific and technological inventions converged to constitute a new scientific paradigm. Castells (1989) points out that the sequential scientific discoveries of the transistor (1947), the integrated circuit (1957), the planar process (1959) and the microprocessor (1971) mean that this new technological paradigm has characteristics which differentiate it from earlier paradigms. In the past, technology transformed processes rather than produced goods or services. The new IT is not only transforming processes but also producing information as an output. IT is also pervasive as it is not confined to the economic sphere of production but is fundamentally changing the social, cultural and political spheres of society at an accelerating rate, through a fundamental technological revolution.

The Russian economist Kondratieff argued that technological change occurred in cycles or waves over about 60 years, and that innovation and the application of new technology to new areas was the trigger to enable economies to emerge out of economic slumps which followed economic booms with remarkable regularity. During the last part of the twentieth century we may be seeing not only the beginnings of Toffler's third wave which represents a paradigmatic shift but the shorter Kondratieff cycle in which the new technologies are providing the innovative thrust to propel the economy out of the slump of the 1980s (Finnegan *et al* 1987).

Applications

IT and computers are now used in homes, schools, hospitals, offices and shops as well as in factories. Microchips control domestic appliances, programmed learning, machinery, banking cashpoints, telephones, aeroplanes and satellites. No type of commercial, service or public organisation has been left untouched. Although the pace of change varies between sectors and organisations, the changes over the last 25 years have revolutionised every aspect of life. In particular, there has been an exponential growth in telecommunications. Microelectronics has made possible the intelligent digital network, satellite communications, cable TV, cellular radio and videotext. All of these are transforming the way people work, where they work, how they receive entertainment, how they shop, how they conduct their financial relationships, how they are educated, and how they communicate with others.

Another dimension of the IT revolution is the international consequences of communication satellites. These make possible the creation of the global village. The international financial market can be accessed from any financial centre in the world. Trader dealings take place continuously and simultaneously throughout a 24-hour period, and a financial movement in any one country can send shock waves around the globe, as it did on Black Friday in 1987. Satellites also make possible the exporting of jobs and the fragmentation of the production process. Component parts can be produced in one area of the world, where labour is cheap, and transported for assembly into a finished product nearer to the main market. Multinational corporations can have their headquarters in one country and their production units spread throughout the world and communicate on a daily basis via internets, e-mail and fax. Meetings are held in airport lounges as managers fly in from all corners of the globe. Thus modern communication systems facilitate organisational flexibility.

Historically, new technology has been met with resistance, as it threatens traditional occupations and skills. Yet in the past new technology has resulted in the creation of jobs and led to increased production, increased wealth and higher standards of living.

Effects

What are some of the effects of the new technology on employment patterns and work processes? As indicated in the previous section, there are different views on the changes taking place, but there is general agreement that IT offers scope for:

- relieving the boredom of repetitive assembly line work
- job enrichment and job enlargement
- new forms of work organisation with flatter hierarchies
- transforming old-style employee relations
- involving workers directly in the decision-making process
- transferring the work base from the office to the home.

All these opportunities have been seized upon to some extent by British industry. The first stage of the transformation from an industrial to an information society has seen the application of new technology to existing work processes and the emergence of new industries, including a computer hardware and software industry. This is setting the pace of the IT revolution as it makes possible new ways of doing things, and new things to do. Computers are eliminating jobs and restructuring organisations as 'informatisation' is developed. Computers make it possible to dispense with clerical systems and create electronic offices. They are replacing brainpower by storing, retrieving, sorting and transforming data into information at phenomenal speeds. In medicine and the law, 'expert systems' are replacing people in taking decisions, whilst bio-technology is extending human control over the body and making new medical interventions possible. Within the public sector, during the 1980s and 1990s, IT facilitated the transformation of the state, which poses new problems for control of 'the automated state' (Snellen 1994; Margetts 1997).

Nilles (1985: page 202) draws a comparison between the microcomputer and the car, and the telephone line and the highway. In industrial society, cars transported workers via the highway to factories and offices. Today it is information that is transported instead of the worker. 'In principle the telecommuter has access to anyone with a computer and with near-zero transit time.' Work styles are being changed significantly through telework and telecommuting. However, as Nilles points out, whilst telecommuting may facilitate geographical mobility, offer flexible patterns of work and solve the problem of urban congestion, it may erode employee loyalty, corporate identity and corporate integration. An alternative view is that telecommuters are becoming part of a peripheral workforce and home-working will provide the sweat shops of the twenty-first century.

It is difficult to predict the future use and the outcome of the application of new technology because of the interrelatedness of the variables in a modern, globalised economy. Technology cannot be divorced from a whole range of factors that affect how it develops and the effect it has on work and society. The impact of technology depends on investment in a telecommunication grid, the reliability of transmissions, and the compatibility of systems both internally and externally. The development of the Internet and the World Wide Web in the last few years indicates what is possible. The present technological revolution is more wide-ranging than any in the past and it is clearly eroding jobs in every sector. Job losses appear to be a significant feature of the 1990s across all sectors of the economy. Job losses, however, are not only the result of new technology but also of over-production, increased competition and falling profits. Business strategy has been to look at ways of reducing labour costs and increasing flexibility which may actually save jobs in the long term.

Miles (1989) suggests that there is no one information society but many possible information societies. Which one will emerge depends on the social choices that are made about the use and application of technology. These decisions are taken in both the public and the private domains and are reflected in public policy and business strategy. There is an ongoing debate about the nature of the technological changes taking place and the social processes facilitating this change. Miles and his colleagues (1988) identify three perspectives. One is the 'transformist' perspective. This argues that there is a synergy between the properties of IT and emerging post-industrial values. The application of IT speeds up value change which, in turn, facilitates further applications of IT. Professional groups within society who are at the forefront of IT, and those societies further down the post-industrial route, provide leadership and act as the vanguard of change. Technology appears in this perspective as a driving force which it is difficult to resist.

The second, 'continuist' perspective is more sceptical about the rate of change and its revolutionary effects. It points to the incremental nature of the change process, including technological change, and to the differential use of the more advanced forms of IT. The adoption and diffusion of IT is slow and pragmatic. The continuists point to the limited changes that have taken place in work processes and in ways of life in the last two decades and the failure of computers to live up to expectations. Change in the future is likely therefore to be gradual, disjointed, incremental, pragmatic and unpredictable.

The third, 'structuralist' perspective shares with the transformists the view that IT represents a revolutionary technology but rejects the idea that it is leading to a new social order. Structuralism sees IT as more likely to facilitate a further development of industrialism or super-industrialism than to lead to its being superseded. In structuralism, elements of continuity and transformation are merged. Technological determinism is rejected in favour of a view of technological development as resulting from social factors on both the supply and demand sides, often called 'technology push' and 'technology pull'. New knowledge and innovations provide the potential for change, but are not all used. There has to be an awareness of them and they have to be perceived to be relevant and appropriate. Whether they are or not depends on management strategies, market conditions and public policies. Equally, a demand for new technology and ways of solving social problems stimulate technological innovation. Thus technology push and technology pull are not exclusive. They feed on each other but both depend on the structural context of organisations and markets.

There is difficulty, therefore, in predicting or forecasting technological change but Miles points to a number of likely trends in the economy and in organisational structures and management:

- employment in the UK will continue to shift from primary and secondary sectors to the tertiary sector
- service, administrative and professional occupations will increase relative to traditional manual and production jobs
- lifetime working hours will decrease
- IT will link operations over long distances
- organisations will both decentralise operations and management activities and centralise co-ordination and strategic control
- IT will provide growing competitive advantage for firms
- IT will be used for scenario-building and to improve decision-making
- information will become a key commodity
- information management will become a key function in firms.

The impact of IT on consumer goods and services and on social behaviour is again difficult to predict but there is likely to be a continuing adaptation of IT to new functions, the development of new IT applications and a greater diffusion of IT-based commodities and services. Education, health and legal services will be transformed as IT enables individuals to access knowledge and information in the home, at resource centres and at terminals in public places, and become their own experts. The 'dark' scenario of the impact on society predicts social isolationism, privatism, increased alienation and breakdown of values. The 'bright' view is one of increased freedom and empowerment, more social time, more communication, more self-service and more and better services, particularly for the sick, the elderly and the disabled. The crucial issues are whether the information society will lead to a more integrated and socially equal community or whether it will lead to new forms of inequality and inequity.

THE SOCIAL CONTEXT

British society has changed more rapidly during the last half-century than at any time in its past. There have been significant changes in its population, social structures, the role of women, social attitudes, culture and the dominant ideas influencing its politics. These are linked to changes in the economic system and in technology but are themselves variables in the total equation of change.

Demography

Britain's population was 58.6 million in 1995, having grown slowly from 50 million in 1951. It will continue to grow to 60 million by 2030, when it is expected that deaths will exceed births and then it will start to fall. There were 28.7 million males and 29.9 million females in 1995. Changes in birth and death rates are important in demographic trends. The birth rate tended to fall in the second half of the twentieth century, although there was a baby boom in the 1960s and another in the late 1980s. There are variations in the birth rates of different ethnic groups within Britain. In 1991, the total period fertility rate for women born in Britain was 1.8 – but 2.5 for women born in the New Commonwealth countries. The latter had fallen from 3.8 in 1971 and there is a continuing convergence between these two groups. A significant recent trend has been the percentage of births outside marriage, which increased from 8 per cent in 1971 to over 33 per cent in 1995. Another trend is the change in the fertility rates amongst different age groups. Whilst women between 25 and 29 are the most likely to give birth, there have been increases in the fertility rates amongst women in their thirties and forties and a decrease in the 20 to 24 age group. These fluctuations are reflected in the age structure of the population (as shown in Table 3), which is also affected by migration and life expectancy.

The declining birth rate has resulted in a fall in the 0–16 age group from over 25 per cent of total population in 1961 to 21 per cent in 1995. This gave rise to talk of a 'demographic time-bomb' in the 1980s, when it was claimed that there would be too few school leavers to meet industry's demand for labour. The onset of recession in 1990 averted that problem and actually resulted in high youth unemployment. At the other end of the age structure, the number of people over 65 is growing both absolutely and relatively. Their number was almost five times greater in 1991 than in 1901 and had grown by 4 million between 1961 and 1991. This group is expected to increase by another 2.4 million by 2021. In 1901, it represented 8 per cent of the population; in 1951, 11 per cent; and in 1995, 16 per cent. By 2031, it is estimated that it will reach 14.5 million (24 per cent) a rise of nearly 40 per cent over 1990 (Social Trends, 1993, 1997).

The labour force is traditionally drawn from the 16–64 age group. This rose from 33.5 million in 1961 to 36.8 million in 1990 but fell to 35.5 by 1996. The economic activity rate is the percentage of the population who are in the labour force. This varies between men and women. Traditionally

Table 3 **Age and sex structure of the UK population for selected years, 1961–95**

	Under 16	16–34	35–54	55–64	65–74	75 & over	All Ages (=100%) (millions)
Mid-Year estimates							
1961	25	24	27	12	8	4	52.8
1971	25	26	24	12	9	5	55.9
1981	22	29	23	11	9	6	56.4
1991	20	29	25	10	9	7	57.8
1995	21	27	26	10	9	7	56.0
Males	22	29	27	10	8	5	28.7
Females	20	26	26	10	9	9	29.9
Mid-Year projections							
2001	20	25	29	10	8	7	59.5
2011	18	24	29	12	9	7	60.05
2021	18	23	26	14	11	8	61.1
2031	17	22	25	13	13	11	60.7
Males	18	22	26	13	12	9	30.01
Females	17	21	24	13	13	12	30.6

Source: *Social Trends 27 1997*

men have constituted the larger part but women now form an ever larger proportion as their participation is increasing whilst that of men continues to fall. In 1971 women made up 38 per cent of the labour force, but that had risen to 45 per cent by 1996 when 71 per cent of women of working age were economically active compared with 85 per cent of men. Because of the ageing profile of the population in general, there is a shift towards the higher age groups in the workforce. In 1986 one in four of the labour force was under 24, but by 2001 only one in six will be under 24, and over one-third of the working population will be over 45. Another trend is an increase in the number of workers above pensionable age who are economically active.

From the 1950s, there was a net influx of Commonwealth immigrants into the UK, first, from the West Indies, then, from the Indian sub-continent and, in the 1970s, from East Africa. A series of laws to restrict immigrants from New Commonwealth countries has resulted in their numbers falling. In 1990, of a total of 52,000 immigrants less than half were from the New Commonwealth and most of those were dependents of people already settled in Britain. There are now 3.3 million people from ethnic minorities born either in Britain or overseas who represent about 6 per cent of the population. Their number has more than doubled since 1971, when they constituted 2.3 per cent of the population. The largest minorities are from India (30 per cent), the West Indies (21 per cent) and Pakistan (16 per cent), with smaller communities from Bangladesh, Africa and the Arab countries, each constituting about 5 per cent.

According to the Department for Employment and Education Labour Force Survey (1996), over 50 per cent of the present ethnic minorities were born inside the UK. There are significant differences in the age structures, of the ethnic minorities. The Pakistan and Bangladesh groups have particularly young age structures with around 75 per cent below 35 and 40 per cent under 16. Nine out of 10 of the ethnic minorities aged under 10 were born in this country, whilst 9 out of 10 under-35s were born abroad. This pattern of past immigration has resulted in Britain's becoming a multiracial society with a rich mix of religions and cultures. Ethnic minorities, however, are not distributed evenly throughout the country but are concentrated in large cities. They also tend to be found in the lowest-paid jobs and are more likely to be unemployed than white people.

Almost 80 per cent of the population of the UK live in urban areas, and amongst the remaining 20 per cent most commute to urban areas to work. There has been a slow but continual migration of population from the north to the south throughout the century, Scotland experiencing an absolute population decline since 1961. The overall pattern is one of net migration from the north-east, Northern Ireland, the north-west and Wales to the south of England. Since the late 1980s the major growth areas have been East Anglia and the south-west. Other significant trends have been suburbanisation, with people moving out of the metropolitan areas to smaller towns and the growth of retirement centres concentrated mainly around coastal areas. Geographical mobility is an increasing social feature of the UK, especially amongst the young and retired.

Social structure

The period between 1945 and the late 1970s was one of relative affluence and social progress. A postwar consensus amongst the major political parties on welfare-Keynesianism, an expanded public sector and high levels of employment and consumption led to rising standards of living for all. There was increased immigration to meet labour shortages and more women entered employment and the labour market. New occupations, and in particular new professions, emerged in the expanded welfare state. These changes resulted in greater social mobility, a more multicultural society and a more complex social structure. The distinctions and boundaries between the classes became blurred as the working class became more affluent and white-collar jobs increased. There was also increased social mobility, merging lifestyles and patterns of consumption. Finally, income and wealth became more evenly distributed.

Class and occupation

There is a debate about the changing class structure which revolves around what is happening to the working class. The concept of working class is itself problematic, since in modern society most people work for a wage or salary. Traditionally, the working class has been associated with blue-collar manual occupations and distinguished from white-collar workers, the professions and self-employed who constitute a middle class. In 1951, about two-thirds of the working population and their families were in manual occupations. Between the 1971 and 1981 censuses the proportion of employed people in manual work fell from 62 to 56 per cent for men and from 43 to 36 per cent for women (Halsey 1986). By 1996, only 30 per cent of the labour force had manual jobs and an increasing proportion of those were females and from ethnic minorities. The traditional working class is therefore smaller than it was and its composition has changed. This is the result of:

- a contraction of the industries in which manual workers were traditionally found – shipbuilding, coal, iron and steel, docks, transport and textiles
- restructuring, automation and the introduction of new technology in industries such as printing and car manufacture
- the transfer of production to countries with cheaper labour and the closure or contraction of British plants.

The middle classes or white-collar occupations, in contrast, grew in the postwar period and now constitute the largest group. They consist of the service group of employees, the professions, managers and the growing number of self-employed. This 'new' middle class is highly fragmented and heterogeneous. It consists of three sub-strata:

- an upper middle class which includes the higher professions, senior civil servants, senior managers and those holding senior technical positions
- a middle middle class which includes the lower professions, middle management and technical grades and the old middle class of small business owners and farmers
- a lower middle class of those in clerical and supervisory positions, minor professionals, para-professionals and white-collar shopworkers.

The middle class has become numerically and socially the most significant social stratum and is predicted to grow between 10 and 14 per cent over the next 10 years (Social Trends 1997). The upper class consists of a small number of interconnected families which own a disproportionate amount of wealth, control and own large parts of industry, land and commerce, and hold the top positions in business, politics and other institutions, thus making up the 'Establishment'. This class is economically dominant and operates through networks which are national and international. 'The core of the class consists of those who are actively involved in the strategic control of the major units of capital of which the modern economy is formed' (Scott, 1982: page 114).

Those who argue that the old class system is coming to an end point to the relatively open and fluid boundary between the middle class and the upper class which enables pop stars, inventors and successful business people to become millionaires, ministers and members of the House of Lords. Equally, they point to the 'new working class' which is now more skilled, more educated and more affluent than the 'old working class', with lifestyles and consumption patterns in common with the professional middle classes. The combination of increased social mobility and the higher status attached to new occupations, it is argued, is levelling the distinctions and blurring the differences.

A closer analysis, however, gives rise to an alternative perspective which has its origins in the work of David Lockwood. He views class membership as largely a function of an individual's market and work situation. The market situation consists of income, degree of job security and opportunity for upward mobility. The work situation refers to 'the set of social relationships in which the individual is involved at work by virtue of his position in the division of labour' (Lockwood 1958: page 15). The latter is reflected in the degree of autonomy, independence and control that an individual has over work and the skills which the work requires. The working class is distinguishable not only by the market situation that workers occupy but also by the work situation, in which workers have little control and no autonomy over the work process.

Though there continue to be differences between the working and middle classes based upon income and types of work, status and qualifications, the changing nature of the work process in many clerical, managerial and professional occupations is leading to a loss of autonomy and job control which is blurring the distinction amongst the classes. Many white-collar, lower middle class workers are being proletarianised and this is reflected in a more instrumental attitude towards work. Another significant factor is that many clerical jobs have become feminised, and this has led to a relative decline in the rewards and status of office work. From this perspective it appears there is a downward merging of the classes and an enlargement of the working class rather than an upward mobility.

Class, income and wealth

Class is more than a group of people with similar jobs or market position. Class is associated with common lifestyles, culture, consumption patterns and command over resources which gives power and status and freedom of choice too. Thus the class structure reflects the distribution of power within society, differential access to resources and relative life chances.

Between 1945 and 1975, there was some evidence of an increase in equality of personal income. The Royal Commission on the Distribution of Income and Wealth, which reported in 1979, showed that there had been some marginal change, with the share of the top 10 per cent falling from 29.4 per cent of total income in 1959 to 26.6 per cent in 1974–75. Over the same period, the share of the top 1 per cent had fallen from 8.4 per cent to 6.2 per cent. However, the bottom 50 per cent only increased their share from 23.1 to 24.2 per cent. So although there was a redistribution amongst the top third of income earners, income distribution in general remained relatively stable. Personal income after tax showed a small degree of equalisation, due mainly to progressive taxation and welfare state redistributive social policies. This trend has been reversed since 1979 and inequality has increased. In 1977, the bottom fifth of households accounted for 4 per cent of disposable income and 9 per cent of post-tax income. The top fifth accounted for 43 and 37 per cent respectively. Between 1979 and 1995 the richest tenth saw their incomes rise by 65 per cent, whilst the poorest tenth saw their incomes fall by 13 per cent in real terms, creating a 78 per cent gap between the richest and the poorest (Labour Research, 1997).

The distribution of wealth has changed slightly more over the postwar period but again the change has been a redistribution within the top 50 per cent which still own over 90 per cent of disposable wealth. The top 1 per cent (some 448,000 people) own 17 per cent of marketable wealth, the top 5 per cent own 36 per cent, and the top 50 per cent own 93 per cent – compared with the bottom 50 per cent, which own only 7 per cent. The distribution does not change significantly when the value of dwellings is excluded but does change marginally when occupational and state pensions are included. Then the most wealthy 1 per cent own only 11 per cent, whilst the least wealthy 50 per cent own 17 per cent. Wealth, then, continues to be very unevenly distributed, even more so than income, and since 1979 the gap has widened.

Townsend (1979) stated that in the late 1970s some 25 per cent of households were in relative poverty. By 1995 that gap had widened and the number of people living below the official poverty line of half average earnings had grown from 5 million to nearly 14 million (Labour Research Department 1997). Furthermore, one in four children lived in poverty, compared with one in 10 in 1979. In 1995, 30 per cent of the population were estimated to be at or below the official poverty line. Of those, some were in work on low wages, others included the unemployed, sick, elderly, one-parent families and ethnic minorities. Lone parents were the most over-represented group, whilst couples without children were the most under-represented.

Amongst this burgeoning strata of poor there is a group described as a new 'underclass'(Dahrendorf 1987). This underclass is distinct from the traditional working class because it is not just poor but marginalised, both economically and politically. It tends to be apathetic and fatalistic or to constitute a criminal subculture, functioning outside the norms and institutions of society. The growth in the underclass is clearly a consequence, in part, of the economic changes taking place in Britain, in particular the falling demand for manual workers and the creation of a dual labour market with low-paid peripheral workers. Government policies of rolling back the welfare state, reducing social benefits and welfare support, and abolishing wages councils, have also contributed. A more controversial explanation of the underclass is found in the writings of Charles Murray (1994) who argues that the 'dependency culture' fostered by the welfare state is the major cause.

Class and consumption

Class based upon occupation, income and wealth is an objective perception, but people's own subjective perceptions and how they assign themselves is often very different. Self-assignment is more often based on patterns of consumption and lifestyle than on market or job position. It is this that has led some writers to suggest that class rooted in production relationships is no longer the most significant social division. They argue that it is changing consumption patterns that explain contemporary political alignments, not economic class (Dunleavy 1980; Hamnett 1989; Saunders 1978; 1984).

Saunders distinguishes between 'collective consumption' and 'private consumption'. The former refers to those goods and services provided by the state and available to the public as a whole, as a citizenship right. Private consumption refers to the purchase of goods and services, by individuals, through the market. There was a great increase in collective consumption after 1945, with the spread of the welfare state. Collective provision of health, education, housing and other community services was associated with a rising standard of living for all and was an important factor in the embourgeoisement of the working classes. Greater personal affluence since the 1960s enabled the working class to consider home ownership and consumer durables similar to those enjoyed by the middle class. There was a convergence of material lifestyles too. However, there was little private consumption of merit goods, such as health and education, except amongst the upper class. Both the middle and working classes received universal services from the state.

Since 1979, there has been a notable shift within both the working and middle classes towards private consumption. Conservative governments between 1979 and 1995 encouraged this, first with the sale of council housing and providing tax incentives to take out private health insurance and educational covenants. Later, changes to the expenditure and organisation of public services persuaded people to look more to the market and to privatised consumption. This change had certain consequences, particularly for those whose market position is weak. Saunders (1984) pointed to the fact that consumption patterns were becoming every bit as important as occupational class in understanding patterns of power, privilege and inequality, in explaining the kaleidoscopic nature of modern social structure, and in accounting for the changing political alignments that occurred during the years of Conservative market-centred governments.

The present class structure consists, then, of an underclass, the new working class, and the salariat and technocrats who largely make up a new middle class. An upper class still tops the social strata, upheld by institutions like the monarchy, House of Lords, aristocracy and honours system. It is divided today between those traditional conservatives, who are often referred to as 'one-nation Tories', and the *nouveau riches* who are 'entryists', part of the business élite and often market liberals. The power and functions of the upper class remain the same, since they combine ownership of property and wealth with strategic control of industry and other major institutions. They are, however, becoming increasingly invisible and globalised.

The enlarged middle classes are the fastest-growing and the most heterogeneous group. They range from the traditional higher professions and salariat of managers and administrators to the new professions and technocrats, para-professionals and small shopkeepers and self-employed. The reconstituted working class is located above the underclass and consists of manual and low-level clerical workers who are distinct from both the apathetic underclass and middle class. Those in the new working class are affluent but not bourgeois. In contrast with the traditional working class, which was class-conscious and politically committed to the trade union and labour movement, the new working class has more instrumental attitudes towards work, unions and politics and they are more privatised in their social lives. They prefer to amass material things, own their own homes and spend time with their families. In the work situation, however, they have little control, are the most vulnerable to economic change, are affected by de-skilling and have the weakest market position. Their numbers are growing as the market situations of lower-grade technical, office and shop workers change. Technological change often downgrades these workers and relegates them to the status of a proletarian working class, whilst upgrading others who gain access to a higher class. The new working class lacks homogeneity but is less heterogeneous than the 'new' middle class.

Gender

Class is not the only basis of inequality in Britain. Another social division cutting across class is gender. Gender differences are socially constructed and reflect the different social expectations and roles which are attached to men and women in society. Just as the changes taking place within the economy are affecting the class structure so they are affecting gender relationships especially, but not exclusively, at work.

In 1901, women accounted for only 29 per cent of the workforce and most were confined to unpaid domestic work within the home. Two world wars saw women called in as a reserve army of labour to do the jobs left by the men mobilised into the armed forces. There was a return to normality after 1918 but in 1945 the welfare state opened up many new jobs for women and, since then, they have formed an increasingly important part of the labour market. Women are entering the labour market at an accelerating rate and are expected to make up half of the workforce by the turn of the century.

The pattern of women's employment is different from that of men in a number of ways. First, women are concentrated in four main areas of employment which account for 80 per cent of all female employment. These are:

- clerical and administrative work
- catering, cleaning and hairdressing
- retailing
- the caring services, including nursing, teaching and social work.

Women's opportunities for work have depended on the growth and expansion of these sectors. After 1945, the expansion of the welfare state and, in the 1970s and 1980s, the growth of service industries provided millions of jobs for women.

Second, in addition to horizontal gender segregation, there is also vertical segregation. Women's jobs are not only different from men's but also concentrated in the lower levels of the occupational hierarchy. Fewer women than men are found in managerial positions, even in those organisations where women are a majority of workers, such as in the NHS. The number of women in management is increasing but they still only represent 33 per cent in the wider economy, and this falls to less than 5 per cent at boardroom level. Their position has improved mostly in the public sector, where they sometimes represent half of the managerial workforce, as in local government (LGMB 1997).

Third, in addition to occupational segregation, women are also found disproportionately in part-time jobs. Part-time paid work was virtually unknown before 1939 but has become an increasingly important feature of the labour market since then. Both during and after the war, the government exhorted employers to provide part-time jobs for women and set an example itself. The increase of women in work over the last 25 years has been almost entirely accounted for by part-time employment. In 1971, there were 5.5 million full-time and 2.8 million part-time female workers. In 1981, the figures were 5.3 and 3.8 million respectively. By 1996 the figures were 6.3 and 4.6 million. Full-time, female workers are more likely to be women without children, without dependent children or professional women. Part-time workers are more likely to be married women with dependent children. 'Part-time employment is particularly appropriate for married women because it enables them to continue to shoulder their dual role – caring for their families and adding to the family income – without radically disturbing the gender divisions of labour within the home' (McDowell 1989: page 165). Women also account for 40 per cent of temporary full-time work.

Women's position in the labour market is reflected in their earnings. In January 1997, average weekly earnings for male workers was £402.30 and for females £292, a relative difference of 27 per cent. Not only is there a difference between gross hourly earnings of around 25 per cent but women's take-home pay is only around 70 per cent of average male income due to both horizontal and vertical segregation. Women are more likely to be in low-paid, low-status, part-time jobs with low levels of responsibility. This has a significant effect on women's career structures and career development.

The reason for this position of women in the labour market is partly a result of social expectations and early socialisation but largely a consequence of the structure of the family and structure of employment itself. Traditionally, the structure and organisation of employment have been based upon male working and career patterns, which take no account of women's role in child-bearing and child-rearing. A continuous working day, week, year and work life are incompatible with the dual role of women in society. Consequently, if women wish to return to work after the birth of a child, they tend to look for part-time employment. An interrupted career inevitably limits the opportunities for promotion and career advancement and results in the smaller number of women in managerial levels or at the top of the professions. Operating in a patriarchy has also meant endemic discrimination against women in all spheres of social activity. Women are under-represented not only in the higher positions of employment but also in politics, the churches, the media and all other major social institutions (Randall 1987; Rees 1992; Witz 1992).

In the 1970s, equal opportunities legislation paved the way for changes in the status of women and has led to some improvement in their economic, political and social conditions. There are a growing number of women in the professions, they constitute 50 per cent of graduates and are breaking into the male bastions of the higher civil service, academic world, police, media and politics. There is evidence that more women are returning to employment after childbirth and many more employers are providing creches, flexitime, annual hours and termtime-only contracts to both attract and retain women. A Business in the Community initiative, Opportunity 2000, launched in 1991 and supported within a year by 141 major employers employing 25 per cent of the workforce, is committed to positive action to change the culture of their organisations and promote equal opportunities for women. Some progress has been made, particularly in public sector organisations such as the police, armed forces and local government. A major event was the election of 116 women MPs in the 1997 election, 101 of these MPs representing Labour. This is the largest number of women ever to enter the House of Commons and was the result of a positive action policy by the Labour party of selecting women candidates in their most winnable seats. There are also four women in the cabinet.

In stark contrast to these positive actions, in the dual labour market which is emerging as a feature of economic reconstruction, women provide the majority of the peripheral workforce. They are also in those clerical occupations, which Gorz (1982) and others see as being proletarianised, and constitute a reserve army of labour which enables employers to adopt numerical flexibility strategies. Women have traditionally been reluctant to join trade unions and are therefore more receptive to calls for individualised systems of employee relations.

The contraction of the welfare state and occupations traditionally associated with the social services affect women disproportionately. The government's community care policy has implications for women in their traditional role as carers of the frail and elderly. As service industries shed labour during the recession in the early 1990s, it was women who were most affected. The changing economic situation offers women employment opportunities but it also exposes women's generally weaker market situation. In addition, women are faced with pressures resulting from the changes in gender roles that are taking place in the family and society generally.

Culture and change

National culture consists of the ideas, values, attitudes and beliefs which influence the way that people perceive the world and themselves in it. It fashions their behaviour, how they relate to others and how they interpret and understand their experiences. Socialisation during childhood, through the primary agencies of the family, kinship and school, has a major influence on the formation of perceptions, attitudes and beliefs. Halsey (1986: page 97) describes the nuclear family of parents and dependent children as 'the reproductive social cell of class, status and of culture'. However, socialisation continues throughout life, and secondary agencies such as the workplace, trade unions, the churches, the army, peer groups and the media may reinforce or challenge earlier influences. People change as a result of their own experiences and observations of their changing environment.

Social change

Society is constantly changing, but there is normally a cultural lag. People are often resistant to change because it threatens their security, their understanding of the world and their status within it. Change is accompanied by uncertainty and threats, although it can also offer opportunities. Older people are usually the most resistant to change, because they have invested so much in the past. Younger people find change easier to cope with, if only because they lack the reference points of the older generations. Also, a rejection of traditional values is seen by the young as a necessary step in asserting their independence.

Britain has experienced rapid change over the last half-century. Halsey (1986) paints a picture of pre-1945 Britain as consisting of a classic industrial economy, a family-centred social structure and a centralised democratic polity. This was the essential triangle within the social order. Men worked and women ran the homes, the economy produced and the family reproduced, and the state protected and administered. After 1945, the social order began to change. The state assumed many of the responsibilities of the family in education, health and the care of the elderly, whilst it supplemented family incomes with benefits and supported the old and the unemployed.

The family began to change as more women, especially married ones, entered paid employment. The size of families declined as contraception enabled women to control their fertility. Marriage itself became less stable as women enjoyed greater economic independence, secular values replaced religious ones and changes in the law made divorce easier. More men became economically inactive, whether by retirement or unemployment, and began to assume domestic responsibilities. This challenged conventional gender roles. More people continued their education beyond school leaving age and a more educated population emerged. Changes in the economy led to changes in occupation and a higher GNP led to higher personal incomes. People worked less and had more leisure time. State expenditure on the welfare state increased, resulting in a rising social wage, more public sector employment and a larger proportion of GNP being spent by government.

From the mid-1970s, the social order began to change again, coinciding with the economic transformation identified earlier in this chapter. The period was one of economic instability, political turbulence and social disruption. In particular, family relationships with the state and the economy have changed. The family now produces and consumes. As women increasingly work, men have assumed domestic roles of parenting and home-working. Work and leisure have become intertwined as people 'do-it-themselves'. Divorce rates have risen to the highest in western Europe, one in two marriages now destined to end in divorce. Serial monogamy has increased and complex networks of unconventional extended families have emerged at the same time that conventional kinship networks are weakened by social and geographical mobility. Further changes in the family have arisen from child-centred, hedonistic approaches to child-raising. Traditional authority relationships have given way as 'familial controls over upbringing were attenuated'. Halsey (1986: page 113) describes a situation in which traditional culture is weakened by these multiple forces of change and, amongst the younger generation, fashionability, hedonism and a desperate individualism serve as substitutes for a securely held morality. The state is withdrawing from its provider role in some areas and families are having to resume responsibility.

Education has come to the fore both as the vehicle for social mobility and changing the nature of the workforce by training people in new skills. Education is no longer restricted to the young, although the participation rate of the 18 to 21 cohort, in further and higher education, has risen dramatically (Social Trends 1997). Adult education and training are being used increasingly as means of changing attitudes to those of an enterprise culture. Education has been at the forefront of government policy throughout the 1980s and 1990s and was given top priority in New Labour's election manifesto in 1997.

Social attitudes

Britain's immediate history, like its past, is characterised by both continuity and change. Continuity is usually associated with stability, tradition and consensus, whilst change is associated with instability, conflict and dissent. How far changes in the last quarter of the twentieth century have affected social beliefs, values, and culture is difficult to assess. One way to monitor people's attitudes is through regular surveys over time. This has been done since 1983 by Social and Community Planning Research (SCPR) which carries out an annual British Social Attitudes Survey (BSAS). This provides a moving picture, portraying how British people see their world and themselves and, through their eyes, how society itself is changing. During the 1990s these surveys have focused on people's attitudes towards: the economy; public spending and the role of government; changes in the family;

and the moral climate. The evidence is that public attitudes have changed and, when plotted against class, gender and age, the results provide a picture of where cultural transformation is accompanying economic change and where traditional attitudes are persisting.

The eighth BSAS (Jowell *et al* 1991) revealed that Britain was divided, although on most issues attitudes were not polarised. Class provided the social roots of economic convictions although disagreements within each class were as common as between the classes. Polarisation, where it existed, tended to occur on moral issues, such as gender roles and homosexuality, but these posed no threat to social stability. The most recent survey published in 1996 (Jowell *et al* 1996) indicated some narrowing of the divide found in earlier surveys. This largely reflects the changing economic geography of the country and the narrowing of the gap between north and south. Although unemployment is still higher in the north than in the south, people's perceptions of the differences between the regions have changed. A significant difference in attitudes is evident in people's economic ideology. Although, in general, those living in the south of England are most likely to adopt a pro-free-market/right-wing stance and those living in Scotland are more likely to take a more anti-free-market/left-wing position, differences in the rest of the country are quite small. These converging attitudes were reflected in voting behaviour in the 1997 general election.

In spite of attacks on the welfare state throughout the period from 1979, there is still a widespread public attachment to it. Throughout the 1980s, 98 per cent of BSAS respondents supported government provision of health care and 97 per cent supported a decent standard of living for the elderly. Although attitudes towards the unemployed were more divided, 68 per cent in 1985 and 60 per cent in 1990 thought the government should provide jobs for those wanting them (Jowell *et al* 1991). In the 1997 election campaign, voters and parties rated unemployment as the most important issue. Support for public provision has not abated during the 1990s. In fact, support for extra spending on education and health was substantially higher in 1995 than in 1983 when the first BSA Survey was undertaken, as indicated in Table 4.

Table 4 **Trends in spending priorities 1983–95**

% support for extra spending on:	**1983**	**1987**	**1991**	**1995**
Health	63	78	74	77
Education	50	55	62	66
Defence	8	4	4	3
Help for Industry	29	11	10	9

Source: *British Social Attitudes the 13th Report SCPR/Jowell et al 1996*

Although there is often an inconsistency in people's attitudes towards social policy and taxation, the vast majority appear willing to pay more tax for health, education and social benefits, whilst a declining number wish to keep taxes the same or to reduce them. In 1983, 63 per cent favoured stable or reduced taxes compared with 36 per cent in 1995. Notably almost 75 per cent opted for more spending on pensions. There is clearly still a widespread consensus on the welfare state and on a positive role for government in dealing with unemployment. Another area of high priority for spending is law and order. In 1995, 72 per cent wanted more spending on policing, although only 40 per cent were willing to pay more taxes to fund it.

There are different interests amongst the classes reflected in the survey. Working class people are especially likely to regard 'the provision of jobs, unemployment benefits and housing for poorer groups as essential government responsibilities, to name social security as a priority for extra spending, and to criticise unemployment benefit as being too low' (Jowell *et al* 1992: page 32). The middle classes, in contrast, favour expenditure on the universal services. They are fortunate in having all-class support for those services such as health, education and pensions of which they make the most use. There is no evidence, however, that rich people are less in sympathy than poorer ones with increases in public spending, even if they are asked to pay a higher share of the tax burden to finance them (Brook *et al* 1996).

Strong support for the welfare state is also matched by positive support for a narrowing of income and wealth inequality. In 1983, 72 per cent thought that the gap between high and low incomes was too large. This has risen consistently throughout the period and stood at 87 per cent in 1995. An analysis of responses by social group and income reveals that concern about inequality has increased the most amongst social groups 1 and 2 who are now in line with the general consensus. The only areas which remain outside the national consensus are benefits for single parents and unemployment benefits, which are still not widely supported.

There is less disagreement about attitudes towards gender roles than in the past. In 1965, nearly four in five women felt that mothers of the under-5s should stay at home. By 1980, that proportion had fallen to around three in five and by 1987, was well under half (Brook *et al* 1989). In 1990, only 27 per cent of the public thought that a woman's job was to look after the home – but when asked whether family life suffered if the woman worked, 47 per cent agreed, 17 per cent were neutral and 36 per cent disagreed. Four in five women between the ages of 18 and 24 felt that it was not the woman's job to look after the home, whilst more than half of women over 65 took the opposing view. Men differ far less in their attitudes to gender roles than women, although there is a class difference, graduates and more educated males tending to adopt more liberal views (Jowell *et al* 1991).

The conclusions drawn by Curtice (1996) from the 13th BSAS were that Britain is less divided than it was in the 1980s and that this reflects its changing economic geography. Differences in economic pessimism and economic ideology were far less pronounced but the legacy of the past is influencing attitudes towards autonomy and devolution. There is convergence about the economic issues of redistribution of wealth and unemployment and a consensus on specific aspects of the welfare state, such as health, education and pensions. Consensus does not extend to unemployment benefits and support for unmarried mothers, and there is also widespread disagreement about moral issues such as extra-marital relationships and pre-marital sex and drugs. On most issues, attitudes are divided but not polarised. Polarisation persists, however, in attitudes towards homosexuality and gender roles. It appears that attitudes towards these two issues become more traditional with age and there is a distinct generation gap. Class does not appear to be the major division in British society today. Although working class people are less divided on economic issues than the middle classes, there is no evidence of a consensus amongst them. Indeed, there is almost as much spread within classes as there is within the population as a whole. Class, therefore, does not appear to be as significant in defining social attitudes, indicating social status or determining political affiliation as it was in the past.

THE POLITICAL CONTEXT

Changes within society stemming from economic, technological and social forces give rise to conflicts. It is these conflicts that are at the root of politics. Politics is the process by which societies resolve and manage conflicts and disagreements about the allocation of resources, distribution of power and the making of the rules which regulate social behaviour. It is about who decides the rules, how the rules are made, and what the rules will be. Not all social behaviour comes within the ambit of politics and there is both a private and public domain. That divide, however, is not fixed but is itself politically determined. The boundary between the public and the private domain became a major political issue in the 1970s and 1980s.

The British political system is primarily concerned with making and implementing the public policies and rules which govern society. In contrast to the market, where individuals themselves take decisions about what to produce and consume, politics is about the collective, authoritative allocation of resources whereby representatives of the people take decisions on their behalf. These decisions are binding and can be enforced by the legitimate exercise of power by the state agencies of the police and the courts.

Britain, like other Western states, is described as a liberal democracy. Liberal democracies have a number of distinctive features including representative governments chosen regularly through open elections by universal suffrage. Parties compete for power offering the electorate manifestos and policies from which they can choose. Civil liberties ensure freedom of speech, freedom of association, freedom of movement and freedom from arbitrary arrest. A free press enables not only the dissemination of ideas but also the opportunity to criticise, challenge and present alternative views to the government in office. An independent judiciary is designed to ensure that governments and public officials are subject to the law and that individual freedoms are protected. Above all, in a liberal democracy, government is limited rather than absolute. It is circumscribed by a constitution as to what it can and cannot do and the ways in which it can exercise its authority (Farnham and Horton 1996).

Governments are also constrained by the need to maintain support within the elected assembly to whom they are accountable, in theory at least. They also need to maintain the support of the electorate if they are to remain in office. They are constrained by the need to ensure the acceptance of their policies by those who have to implement them. Governments are further limited by the availability of resources, their involvement in international organisations, such as the EU, the UN and GATT (General Agreement on Tariffs and Trade), and by their inability to control their own external environment.

Political systems only ever approximate political models like that of liberal democracy, and Britain is no exception. Politics evolve and change over time and the absence of a written constitution has enabled the British system to change more easily than most, although it is marked by continuity and tradition, as well as by innovation and modernity. Those same features are to be found in the British political culture as well as its political institutions.

Political change

One of the main characteristics of the British political system has been its dominance by two main political parties. In all general elections between 1945 and 1974, the Conservative and Labour parties between them never won less than 87 per cent of the vote, and they dominated the House of Commons. Since then that pattern has changed. Table 5 shows that since 1974 there have been significant changes in support for the two main parties and a realignment of the electorate. Third parties have taken approximately 25 per cent of the vote. Another trend has been a fall in the electoral turnout. These changes in the political system have coincided with the changes in the economy identified above.

Table 5 **UK electoral statistics 1945–97**

	Electoral Turnout %	Conservatives % votes		seats	Labour % votes		seats	Liberals[1] % votes		seats	Welsh & Scottish Nat. % votes		seats	Other % votes		seats
1945	73.3	39.8	-	213	48.3	-	393	9.1	-	12	0.2	-		2.5	-	22
1950	84.0	43.5	-	299	46.1	-	315	9.1	-	9	0.1	-		1.2	-	2
1951	82.5	48.0	-	321	48.8	-	295	2.5	-	6	0.1	-		0.6	-	3
1955	76.8	49.7	-	345	46.4	-	277	2.7	-	6	0.2	-		0.9	-	2
1959	78.7	49.4	-	365	43.8	-	258	5.9	-	6	0.4	-		0.6	-	1
1964	77.1	43.4	-	304	44.1	-	317	11.2	-	9	0.5	-		0.8	-	0
1966	75.8	41.9	-	253	47.9	-	363	8.5	-	12	0.7	-		0.9	-	2
1970	72.0	46.4	-	330	43.0	-	288	7.5	-	6	1.3	-	1	1.8	-	5
1974 Feb	78.1	37.8	-	297	37.1	-	301	19.3	-	14	2.6	-	9	3.2	-	14
1974 Oct	72.8	35.8	-	277	39.2	-	319	18.3	-	13	3.5	-	14	3.2	-	12
1979	76.0	43.9	-	339	37.0	-	269	13.8	-	11	2.0	-	4	3.3	-	12
1983	72.7	42.4	-	397	27.6	-	209	58.4	-	23	1.5	-	4	3.5	-	17
1987	75.3	42.3	-	376	30.8	-	229	22.6	-	22	1.7	-	6	2.8	-	17
1992	77.7	41.9	-	336	34.4	-	271	17.8	-	20	2.3	-	7	3.5	-	17
1997	71.4	31.5	-	165	44.4	-	419	17.2	-	46	2.5	-	10	4.4	-	19

[1] 1945–1979 Liberals; 1983–7 Lib-SDP Alliance; 1992 Liberal Democrats

Source: Butler, D. and Kavanagh, D. *The British General Election of 1992, Labour Research 1997 June*

Traditionally, class appeared to be the dominant factor in the way people voted. The Labour party, created by the trade unions to represent working class interests in Parliament, traditionally attracted the majority of the working class vote, although never all of it. The Conservative party, seen as the party of the privileged, propertied and business classes, attracted the votes of the upper and middle classes and some working class deferential voters. The two main parties tended to present issues in class terms, although they also claimed to be acting in the national interest. Whilst class voting was the norm, throughout most of the century substantial minorities – both of the middle and working classes – have voted against their supposedly natural class interests. About one third of the working class have regularly voted Conservative and about 20 per cent of the middle class have voted Labour (Nordlinger 1967; McKenzie and Silver 1968).

Since 1974, however, the electorate appears to be fragmenting politically along unfamiliar lines and political scientists have sought to explain this partisan dealignment. One view, before the last election, was that there is a shrinking working class and that this explains the decline in Labour voting (Heath *et al* 1985). Another view is that voters are more discriminating now and vote for the party which they think will run the economy most efficiently (Crewe 1984). A more radical approach to explaining changes in voting patterns, linked to ideology and the media, is developed by Dunleavy and Husbands (1985).

Clearly, the main beneficiaries of the changes in voting patterns since 1974 have been the centrist and nationalist parties. Their support is drawn equally from all classes and their images and ideologies are not class-based. Their electoral support however has not been able to break the mould of British politics because the electoral system does not translate votes proportionately into seats in the House of Commons, as shown in Table 5. Britain remains an essentially two-party system which after 18 years of Conservative governments returned a Labour government in May 1997. The evidence from the BSA Surveys since 1983 suggest that major changes in the ideologies and policies of the main political parties are important influences upon voting behaviour and these, in turn, are responses to the economic and social changes occurring within society itself.

The postwar settlement

All governments elected between 1945 and the 1970s were broadly agreed on policy objectives, although there were differences of emphasis on means and priorities. This came to be called the postwar consensus. It comprised three interrelated elements:

- support for a mixed economy, incorporating Keynesian demand management
- support for a welfare state, with universal services including health, education, housing, social insurance and old age pensions

- acceptance of a social democratic framework within which people had both civil and social entitlements and rights.

Within this consensus, minority interests were acknowledged and major interests were incorporated into the policy-making process. In particular, industry and labour, represented by the CBI and the TUC, joined with government to form a tripartite structure for discussing economic policy (Farnham and Horton 1996). Gamble (1988) observes that the postwar consensus provided a political context compatible with an economic system based on the Fordist principles of mass production and mass consumption. Commitment of all governments to the four economic goals of full employment, economic growth, low inflation and a stable currency – and the use of Keynesian economic techniques – ensured a high and constant level of aggregate demand and the transfer of many of the social costs of capital accumulation to public agencies. As a result, public expenditure increased, the public sector expanded and large public bureaucracies became the monopoly suppliers of both social services and public utilities. Initially this was funded by a constantly rising GNP, but by the 1970s the state was consuming almost 50 per cent of GNP and accounted for almost 30 per cent of the labour force (see Chapters 1 and 4).

In the 1970s, cracks began appearing in the political consensus, largely because Keynesian demand management of the economy, so apparently successful in the 1950s and early 1960s, was no longer working. Growth was slowing down, unemployment was rising, inflation was proving difficult to control and there were recurrent balance-of-payments crises. Britain was losing its share of world markets and import penetration by its main competitors was encroaching on domestic markets. Keynesianism as an economic strategy came under attack, but so too did the welfare state (Dearlove and Saunders 1991). High public expenditure on the welfare state was seen as a root cause of Britain's economic problems because it was sustained by high taxation, high borrowing and high interest rates. All of these, it was claimed, discouraged investment, choked off consumption and led to economic stagnation.

There were many critics and critiques of the postwar settlement, from both the left and the right of the political spectrum, but it was the New Right that came to the fore and exploited some people's fears of a large-spending, social welfare state (Farnham and Horton 1996).

The New Right

A new ideology, often referred to as the 'New Right', advocated the primacy of the market over politics, both as a means of producing and distributing goods and services in society and as an institutional arrangement for providing social organisation and social control. It argued that markets offer freedom of choice, result in the most efficient use of resources, and give opportunities for inventiveness, creativity and enterprise. Politics, in contrast, restricts, constrains, denies choice and results in inefficiency and a misallocation of resources. New Right critics also challenged the welfare state as creating dependency, weakening individual responsibility, denying people freedom of choice and empowering professional interests.

These ideas came to dominate the Conservative Party, especially under the leadership of Margaret Thatcher, and they were evident in the policies pursued by consecutive Conservative governments following the elections of 1979, 1983, 1987, and 1992. Conservative governments sought to reverse Britain's relative economic decline, improve the efficiency of the economy, create the conditions for continual economic prosperity, reassert Britain's role in the world and 'destroy socialism'. The strategies adopted were to 'roll back the state', reduce public expenditure, cut taxation and state borrowing, privatise the nationalised industries and other parts of the public sector and deregulate the economy, including the labour market.

Quasi-markets and new management systems were introduced into the public sector aimed at increasing the economy, efficiency, effectiveness and value for money of public organisations. Keynesianism was replaced by monetarism and supply-side economics, and the major economic priority of government became controlling inflation. Efforts were made to change public expectations and to wean people from supporting the welfare state to supporting 'popular capitalism' and an 'enterprise culture'. A property-owning democracy was engineered by the forced sale of council houses, the sale of public industries and encouraging share ownership schemes and profit-sharing in the private sector. Compulsory competitive tendering (CCT) in local government, the NHS and the civil service broke down the barriers between the public and private sectors, and deregulation afforded opportunities for businesses, old and new, to compete in public transport, telecommunications, hospitals, residential nursing homes and ophthalmic services. Gradually CCT, or market testing as it became known, was extended throughout the whole of the public sector. Labour market deregulation was accompanied by attacks on the trade unions. A programme of legislation curbing the powers of trade unions sought not only to free up the labour market but also to undermine collectivism in favour of individualism at work (see Chapters 7 and 10).

For 18 years successive Conservative governments pursued their objectives taking it as axiomatic that market decision-making was inherently superior to political decision-making, and that free markets, free enterprise and free trade were the panaceas for Britain's economic problems. They consistently sought to bring inflation down in the belief that a stable medium of exchange and store of value is essential for the market to function efficiently. They achieved low inflation and Britain's competitive position in international trade improved, although at the cost of high unemployment rates and growing inequality. Income tax fell, although overall taxes increased. Financial, product and labour markets were deregulated, which resulted in increased competition but also instability. The success rate of new businesses was low, fewer than 60 per cent surviving more than a year. Government failed to reduce public expenditure, which was the same proportion of GNP in 1996 as it had been in 1979 and neither did it con ted £33 billion, was hig

New Labour

During this long period of Conservative domination of British politics the Labour Party undertook a major review of its own ideology. After its fourth electoral defeat in 1992, New Labour emerged under a new leadership and with a new set of ideas aimed at getting the party into power at the next general election. The conception, however, goes back to the late 1980s under the leadership of Neil Kinnock. Between 1987 and 1997 Labour changed and modified its political values and made itself more attractive to the electorate and more relevant to the problems confronting the country. New Labour moved to the centre of British politics and effectively ceased to be a democratic socialist party to the left of the political spectrum. First, it reformed the internal structures and procedures of the party, weakening its close links with the trade unions and expelling the more extreme socialist elements within it. Second, it abandoned its Clause IV commitment to the socialisation of the means of production. Third, it elected a new leader who adopted a strategy of embracing many of the changes introduced by successive Conservative governments since 1979 but offering a fairer and more just distribution of resources. Focusing on people's concerns about unemployment, declining education and health services, it made an appeal to voters from all sections of society and all classes. In doing this, it became a social democratic party, to the centre of the political spectrum.

Mandelson and Liddle (1996) trace the emergence of New Labour and identify the major attitudinal differences between old and new Labour in seven key areas: the private sector, public ownership, trade unions, the role of the state, public expenditure, Europe, and personal incentives. These were spelt out in the Labour Party's election manifesto (1997: *passim*):

> The old left would have sought state control of industry. The Conservative right is content to leave all to the market. Government and industry must work together to achieve key objectives aimed at enhancing the dynamism of the market not undermining it.

> We have rewritten our constitution, the new Clause IV, to put a commitment to enterprise alongside the commitment to justice ... in the utility industries we will promote competition [and] ... pursue tough, efficient regulation ... which is fair both to consumers and shareholders and at the same time provides incentives to managers to innovate and improve efficiency.

> We have put our relations with the trade unions on a modern footing where they accept they can get fairness but no favours from a Labour government ... In industrial relations there will be no return to flying pickets, secondary action, strikes without ballots or trade union law of the 1970s. There will instead be basic minimum rights for the individual at the workplace, where our aim is partnership not conflict between employers and employees.

> We will give Br ... ieed ... [but on the ... e to be satisfied be ... the Cabinet would ... ould have to say 'Yes' in a referendum.

> We will be the party of welfare reform ... we will design a modern welfare state based on rights and duties going together ... get the unemployed from welfare to work ... save the NHS ... be tough on crime and causes of crime ... strengthen family life ... help get more out of life ... the best way to tackle poverty is to get people into jobs – real jobs ... we will stop the growth of an 'underclass'

> We will examine the interaction of tax and benefits systems so that they can be streamlined ... and fulfil our objectives of promoting work incentives, reducing poverty ... and strengthening community and family life ... There will be no return to the penal taxes ... to encourage work and reward effort, we pledge not to raise the basic or top rates of income tax throughout the parliament.

It was on the basis of this new ideology and its 10 commitments, covering a range of policy pledges in its manifesto, that New Labour was elected with a landslide majority of 146 seats over all other parties on 1 May 1997.

It is too soon to assess how far its election commitments and its espoused New Labour philosophy will translate into practice, but in its first three months of office the Labour government introduced new policies on education, health and unemployment. In the first budget in July it committed £1.2 and £1.0 billion increased expenditure to health and education respectively, and £3.5 billion for the Welfare to Work programme. These were to be paid for by a windfall tax imposed on the privatised utilities raising a total of £5.2 billion. Other than increases in excise tax on cigarettes, beer, wine and the road tax and a reduction in mortgage interest relief, there were no other changes affecting the incomes and expenditure of the general public. Major changes in the constitution were already being planned, the UK agreed to sign the European Social Chapter, and a committee was set up to report on a level for a national minimum wage.

TRADITIONAL AND EMERGING PATTERNS OF EMPLOYEE RELATIONS MANAGEMENT

Figure 10 sums up the main traditional and emerging economic, organisational, social and political contexts within which employers and managements have operated and are operating, especially but not exclusively in Britain. The elements within each of these contexts are derived from the analyses provided in the earlier parts of this chapter. These are obviously 'pure' typologies and, in the 'real world' of personnel and development, the traditional and emerging contexts of employee relations management are rarely as clear-cut as Figure 10 implies. These typologies are identified and used merely as tools of analysis and for the purposes of description rather than of prescription. What is clear, however, is that the traditional contexts, which were established largely in the immediate postwar period, no longer apply universally. Above all, the 1980s were and the 1990s are a period of immense change, uncertainty and transition, economically, socially, politically and organisationally. Whilst, in practice, elements of the traditional contexts remain, they are being challenged and counterbalanced by the forces of change, as indicated in the emerging contexts outlined in Figure 10.

Figure 10 **The contexts of British employee relations**

Traditional contexts	Emerging contexts
The Economy	
protected economy	open economy
strong national markets	globalised markets
industrialisation	de-industrialisation
strong manufacturing base	dominant service base
national ownership	multinational ownership
large public sector	smaller public sector
mass consumption	customised consumption
steady growth	variable growth
regulated labour market	de-regulated labour market
Work Organisation	
Fordist	post-Fordist
bureaucratic/hierarchic	organic/flat
mechanical technology	information technology
mass production	batch production
full-time employment	flexible employment
male employment	growing female employment
single skills and unskilled work	multi-skills and de-skilled work
task-based work	team-based work
The Social Structure	
young population	ageing population
nuclear family structure	multiple family structure
large working class	small working class
small middle class	large middle class
strong class identities	interest-based identities
class subcultures	diverse subcultures
growing equality	growing inequality
stable society	dynamic society
The Polity	
two-party system	multi-party system
partisan voting	issue-based voting
consensus politics	conviction politics
corporatist policy-making	governmental policy-making
national sovereignty	Europeanisation
strong collectivist/welfare state culture	strong individualist/enterprise culture
Keynesian policies	monetarist/supply-side policies
state support for collective bargaining	state support for individual contracts

These external contexts, in turn, are impinging on the patterns of employee relations management currently being practised in Britain, as shown in Figure 11. Traditional patterns of employee relations management, based on collectivism, managing relatively high levels of organised industrial conflict and 'personnel management' strategies, now co-exist with emerging patterns of employee relations management – sometimes in the same organisation, sometimes in different organisations. The 'new employee relations' and the emerging patterns of employee relations management, in contrast, are based on individualism, low levels of organised industrial conflict and 'human resources management' strategies. There are clearly hybrid forms of employee relations management, which draw on elements of both the traditional and emerging models outlined in Figure 11. But the important factor to recognise is that the pattern which predominates, whether nationally or organisationally, evolves largely from the contexts which have been examined in this chapter. When these contexts change, as they inevitably do, so do the dominant patterns of employee relations management. No one pattern of employee relations management is either self-evident or axiomatic at any one time, or over time. It is a function of management choice, taking account of the economic, organisational, social and political contexts in which contemporary employers operate.

Figure 11 **Patterns of British employment relations (ERL) management**

Traditional patterns	Emerging patterns
strong unions	weak unions
collective bargaining	employee involvement
jointly driven ERL	management-driven ERL
policy focused on groups	policy focused on individuals
collective agreements	personal contracts
standardised payments	payment by performance
narrow wage differentials	wider wage differentials
common employee benefits	packaged employee benefits
employment security	employment insecurity
high levels of organised industrial conflict	low levels of organised industrial conflict
personnel management strategies	human resources management strategies

ASSIGNMENTS

(a) What are the major changes that have occurred in the British economy since 1976?

(b) Read the latest edition of *Social Trends* and identify three major features that could be having an effect upon employee relations in your organisation.

(c) What are the main characteristics of pre-industrial, industrial and post-industrial societies? What causes a change from one to another?

(d) Read Murray, 'Fordism and post-fordism', in Hall and Jaques (1989) and argue the case for a new model of political economy.

(e) Divide into groups and examine one of the four theoretical perspectives of social and economic change in Britain – Fordism, post-industrialism, post-modernism and globalisation. Discuss the similarities and differences between them, and their implications for employee relations management.

(f) Consider the major differences between the old technologies and IT.

(g) Within groups, discuss whether class is still the major division in British society.

(h) What are the most significant observations of the latest British Social Attitudes Survey?

(i) What are some of the implications of the changing role of women both within society and the work organisation?

(j) Read Allen *et al* (1992: pages 357-368) and examine the 'modernist dilemma'.

(k) What light do theories of flexibility shed on the major transformation in the gender composition of the workforce?

(l) Read Chapter 7 of Miles *et al* (1988). Debate the optimistic and pessimistic scenarios of the future effects of technology in the UK. How relevant are they 10 years on?

(m) What do you consider to be the main economic, social, technological and political factors affecting the management of employee relations in recent years?

(n) What evidence is there that the human resources control strategies that management adopt are changing in line with changes in the structure and organisation of work?

(o) How would you categorise your organisation's current patterns of employee relations management?

(p) What difference, if any, is the New Labour government having on employee relations?

REFERENCES

AGLIETTA, M. 1979. *A Theory of Capitalist Regulation: the US Experience.* London: Verso.

ALLEN, J., BRAHAM, P. *and* LEWIS, P. 1992. *Political and Economic Forms of Modernity.* Oxford: Polity.

ATKINSON, J. 1985. 'Flexibility: planning for an uncertain future'. *Manpower Policy and Practice.* 1, Summer.

BAUDRILLARD, J. 1988. *Selected Readings.* Ed Poster, M. Cambridge: Polity Press.

BELL, D. 1973. *The Coming of Post-Industrial Society.* NY: Basic Books.

BELL, D. 1980. 'Beyond Modernism. Beyond Self'. *Sociological Journeys: Essays 1960-1980* London: Heinemann.

BELL, D. 1987. 'The World and the United States in 2013'. *Daedalus.* 116.

BEST, S. *and* KELLNER, D. 1991. *Postmodern Theory.* London: Macmillan.

BOYER, R. 1990. *The Regulation School: A critical introduction*. NY: Columbia University Press.

BROOK, L., JOWELL, R, *and* WITHERSPOON, S. 1989. 'Recent trends in social attitudes'. *Social Trends 19*. London: HMSO.

BROOK, L.,HALL, J. *and* PRESTON, I. 1996. 'Public spending and taxation' in Jowell R. *et al, British Social Attitudes: The 13th Report*. Aldershot: SCPR/Dartmouth Publishing.

CASTELLS, M. 1989. *The Informational City*. Oxford: Blackwell.

COOMBES, R. *and* JONES, B. 1988. 'Alternative successors to Fordism'. Paper presented at the Conference on Society, Information and Space, Swiss Federal Institute of Technology, Zurich. Mimeo: UMIST and Bath University.

CREWE, I. 1984. 'The electorate: partisan dealignment 10 years on'. In Berrington, H. (ed.), 1984, *Change in British Politics*. London: Frank Cass.

CURTICE, J. 1996. 'One nation again' in Jowell, R. *et al, British Social Attitudes: The 13th report*. Aldershot: Dartmouth.

DAHRENDORF, R. 1987. 'The erosion of citizenship and its consequences for us all'. *New Statesman*. 12 June.

DEARLOVE, J. *and* SAUNDERS, P. 1991. *Introduction to British Politics*. Oxford: Polity.

DEPARTMENT OF EDUCATION AND EMPLOYMENT (1996). *Labour Force Survey*. London: HMSO.

DUNLEAVY, P. 1980. *Urban Political Analysis: The politics of collective consumption*. London: Macmillan.

DUNLEAVY, P. *and* HUSBANDS, C. 1985. *British Democracy at the Crossroads*. London: Allen and Unwin.

FARNHAM, D. *and* HORTON, S. 1996. 'Politics and power' in Farnham, D. *The Corporate Environment*. London: IPD.

FARNHAM, D. *and* HORTON, S. (eds). 1996. *Managing the New Public Services*. Basingstoke: Macmillan.

FINNEGAN, R, SALAMAN, G. *and* THOMPSON, K. (eds). 1987. *Information Technology: Social Issues. A Reader*. Sevenoaks: Hodder and Stoughton.

FOUCAULT. M. 1970. *The Order of Things: An archaeology of the human sciences*. London: Tavistock Publications.

FOUCAULT, M. 1980. *Power/Knowledge*. London: Tavistock.

FORESTER, T. (ed.) 1985. *The Information Technology Revolution*. Oxford: Blackwell.

FRISSEN, P. 1994. 'The virtualization of informatization of public administration ', *Informatization and the Public Sector*. Vol. 3, Nos. 3/4.

GAMBLE, A. 1988. *The Free Economy and the Strong State*. Basingstoke: Macmillan.

GIDDENS, A. 1985. *The Nation State and Violence*. Cambridge. Polity Press.

GIDDENS, A. 1990. *The Consequences of Modernity*. Cambridge: Polity Press.

GIDDENS, A. 1996. *In Defence of Sociology*. Cambridge: Polity Press.

GORZ, A. 1982. *Farewell to the Working Class*. London: Pluto Press.

HALL, S. *and* Jacques, M. (eds) 1989. *New Times*. London: Lawrence and Wishart.

HALSEY, A. 1986. *Change in British Society*. Oxford: Oxford University Press.

HAMNETT, C. 1989. 'Consumption and class in contemporary Britain'. In HAMNETT, C., McDowell, L. and Sarre, P. (eds) 1989, *The Changing Social Structure*, London: Sage.

HARRIS, L. 1988. 'The UK economy at a crossroads'. In Allen, J. and MASSEY, D. (eds) 1988, *The Economy in Question*, London: Sage and the Open University.

HEATH, A., JOWELL, R. *and* CURTICE, J. 1985. *How Britain Votes*. Oxford: Pergamon.

HIRST, P. *and* ZEITLIN, J. 1991. 'Flexible specialisation versus post-Fordism: theory, evidence and policy implications'. *Economy and Society*. 20(1), February.

HOBSBAWN, E. 1968. *Industry and Empire*. NY: Weidenfeld and Nicolson.

JAMESON, F. 1992. *Postmodernism or The Cultural Logic of Late Capitalism*. London: Verso.

JESSOP, B. 1989a. *Thatcherism: The British Road to post-Fordism*. Essex Papers in Politics and Government No 68. Department of Government: University of Essex.

JESSOP, B. 1989b. 'Conservative regimes and the transition to post-Fordism: the cases of Britain and West Germany'. In Gottdiner, M. and Komninos, N. (eds) 1989, *Capitalist Development and Crisis Theory: Accumulation, regulation and spatial restructuring*, London: Macmillan.

JOWELL, R., BROOK, L. *and* TAYLOR, B. (eds) 1991. *British Social Attitudes: The 8th Report*. Aldershot: Dartmouth.

JOWELL, R., BROOK, L., PRIOR, G., *and* TAYLOR, B. 1992. *British Social Attitudes. (9th Report.)* Aldershot: Dartmouth.

JOWELL, R., CURTIS, J., PARK, A., BROOK, L. *and* THOMSON, K. 1996. *British Social Attitudes. (13th Report.)* Aldershot: Dartmouth.

KUMAR, K. 1995. *From Post-Industrial to Post-Modern Society*. Oxford: Blackwell.

LABOUR PARTY MANIFESTO. 1997. *New Labour: Because Britain deserves better*. London: Labour Party.

LABOUR RESEARCH DEPARTMENT. 1997. *Editorial*. May. Vol. 86, No. 5.

LACLAU, E. 1990. *New Reflections on the Revolution of our Times*. London: Verso.

LASH, S. *and* Urry, J. 1987. *The End of Organised Capitalism*. Oxford: Polity.

LIEPITZ, A. 1985. *The Enchanted World: Money, Finance and the World Crisis*. London: Verso.

LIEPITZ, A. 1988. *Mirages and Miracles: The crisis of global Fordism*. London: Verso.

LIEPITZ, A. 1992. *Towards a New Economic Order*. Oxford: Polity.

LOCAL GOVERNMENT MANAGEMENT BOARD. 1997. *Flexible Working in Local Authorities*. Luton: LGMB.

LOCKWOOD, D. 1958. *The Blackcoated Worker*. London: Allen and Unwin.

MANDELSON. P. *and* LIDDLE, R. 1996. *The Blair Revolution: Can New Labour Deliver?* London: Faber and Faber.

MARGETTS, H. 1997. 'The Automated State' in Massey, A., *Globalization and Marketization of Government Services*, Basingstoke: Macmillan.

McDowell, L. 1989. 'Gender divisions'. In Hamnett, C., McDowell, L. and Sarre, P. (eds) 1989. *The Changing Social Structure*, London: Sage.

McKenzie, R. *and* Silver, A. 1968. *Angels in Marble*. London: Heinemann.

Miles, I. 1989. *Information Technology and Information Society: Options for the future*. Programme on Information and Communication Technologies (PICT). Policy Research Paper No. 2. ESRC: London.

Miles, I., Rush, M., Turner, K. *and* Bessant, J. 1988. *Information Horizons: The long-term implications of new information technologies*. Aldershot: Edward Elgar.

Murray, C. 1994. *The Underclass: The crisis deepens*. London: Institute of Economic Affairs.

Murray, R. 1989. 'Fordism and post-Fordism'. In Hall, S. and Jaques, M. (eds), 1989, *New Times*, London: Lawrence and Wishart.

Naisbitt, J. 1982. *Megatrends*. NY: Warner Brothers.

Nilles, J. 1985. 'Teleworking from home'. In Forester, T. (ed.), *The Information Technology Revolution*, Oxford: Blackwell.

Nordlinger, E. 1967. *Working-Class Tories*. London: MacGibbon and Kee.

Parsons, T. 1966. *Societies*. Englewood Cliffs: Prentice Hall.

Piore, M. *and* Sabel, C. 1984. *The Second Industrial Divide*. NY: Basic Books.

Randall, V. 1987. *Women and Politics*. London: Macmillan.

Rees, T. 1992. *Women and the Labour Market*. London: Routledge.

Robertson, R. 1992. *Globalization: Social theory and global culture*. London: Sage.

Rose, M. 1988. *Industrial Behaviour*. London: Penguin.

Sabel, C. 1982. *Work and Politics: The division of labour in industry*. Cambridge: Cambridge University Press.

Saunders, P. 1978. 'Domestic property and social class'. *International Journal of Urban and Regional Research*. 2.

Saunders, P. 1984. 'Beyond housing classes'. *International Journal of Urban and Regional Research*. 8.

Scott, J. 1982. *The Upper Classes: Property and Privilege in Britain*. London: Macmillan.

Smart, B. 1993. *Postmodernity*. London: Routledge.

Snellen, I. 1994. 'ICT: a revolutionizing force in public administration'. *Information and the Public Sector*. Vol. 3. No. 3/4.

Social Trends 22. 1992. London: HMSO.

Social Trends 23. 1993. London: HMSO.

Social Trends 27. 1997. London: HMSO.

Taylor, F. W. 1947. *The Principles of Scientific Management*. NY: Harper and Row.

Taylor-Gooby, P. 1991. 'Attachment to the welfare state'. In Jowell, R. *et al*, 1991, *British Social Attitudes: The 8th report*. Aldershot: Dartmouth.

Thompson, G. 1989. 'Strategies for socialists'. *Economy and Society*. 18(4), November.

Toffler, A. 1980. *The Third Wave*. NY: Bantam Books.

TOURAINE, A. 1974. *The Post-Industrial Society: Tomorrow's social history*. London: Wildwood House.
TOWNSEND, P. 1979. *Poverty in the United Kingdom*. Harmondsworth: Penguin.
TURNER, B. (ed.) 1990. *Theories of Modernity and Post Modernity*. London: Sage.
WATER, M. 1995. *Globalization*. London: Routledge.
WEINER, M. 1981. *English Culture and the Decline of the Industrial Spirit 1850-1980*. Cambridge: Cambridge University Press.
WITZ, A. 1992. *Professions and Patriarchy*. London: Routledge.
WOOD, S. (ed.). 1989. *The Transformation of Work*. London: Unwin Hyman.

7 The state and employee relations

The state consists of those institutions and offices of state which provide the machinery of government. In Britain, these include:

- the cabinet and government ministers who comprise the executive authority of the state
- Parliament, which is a representative assembly that makes law, raises revenue and is a scrutinising body
- central government departments, governmental agencies, public bodies, public enterprises and the local authorities which administer governmental policies
- the state's agencies of law enforcement and adjudication such as the courts, tribunals and the police.

In contemporary capitalist states, like those of western Europe, North America and Australasia, because relations between employers and employees have become part of the public domain, the state is also an employee relations policy-maker. Public policy in this area relates to the ways in which the state seeks to influence the parties, processes and outcomes of employee relations. The state acts in a number of roles including:

- as an actor in the labour market and in the determination of wages and employment
- as a regulator of industrial conflict
- as an employer
- as a law maker and law enforcer.

It is these issues of state employment policy that are addressed in this chapter.

EARLY PUBLIC POLICY: *LAISSEZ-FAIRE* AND THE EMERGENCE OF COLLECTIVE *LAISSEZ-FAIRE*

An embryonic modern public policy on employee relations in Britain developed in the early nineteenth century and was rooted in the ideas of *laissez-faire*. *Laissez-faire* was based on the assumption that market decisions were preferable to political fiats in determining the allocation, distribution and exchange of economic resources. As applied to the free labour market, *laissez-faire* policy meant that market freedoms took precedence over political decisions in determining the procedural arrangements and the substantive outcomes of the wage bargaining process. The state's role was a minimalist one of providing a framework of contract law within which the primary parties to the wage–work bargain conducted themselves. Wage-fixing was regarded as a private matter, between the individual 'master' and individual 'servant', in which there was no role for the state or state institutions to intervene.

The state's attitude to trade unions in the early part of the nineteenth century was one of outright hostility and opposition. Unions were seen by both the state authorities and employers as 'criminal conspiracies' and illegitimate combinations acting 'in restraint of trade' (Pelling 1987). Unions, it was argued, distorted the workings of the free labour market and took away the freedoms of the primary parties to negotiate terms and conditions individually, in pursuit of their own advantage and self-interest. Accordingly, both Parliament and the judges declared unions to be criminal combinations. It was only after Parliament relaxed its outright ban on unions in 1824 and after emancipatory statutes were enacted – in 1859, 1871 and 1875 – that trade unions were relieved from the worst consequences of criminal liability. The judges then turned to the development of civil liability which, in turn, was only relieved by the Trade Disputes Act 1906 (see Chapter 4). This gave trade unions blanket immunity from liability in tort, provided immunities to individuals inducing breaches of contracts of employment and legitimised peaceful picketing.

By the early twentieth century, trade unions were well established as collective wage-bargaining agencies, covering a number of well-organised trades and industries (Clegg, Fox and Thompson 1964). But whilst Parliament had legitimised trade union activities, the state excluded itself from the joint wage-fixing process between autonomous employers and independent unions – just as it had done in the individual wage bargain between master and servant and employer and workman. Collective agreements were negotiated voluntarily between the secondary parties to employee relations, they were legally unenforceable and there was no legally binding, national minimum wage. A policy of collective *laissez-faire* and 'voluntarism' – embodied in the concepts of 'free collective bargaining' and the exclusion of the judges and the courts from relations between employers and trade unions – began to replace individual *laissez-faire* as the dominant ideology underpinning British employee relations. It was a 'public' policy which suited government, employers and trade unions alike.

Gradually, however, the policy of collective *laissez-faire* incorporated a series of incremental, interventionist policies by the state. First, the state found that it could not stand aside when standards of cleanliness, overcrowding, ventilation and working conditions in factories and mines, especially those affecting women and children, were unsatisfactory, dangerous to health and safety or offensive to 'public morality'. Accordingly, there was the piecemeal enactment of a series of factory and safety legislation, starting as early as the Factory Act 1833, which aimed to deal with these matters on a trade-by-trade and industry-by-industry basis.

Second, the state also found that it could not stand aside when disruptive industrial conflict appeared to threaten either social stability within the community or the established political order. In 1896, the Conciliation Act was passed, enabling provision to be made for the registration of boards of conciliation and arbitration and for the Board of Trade to inquire into the causes and circumstances of a trade dispute, or nominate a person to do so, or appoint conciliators or arbitrators to try to resolve it. This was followed by the Industrial Courts Act 1919 which extended the provisions for voluntary arbitration in Britain beyond those embodied in the 1896 Act (Wedderburn and Davies 1969). This effectively provided the legal basis for state intervention in the regulation of industrial conflict until ACAS was created by the Employment Protection Act 1975.

Third, the state also found itself having to intervene to protect the terms and conditions of employment of those in the labour market unable to look after themselves and who were likely to be exploited in the wage-bargaining process by unscrupulous, greedy employers. There was particular concern about the so called 'sweated trades' at the beginning of this century. Sweating was associated with home workers who had very low wage rates, excessive hours of work and insanitary working conditions. It was the Trade Boards Acts 1909 and 1918, followed by Wages Councils Acts after 1945, which sought to remedy these abuses. These Acts set up wage-fixing bodies, comprised of equal numbers of employers and worker representatives with independent members, to establish minimum, legally enforceable, hourly wage rates and other conditions of employment for workers in trades and industries where wages were low and there was no collective bargaining. The intentions were, initially, to protect the low paid and, later on, to encourage the development of collective bargaining in unorganised industries (Bayliss 1959).

THE EMPLOYEE RELATIONS CONSENSUS 1945-79

The interwar years, from 1919 to 1939, were a watershed in the development of public policy on employee relations, when deep economic recession and high unemployment resulted in hard labour markets, weakened trade unions and the strengthening of the right to manage in the workplace. However, with the steady growth in the scope and size of the state and of state activity in economic and social affairs in the twentieth century, government could no longer abstain from employee relations decision-making as it had done for much of the nineteenth century. This was especially the case during the First World War, the Second World War and after 1945. During the two world wars, for example, the state developed active labour market and wages policies. These were necessary to ensure that labour was allocated and directed to essential industries and occupations, to maximise industrial output and to gain the collaboration of the unions and their members in the war effort.

The state built on these policies in the postwar period, after 1945. Besides the policy of being a 'model' and 'good practice' employer (see below) and, after 1965, of developing a statutory floor of employment protection rights (see Chapter 4), Britain's postwar governments up to 1979, with the major exception of the Heath government 1971-74, tried to develop a consensus on employee relations policy, acceptable to employers, trade unions, their members and the wider community. This policy comprised three interrelated elements:

- maintaining full employment in the labour market
- searching for an incomes policy
- supporting voluntary collective bargaining.

The attempt to achieve an employee relations consensus incorporated a policy, where trade union power was strong, based on *free collective bargaining*. This was modified at other times by a policy of *bargained corporatism* (see Chapter 1), when the state authorities tried to constrain union wage-bargaining power, in conditions of full employment, by making concessions to the unions and their members on social policy, economic policy and employment law. An attempt was made to move away from a liberal state organised on free market principles to a more corporatist state. Corporatism is where the state authorities try to integrate the interests of capital, labour and government through centralised political institutions so that wage, economic and related policy issues are discussed centrally (Schmitter and Lehmbruch 1979).

Maintaining full employment

Market *laissez-faire* economic policies in the interwar years resulted in mass unemployment, widespread poverty and social deprivation (Taylor 1965). The popular demand at the end of the Second World War for 'full employment', which had been an economic reality from 1939 to 1945, was in part a reaction by the British people to the economic and social distress experienced by millions of them a decade earlier.

The rationale for full employment

With the extension of the political franchise and the gradual democratising of society during the twentieth century, the democratic imperative began to challenge the market imperative as the motivating influence on state policy in both economic affairs and employee relations. After the second world war, the democratic imperative became even more pressing.

One impact of the democratic imperative was from below. It arose from the fact that a generation of workers emerged – from 1945 till the mid-1970s – with the expectation that governments would pursue, amongst other measures, a labour market policy of full employment. The power of the ballot box now meant that the electorate could replace any government failing to deliver the policy objective of full employment and the extension of a comprehensive welfare state. This political fact was not lost on government ministers and public policy-makers in determining their economic, employment and labour market priorities after 1945.

A second impact of the democratic imperative immediately post-1945 was from above. This derived from the demands of certain political reformers, social theorists and democratic forces, especially within the Labour party. They attacked the five pre-war social evils of 'Want, Disease, Ignorance, Squalor and Idleness' and wanted 'full employment in a free society'. They not only accepted the principle but also wished to implement the policy of full employment in practice. Indeed, by the 1950s, full employment had become a bipartisan policy to which both major political parties, the Conservatives and Labour, were committed. The reasons for this bipartisanship were partly political. The realities of democratic politics meant that unless cabinets and ministers actively pursued full employment as a policy goal, neither they nor the government of which they were members would be re-elected at the next general election.

There were also intellectual reasons for governments to support the policy of full employment, since the arguments supporting the full employment agenda had been put and won earlier by individuals such as Keynes (1936) and Beveridge (1944). For Beveridge (1944: pages 15-16) unemployment was an 'evil'. But the greatest evil of all 'is not physical but moral, not the want it may bring but the hatred and fear which it breeds'. In his view, to look to individual employers to maintain aggregate demand and full employment was absurd. They were not within the power of employers to determine. 'They must therefore be undertaken by the State, under the supervision and pressure of democracy, applied through . . . Parliament.'

By full employment, Keynes, Beveridge and their supporters did not mean 'no unemployment' at all but unemployment being reduced to a minimum and for as short a time as possible. This required government stimulating aggregate demand in the economy (Chapter 4) and ensuring that those seeking jobs would be certain that they would be re-employed after only a short period of being out of work. To facilitate the transition between jobs, the unemployed would receive unemployment benefit whilst looking for new employment, and be provided with state funded employment services to assist them in doing this. Using combinations of fiscal and incomes policies, successive governments, both Conservative and Labour, fine-tuned the economy for some 30 years – 1945-75. This ensured, certainly until the early 1970s, that unemployment in Britain remained low at some 2-3 per cent of the working population or around 300,000 to 500,000 unemployed persons.

The consequences of full employment

The government's economic policy goal of full employment had three main consequences for employee relations. The first was that with the economy expanding, private sector employers were often faced with labour shortages, particularly of skilled, trained workers. Employers normally responded to this by bidding up wage rates, or by supplementing the earnings of their workforces locally, in order to compete in local labour markets with other employers. The result was 'wages drift' or a gap between nationally negotiated wage rates and what was actually earned by workers at workplace level.

Furthermore, when government dampened down the economy, because of inflationary pressures, employers would hoard labour, rather than lose it to other employers. This was in the expectation that when the economy began to take off again, they would have the necesssary labour resources to enable them to deal with rising demand for their products or services.

The second, related consequence of soft labour markets was the increased wage-bargaining power provided to trade union negotiators. Local labour market shortages also undermined the regulative authority of national, multi-employer collective agreements. This resulted in the spread of plant or workplace bargaining, led from the union side by local, autonomous shop stewards, accountable largely to their members at plant level (see below). They often bargained toughly with local managers and were generally more willing than full-time union officers to threaten and use industrial sanctions in the wage-bargaining process. In consequence, during the 1960s, there was an increase in the number of unconstitutional strikes (in breach of agreed negotiating procedures) and unofficial strikes (not supported by the unions nationally). Governments became increasingly concerned about the economic efficiency and efficacy of British collective bargaining arrangements, processes and outcomes.

A third, knock-on effect of tough wage bargaining in the private sector was that these wage increases provided the benchmarks by which the public sector unions made their wage claims to the employers. This provided governments with a series of dilemmas. Resisting such wage claims could result in industrial conflict amongst the state's workforce, damage to the state's reputation as a fair employer or the loss of staff to the private sector. On the other hand, conceding such claims could result in: large rises in public spending, and therefore in taxation and/or public borrowing; wage-price-wage inflation; and state employers being seen as weak, ineffective parties in the wage-bargaining process, providing a bad model for private sector employers to follow.

Searching for an incomes policy

The potentially inflationary effects of collective bargaining in conditions of full employment led postwar governments to search for an industrial consensus on the levels of annual wage increases compatible with price stability, economic growth and balance-of-payments equilibrium. The first attempt was that of the Labour government in 1948, following an economic crisis during summer 1947. It issued a White Paper (Cmd 7321, 1948) arguing for no general increase in money incomes, unless justified by labour shortages. The TUC, though initially sceptical, gave the policy its qualified approval, but its annual Congress in 1949 voted for an end to wage restraint and the policy ceased to have effect during 1950. The last attempt at an agreed incomes policy was at the beginning of 1979. The Labour government and the TUC published a joint statement which, whilst placing no limits on wage increases, expressed a joint commitment to reduce inflation to the level of Britain's overseas competitors over the following three years.

With the return to power of a Conservative government, led by Margaret Thatcher, in May 1979, the policy lapsed.

Between 1950 and 1979, there were over 20 attempts to create a wage-bargaining consensus acceptable to employers and unions (ACAS 1980). Some were unilaterally initiated and imposed by government for given periods such as between 1966 and 1969 and, under the Counter Inflation Act 1972, between 1972 and 1974. Other attempts, for example in the mid-1960s, sought the voluntary support both of the unions, through the TUC, and of the employers, through the CBI. Yet others, such as the 'social contracts' between the Labour government and the TUC between summer 1975 and August 1977, were jointly monitored, government-union attempts at limiting wage increases for limited periods.

The nub of the incomes policy issue was trying to get a central agreement on annual wage increases. This involved developing a wages consensus amongst government, the unions and the employers, by which the economic outcomes of voluntary collective bargaining (increasingly conducted at company and factory levels in the private sector) would be broadly in line with annual increases in national productivity and output.

If wage negotiators could not be persuaded to agree to limit their members' money wage increases in line with rises in real productivity at factory level, this would have a number of effects. First, private sector employers which conceded such wage rises would have to increase their product prices to remain profitable. This would contribute to wage-price or cost-push inflation. Second, these wage increases, in turn, would provide benchmarks for other wage bargainers to follow in the private sector, especially those operating in the same external labour markets. Unless the outcomes of these wage bargains were in line with productivity increases, these too would add to wage-price inflation. Third, the rates of increase in private sector wages provided reference points for union negotiators in the public sector. Where these were conceded, without productivity strings being attached, these in turn would fuel wage-cost inflation, creating demands for even higher wage increases by wage bargainers in the next pay round.

In these circumstances, there were few incentives for union wage bargainers to restrain their members' wage claims for any substantial period. If union leaders failed to satisfy their members' wage expectations, their members might take unofficial industrial action anyway. Employers, too, were unlikely to be convinced of the merits of wage restraint by resisting the wage demands of their unionised workforces. They would generally want to avoid expensive and disruptive industrial action and would also be concerned that they might lose some of their labour force, if their company's wages were uncompetitive with those of other employers. And in any case, they were able to pass on rises in wages costs to their customers, in the form of higher product prices, in soft product markets. The only set of employers likely to resist excessive wage claims were public sector ones. They needed to set examples to the private sector and to keep public spending under control but they employed only a minority of the labour force.

It is clear, in retrospect, that in the period of the employee relations consensus, the one area of public policy where consensus proved to be elusive was in constraining wage bargaining 'in the national interest'. After 1965, the efforts were virtually continuous and a number of approaches were tried. These included voluntary and statutory pay norms (see Chapter 4) but none were successful in restraining wage increases for any length of time. With strong trade unions operating in conditions of full employment, various attempts by governments to adopt a policy of 'bargained corporatism' (see Chapter 1) failed to persuade union leaders, and their members, to accept any variant of public wage policy other than that of 'voluntary collective bargaining'. When national pay guidelines existed, national union leaders lacked the authority and control to get local shop stewards and full-time officers to comply with pay norms, other than in the short term. Unlike the Swedish and German experiences at this time, attempts at designing effective incomes policies in Britain failed miserably to deliver what was intended.

Supporting voluntary collective bargaining

State support for voluntary collective bargaining, or collective laissez-faire, as a process for determining the outcomes of the market relations between employers and employees, can be traced back to the late nineteenth century. Indeed the final report of the Royal Commission on Labour Laws (1894) had supported the growth of strong, voluntary organisations of employers and employees, industry-level collective bargaining and a role for government in helping to minimise and settle industrial disputes. It was during the period 1945-79 that this policy reached its apotheosis.

Whitleyism

The Whitley Committee (1916–18) reinforced state support for voluntary collective bargaining as a method of conducting employee relations. During the First World War there had been a great expansion, reorganisation and flexibility expected in manufacturing industry, in response to the demands of the war economy. There had been a significant growth in the numbers and powers of local shop stewards who had challenged the authority of full-time union leaders, had used local bargaining to undermine national wage agreements and had made demands for 'workers' control' of industries and factories.

In the light of these pressures for change, the Committee recommended the establishment of standing joint councils of voluntary employers' associations and union organisations at industry, district and workplace levels. Whilst power was to be concentrated at national level, it was recommended that the machinery should concern itself with a wide range of issues. These included:

- determining wages
- agreeing terms of employment
- promoting efficiency
- encouraging 'joint co-operation' between employers and workers at all levels.

To encourage the development of collective bargaining, the Committee further recommended the setting up of a permanent, voluntary arbitration body and inquiry machinery (Farnham 1978).

In the interwar years, Whitley councils were established in a number of private and public industries. These included the civil service, electricity, gas, building and printing – largely where collective bargaining had not existed previously (Charles 1973). With the encouragement of the Ministry of Labour and National Service, further joint industrial councils, or similar bodies, were established or re-established in the period immediately following the second world war. These included the NHS, local government, the railways and the water supply industry. Furthermore, with full employment, steady economic growth and rising union membership, the numbers of workers whose terms and conditions of employment were directly determined by collective bargaining increased, mainly through industry-level, multi-employer bargaining. By the mid-1960s, the Ministry of Labour (1965) estimated that upwards of 18 million employees, out of a workforce of 24 million, had their terms and conditions of employment determined by voluntary collective bargaining or statutory wage-fixing machinery.

The Donovan Commission

Between 1965 and 1968, the Royal Commission on Trade Unions and Employers' Associations (the Donovan Commission) undertook an examination of British employee relations, at a time when collective bargaining was being conducted in conditions of full employment and strong union bargaining power. Its report epitomised the support that the liberal state wished to give to voluntary collective bargaining. It concluded (Donovan 1968: page 50) that:

> Collective bargaining is the best method of conducting industrial relations. There is therefore wide scope in Britain for extending both the subject matter of collective bargaining and the number of workers covered by collective agreements.

Donovan's analysis concentrated on what was happening in private manufacturing industry. The Commission identified the central defects in British employee relations at that time as the disorder in employer-union relations, pay structures and collective bargaining procedures within factories. This was the result of the conflict between formal, industry-wide bargaining at multi-employer level and informal, factory bargaining at company or plant level. The formal system purported to settle the terms and conditions of employment of workers. But in practice it was fragmented, competitive, wage bargaining within factories between managers and shop stewards, outside the control of employers' associations and national trade unions, which determined actual earnings. This bargaining provided local additions to national wage rates, such as piecework, bonus and overtime payments. In the Commission's view, moreover, companies lacked effective internal procedural arrangements to curtail unofficial and unconstitutional industrial action by their workforces.

The Commission's main recommendations (pages 262-64) for the reform of collective bargaining were:

- collective agreements should be developed within factories to regulate actual pay and procedural matters at this level, whilst industry-wide agreements should be limited to those matters which they could effectively regulate
- at corporate level, boards of directors should develop comprehensive collective bargaining machinery and joint procedures for the settlement of grievances, discipline, redundancy and related issues
- companies with over 5,000 employees, including the public sector, should be required to register their procedural agreements with the Department of Employment and Productivity
- a Commission on Industrial Relations (CIR) should be established which (a) would investigate and report on problems arising out of the registration of procedural agreements and (b) would consider problems referred to it concerning companies not large enough to be covered by the registration arrangements.

The Royal Commission also argued that new measures were needed to encourage the extension of collective bargaining in Britain. Its main recommendations here were:

- any stipulation in a contract of employment that an employee was not to belong to a trade union should be void in law
- the CIR should deal with problems of trade union recognition, where employers refused to negotiate with unions
- wages councils legislation should be amended to encourage the development of voluntary collective bargaining machinery
- legislation under which an employer was required to observe relevant terms and conditions for an industry should be amended
- unilateral arbitration should be available on a selective basis, where it could contribute to the growth or maintenance of sound collective bargaining machinery.

Donovan's prescriptions for change epitomised the state's support for the development of voluntary collective bargaining in Britain and for extending its scope. Whilst voluntary reform proceeded on a piecemeal basis after Donovan, its proposed programme of legislation to promote voluntary collective bargaining was not acted upon immediately. This was because the Labour government that had established the Commission lost the general election of 1970 and, even before then, it had difficulty getting its post-Donovan White Paper accepted by the TUC and Parliamentary Labour Party (Jenkins 1970). The Heath government which replaced it was committed to major reforms of the law on employee relations. Although the

Industrial Relations Act 1971 claimed to promote the principle of collective bargaining freely conducted between workers' organisations and employers, in fact, it sought to extend the influence of the law on employer and union behaviour but markedly failed to do so (Weekes *et al* 1975). Its principles challenged those of the employee relations consensus and, largely as a result of this, the vast majority of employers and unions ignored the Industrial Relations Act 1971. They continued to conduct their employee relationships as they always had done, through voluntary collective bargaining.

The Employment Protection Act 1975

With the Labour party re-elected to office in 1974, state support for the reform and extension of voluntary collective bargaining continued and, in retrospect, reached its highest point. It was facilitated by the Employment Protection Act (EPA) 1975, the Employment Protection (Consolidation) Act (EPCA) 1978 and related legislation. Part I of the EPA 1975 focused on the machinery for promoting the improvement of employee relations, within which ACAS had a pivotal role, whilst the EPCA 1978 consolidated the employment protection rights of individual employees, including those of trade unionists. In establishing ACAS, the EPA 1975, section 1(1), stated:

> [ACAS] shall be charged with the general duty of promoting the improvement of industrial relations, and in particular of encouraging the extension of collective bargaining and the development and, where necessary, reform of collective bargaining machinery.

The legislation drafted to do this was aimed at:

- *Encouraging trade union membership and activities.* Employees were given statutory protection from being prevented or deterred by employers from joining or taking part in the activities of an independent union or being compelled to join a non-independent union. Where employers infringed these provisions, employees had the right to go to an industrial tribunal.
- *Providing statutory time off work for those involved in trade union duties.* Officials of independent, recognised trade unions were given the right to time off work with pay for undertaking certain union duties, such as approved training, and time off without pay for certain union activities. Where these rights were infringed by employers, individuals could make a claim to an industrial tribunal.
- *Facilitating trade union recognition by employers.* Under the Section 11 procedure of the EPA 1975 (repealed by the Employment Act 1980), independent trade unions could approach ACAS where an employer refused to recognise them. It was ACAS's duty to examine the issue, consult with the parties, conduct inquiries and to report its findings. Where ACAS recommended recognition and an employer refused to comply with it, the Central Arbitration Committee (CAC) could make an award on terms and conditions, which became incorporated as implied terms in the

contracts of employment of individual workers. This was a form of compulsory arbitration but there was no legal enforcement of union recognition.

- *Obliging employers to consult with and provide information to recognised independent unions.* Independent recognised trade unions were provided with statutory rights to be consulted on proposed collective redundancies and occupational pensions. They were also entitled to be provided with information by employers where it would be in accordance with good practice to disclose or where it would assist in the conduct of collective bargaining. There was, additionally, a statutory duty on employers to consult with independent recognised unions on health and safety matters. These included: the appointment of safety representatives; the appointment of safety committees; and the provision of information to safety representatives.
- *Providing legal procedures for extending terms and conditions of employment where unions were not recognised.* Schedule 11 of the EPA 1975 (repealed by the Employment Act 1980) enabled claims to be made to ACAS by independent unions (or employers' associations) that an employer was observing terms and conditions of employment less favourable than the recognised terms and conditions or, where there were no recognised terms and conditions, less favourable than the general level in any trade, industry or district. Failing settlement by ACAS, the CAC, if it found the claim to be well founded, could make an award for the appropriate terms and conditions to be observed as implied terms in the contracts of employment of workers. This too was a form of compulsory arbitration.

PUBLIC POLICY 1979-97: THE CHALLENGE TO COLLECTIVE *LAISSEZ-FAIRE*

Between 1979 and 1997, successive Conservative governments rejected Keynesian economic theory and Beveridge social welfare principles (see Chapter 4). This had considerable implications for public policy on employee relations, which shifted from one focused on *voluntary collective bargaining*, in conditions of full employment and strong trade unions (with attempts at *bargained corporatism* through 'social contracts') to a policy of neo-*laissez-faire*. It was a policy rooted in market liberal economic principles and weak trade unions (see Chapter 1).

The *employee relations consensus* emphasised:

- state intervention in the labour market
- state support for employee relations collectivism, whilst using the law as a 'prop' to promote collective bargaining
- excluding the courts and the judges from intervening in the internal affairs of trade unions and the regulation of industrial conflict.

Neo-*laissez-faire*, in contrast, emphasised:

- deregulating the labour market
- individualising employee relations, with the legal props to collective bargaining being loosened or removed and legal restrictions on trade unions being enacted
- depoliticising the trade unions.

The policy instruments used included: legislation, economic measures, government example in its own spheres of responsibility, the creation of the Commission for the Rights of Trade Union Members (Farnham 1990), and the appointment of a Commissioner for Protection Against Unlawful Industrial Action.

The theoretical and moral underpinnings of economic, social and employee relations policy after 1979 were rooted in market economics and liberal individualism, or 'market liberalism'. Market economics assumes that supply and demand in the market place, acting through the price mechanism, are preferable to political rationing by politicians in deciding what to produce in an economy, how to produce it and how goods and services are to be distributed amongst the population. Liberal individualism pinpoints the individual, not interest groups or pressure groups, as the prime decision-making authority, with the freedoms and natural rights of the individual being inalienable and non-negotiable. Free markets lead to economic efficiency and equity, it is argued, whilst free-thinking individuals in doing what is best for themselves maximise economic welfare generally.

The market economic model makes three assumptions about the relationship of the market to the individual:

- that individuals act rationally in pursuing their own self-interest in the market place
- that the free play of impersonal, decentralised market forces is the best way of increasing the prosperity and welfare of the individual and of the wider community
- that the individual consumer is sovereign in the market place because of freedom of consumer choice and market competition amongst producers.

For market liberals, because the individual is central to economic decision-making, and because it is assumed that he or she knows what is best for him or herself, the role of government is limited to providing an economic and constitutional framework for individuals to pursue their own self-interest. The state intervenes only to protect the individual's rights to property, liberty and access to free markets. Market liberal – or neo-*laissez-faire* – economic, social and employee relations policy, in short, aims at optimising market efficiency, minimising government intervention in private affairs and protecting individual rights against vested interests.

Deregulating the labour market

There is some debate whether there is 'a' labour market in Britain or a series of 'segmented' labour markets. Market liberal macro-economists emphasise the contexts of the general labour market, whilst market liberal micro-economists try to explain how rational agents in disaggregated labour markets produce different responses to changes in wage levels and unemployment. The macro-economists focus on how factors independent of the labour market – such as inflation, the exchange rate and mortgage interest tax relief – are likely to influence wages and unemployment; the micro-economists try to evaluate the influence of institutional factors affecting them. To simplify the market liberal analysis, this section focuses on the micro-issues of labour market policy, rather than the macro-issues.

The micro-issues

Labour market deregulation was a central plank of government policy from 1979. Given that labour services are commodities which are bought and sold by rational employers and rational workers in the market place, market liberals argue that levels of wages and employment are determined by the forces of supply and demand in the market. In a free labour market, the quantity of labour supplied equals the quantity demanded at the market wage. Unemployment is symptomatic of labour market rigidity and means that the price of labour is too high, so that wages need to be adjusted downwards if the labour market is to clear. Where there are barriers to a freely operating labour market, it is necessary to deregulate it to make it more competitive. This, it is argued, is in the interests of economic efficiency and individual freedom.

One cause of unemployment and labour market rigidity identified by market liberal economists is institutional. Where, for example, employers have to take account of the costs of compensation for unfair dismissal, they are deterred, it is claimed, from increasing demand for new employees. Extending employment protection rights thus has the overall effect of bringing about a fall in labour demand and increasing unemployment. Second, fiscal factors, such as changes in taxation and social security, are also claimed to increase unemployment. This is because higher taxes reduce labour supply, whilst higher social security payments result in people being unemployed longer, with more time being spent in job searches.

A third cause of unemployment, in the view of market liberals, is collective action by workers organised into trade unions. Unionised workers are viewed as restricting labour supply and limiting access to jobs for non-union workers who are likely to drive wage rates down. A rise in demand for unionised labour results in higher wages but not in higher employment, because the supply of labour is fixed in the short term. Indeed, market liberals argue that trade unions actually contribute to higher unemployment because they restrict labour supply, whilst union wage rates do not reflect changes in labour supply or labour demand. More than that, the unionised sector is the benchmark for the whole economy, setting wage norms for other workers to follow. In the non-unionised sector, in contrast, labour supply is seen as being responsive to changes in wage rates. And an increase in labour demand there will be reflected in both higher wages and higher levels of employment.

The policy prescriptions

According to market liberals, government can reform and deregulate the labour market by improving the supply side of the market. It can do this in four ways. First, it can reduce the time spent unemployed and in job searches by reducing the rates of social security payments. Second, government can increase labour supply by reducing personal taxation rates. These two measures aim to increase incentives to work, so that more people make themselves available for employment and join the labour market. A third measure is removing wages councils and minimum wages legislation, since these are likely to increase the price of labour to employers thus resulting in a fall in labour demand. The fourth way in which government can act is by reforming trade union immunities. The aim here is to make it more difficult for trade unions to take lawful industrial action, without incurring severe financial costs in doing so. All these measures were, to varying degrees, adopted by Conservative governments during the 1980s and 1990s by a series of legislative and economic initiatives.

Individualising employee relations

The necessary conditions for employee relations collectivism are:

- freedom of association for workers to join trade unions
- 'free' trade unions independent of employers and the state
- employer recognition of trade unions
- bargaining in good faith.

Between 1979 and 1997, one plank of public policy aimed at the decollectivisation of employee relations, with employers being encouraged to use more individualist methods of determining and implementing the wage-work bargain. This policy, stemming from the precepts of market liberalism, took three main forms, with government attempting to:

- weaken union organisation
- strengthen the right to manage
- discourage union militancy.

Weakening union organisation

Whilst freedom of association and independent trade unions continued to exist in Britain, union organisation was weakened dramatically after 1979 in at least three respects. First, union density, normally expressed as the percentage of the potential workforce who are union members, fell drastically, especially in the private sector (see Chapter 8). This was largely as a result of structural reorganisation of the economy and high levels of unemployment during the 1980s and 1990s (Daniel and Millward 1983; Millward and Stevens 1986; Millward *et al* 1992). Smaller employment units and the reduction in size of the manufacturing sector adversely affected union organisation. High unemployment also weakened union bargaining power with employers and made the retention of union members more problematic and the recruitment of new members a more difficult task for union organisers (Martin 1992).

Second, as a result of a series of changes in employment law in the 1980s and 1990s, closed shop agreements, or union membership agreements (UMAs), between employers and trade unions were made unlawful. A UMA is any arrangement by which employees are required to be members of a union as a condition of employment. Pre-entry closed shops are where jobs are restricted to individuals who are already members of the appropriate union, whilst post-entry closed shops require employees to join a specified union within a set period of starting work. Where individuals claim that their legal right not to belong to a union is infringed, they have a right to make an application to an industrial tribunal and seek compensation.

Outlawing the closed shop weakened union organisation. UMAs covered some quarter of the employed workforce in the late 1970s (Dunn and Gennard 1984). Although it is difficult to calculate the extent of the closed shop currently, and despite the continuance of some informal closed shop arrangements, current legislation both ended the enforcement of the practice and debilitated union organisation.

Third, other legal measures, originally incorporated in the Employment Act (EA) 1988 and the Trade Union Act (TUA) 1984 and now embodied in the Trade Union and Labour Relations (Consolidation) Act (TULRCA) 1992, as amended, provided rights for union members to elect union executive committees and union leaders by postal ballot, at least once every five years. These legislative changes in union election procedures, outlined in a Green Paper in 1983, stemmed from the government's desire to ensure that trade union members are truly representative of their memberships. Because the unions had not reformed themselves voluntarily, the government claimed that it 'had reluctantly come to the conclusion that some legislative intervention is necessary' (Department of Employment 1983: page 16). Another interpretation of these provisions, however, is that they were seen by government as a further means of weakening collective links amongst trade unionists, and between union members and the union, thus loosening union cohesion and collective solidarity (see Chapter 8).

Strengthening the right to manage

The right to manage is that area of corporate decision-making which management considers to be its alone and is not constrained by collective bargaining or the law (see Chapter 3). The boundaries of the right to manage are the interface between unilateral management control and the ability of employees, individually or collectively, to influence or counterbalance those decisions most affecting their working lives. Given government commitment to the enterprise culture and the free market economy between 1979 and 1997, one policy goal was to strengthen the right to manage. Its rationale was to provide managers, in both the private and public sectors, with more autonomy in organisational decision-making and to restrict union activity and collective action. It was aimed at enabling employers to react more swiftly to changing product markets, to obtain greater flexibility from their human resources and to have more control over worker productivity. Companies and public sector organisations, in turn, would then become more efficient, effective and competitive, thus boosting the economy, economic growth and employment.

The pressure for employers to recognise unions for collective bargaining purposes was considerably weakened after 1979. One of the first measures taken by the government was to repeal, in the EA 1980, the Section 11 procedures embodied in the Employment Protection Act (EPA) 1975. This means that ACAS no longer has a statutory duty to investigate and make recommendations on union recognition. ACAS's only remaining duty is to conciliate on trade union recognition claims, on a voluntary basis. The number of requests for this has fallen dramatically in the past two decades (ACAS Annual Reports).

The powers of wages councils to set wage rates for those aged under 21 and other conditions were abolished by the Wages Act 1986, which limited wages councils to setting minimum adult hourly rates and overtime rates. Subsequently, the Trade Union Reform and Employment Rights Act 1993 abolished the remaining 26 wages councils completely. Fair Wages Resolutions (see below) were rescinded and the comparable terms and conditions procedure – Schedule 11 of the EPA 1975 – repealed. Where 10-99 employees are to be made redundant, the minimum period for trade union consultation has been reduced. Further, union-only or union recognition clauses in commercial contracts are now void in law. It is also unlawful to discriminate against or victimise contractors on these grounds.

All the above public policy changes enabled employers to be more flexible and autonomous in determining the terms, conditions and working arrangements of their employees. The emphasis was on strengthening the right to manage, at the expense of employee and union rights, and weakening the legal props to collective bargaining.

Discouraging union militancy

Changes in collective labour law by Conservative governments during the 1980s and 1990s were aimed at reducing union ability to take part in lawful trade disputes (see Chapter 4). Legal immunities, the legal definition of a trade dispute and industrial action ballots are at the root of the issue. Where employees take industrial action, they are normally in breach of their contracts of employment. Under common law, it is unlawful to induce people to break a contract, to interfere with the performance of a contract or to threaten to do so. Without legal immunities, unions and their officers could face legal action for inducing breaches of contract when organising industrial action. Legal immunities provide protections for unions and individuals so that they cannot be sued for damages for inducing breaches of contract when furthering industrial action in certain circumstances (see Chapter 1). The Employment Acts 1980 and 1982, however, withdrew immunities from certain types of industrial action, opening up the possibility of unions and individuals having injunctions issued against them, or being sued, where their actions are unlawful. These legal provisions are now incorporated in the TULRCA 1992.

The law also provides that those organising industrial action are only protected when acting 'in contemplation or furtherance of a trade dispute'. To remain within the law, those calling industrial action must be able to show that there is a dispute and that the action is in support of it. Lawful disputes are those between workers and their own employers and must be concerned with matters 'wholly or mainly' connected with terms and conditions, negotiating machinery and so on. The following types of disputes are now *unlawful*:

- inter-union disputes
- 'political' disputes
- disputes relating to matters occurring overseas
- disputes with employers not recognising unions or employing non-union labour
- 'secondary' or 'sympathy' disputes between workers and employers other than their own.

Where unions act unlawfully, they lose their legal immunity (see Chapter 11).

Unions are also required to ballot union members involved in a trade dispute, before authorising the action. Under the TUA 1984 (now incorporated in the TULRCA 1992), it became a condition of legal immunity that, before organising industrial action, the union holds a secret ballot in which all those about to take the action are entitled to vote. The action is only lawful where a majority of those voting support it. The EA 1988 went further by providing union members with the right to apply to the courts for an order restraining their union from inducing them to take industrial action without a properly conducted ballot. The Trade Union Reform and Employment Rights Act 1993 requires unions to give seven days' notice to the employer of their intention to hold an industrial action ballot, which must normally be a full postal ballot and be independently scrutinised. Where an unlawful act is authorised by a union official, or by a committee to which such officials report, the union is liable unless it disowns the unlawful act in writing.

The effect of removing legal immunities from certain industrial action is to provide those damaged by the action, such as employers or union members, with the right to take civil proceedings against the union, or in some cases the individual, responsible. The remedies are:

- seeking an injunction to prevent or stop the action
- claiming damages from the union for conducting unlawful action.

Under the TULRCA 1992 and the Trade Union Reform and Employment Rights Act 1993, union members have the statutory right not to be unjustifiably disciplined by their union. It specifies the actions that count as discipline and the conduct for which discipline is justifiable. Conduct incurring unjustifiable discipline for union members includes:

- refusing to take part in balloted industrial action
- crossing a picket line
- refusing to pay a levy for supporting a strike or other industrial action
- failing to agree or withdrawing from an agreement with an employer regarding deductions of union dues
- working or proposing to work with members of another union or with non-union members
- working or proposing to work for an employer who employs non-union members or members of another union.

Depoliticising trade unions

Union political activity, though difficult to define in practice, has always been a sensitive and ambivalent issue for the Conservative Party to deal with. On the one hand, the Conservatives want the votes of trade union members in local, national and European elections. On the other hand, there are many in the Conservative Party who are distinctly hostile to unions on not only political but also economic grounds. The political objections of many Conservatives to the trade unions are to the close political affiliations of some unions to the Labour Party. Trade unions affiliate members to the Labour Party, support Labour Members of Parliament financially and participate in Labour Party decision-making. The economic objections of many Conservatives to the trade unions are that they distort the working of the free labour market, inhibit economic efficiency and weaken management authority in the workplace.

The underlying assumption of Conservative public policy-makers in seeking to depoliticise the trade unions is that the economic and political roles of trade unions can be dissociated. This analysis accepts the unions' economic role as legitimate, up to a point, but asserts that their political role needs to be circumscribed, by law. This is necessary, market liberals argue, on the grounds that it makes politicians democratically accountable to their constituents, not to special interest groups such as trade unions, and second that the unions can concentrate on their more rightful and more legitimate role of protecting their member's employment interests in the labour market. Depoliticising the unions could also facilitate an ideological change on the part of the unions and their members, enabling them to identify more closely with the goals of a dynamic effective capitalism, operating in a competitive enterprise culture.

Political strikes

The definition of a trade dispute in the TULRCA 1992 now requires trade disputes to 'relate wholly or mainly to' the subjects listed. This raises doubts about the lawfulness of any dispute having political elements. This change in the legal definition of a trade dispute, in seeking to exclude those with a political element, effectively restricts some types of actions aimed at defending or improving terms and conditions of employment. An example is where workers decide to take industrial action in protest at their industry or organisation being privatised.

Political fund review ballots

The TULRCA 1992, as amended, requires unions with 'political objects' and political funds, which are normally used to support the Labour Party and to conduct political campaigns, to ballot their members, at least once every 10 years, on whether they wish their union to continue to spend money on political matters. Ballots must be by post and are subject to independent scutiny. The scrutineer has access to a union's membership register and must inspect the register or a relevant copy where it is felt appropriate to do so. The distribution, counting and storage of voting papers must be undertaken by independent scrutiny. If these ballots are not held, the authority to spend money on political objects lapses.

Privatisation

This was a leading policy initiative of the Thatcher and Major administrations. Privatising substantial parts of the public sector, and contracting out certain services in public sector organisations, has transferred large numbers of workers out of public employment (see below). This means that government is no longer their employer. These businesses cannot therefore call upon government to increase public spending to finance their wage settlements with their employees. They are now required to have regard to market and financial considerations when responding to terms and conditions claims. This takes wage determination in these sectors out of politics, thus in effect depoliticising their wage bargaining process.

Settling trade disputes

Between 1979 and 1997, successive Conservative governments publicly rejected any role in industrial peacekeeping. Government ministers abstained from directly intervening, by conciliating or mediating, in intractable trade disputes, even in the public sector, no matter how bitter the disputes were. This approach assumed that dispute resolution should be left to the direct employers and trade unions to settle themselves. The outcome could then be determined by strong employers relying on market forces to generate financially prudent wage settlements and a sense of economic reality amongst the workforce and their union leaders in the wage bargaining process.

Rejecting corporatism

The Conservative governments' public policy after 1979 resulted in exclusion of the TUC from industrial policy-making. Governments refused to consult directly with the TUC on economic, employment or social policy decisions and they have abandoned top-level meetings with TUC officials. A succession of government Green Papers on trade union law reform, for example, was not used for consultative purposes but as draft legislation which was enacted subsequently in virtually the form in which it had been presented. Indeed, the only remaining corporatist body, the National Economic Development Council, was formally wound up in 1991.

NEW LABOUR, NEW DEAL FOR PEOPLE AT WORK?

Shortly after being elected by a landslide majority in the general election of 1997, New Labour's policy on employee relations was, to some extent, indeterminate. The central issue was to what extent was it likely to be a continuation of existing policy, a return to Labour's traditional policy or a 'new' policy in its own right? By autumn 1997, the exact direction of New Labour's policy was still not apparent but there were indicators of where the party was going in terms of a 'new deal' on employee relations and regulation of the employment relationship. In essence, its policy direction appeared to be moving away from not only its former voluntary, collectivist approach (and the bargained corporatist model) but also the Conservative's anti-union, neo-laissez-faire approach.

In outline, New Labour is shifting to a policy which appears to be based on three fundamental pillars: encouraging employment flexibility, supporting partnership at work, and protecting minimum employment standards. The main policy instruments to be used in furthering its objectives are legal enactment and signing up to the Social Chapter. New Labour's, 'new deal' on employee relations, therefore, appears to be incorporating support for a flexible labour market, underpinned by a limited range of legal protections at work, largely for individuals but, to a lesser degree, for trade unions also.

Encouraging employment flexibility

The starting-point for New Labour's new employment policy (Labour Party 1997: page 150) is that healthy profits are 'an essential motor of a dynamic market economy'. But these depend on 'quality products, innovative entrepreneurs and skilled employees'. Since many fundamentals of the British economy remain weak – such as low pay, low skills and low-quality jobs – there is no future, in New Labour's view, in Britain's following this pathway, since she cannot compete with countries paying 'a tenth or a hundredth of British wages' in free market economies. Instead Britain 'needs to win on higher quality, skill, innovation and reliability'. Labour therefore wants British and inward investors to find the UK an attractive and profitable place in which to do business.

Accordingly, New Labour 'believes in a flexible labour market that serves employers and employees alike'. But, New Labour argues, flexibility is not enough; what is needed is '*flexibility plus*':

- *plus* higher skills and higher standards in our schools and colleges
- *plus* policies to ensure economic stability
- *plus* partnership with business to raise investment in infrastructure, science and research to back small firms
- *plus* new leadership from Britain to reform Europe, in place of the ... policy of drift and disengagement from our largest market
- *plus* guaranteeing Britain's membership of the single market – indeed opening up further markets inside and outside the EU – making Britain an attractive place to do business in
- *plus* minimum standards of fair treatment, including a national minimum wage
- *plus* an imaginative welfare-to-work programme to put the long-term unemployed back to work and to cut social security costs.

To sustain economic opportunity and prosperity in a global economy, therefore, New Labour argues that Britain needs to use the talents of its workforce fully. With leading-edge companies recognising that high performance is directly associated with maximising the potential of every employee, New Labour believes that 'the way to achieve this is through trust, consultation, teamworking and offering people [at work] real security' and 'a highly educated and skilled workforce able to succeed in the labour market'. Labour further 'recognises [that] competitive success is achieved through partnership between employers and employees', not confrontation, with business success depending upon avoiding rigidity in labour market regulation and 'promoting the flexibility we require' (Labour Party 1997b: page 1). As a result of this approach:

> There will be no blanket repeal of the main elements of the 1980s' legislation. What there will be is a new deal for people at work, which will avoid rigidity but give people a decent threshold of fair treatment, recognising that social partnership is at the heart of the successful company of the future.

New Labour thus believes that the labour market of the 1990s and 2000s, with its growing emphasis on the importance of flexibility, can bring positive, fresh opportunities for people at work in ways which better suit their own needs. This means, for example, that they can combine atypical work with caring for children or elderly relatives, or they can learn new skills and take on new responsibilities. New Labour supports, too, the Social Chapter of the EU and seeks to deploy its influence in Europe to ensure that it develops so as to promote employability and competitiveness, not inflexibility.

Supporting partnership at work

New Labour's enthusiasm for partnership at work focuses on two key areas: partnership between employers and employees and partnership between employers and unions. As its 1997 manifesto puts it (Labour Party 1997a: page 17):

> The best companies recognise their employees as partners in the enterprise. Employees whose conditions are good are more committed to their companies and are more productive. Many unions and employers are embracing partnership in place of conflict.

The implications of adopting this approach to the employment relationship are, first, that the Labour government is keen to encourage a variety of forms of partnership and enterprise, by spreading ownership and encouraging more employees to become owners through employee share ownership plans and co-operatives. Second, it is assumed that by promoting more conflict-free employer-union relations, the need for damaging and costly strikes and other forms of industrial action can be avoided.

Incorporated within its 'partnership at work' perspective is New Labour's commitment to supporting the right of unionised workers to have their union recognised by non-union employers who refuse recognition. Whilst up to 85 of Britain's top 100 companies negotiate pay and conditions with unions, the proportion of workplaces where unions are recognised has fallen from around two-thirds in 1979 to under 40 per cent in the mid-1990s. Amongst firms refusing union recognition are Marks & Spencer, IBM, McDonalds, Honda, United Utilities and the Body Shop. Labour's proposal is that 'the union should be recognised' where 'a majority of the relevant workforce vote in a ballot for the union to represent them' (Labour Party 1997a: page 17). This, it believes, will promote stable and orderly employee relations. At the time of writing, the exact form that this legal recognition procedure will take is unknown but Labour has said that there will be full consultation on the most effective means of implementing this proposal.

Protecting minimum employment standards

New Labour also argues (page 17) that 'there must be minimum standards for the individual at work, including a minimum wage, within a flexible labour market.' With weakened trade unions, a changing labour market and a shift to service-sector employment, the most effective way in which minimum standards of employment practice can be enforced is through the law. New Labour wants a sensible balance in employment law, where 'rights and duties go together'. To this end, 'the key elements of the trade union legislation of the 1980s will remain – on ballots, picketing and industrial action.' But people should be free to join or not to join a union and 'every person at work should be entitled to basic minimum standards of fairness, properly enforced', based largely on the notion of individual rights (Labour Party 1997b: page 1).

A national minimum wage

Labour believes that there should be a statutory wage level beneath which pay should not fall. Most other OECD countries have a wages floor, including the United States, Japan and France, but apart from agriculture Britain has had none since abolition of the last wages councils in 1993. Labour argues that the minimum wage should not be decided by a rigid formula but according to the economic circumstances of the time, with the advice of an independent low pay commission, chaired by Professor George Bain, and including representatives of employers, small businesses and employees. Introduced sensibly, Labour believe, a statutory minimum wage will remove the worst excesses of low pay, particularly benefiting women, whilst cutting some of the benefits budget by which taxpayers subsidise companies paying very low wages.

Those opposed to a statutory minimum wage argue that it would result in job losses, would raise employment costs and therefore result in price rises, and would have a knock-on impact on pay differentials. Those favouring the introduction of a statutory minimum wage, on the other hand, argue that Britain has amongst the fewest basic legal standards to protect the working conditions of employees. New Labour's objective is (page 3) 'to establish a framework of minimum standards in the labour market and at the workplace which seeks to support proper flexibility and provide protection against unfair treatment'. The minimum wage issue fits this agenda and forms a central plank in Labour's attempts to set basic standards at work, 'which should be regarded as part of fundamental citizenship' and 'as natural as the rule of law.'

Research by the TUC (1995) into the arguments for introducing a statutory minimum wage in Britain demonstrates that:

- women are twice as likely to be low paid as men
- more than half of those paid less than £2.50 an hour are part-time workers
- 85 per cent of those on less than £2.50 an hour work in the private sector
- income inequality has increased dramatically in the past 25 years
- basic hourly rates have fallen in all industries previously covered by wages councils
- the cost of means-tested benefits for people in work is estimated to be £2.4 billion per year
- more than a third of those who would benefit from a national minimum of £3.00 an hour live in the poorest 10 per cent of households.

Further, although the case for a minimum wage has been dominated by economic arguments, for and against it, there is also a moral case for raising minimum pay levels.

Age discrimination

New Labour also believes that all people at work should be treated fairly, building on existing entitlements. It sees the case for employing a balanced workforce, including older and younger workers, as an overwhelming one. This mixes skills and experience and brings a wealth of accumulated talent to employers, enabling older employees to assist in the development of younger staff. Labour therefore intends to strengthen existing safeguards and end age discrimination at work.

Health and safety

Labour is committed to continue working with employers and employees to promote best practice throughout industry and the service sector. It intends working with employers' and employees' organisations to improve occupational health, reduce absenteeism and ensure that independent advice and support is available to those wishing to improve the situation in their workplaces. Labour also believes that health and safety protection at work is an area where partnership between employers and employees has been successful in setting minimum standards. This social partnership approach can be extended with positive benefits for companies, employees and all concerned. There is an overwhelming economic case for high standards of occupational health-care, with 31 million working days lost through work-related illness, 23 million of them because of industrial injury.

The Social Chapter

The Social Chapter, or Social Policy Agreement, is a protocol to the Treaty of Maastrict 1992 which sets out broad objectives on improving working and living conditions in member states of the EU. Labour is pledged to sign the Social Chapter, as part of the package of measures which have been incorporated into the Treaty of Amsterdam 1997. Only two Directives have been introduced so far. One gives workers in multinational companies the right to be informed of corporate changes through European works councils. A second is the parental leave ruling, which member states have to enforce by June 1998. This gives both parents the right to a minimum of three months unpaid leave but is not to be confused with maternity leave. The Labour government says that all future proposals for legislation under the Social Chapter will be measured against their impact on competitiveness.

THE STATE AS AN EMPLOYER

As the role of the British state expanded during the twentieth century, so the number of people employed by state agencies also increased, until the late 1970s. An outline summary of the structure of state employment by major sectors, since 1961, is provided in Table 6. From this, it can be seen that state employment rose steadily until 1979, when it reached a peak of almost

8 million employees. By 1996, employment in the public sector had fallen to its lowest level in the the postwar period: just over 5 million. Between 1961 and 1996, employment in the nationalised industries had fallen by almost 2 million. In central government, employment had fallen to under 1 million by 1996, compared with over 2 million in the late 1970s, with the civil service having only just over half a million staff in 1996 and the armed services just over 200,000. Another significant change was the proportion of the NHS working in public corporations (NHS trusts) in 1996, since NHS personnel were formally classified as central government employees. The numbers employed in local authorities, in contrast, were relatively more stable between the late 1970s and 1996, although there were redistributions of staff within this sector, the numbers employed in education and social services slowly falling and those in the police steadily rising.

Table 6 **Numbers employed in the public sector 1961, 1974, 1979, 1991 and 1996**

(thousands)

	1961	1974	1979	1991	1996
Public corporations					
Nationalised industries	2152	1777	1849	516	335
NHS trusts	–	–	–	124	1102
Other	48	208	216	107	75
Total	2200	1985	2065	747	1512
Central government					
Armed services	474	345	314	297	221
NHS	575	911	1152	1092	90
Civil service	672	705	738	580	534
Other	69	179	183	208	142
Total	1790	2140	2387	2177	987
Local authorities					
Education	785	1453	1539	1416	1183
Social services	170	272	344	414	408
Construction	103	135	156	106	79
Police	108	160	176	202	207
Other	703	762	782	810	774
Total	1869	2782	2997	2948	2651
Grand Total	5859	6907	7749	5872	5150

Source: derived from *Economic Trends*

The state as a model and good-practice employer

One of the traditional roles of the state in employee relations, from the late nineteenth century till the late 1970s, was to be a 'model' and 'good-practice' employer. Although the concepts overlap, they may be distinguished analytically. As a 'model' employer, the state adopted what it deemed to be progressive employment practices, such as encouraging union membership and recognising trade unions, in order to enhance 'best practice' in the public sector and to act as an example for the private sector. As a 'good-practice' employer, in contrast, the state adopted certain of the employment practices of the best private sector companies, such as wages comparability, so as to be able to recruit, retain, reward and motivate high-quality staff in the public sector. As a 'model' employer, the state played a 'lead' role in employee relations, whilst as a 'good-practice' employer, the state had a 'following' role (Farnham and Horton 1993 and 1996).

The model employer concept of the public sector can be traced back some 100 years. In 1893, for example, the House of Commons passed a resolution stating that 'no person in Her Majesty's Naval Establishments should be engaged at wages insufficient for proper maintenance.' It added that 'the conditions of labour as regards hours, wages, insurance against accidents, provisions for old age, sickness, etc., should be such as to afford an example to private employers throughout the country' (White 1933: page 156). Examples of model employment practices adopted by public sector employers after 1945, and earlier in some cases, include:

- job security
- jointly agreed employee relations procedures with the public sector unions for handling grievances, discipline, dismissal and redeployment
- equal opportunities and equal pay
- occupational pensions
- training and career development
- the recruitment of disadvantaged workers.

To varying degrees, these model practices applied across the public sector. When compared with private employers, the public sector demonstrated a rich pattern of relatively homogeneous, consistent and standardised employment practices, aimed partly at influencing 'bad' practices in the private sector (Beaumont 1981).

A prime example of a model employment practice was in relation to 'fair wages' principles, linked with union membership. The Fair Wages Resolutions of the House of Commons (1891 and 1946, but rescinded in 1983) obliged private contractors, supplying goods to public organisations, to pay 'fair wages' to their employees and to recognise their rights to be union members. The principle underlying these resolutions was that it was the government's duty to use its bargaining position with private contractors to ensure that they observed at least minimum standards of fairness in the terms and conditions of employment provided to their employees. The outcome of collective bargaining was acknowledged to be the relevant standard of fairness to be met by the contractors' terms and conditions of employment (Beaumont 1992). These arrangements, it was believed, would eliminate unfair wage-cutting amongst government contractors and influence the development and growth of union organisation and collective bargaining in these parts of the private sector.

One facet of being a good-practice public employer meant providing terms and conditions of employment comparable with those provided by the best private employers. As the Priestley Commission wrote regarding Civil Service pay (Priestley 1955: para. 172):

> We consider that the Civil Service should be a good employer in the sense that while it should not be among those who offer the highest rates of remuneration, it should be among those who pay somewhat above the average . . . the Civil Service rate should not be lower than the median but not above the upper quartile.

This principle of 'pay comparability' was incorporated in guidelines provided to the Civil Service Pay Research Unit, set up as a result of the Priestley Commission. It was a principle legitimised more generally in the public sector in the late 1970s by the Standing Commission on Pay Comparability (SCPC). Although abolished in 1981, the SCPC, set up by the Prime Minister, James Callaghan, in March 1979, had a distinctive role. Its remit was to examine the pay and conditions of employment of groups of public sector workers referred to it by the government, with the agreement of the employers and unions concerned, and to report on these. In each case, the SCPC had to make recommendations 'on the possibility of establishing acceptable bases of comparison with terms and conditions for other comparable workers and of maintaining appropriate internal relativities' (Standing Commission on Pay Comparability 1981: iii).

The related roles of the model and good-practice employer in the public sector were not always compatible. One example was public sector employers acting as leaders of wage restraint in their own sector, during periods of incomes policy, but at other times acting as followers of private sector wage levels in order to recruit and retain staff. However, providing a lead in some employment practices and in others following the best private employers were crucial elements in the employment policy of the state to its employees, certainly up to 1979.

The reasons for state employers adopting these policies were partly practical and partly ethical. First, they had the relative freedom to develop innovative employment policies and practices because they were unconstrained by the short-term pressures of profit-making and financial stewardship that acted on private employers. Second, such practices were seen as contributing to public sector efficiency by attracting the right staff, minimising industrial conflict and retaining a quality workforce. Third, the government considered that public employers had a social duty to provide examples of model and good employment practices which might be copied by less progressive private sector employers.

Converging with the private sector?

Since 1979, although the changes must not be exaggerated, public sector employment policies and practices have shifted as a result of government initiatives. Put briefly, rather than public sector employment practices being used by state employers to influence the private sector, a number of private sector employment practices – such as performance-related pay, personal contracts, the removal of wage-bargaining procedures and compulsory competitive tendering – are being introduced into the public sector. There is thus increasing convergence between the public and private sectors, but with the public sector following the lead of some leading private employers, rather than vice versa. These changes in employee relations policies and practices in public sector organisations are complementary to the changes in macro public policy – based on neo-*laissez-faire* principles – since 1979.

Compared with the private sector, the specialist personnel management function came into the public sector relatively late. It was not until the 1970s, partly as a result of local employee relations problems, that the establishment function, certainly in the Civil Service, NHS and local government, began to be superseded by specialist personnel managers. Although part of the management structure, personnel managers also saw themselves as mediating between employers and employees, and seeking to accommodate both the management needs for efficiency and fairness and the employee needs for fairness and job satisfaction. Since the 1980s and in the 1990s, this traditional personnel management role, in turn, is being challenged by an increasing emphasis on styles of management and employee relations more associated with those of the private sector – HRM.

There is a lively academic debate about the differences between personnel management and HRM (Guest 1987, Storey 1989, Torrington and Hall 1991, Beardwell and Holden 1994). However, it is generally recognised that HRM differs from traditional personnel management in a number of ways:

- HRM focuses on employees as resources which, like other resources, need to be used efficiently.
- Employees are viewed as a key resource, with employers actively pursuing employee commitment to corporate goals and values. Only through a systematic set of policies on recruitment, rewards for performance, staff appraisal, training and development, and effective communication, it is argued, can commitment and excellence be achieved.
- HRM assumes that personnel management is the responsibility of all line managers rather than of personnel specialists.
- There is a preference for management communication with employees individually, rather than relying on collective forms of information exchange through trade unions.
- HRM assumes a unitary model of employee relations, in contrast with the pluralist model underpinning traditional personnel management.

A central focus of HRM, compared with traditional personnel management, is improving employee performance. This necessitates selecting the 'right' people to do the job, rewarding them accordingly, appraising their performance and training and developing them to do their existing and future jobs better and more efficiently. As in the private sector, public sector employers are responding to these issues in a number of ways (Farnham and Horton 1993 and 1996).

Recruitment and selection

In parts of the public sector, responsibility for recruitment is being decentralised, innovations are reducing the time taken to recruit and better selection techniques are being introduced. 'Head hunters' and assessment centres are now being used and greater use is being made of psychometric testing, bio-data sifting and wider sources of potential recruitment. The latter is being achieved by opening up competition to top posts, recruiting from the private sector and using short-term contracts. Another recruitment and employment strategy, borrowed from the private sector, is that of implementing more flexible working arrangements (Management and Personnel Office 1987). These challenge the public sector model of lifetime employment, enabling public employers to reduce costs, improve productivity and compete with the private sector for some of their staff.

Rewarding performance

One of the most significant HRM innovations in the public sector since the mid-1980s has been the introduction of performance-related pay (PRP). PRP is an individualised form of payment providing for periodic rises in pay that reflect assessments of individual performance and personal value to the organisation. Such increases may determine the rate of progression through pay scales or be increments added to existing pay scales or lump sums. Copied from the private sector, PRP is predicated on the belief that rewarding 'high performers' by paying them more helps to focus attention on achieving corporate objectives, improves performance and encourages 'a more decisive, competitive and entrepreneurial spirit' (Murlis 1987: page 27). PRP was first introduced into the Civil Service in 1985 and has been extended radically since then. In the NHS, the recommendations of the Griffiths Report (Department of Health and Social Security 1983) resulted in the introduction of PRP for general managers and, in the 1990s, there were plans to extend PRP to other professional groups.

Staff appraisal

With increased emphasis on improved performance in the public sector, staff appraisal systems are becoming widespread for many groups of staff. Based on private sector practice, staff appraisal was triggered in the NHS by the Griffiths Report and led to the introduction of an 'individual performance review' for some senior staff. The emphasis was on sharply defined individual responsibilities for achieving objectives, combined with the need to develop a stock of potential general managers from within the service. As in other parts of the public sector, staff appraisal is seen as playing a key role in redefining roles, generating clarity of purpose and building commitment to a new sense of corporate identity. Performance appraisal, together with staff development (see below), is being used by government as an instrument for inducing cultural change, measuring performance and introducing flexible reward systems in the public sector, based on private sector experience (Farnham and Horton 1993).

Staff development

Part of the drive to enlarge the training function in the public sector since the 1980s has derived from the need to provide staff with the skills and competences necessary for operating the new management systems being introduced. In the Civil Service, NHS and local government, many of these new systems are computer-based, and staff therefore need appropriate training.

New management development programmes have been introduced in the Civil Service, some of them offered jointly with private sector organisations. In the NHS, the National Health Service Training Agency was established in 1985 to provide health authorities with leadership and support 'as they develop, implement and manage education and training programmes to help achieve the goal of cost-effective high-quality health services' (Annandale 1986). In local government, a key role has been taken on by the Local Government Management Board, which resulted from a merger between the Local Government Training Board and the Local Authorities Conditions of Service Advisory Board. In an attempt to raise the quality of public service provision, public organisations are also using another 'big idea' borrowed from the private sector – 'total quality management' – and training their staff to implement it (see Chapter 10).

Relations with employees

The new employee relations in the public sector since 1979 have manifested themselves in a number of ways. Wage negotiating machinery was removed from nurses and the NHS professions allied to medicine in 1983, and from school teachers in 1987. As a result, about half the staff in the NHS have their pay determined by pay review bodies, and about 400,000 teachers in England and Wales now have no national wage bargaining arrangements. The principle of comparability of public sector pay with that of the private sector, as embodied in the Priestley Commission (1955), was effectively destroyed by the abolition of the Civil Service Pay Research Unit in 1981. Since then, the ability of the employer to pay, value for money and market forces have become the dominant criteria for determining collective pay increases in all parts of the public sector. National collective bargaining came under further attack in 1990 when the government signalled its intention to encourage decentralised wage bargaining in the public sector, modelled on private sector practice. Structural changes in the Civil Service, NHS and education provide the opportunity for changing bargaining structures (see Chapter 9), with likely changes in local government to follow. NHS trusts are free to set their own terms and conditions for staff, whilst 'Next Steps' agencies in the Civil Service are likely to break away from Whitleyism.

Compulsory competitive tendering

Compulsory competitive tendering (CCT) and 'contracting out' are not new to the public sector. But previously, under the Fair Wages Resolutions (FWRs), any private employer subcontracting to the public authorities had to ensure that its terms and conditions of employment were not less favourable than those existing in the public sector, or those which were the norm in the industry through collective bargaining. With the rescinding of the FWRs in the 1980s, there was a general deterioration of the terms and conditions for those workers covered by CCT arrangements.

Until the Trade Union Reform and Employment Rights Act 1993, there appeared to be no legal protection for such workers. The government claimed that the European Commmunity's Acquired Rights Directive, implemented in Britain through the Transfer of Undertakings Regulations 1981, applied only to commercial undertakings. In the European Court of Justice in 1992, however, the Redmond case confirmed that the Directive applies to employees in both the private and public sectors. This decision was incorporated in the 1993 Act. This means, in any transfer of undertakings, that: contracts of employment are transferred to the new employer, together with existing terms and conditions; collective agreements, where they exist, are transferred; union recognition is transferred; and dismissals that result from such transfers are automatically unfair.

ASSIGNMENTS

(a) Why did 'free collective bargaining', or collective *laissez-faire*, have such an appeal to employers, the unions and the state? Does it still do so?

(b) Read Wedderburn (1986) pages 21-25 and examine why legal immunities, rather than positive legal rights, became incorporated in the English legal system affecting employee relations.

(c) Critically examine the Donovan Commission's presumption (1968: page 54) that: 'properly conducted, collective bargaining is the most effective means of giving workers the right to representation in decisions affecting their working lives, a right which is or should be the prerogative of every worker in a democratic society.' What are some of the implications of this statement for managing employee relations?

(d) Read Farnham (1978) and analyse the main characteristics of Whitleyism as a model of employee relations practice.

(e) What were the goals of neo-*laissez-faire* public policy on employee relations between 1979 and 1997? Evaluate the effectiveness of this policy and examine some of its implications for employee relations management.

(f) Interview a number of public sector employees and find out why they joined public sector organisations. Ask them what they understand by the terms 'model' employment practices and 'good' employment practices, with examples of each. Ask them what they regard as the main differences between public sector employment practices and those of the private sector.

(g) What features of state policy on employee relations, in the 1980s and the 1990s, have influenced the emergence of 'human resource management' practices amongst British employers? How have these HRM practices manifested themselves?

(h) How is New Labour's employee relations policy similar to and different from (1) the 'employee relations consensus' and (2) the Conservatives' neo-*laissez-faire* approach?

REFERENCES

ADVISORY, CONCILIATION AND ARBITRATION SERVICE. 1980. *Industrial Relations Handbook*. London: HMSO.

ADVISORY, CONCILIATION AND ARBITRATION SERVICE. 1981-1992. *Annual Reports*. London: ACAS.

ANNANDALE, S. 1986. 'The four faces of management development'. *Personnel Management*. July.

BAYLISS, F. 1959. *British Wages Councils*. Oxford: Blackwell.

BEARDWELL, I. *and* HOLDEN, L. *Human Resource Management: A contemporary perspective*. London: Pitman.

BEAUMONT, P. 1981. *Government as Employer – Setting an example?*. London: Royal Institute of Public Administration.

BEAUMONT, P. 1992. *Public Sector Industrial Relations*. London: Routledge.

BEVERIDGE, W. 1944. *Full Employment in a Free Society*. London: Allen and Unwin.

CHARLES, R. 1973. *The Development of Industrial Relations in Britain 1911-1945*. London: Hutchinson.

CLEGG, H., FOX, A. *and* THOMPSON, A. 1964. *A History of British Trade Unions since 1889. Volume 1 1889-1910*. Oxford: Clarendon.

CMD. 7321 1948. *Personal Incomes, Costs and Prices*. London: HMSO.

DANIEL, W. *and* MILLWARD, N. 1983. *Workplace Industrial Relations in Britain*. London: Heinemann.

DEPARTMENT OF EMPLOYMENT. 1983. *Democracy in Trade Unions*. London: HMSO.

DEPARTMENT OF HEALTH AND SOCIAL SECURITY. 1983. *NHS Management Inquiry (the Griffiths Report)*. London: HMSO.

DONOVAN, Lord 1968. *Royal Commission on Trade Unions and Employers' Associations: Report*. London: HMSO.

DUNN, S. *and* GENNARD, J. 1984. *The Closed Shop in British Industry*. London: Macmillan.

EMPLOYMENT PROTECTION ACT 1975.

FARNHAM, D. 1978. 'Sixty years of Whitleyism'. *Personnel Management*. July.

FARNHAM, D. 1990. 'Trade union policy 1979-89: restriction or reform?'. In

Savage, S. and Robins, L. (eds), *Public Policy under Thatcher*, Basingstoke: Macmillan.

FARNHAM, D. *and* HORTON, S. 1993. 'Human resources management in the public sector: leading or following the private sector?'. *Public Policy and Administration*. Special edition, Spring.

FARNHAM, D. *and* HORTON, S. 1996. *Managing People in the Public Services*. London: Macmillan.

GUEST, D. 1987. 'Human resource management and industrial relations'. *Journal of Management Studies*. 24(5).

JENKINS, P. 1970. *The Battle of Downing Street*. London: Knight.

KEYNES, J. M. 1936. *The General Theory of Employment, Interest and Money*. London: Macmillan.

LABOUR PARTY 1997a. *New Labour: Because Britain Deserves Better*. London: Labour Party.

LABOUR PARTY 1997b. *Building Prosperity: Flexibility, Efficiency and Fairness at Work*. London: Labour Party.

MANAGEMENT AND PERSONNEL OFFICE. 1987. *Working Patterns*. London: MPO.

MARTIN, R. 1992. *Bargaining Power*. Oxford: Clarendon.

MILLWARD, N. *and* STEVENS, M. 1986. *British Workplace Industrial Relations 1980-1984*. Aldershot: Gower.

MILLWARD, N., STEVENS, M., SMART, D. *and* HAWES, W. 1992. *Workplace Industrial Relations in Transition*. Aldershot: Dartmouth.

MINISTRY OF LABOUR 1965. *Written Evidence of the Ministry of Labour to the Royal Commission on Trade Unions and Employers' Associations*. London: HMSO.

MURLIS, H. 1987. 'Performance-related pay in the public sector'. *Public Money*. March.

PELLING, H. 1987. *A History of British Trade Unionism*. Harmondsworth: Penguin.

PRIESTLEY REPORT 1955. *Royal Commission on the Civil Service*. London: HMSO.

ROYAL COMMISSION ON LABOUR LAWS 1894. *Final Report of the Commission 1991-94*. (Chairman: Duke of Devonshire). London: HMSO.

SCHMITTER, P. *and* LEHMBRUCH, G. 1979. *Trends Towards Corporatist Intermediation*. London: Sage.

STANDING COMMISSION ON PAY COMPARABILITY. 1981. *Final Report*. London: HMSO.

STOREY, J. 1989. *New Perspectives on Human Resource Management*. London: Routledge.

TAYLOR, A. J. P. 1965. *English History 1914-45*. Oxford: Clarendon.

TORRINGTON, D. *and* HALL, L. 1991. *Personnel Management*. London: Prentice Hall.

TRADE UNION REFORM AND EMPLOYMENT RIGHTS ACT 1993.

TRADE UNION AND LABOUR RELATIONS (CONSOLIDATION) ACT 1992.

TRADES UNION CONGRESS 1995. *Arguments for a National Minimum Wage*. London: TUC.

WEDDERBURN, LORD. *The Worker and the Law*. 1986. Harmondsworth: Penguin.

WEDDERBURN, LORD *and* DAVIES, P. 1969. *Employment Grievances and Disputes Procedures in Britain*. Berkeley: University of California Press.

WEEKES, B., MELLISH, M., DICKENS, L. *and* LLOYD, J. 1975. *Industrial Relations and the Limits of the Law*. Oxford: Blackwell.

WHITE, L. 1933. *Whitley Councils in the British Civil Service*. Chicago: Chicago University Press.

WHITLEY COMMITTEE 1917-18. *Reports*. London: HMSO.

8 Management and trade unions

Voluntary collective bargaining, with management dealing with trade unions and employee representatives, on labour market and certain managerial issues, remains an important employee relations process in Britain. The Workplace Industrial Relations Survey (WIRS) estimates that in 1990 the proportion of employees covered by collective bargaining was 54 per cent of all establishments in its representative sample. Although this was considerably less than the 71 per cent coverage identified in an earlier survey in 1984, in 1990 80 per cent of the establishments surveyed still recognised trade unions, compared with 89 per cent in 1984 (Millward *et al* 1992). Union recognition, and therefore coverage of collective bargaining, has continued to decline since then, however, and it is estimated that in 1995 only 49 per cent of establishments in private manufacturing recognised unions. This compared with 88 per cent in public administration, 83 per cent in education and 64 per cent in the health sector in the same year (Cully and Woodland 1996). It is in agriculture and private sector services that collective bargaining is particularly under-represented – 13 per cent in agriculture, 14 per cent in hotels and restaurants, and 23 per cent in the wholesale and retail trade.

The conditions necessary for effective collective bargaining to take place include:

- freedom of association for workers to organise into independent trade unions
- the willingness of workers to join and participate in the activities of independent trade unions
- the ability of the unions to recruit, retain and service their members effectively
- employer recognition
- a fair balance of bargaining power between employers and unions in the bargaining process.

To deal with trade unions effectively, therefore, managements need to understand the nature of trade unions, their employee relations activities, preferred methods of operating and the values and purposes for which they stand. They also need to be aware that whilst unions collectively share certain common principles and ideologies, each individual union, in turn, has its own institutional characteristics, employment policies and responses to employee relations problems.

In Britain, employer recognition of trade unions depends, to a large extent, on the ability and voluntary efforts of trade unions in recruiting, retaining and providing services to their members effectively. It also reflects the level of economic activity and structure of the economy at any one time. The willingness of employers to recognise trade unions is a function of:

- the balance of bargaining power between the secondary parties, when unions demand recognition for the first time
- the perceived benefits of recognition to the employer in each case
- the role of the law in determining union recognition.

With the economy expanding and the demand for labour rising, union recognition is more easily achieved by the unions and more likely to be agreed to by managements. With the economy in recession and with excess labour supply, union recognition is less easily achieved and more likely to be resisted by management. In these circumstances, derecognition may be a more attractive option for some employers to adopt.

DEVELOPMENTS IN TRADE UNIONS

Membership trends

Union membership in Britain is in the form of a Pareto distribution. This means that there is a small number of very large unions and a large number of very small ones, with the small number of very large unions making up over 80 per cent of total union membership. In 1995, for example, the Certification Office listed 17 unions each having over 100,000 members and another 231 unions each with less than 100,000 members. The 17 largest unions comprised some 6 million members and the 231 other unions only had about 1.7 million members distributed amongst them. This compared with 23 unions with over 100,000 members and a total of 8 million members in 1990 and 264 with under 100,000 members and a total of 1.8 million members (Certification Office 1992 and 1997).

Table 7 shows that in 1960 there were 15 major trade unions in Britain, with more than 100,000 members each, comprising a total of over 6 million members. By 1980, there were 26 such unions, totalling over 10 million members. In 1990 this had fallen to 24 unions of this size, including the Police Federation, which is not listed by the Certification Office, with a total of 8 million members. In other words, total union membership in Britain's largest unions in 1990 was about 2 million members less than it had been in 1980. This total membership, however, was still some 2 million members higher than amongst similar unions in 1960. In 1995, there were 17 major unions each with over 100,000 members, totalling about 6.5 million members, which was about the same total union membership as in 1960.

Table 7 **Union membership in Britain's largest unions in 1960, 1980, 1990 and 1995**

(000s)

	1960	1980	1990	1995
UNISON – the public service union	*	*	*	1355
Transport and General Workers Union (TGWU)	1302	1887	1224	897
Amalgamated Engineering Union (AEU)[1]	973	1166	702	726
GMBU[2]	796	916	865	740
National Union of Mineworkers (NUM)	586	370	116	*
Union of Shop Distributive and Allied Workers (USDAW)	355	450	362	283
National Union of Rail Maritime and Transport Workers (NURMTW)[3]	334	167	101	*
National and Local Government Officers Association (NALGO)***	274	782	744	*
National Union of Teachers (NUT)	245	272	218	248
Electrical Electronic Telecom-munication and Plumbing Union (EETPU)[4]	243	405	367	*
National Union of Public Employees (NUPE)***	200	699	579	*
Manufacturing Science and Finance Union (MSFU)[5]	*	491	653	446
Union of Construction Allied Trades and Technicians (UCATT)[6]	192	312	207	108
Confederation of Health Service Employees (COHSE)***	*	216	203	*
Communication Workers Union (CWU)[7]	166	203	203	275
Society of Graphical and Allied Trades (SOGAT)[8]	158	200	169	*
Iron and Steel Trades Confederation (ISTC)	117	104	*	*
Civil and Public Services Association (CPSA)[9]	140	216	123	121
Graphical Paper and Media Union (GPMU)	*	*	*	217
Royal College of Nursing (RCN)	*	181	289	303

Banking Insurance and Finance Union (BIFU)	*	141	171	124
Association of Professional Executive and Computer Staff (APEX)[10]	*	140	*	*
National Communications Union (NCU)[11]	*	131	155	*
National Association of School Masters/ Union of Women Teachers (NAS/UWT)	*	156	169	234
Amalgamated Society of Boilermakers (ASB)[12]	*	124	*	*
Association of Teachers and Lecturers (ATL)	*	*	139	171
National Graphical Association (NGA)[13]	*	116	130	*
Police Federation (PF)	*	112	180	200
National Union of Civil and Public Servants (NUCPS)[14]	*	109	114	102
	6332**	10066	8183	6550

* Not applicable

** This total includes two other unions, the National Union of Agricultural Workers and the National Union of Garment and Tailoring Workers, with 135,000 and 116,000 members respectively in 1960.

*** Merged to form UNISON in 1993.

1. Known as the Amalgamated Union of Engineering Workers in 1980; became the Amalgamated Electrical and Engineering Union in 1992, after a merger with the EETPU.
2. Known as the General and Municipal Workers Union in 1960 and 1980.
3. Known as the National Union of Railwaymen in 1960 and 1980.
4. Known as the Electrical Trades Union in 1960.
5. Known as the Association of Scientific Technical and Managerial Staff in 1980. It merged with the Technical Administrative and Supervisory Section of the AEU to form the MSFU in 1988.
6. Known as the Amalgamated Society of Woodworkers in 1960.
7. Known as the Union of Post Office Workers in 1971. CWU was formed in 1995, following a merger between the Union of Communication Workers and the National Communications Union.
8. Known as the National Union of Printing Bookbinding and Paper Workers in 1960. Became the SOGAT in 1975 and merged with the NGA in 1991 to form the Graphical Paper and Media Union.
9. Known as the Civil Service Clerical Association in 1960.
10. Merged with the GMBU in 1989.
11. Known as the Post Office Engineering Union in 1960 and 1980. See also footnote 7.
12. Merged with the General Municipal Workers Union in 1982.
13. See note 8 above.
14. Known as the Society of Civil and Public Servants in 1980.

Source: TUC and Certification Officer *Annual Reports*

Table 7 also shows that of the 15 largest unions listed in 1960, only three had smaller memberships in 1980. These were the NUM, NURMTW and ISTC. By 1980, these 15 largest unions had been joined by 11 others: MSFU (then known as ASTMS); COHSE; RCN; BIFU; APEX; NCU;

NAS/UWT; ASB; NGA; PF; and NUCPS. The decline in the absolute and relative size of some of the old 'smokestack' unions, such as the NUM, NURMTW and ISTC, and the rise to greater prominence of 'white-collar' unions in the public and private services by 1980 reflected, in part at least, the changing industrial and employment structures in Britain during the 1960s and 1970s (Bain 1970).

Between 1980 and 1990, as also shown in Table 7, this trend continued. During this decade, whilst there was a decline in the absolute memberships of all the largest unions recruiting amongst manual workers (except the NGA), and even amongst some white-collar unions in the public sector, such as the NUT, NALGO and CPSA, there were rises in membership in other white-collar unions recruiting professional, technical and administrative workers in parts of the private and public sectors. The large unions gaining members during these years were: MSFU; RCN; BIFU; NCU; NAS/UWT; AMMA; and NUCPS. Some of this growth in the memberships of these unions can be accounted for by union mergers, such as those involving the MSFU. In other cases it arose from expanding recruitment opportunities for unions such as the RCN and BIFU or for the NAS/UWT and AMMA which were taking members from established organisations in their own sector, such as the NUT. Further evidence of the relative decline amongst some of the large private sector unions during the 1980s is provided by the absence of the ISTC, ASB and APEX from those organisations with over 100,000 members each in 1990. By this time, the ISTC's membership had fallen to around 40,000, the ASB had merged with the General and Municipal Workers' Union in 1982 to form the GMBU and APEX, in turn, had merged with the GMBU in 1989.

By 1995, as shown in Table 7, there were 17 large unions, each with over 100,000 members. Between 1990 and 1995, decline in the membership of manual workers' unions continued, except in the AEU, and in white-collar unions such as MSFU, CPSA, BIFU and NUCPS. The professional and technical unions that increased their memberships during these years were in the public sector, such as the NUT, RCN, NAS/UWT, ATL and Police Federations, and in the utilities such as CWU.

It is likely that the trend towards more union amalgamations and mergers will continue in the 1990s and the 2000s. The AEU and EETPU amalgamated in 1992 to create the Amalgamated Engineering and Electrical Union, with over a million members. NUPE, NALGO and COHSE also merged, in 1993, to form the largest public sector union in the world, UNISON, with some 1.5 million members. And discussions are reported to have taken place between the TGWU and GMBU about future working arrangements between them. In the mid-1990s there was a spate of union transfers of engagements from smaller to larger unions such as the Scottish Health Visitors' Association to UNISON, the Rossendale Union of Boot, Shoe and Slipper Operatives to the National Union of Knitwear Footwear and Apparel Trades and the Northern Ireland Bakers' and Confectioners' Union to the Bakers' Food and Allied Workers Union (Certification Office 1997).

Table 8 **TUC membership, TUC affiliations and non-TUC membership 1978-95**

Year	Membership of TUC	Numbers of TUC-affiliated unions	Membership of non-TUC unions
1978	11,865,390	112	1,188,206
1979	12,128,078	112	1,084,276
1980	12,172,508	109	463,847
1981	11,601,413	108	709,821
1982	11,005,984	105	738,406
1983	10,510,157	95	789,722
1984	10,082,144	89	691,809
1985	9,855,204	91	963,745
1986	9,580,502	89	1,017,506
1987	9,243,297	87	1,236,853
1988	9,127,278	83	1,259,960
1989	8,652,318	78	1,391,288
1990	8,405,246	78	1,404,773
1991	8,192,664	74	not available
1992	7,786,885	72	1,142,017
1993	7,647,443	70	1,018,501
1994	7,117,436	69	1,113,109
1995	6,894,604	67	1,136,722

Source: TUC, *Annual Reports* and CO, *Annual Reports*

Another way of examining recent union membership trends is by analysing membership in unions affiliated to the TUC (see Chapter 2) and that in unions which are not TUC-affiliated, as shown in Table 8. This shows, first, that total union membership in Britain peaked at an all-time high of 13.2 million members in 1979, comprising 12.1 million members in TUC-affiliated unions and just over 1 million in non-TUC unions. By 1990, the overall level of union membership had fallen to 9.8 million members, consisting of some 8.5 million in TUC-affiliated organisations and some 1.4 million in non-TUC unions. This represented a fall of 26 per cent in overall membership, a fall of 30 per cent in the membership of TUC unions and a rise of 30 per cent in the membership of non-TUC unions for the period 1979-90. Between 1990 and 1995, however, these relative decreases in union membership levelled out, with a further fall of 18 per cent in overall union membership, 18 per cent in TUC affiliated membership and 19 per cent in non-affiliated union membership.

Second, between 1978 and 1995, the number of unions affiliated to the TUC declined from 112 to 67. This reduction in the number of TUC-affiliated unions is largely accounted for by the series of amalgamations and mergers taking place amongst TUC unions after 1980. Yet whilst membership in TUC-affiliated unions fell steadily during the 1980s and early 1990s, that in non-TUC unions grew slowly from 1981, after it had fallen dramatically by over 600,000 members between 1979 and 1980. The effect was that between 1981 and 1990, membership in non-TUC unions rose by almost 100 per cent from about 709,000 to 1.4 million. Between 1990 and 1995, however, membership in non-TUC unions fell by some 250,000.

Union structure

Union structure focuses on the recruitment and membership bases of trade unions, which are organised on occupational (or craft), industrial or general lines. Occupational, 'craft' or 'trades' unions are exclusive bodies and were the first type of employee organisation to emerge in Britain (during the nineteenth century). One of their main recruiting devices was the pre-entry closed shop (Gennard 1990). Today few occupational unions exist and those that do are relatively small in size. This is because of changing occupational boundaries, the widening scope of occupational classifications, the de-skilling of craftwork due to technological changes, the growth of multi-skilling and the breakdown of traditional craft sectors of employment. Unlike industrial unions which recruit vertically within an industry, occupational unions recruit horizontally across industries.

Current examples of occupational unions include the British Actors' Equity Association, British Medical Association, British Airline Pilots' Association and Professional Footballers' Association. The main structural feature of occupational unions such as these is that they recruit members selectively, on a job-by-job basis, irrespective of where they work. It is the worker's occupational status, job skills and qualifications or training that determine whether or not individuals qualify for membership of a particular occupational union, not the industry or the organisation that employs them.

Industrial unions recruit selectively but less exclusively than occupational unions. They seek members vertically from amongst all employment grades, normally including both manual and non-manual workers, within a single industry. The best examples of industrial-based unions are in Germany, where there are 16 industrial unions with about 8 million members, all of which are affiliated to the DGB. These unions cover:

- the metal industry
- public services
- chemicals
- postal services
- construction
- food, drink and tobacco
- textiles and clothing
- education and science
- media
- police
- wood and plastics
- agriculture
- leather
- mining and energy

- rail
- commerce, banking and insurance.

With reunification of western and eastern Germany, demarcation disputes between certain industrial unions have emerged and some reorganisation within the DGB took place, such as between the chemicals and mining and energy sectors (Jacobi *et al* 1992).

In Britain, in contrast, because of the continually dynamic and constantly evolving structure of industry, the difficulty of defining industrial boundaries with precision, and the growth of multi-occupational and multi-industry unions, there are very few single-industry unions left. The best remaining examples are the NUM and the ISTC, with the NURMTW and the Broadcasting Entertainment Cinematograph and Theatre Union retaining some features of industrial unionism. Yet even in these cases, there are other unions competing for members in these sectors, thus weakening the exclusivity of the industrial union base.

General or 'open' unions, in contrast to occupational and industrial unions, are 'all-comers' organisations with four main membership characteristics. They draw their members:

- non-exclusively
- from amongst both manual and non-manual workers
- horizontally across industries
- vertically within industries.

For a number of historical and structural reasons, general unions have become the dominant model of British trade unionism.

Because of the financial pressures on them, substantial membership leakages in the 1980s and 1990s and changes in the economy, British trade unions have had to adapt their recruitment strategies and institutional structures to these circumstances. The essential issues facing British unions in recent years have been employer hostility, financial viability and membership retention. Consequently, most craft unions have opened up their boundaries to less skilled workers; industrial unions have continued to diversify their memberships – sometimes across industrial sectors; and general unions have sought to retain and extend their membership boundaries to maintain their influence and power in the trade union movement.

The net result has been a series of union amalgamations and mergers since the early 1980s. This has strengthened general unionism in Britain at the expense of occupational and industrial unions. These mergers have often been driven by the political allegiances of union leaderships or the search for stronger union membership bases, rather than by the desire to create rational union structures. There are four main consequences of this:

- There has been a shift towards the creation of a few 'super' unions whose membership boundaries overlap, resulting in competitive membership recruitment amongst them.

- These amalgamations and mergers have not mitigated the problems associated with multi-unionism at industry, employer and workplace levels and in dealings with employers.
- The role of the TUC has to some degree been weakened, since larger unions feel less need for the services and support of an umbrella organisation at central level like the TUC and are sometimes more critical of its co-ordinating functions.
- At the same time, the TUC (1995: page 12) has been forced to become a more crusading body, seeking to be:

> A high profile organisation which campaigns successfully for trade union aims and values, assists trade unions to increase membership and effectiveness, cuts out wasteful rivalry and promotes trade union solidarity.

TRADE UNION POLICY

The essence of trade union policy is to protect the employment interests of their members, as individual workers, by dealing with employers collectively. As Hyman (1975: page 64) writes, the central purpose of a trade union 'is to permit workers to exert, collectively, the control over the conditions of employment which they cannot hope to possess as individuals'. They do this largely 'by compelling the employer to take account, in policy- and decision-making, of interests contrary to [its] own'.

Any general analysis of union policy starts by examining their functions and roles as economic and political agents, acting on behalf of employees in their market and managerial relations with employers. Such an analysis clearly highlights the essential divergences between union policy and employer policy on many employee relations issues. Employer policy is normally aimed at achieving profitability, economic efficiency and management control of employee behaviour, achieved through corporate hierarchies. Union policy, on the other hand, is aimed at achieving 'fair' terms and conditions of employment, participation in corporate decision-making and power-sharing with management, achieved through collective bargaining, other employee relations processes and internal union democracy.

It is these differences in organisational rules and values, stemming from this dichotomy between purpose and method, which give rise to conflicts of interest in employee relations between employers and unions, where trade unions are recognised. This dichotomy also explains why some employers resist union organisation and recognition in their workplaces.

The labour market function

The classical analysis of the trade union function is provided by the Webbs. It was they who first described, analysed and evaluated the purposes and methods of trade unions. For the Webbs, unions exist to enforce 'Trade Union Regulations' on employers for the workers they represent. There is no 'Trade Union Rate of Wages' nor 'a Trade Union Working Day' but many different rates and hours of work which vary from occupation to occupation. (Webbs 1913: page 560) Trade unions are thus seen by the Webbs as bodies defending sectional economic interests, rather than working class interests as a whole. Whilst all unions have broadly similar purposes, and use largely the same methods to achieve them, each union has its own unique purposes and uses those methods most appropriate to its particular circumstances.

Seven trade union regulations are identified by the Webbs. These are:

- the Standard [wage] Rate
- the Normal [working] Day
- Sanitation and Safety [at work]
- New Processes and Machinery
- Continuity of Employment
- the Entrance into a Trade
- the Right to a Trade.

At the core of the Webbs' analysis is their conclusion that: 'in the making of the labor contract the isolated individual workman, unprotected by any combination with his fellows, stands in all respects at a disadvantage compared with the capitalist employer' (page 658). Whilst workers strive to get the best terms they can from their employers, the employers, in turn, 'are endeavouring, in accordance with business principles, to buy their labor in the cheapest market' (pages 658 and 184). Workers combine together, therefore, to be better able to enforce the regulations of their trade upon employers.

Unions use two 'economic devices' to do this: 'the Device of the Restriction of Numbers' and 'the Device of the Common Rule' (Part III: Chapter III). The device of the restriction of numbers is concerned with labour supply. It involves unions using apprenticeships, excluding new competitors from the trade and asserting 'a vested interest in a particular trade' in order to influence the labour market. In these ways, unions can make a better bargain with the employers, insisting on adequate wages, better conditions of employment and shorter hours of work for their members.

The device of the common rule is the enforcement of minimum standards of employment on employers below which no employer may fall. It is not a maximum standard, since some employers may provide terms and conditions better than the minimum. The Webbs go on to analyse the 'three distinct instruments or levers' used by unions to enforce the regulations of their trades. These are: 'the Method of Mutual Insurance, the Method of Collective Bargaining, and the Method of Legal Enactment' (page 150).

Mutual insurance

The method of mutual insurance is the provision of funds by trade unionists, through collective subscriptions, to insure their members' incomes against the economic misfortunes of unemployment, sickness and accidents.

According to the Webbs, 'until Collective Bargaining was permitted by the employers, and before Legal Enactment was within the workman's reach, Mutual Insurance was the only method by which Trade Unionists could lawfully attain their end.' The existence of 'friendly [society] benefits' enables unions to maintain discipline over members who break union rules and to enforce upon all members the decisions of the majority.

Where differences arise between an employer and its employees, unions using the method of mutual insurance can apply economic pressure on employers, through what the Webbs describe as the 'Strike in Detail'. This is the process, if an employer refuses to conform to the regulations of the trade, by which union members leave the employer's employment, one by one, and are sustained by 'Out of Work' benefit from the union. But, as the Webbs state, 'as a deliberate Trade Union policy, the Strike in Detail depends upon the extent to which the union has secured the adhesion of all the component men in the trade' and their capacity to pursue their common ends collectively (pages 166 and 169).

Collective bargaining

The method of collective bargaining enables joint machinery to be established between employers and unions to settle the employment rules within a trade (Part II: Chapter II). Collective bargaining prevents wage undercutting by both employers and employees, maintains 'industrial peace' and enables distinctions to be made between the negotiating arrangements for concluding new agreements and those for interpreting existing ones. Also (page 209):

> When the associated employers in any trade conclude an agreement with the Trade Union, the Common Rule thus arrived at is usually extended by the employers, as a matter of course, to every workman in their establishment, whether or not he is a member of the union.

Determining the common rules of the trade through collective bargaining is a very flexible union method, since agreements can be made at 'shop', 'district' and 'whole industry' level, with 'impartial umpires' or conciliators being available, acceptable to both sides, where collective agreement cannot be reached. For the Webbs (page 218), this joint method for settling the terms and conditions of employment, 'neither by the workmen nor by the employers [alone], but by collective agreement', was attracting 'a growing share of public approval' and support at the time. This was because of the compromises and concessions required of the two sides in the negotiating process and the benefits to both sides in adopting it.

Legal enactment

The method of legal enactment enforces the regulations of the trade through Act of Parliament. For the Webbs, legal enactment is a method about which trade unionists are ambivalent. On the one hand, before unions can get a common rule enforced by the state, they must convince the community at large 'that the proposed regulation will prove advantageous to the state as a whole, and not [be] unduly burdensome to the consumers'. Further, what Parliament enacts might not be the full measure asked for. On the other hand, Acts of Parliament apply uniformly to all districts, whether unions are strong or weak, and to all employers. Legal enactment, therefore, is 'the ideal form of Collective Bargaining, a National Agreement made between a Trade Union including every man in the trade, and an Employers' Association from which no firm stands aloof'.

The Webbs saw the TUC as the body for obtaining, by Parliamentary action, particular measures desired by its constituent unions. But, as the Webbs warned, once the TUC 'diverges from its narrow Trade Union function, and expresses any opinion, either on general social reforms or party politics, it is bound to alienate whole sections of its constituents' (Part II: Chapter IV).

Summary

For the Webbs, then, all trade union regulations are based on the assumption that, in the absence of common rules, the determination of terms and conditions of employment are left to the free labour market, placing workers at an economic disadvantage *vis-á-vis* employers.

> . . . this always means, in practice, that they are arrived at by Individual Bargaining between contracting parties of very unequal economic strength. Such a settlement, it is asserted, invariably tends, for the mass of the workers, towards the worst possible conditions of labor – ultimately, indeed, to the barest subsistence level – whilst even the exceptional few do not permanently gain as much as they otherwise would (page 560).

In the Webbs' analysis, the essence of trade union policy is to remedy and offset this imbalance in labour market power, through the use of appropriate economic devices and methods. For everything beyond 'the National Minimum', wage earners must depend on the method of collective bargaining. But for those regulations and rules based on enduring considerations, such as the health and efficiency of workers, legal enactment is to be preferred (pages 796-806).

The participatory function

It was Flanders who took the Webbs' analysis of union policy and the union function a stage further. In his view, the value of a union to its members is less in its economic achievements than in its capacity to protect their dignity. Whilst union members are interested in labour market regulation and how labour is managed, because these define their rights, status and security, they are also interested in making and administering employment rules and having a voice in shaping their own destiny. To secure membership allegiance and support, unions must provide services to their members and 'this is made possible by [union] participation in job regulation'. They do this primarily through collective bargaining. Yet since collective agreements are a body of jointly agreed rules, and the process of negotiation 'is best conceived as a diplomatic use of power, trade unions operate primarily as political, not economic, institutions' (Flanders 1968a: pages 238-40).

The constant underlying purpose of trade unions, then, is participation in job regulation. 'But participation is not an end in itself, it is a means of enabling workers to gain more control over their working lives' (Flanders 1968b: page 42). The issue that concerns Flanders is the slow rate of progress made by trade unions in advancing this social purpose, especially, when he was writing, under conditions of full employment. For him, one of the weaknesses of trade unions is that a lot of their energies are absorbed in the struggle for 'more money' for their members, whilst the struggle for their members' status in the workplace receives far less attention. In this view this is remediable, where unions refuse to accept any final definition of exclusive managerial functions: 'They have recognised that the frontiers of union control are shifting frontiers, that any decision that affects the life and well-being of their members can be their concern' (Flanders 1961: page 23). Participation by unions jointly with management in non-wage issues is clearly legitimate where their members' employment interests are affected.

TRADE UNION PRACTICE

Trade union practice derives from trade union policy. Given the essential role of trade unions in providing the collective representation of employees in their relations with employers, trade union practices are directed towards any area of common concern to their members, their employment status or occupational interests. Union practices are reflected in the objectives, means and methods of trade unions. These vary by union and according to the circumstances facing any group of trade unionists at any one time. A number of contingent factors affect whether or not these objectives are achieved and whether or not the means and methods used are effective. These include (see also Chapters 6 and 7):

- the state of labour markets
- employer policy
- management style
- the law
- public policy.

Objectives

Because of the sectionalised nature of British trade unionism, it is very difficult to provide a definitive set of universal trade union objectives, applicable to all unions at all times, and it is significant that neither the Webbs nor Flanders tried to do so. A prescriptive analysis of the 'permanent objectives' of unions is provided by the TUC in its evidence to the Donovan

Exhibit 21 **The TUC's union objectives**

- improved terms of employment
- improved physical environment at work
- security of employment and income
- industrial democracy
- fair shares in national income and wealth
- full employment and national prosperity
- improved social security
- improved public and social services
- a voice in government
- public control and planning of industry.

Commission. The objectives distinguished by the TUC (1966) are of different kinds. Some are substantive, some procedural and others do not concern employment as such. They are seen as complementary to one another and as providing choice for unions, enabling them to place lesser or greater emphasis on any one or more of them at any given time. The union objectives outlined by the TUC are illustrated in Exhibit 21.

Of these 10 objectives, only the first four are direct employee relations objectives. The next three are macro-economic and the last four are political objectives. It is some measure of the difficult environment facing trade unions in the 1990s that only the first three of the above objectives are likely to be aimed at by trade unions in Britain currently.

A modified analysis of union objectives was provided by the TUC (1974: pages 6-7) a few years later. It is through the unions, the TUC argues, that employees set the key objectives for advancing their interests. These provide rights at work including:

- *Establishing terms of employment.* Bargaining with employers about pay, hours and working conditions, including equal pay, allowances, retirement and pensions, redundancy, safety and health, and training, for all workers who are employed, part-time as well as full-time.
- *Fair representation.* Representing members to ensure the implementation of all rights that flow from agreements and from the law – eg maternity pay; safety requirements; protection against unfair disciplinary action or dismissal; protection against race or sex discrimination.
- *Influencing employer decisions.* Working together with employers to ensure the future of the enterprise and to safeguard jobs, and to that end to improve productivity.

Over and above this, however, workers' standards of living depend on actions taken by governments. These include:

- how the government manages the economy
- the priorities given to welfare and public services

- how taxes are raised and used
- what government does to ensure that unions are not at a disadvantage given the enormous power of many modern businesses.

The union role, then, is to protect and advance the standards of living of workers in any way which is appropriate.

The TUC is always updating its approaches to fulfilling this role and protecting workers' interests in employment. Following the continual challenges posed to trade union organisation in the past two decades, and reorganisation within the TUC itself, it 'relaunched' itself in 1994 and made a commitment to turn itself into a high-profile campaigning organisation for trade union goals and values. As its general secretary, John Monks, reported in 1995: 'Our priorities are firmly rooted in the world of work. Full employment remains our central objective. But alongside this we are also campaigning for minimum standards at work.' The TUC's stated purpose regarding its new role is 'to bring workplace relations out of the feudal era and into a new age of industrial enlightment' (TUC 1995: page 8). The chief characteristics of this 'new "campaigning" unionism' are:

- concentrating on priorities on world of work issues
- giving voice to the common concerns that people have in the world of work, as well as those specific to union members
- setting out to address new audiences
- taking the TUC's and the unions' arguments to all main political parties
- arguing the benefits of unions' working as social partners at workplace and national levels.

In its early 'new' campaigning role, the TUC focused on four key results areas: campaigning through task groups, raising current issues, campaigning for equality, and campaigning in Europe. TUC task groups, for example, have specific remits and a clear timetable. Four task groups were initially created:

- representation at work
- full employment
- minimum standards and national minimum wage
- part-time working.

Nine other current campaigning initiatives were also raised by the TUC in its 'relaunch':

- top pay, corporate governance and standards in public life
- public services
- benefits and the world of work
- pensions
- training;
- repetitive strain injuries

- industry/sectoral work
- technology and employment.

In its campaign for equality, the TUC identified four immediate areas demanding attention:

- women workers
- uniting against racism
- disability
- lesbian and gay rights.

Finally, campaigning in Europe focused on three main issues:

- economic policy and employment
- social policy
- European Works Councils.

Means and methods

For the TUC (1966: page 43), trade union 'means' are interdependent with trade union 'methods'. 'It is impossible to bargain without anything to bargain with. This is the distinction between trade union means and trade union methods.' The choice between means and methods is a practical one, with union practice reflecting the circumstances in which a particular group of workers finds itself. But the basis of trade union effectiveness is 'combination' and this involves a number of means. Exhibit 22 illustrates the union means, listed by the TUC.

Exhibit 22 The TUC's union means

These include:

- organisation
- 100 per cent membership
- national and local co-ordination
- income
- union competence.

Without high levels of membership, sound organisation and responsive leadership, a union's ability to perform its representative functions on behalf of employees is seriously impaired.

Union methods, in turn, are related to their objectives and means. The TUC argues that the dividing lines between the various methods are imprecise, they are diverse and their emphasis varies according to circumstances. The union methods that the TUC distinguishes are illustrated in Exhibit 23.

Exhibit 23 **The TUC's union methods**

These include:

- collective bargaining
- joint consultation
- autonomous job regulation
- services for members
- influencing government
- political action
- international activities.

The challenges to the unions

It is clear that by the 1990s the 'permanent objectives', means and methods of trade unions had been weakened by labour market factors, the employee relations strategies of some employers and Conservative government policy. Trade union practice is obviously affected by high levels of unemployment, when more emphasis is placed by some employers on soft forms of joint consultation or non-union forms of employee involvement, and when other employers use more direct methods – dealing with employees on an individual rather than on a collective basis (see Chapter 10). Union effectiveness also suffers when government policy is directed towards deregulating the labour market and excluding the unions from the political process. As a result, since the mid-1980s, trade union practice, membership recruitment patterns and membership attitudes have been adversely affected by a number of contextual and employee relations factors.

Contextual changes

The 1980s and the 1990s were a period of immense economic, technological, social and political change in the Western world but especially in Britain (see Chapter 6). There were significant changes in the social structure, with an ageing population, a larger proportion of women workers in the labour market and the weakening of traditional class allegiances. Working methods and working practices were dramatically affected by technological change, whilst the 'information technology' revolution had left few occupational groups unaffected by its impact on employment, job tasks and the work environment (Daniel 1987).

For over a decade, there have been persistent and very high levels of unemployment and radical changes in the structure of the economy, with shifts in the balance between manufacturing and services, and the private and public sectors. The international economic environment has been continuously turbulent and unstable. Large flows of finance capital have been transferred across national frontiers, with the purpose of gaining the highest possible returns from it, resulting in the weakening of national employment bases and traditional patterns of employment. Further, the move towards a single European market has not always resulted in the economic stability and economic potential expected of it by some British companies.

The election to power of four consecutive Conservative administrations, in 1979, 1983, 1987 and 1992, resulted in public policies on employee relations which were generally recognised as being unsupportive of the trade union function. The result was a set of labour market policies, employment legislation and government strategies that weakened union bargaining power, outlawed inter-union solidarity action and denied the unions any role in influencing public policy (see Chapters 3 and 7).

What the impact of the election to office of a New Labour government in May 1997 will have on the trade union function is, at the time of writing, uncertain. However, prima facie, New Labour seems more likely to be favourable than unfavourable to working people's interests and more receptive to taking account of them than previous Conservative administrations in the 1980s and 1990s did. The leader of the Labour Party and Prime Minister, Tony Blair, for example, has argued for 'fairness' for the unions and their members, although he promised them 'no favours'. Further, Labour's 1997 election manifesto committed the government to supporting union recognition, 'where a majority of the relevant workforce vote in a ballot for the union to represent them' (Labour Party 1997; page 17). Similarly, both the TUC and New Labour government support the concept of 'partnership at work'. Indeed, the TUC has argued strongly for a 'new approach' being needed in relationships at work 'based on the development of a world class workforce', with 'skills to produce high-quality, high-value-added products' and 'to respond to rapid technological change'. For the TUC, this new approach 'can best be achieved through a partnership between employers and trade unions', a key element of which is 'a commitment by employers to security of employment' (Trades Union Congress 1994: page 5). This mirrors the Labour party's statement, in its 1997 election manifesto, that the 'best companies recognise their employees as partners' in their enterprises and that many employers and unions are embracing 'partnership in place of conflict' in the workplace. 'Government should welcome this.'

In summary, the changes outlined above have not generally benefited the trade unions. Many employment units have become smaller, mass redundancies have resulted in large membership leakages from the unions and recruitment of new members from the 'new' service sector has proved to be problematic for trade unions. The occupational structure, the nature of labour markets and the content of job tasks have changed, weakening traditional union membership bases and patterns of union recruitment. The impact that New Labour's new employee relations policy is likely to have on these factors has yet to be determined (Chapter 7).

Employer policies

With private sector employers facing increasingly competitive open markets, and the public sector being privatised or deregulated, there has been a shift towards employment flexibility. This has resulted in the growth of short-term contracts, part-time working and changing patterns of shift work. These new working arrangements are generally not conducive to employment stability and membership retention in the trade unions. According to the third Workplace Industrial Relations Survey (WIRS) (Millward *et al* 1992: page 74), whilst there is little evidence of full union derecognition in Britain in recent years, which amounts to 'just over 1 per cent of all workplaces in 1990', its limited data on the timing of derecognition 'was suggestive of a growing phenomenon', with a substantial concentration of the practice in 1989.

WIRS 3 also concludes that although new consultative arrangements created by management normally supplement rather than replace collective bargaining, there is evidence of management initiatives 'aimed at increasing employees' involvement at work' which took place with 'increasing frequency throughout the 1980s' (page 362). In these circumstances, it is possible that some employees see the union role of participating in 'job regulation' as being less important, especially where managements adopt proactive employee relations practices of these sorts. Indeed, the TUC claims (1988: page 6), union influence is being further challenged in organisations because of trends 'such as the increasing management emphasis on winning the commitment of the individual employee ("human resources management") and the continued decentralisation of collective bargaining'.

Later research conducted by the TUC (1994: page 6), however, using WIRS 3 data, concludes that 'HRM in practice is rarely applied as a comprehensive package' and that 'fragments of HRM' are more likely to be found in unionised rather than non-unionised workplaces. Its findings suggest that:

- multiple channels of communication are more likely to be used in unionised workplaces
- non-union workplaces are characterised by authoritarian and hierarchical management practice
- non-unionised workers have few opportunities to influence their working lives
- workers in unionised companies receive more information from their employers than workers in non-unionised firms
- financial participation is as common in unionised as in non-unionised companies
- the most anti-union employers are least likely to offer financial participation schemes
- single status is found as frequently in unionised as in non-unionised companies
- the more anti-union an employer, the less likely single status applies.

The TUC concludes therefore that there is no correlation between anti-unionism and HRM. Indeed, 'the more anti-union the employer, the less likely it is that HRM techniques are being used'.

Inter-union competition

Differences between unions arise from a number of factors. These include:

- membership recruitment
- job demarcation
- recognition and bargaining rights
- wages policy
- contribution levels and services to members.

In the majority of inter-union disputes involving TUC affiliates, the TUC has been the final arbiter through the device of TUC disputes committees. In the early and mid-1980s, however, the so called 'Bridlington Principles', which aim to regulate inter-union membership competition and poaching amongst affiliated unions, came under increasing stress. This was the result of:

- the pressure on unions to recruit new members in competing areas because of membership leakages after 1980
- the multi-occupational and multi-industry structure of British unions
- the emergence of 'single-union agreements' on greenfield sites that exclude other unions with members in the unit from employer recognition
- controversy over the 'no-strike' provisions in such agreements.

(See TUC 1988.)

However, the pressures for inter-union competition are likely to become more intense, now that the Trade Union Reform and Employment Rights Act 1993 provides trade union members with a statutory right to decide for themselves which union to join, even in multi-union situations. This effectively removes the Bridlington arrangements for dealing with disputes over membership amongst TUC unions.

It was the issue of single-union or 'new-style' agreements that caused particular differences amongst TUC affiliated unions and led eventually to the expulsion of the EETPU from Congress in September 1988. The decision to expel the EEPTU from the TUC arose from a complaint by the GMBU, TGWU and USDAW that the EEPTU had acted in contravention of the TUC's Disputes Principles and Procedures by signing a single-union deal with Christian Salvesen at its Warrington and West Cross depots. The disputes committee decided, on the evidence presented, that the complainant unions should have been consulted by the EEPTU, before it entered into a sole negotiating agreement with the company at the two depots. The EEPTU's failure to accept the decision of the committee placed it in direct conflict with Congress who heard the union's appeal on 5 September, which was lost (TUC 1989).

TRADE UNION STRATEGY

Trade union strategy is the ways in which unions adapt their policies and objectives and adjust their means and methods in response to economic and social factors, employer initiatives and the framework of public policy within which employers and unions operate. As voluntary associations promoting the employment interests of their members, trade unions are a mixture of 'movement and organisation' (Flanders 1968b). Members of a movement combine together because they share the same sentiments, values and ideas and want to achieve common goals collectively. To survive as organisations, however, unions must have effective means for translating their goals into practical outcomes for their members. By their very nature, unions have to be dynamic organisationally, whilst maintaining the values and ideas for which they stand. They 'need organisation for their power and movement for their vitality, but they need both power and vitality to advance their social purpose' (page 44). As indicated above, this dual measure of trade union effectiveness has been severely tested in recent years. The main responses of the unions to these challenges are discussed below.

The collective bargaining agenda

Objectives

During the 1990s, trade unions have developed and are developing a number of positive and developmental responses to the economic, technological, social and political problems facing them and their members. The TUC (1991a: pages 12-13) has outlined some of these main developments in what it describes as the 'New Bargaining Agenda' of trade unions. It provides examples of attempts by some unions to 'raise the negotiating horizon beyond immediate pay concerns to embrace [a] wide range of longer-term developmental considerations'. The emerging themes, identified by the TUC, at which the unions are aiming, are illustrated in Exhibit 24.

Exhibit 24 **The bargaining agenda for TUC unions in the 1990s**

- building for the future in terms of job security, job creation, the attainment of full employment and the elimination of under-employment
- focusing on job development, training and career prospects to give more workers control over their working lives and to provide them with more satisfying, fulfilling and rewarding jobs
- emphasising 'fair play' policies, such as: improving the jobs, careers, status and pay of low paid workers; upvaluing the jobs of women; providing equal opportunities for disadvantaged groups; and providing developmental opportunities for those doing part-time, temporary and sub-contract work
- giving priority to environmental and quality of life objectives and essential working conditions, such as: health and safety; the working environment; leisure; sickness benefit; occupational pensions; and family provisions.

In the TUC's view, the more the unions talk about employee development issues of this sort, and about the devolution of management responsibilities to their members, the more they will find themselves questioning existing management prerogatives.

The GMBU and CWU (1991: page 1) have suggested a similar 'New Agenda' that Britain's unions should adopt in the 1990s. In their view, 'it is essential that Britain's unions abandon traditional reactive stances . . . set an Agenda which confronts the new issues of the 1990s . . . [and take] collective bargaining into territory that we have barely explored before.' They argue that unions need to work together with employers and government to create successful industry, a strong economy and a 'caring, sharing society'. In these unions' analysis, the new circumstances facing employers, unions and government in the 1990s are:

- the European Union
- rising expectations amongst consumers and employees
- the role of women in the workforce
- environmental concerns
- restructuring within industry.

The GMBU and CWU argue that this situation should involve a joint response by unions and employers, with government support, aimed at matching productivity levels abroad and at negotiating ways of working which ensure that new skills and new plant are brought to bear on the productivity gap separating Britain from its foreign rivals.

In response to these challenges, the GMBU and CWU want unions to talk 'to Britain's employers about how to achieve quality performance, cost and price competitiveness and a fairer society'. The collective bargaining agenda would include issues such as training, investment, new product development, work restructuring, equal opportunities and health and safety issues. 'The New Agenda would make the quality of output rather than the price of inputs the centrepiece of talks between trades unions and employers.' Pay would be on the bargaining agenda 'but work organisation, training and quality should form the focus' (page 8). Unions should press management to discuss how they intend to develop the talents of their workforces, the investment they propose to make and how they can encourage employees to ever higher standards of customer service.

The negotiating framework

The TUC identifies enterprise-level bargaining as the obvious focus for employee relations decision-making, although it does not rule out industry and sector bargaining for some matters. Indeed, the TUC emphasises the importance of national framework agreements for establishing minimum rates for jobs or a floor of pay below which no employee may fall. It also supports single-table bargaining so that the entire job and pay structure can be taken into account in union-employer negotiations. On a wider front, the

TUC believes that there is need for co-ordination at a European level – 'initially in terms of exchanges of information on . . . performance comparisons and agreement on principles' (TUC 1991a: page 14). This international role is likely to expand in the future but, in the short term, is focused on agreeing bargaining objectives amongst European unions. There is also a case for establishing 'independent comparability arrangements', providing an agreed database for negotiators, especially but not exclusively for public sector unions.

The 'new unionism'

Prior to the 1997 general election, the TUC (1996a: page 1) argued that 'we need a New Unionism so that unions and employers can work together in partnership to make Britain's industries and services more efficient and competitive and to protect people at work.' This new unionism is rooted in the concept of 'social partnership'. For the TUC, social partnership in the workplace means employers and unions working together to achieve common goals, such as fairness and competitiveness. At national level, it means government discussing issues with employers and unions on an open and fair basis, where a common approach can result in benefits such as attracting inward investment and promoting training and equal opportunities.

The TUC's priority is jobs: good-quality, well rewarded and secure ones. In the private sector, this implies firms which are prosperous, profitable and competitive. In the public sector, it implies good-quality, secure jobs providing high-quality public services, held in esteem by those using them and wanting to use them. The TUC (page 5) sets out an agenda for achieving this, underpinned by the belief that 'the new Government's early actions must lay the foundations for economic success and to create a greater spirit of national common purpose'. It adds that 'the more trade unions can be seen as part of the solution, the more Government and employers will take up their ideas.'

Medium-term principles and priorities

In the TUC's view, economic priority must be to return to full and fair employment, based on:

- active economic policy by government
- active labour market policies regarding training, the long term unemployed and helping individuals cope with unemployment
- building social partnership between employers and trade unions, and delivering investment in people, greater job security and best practice to secure quality products and services
- increased public investment in social housing, urban regeneration and environmental improvement
- providing help for the long-term unemployed and the young
- promoting workplace skills and security.

As sustainable growth continues, the TUC argues, more resources will be released to support the drive towards full employment, without risking the stability of public finances.

Jobs

Here the TUC is keen to promote the concept of 'best practice' and show how unions and employers can develop the most effective models of work organisation, with the aim of enhancing productivity and competitiveness and protecting individuals. Another area is the organisation of working time and enriching job content to alleviate the problem of monotonous, unchallenging jobs. The TUC would also like to encourage the social partners to explore the scope for 'job security' collective agreements. Another proposal is for public sector bodies to set best practice in terms of job objectives. Action to which the public sector could contribute includes:

- helping combat sex, race, disability and age discrimination at work
- setting the pace in terms of single-status collective agreements to remove discrimination against the low paid, women and manual workers
- creating employment and training opportunities for young people
- promoting youth training and modern apprenticeships which offer high-quality training for young people
- targeting the long-term unemployed
- incorporating an Employment Chapter in the Treaty of Amsterdam and signing up to the Social Chapter.

The TUC also believes that decentralised bargaining has not achieved both low inflation and high employment. In its view (page 11), 'a national framework, and bargaining arrangements for minimum standards can help reconcile the need for local flexibility and national standards.'

Investment

To ensure the foundations for steady growth, the TUC believes that economic policy should aim at limiting consumption growth to a slightly lesser rate than growth of GDP. This is to ensure that resources are available for investment and exports. The priority investment areas identified by the TUC are: transport; information technology; social housing; and health and education. Whilst acknowledging that government is still a major player in the field, the TUC supports the injection of private finance and development of private/public partnerships, which offer ways of protecting public investment and, at the same time, promote additional investment.

Training and education

The TUC's view (page 14) is that 'Britain will only be able to exploit new investment if it becomes a learning society; that is why education has to be a priority of a new Government.' The TUC therefore supports life-long learning and the integration of education and training into a single system. It also argues that employers which involve unions in their training decisions are the most successful in managing change. In this sense, unions can be part of the solution to closing the skills gap experienced by employers.

The new unionism and new industrial relations

For the TUC, given the immense labour market, product market, legal and technological changes over the past two decades, strong trade unions are needed to ensure that the most vulnerable at work benefit from a national minimum wage, through either collective bargaining or a statutory minimum. This is to achieve minimum standards in the labour market. Further, inherent in the social partnership model is the need to minimise industrial disputes and encourage unions and employers to reach employment security agreements. The TUC concludes (page 22) that:

> By acting in partnership with employers on matters such as jobs, training, investment and ... minimisation of industrial disputes, trade unions will ensure that they can help tackle the problems the new Government will face .... trade unions can be part of the solution.

Quality in the public services

With new approaches to public sector management being introduced into public organisations in recent years (Farnham and Horton 1996a and 1996b; Storey 1992), and increasing emphasis being placed on 'service quality', the TUC is becoming increasingly conscious of the need for the unions to address quality as an issue. It distinguishes three approaches to service quality in the public services (TUC 1992a). These are:

- 'quality management', which requires all members of staff to clarify their products and services, so as to identify their customers, and to be given measurable goals to achieve that are monitored on a regular basis (see Chapter 10)
- 'customer care', which clarifies the provider-user relationship by setting out the quality of service to be provided and the rights of redress
- 'quality assurance', which attempts to improve the quality of standards through the application of the British Standards Institution quality assurance standard BS 5750 (now BS EN ISO 9000).

Each of these demands union responses to the search for quality in the public services.

Union participation

The unions argue that most quality programmes are management-driven; consequently they are not designed to accommodate union involvement. The TUC proposes, therefore, that if service quality is to be significantly improved, it requires more direct involvement of employees in decision-making about the way services are provided and managed. According to the TUC, a key challenge for the unions 'is to confront the call for more open communications, devolved self-management and active employee participation'. The unions claim that quality agendas are set by management, with the strategy for enhancing employee involvement designed and executed with minimum consultation with staff. Similarly, employee empowerment is often more concerned with the obligations and duties of individual employees rather than with collective rights and representation. 'The main objective is usually to tie the employee's performance more closely to [the] overall goals of the organisation.' What public service unions are arguing for is the benefits of a 'partnership approach to improving quality service', especially at workplace level, with the key to responsive and effective public services being a well-trained workforce (TUC 1992a: pages 20-22).

A Quality Work Assured (QWA) servicemark

The public service unions want to raise the union profile and articulate more precisely the commitment of staff to quality and what improving service quality means from the workers' perspective. They believe that it is important to grasp the language of service quality and to stress their commitment to partnership, openness, accessibility, flexibility and choice. But the unions also want to formulate a mechanism for identifying the quality component in service provision in relation to the quality of working conditions and the quality of the workforce. The aims of the TUC's QWA servicemark are to (TUC 1992a: page 26):

- increase citizen and customer awareness and evaluation of the conditions and way in which a service is provided
- expose the competence and commitment of the workforce and management
- illustrate best practice in terms of employee participation and involvement
- identify the employer's commitment to training and equal opportunities
- facilitate a close relationship and understanding between staff and service users
- ensure compliance with health and safety and other employment legislation
- increase employee awareness of good management practice
- inform users of an employer's industrial relations record
- help develop quality standards at work
- widen choice and preference
- inform users of staff behaviour and attitudes
- identify labour costs for a public service.

It is hoped, in short, that the QWA servicemark will provide a benchmark by which quality of public service inputs and outcomes might be measured, for the benefit both of users and providers.

The union response

The key 'quality' objective identified for public service unions in the 1990s is to exert a positive influence on the development of public services to the benefit of users and producers. It is suggested that unions will have to work much closer together and that further consideration needs to be given, in managing quality, to union relations with management and service users. The unions are stressing the importance of education and training programmes to equip staff, and union officials, to deal with demands for high-quality services and to ensure that programmes of performance measurement and appraisal are implemented in a fair and systematic way. In campaigning for quality, the unions are arguing that their 'vision is a high-quality workforce producing high-quality services' (TUC 1992b: page 3).

Inter-union disputes

In 1988, the TUC amended its rules on inter-union relations and a new code of practice was approved by Congress to mitigate inter-union rivalry, as a result of the recommendations by a Special Review Body appointed after the 1987 Congress.

The amendments to 'Principle 5' provide that no union is to organise where another union has the majority of workers employed and negotiates terms and conditions, unless by arrangement with that union. Where a union has members, but not a majority and does not negotiate terms and conditions, another union seeking to organise should consult with the existing union. If there is no agreement, the matter should be referred by either union to the TUC. Where a disputes committee adjudicates, it will take into account:

- the efforts that the union opposing entry of another union is making to retain membership and the degree of organisation over this period
- any existing collective bargaining arrangements
- the efforts that the union seeking entry is making to secure majority membership
- the provisions of the code of practice.

The code of practice, which is annexed to the TUC's Disputes Principles and Procedures, is designed to set standards for affiliated unions organising and seeking recognition with an employer on new sites. It requires affiliated unions that are negotiating single-union agreements to give prior notification to the TUC of their intention to do so. The code goes on to say that (TUC 1988: page 19):

> Unions must not make any agreements which remove, or are designed to remove, the basic democratic lawful rights of a trade union to take industrial action in advance of the recruitment of members and without consulting them.

Unions are also expected to co-operate with any procedures operated by the TUC and related bodies concerning inward investing authorities. This is to avoid inter-union competition which could damage the attractiveness of the area. When negotiating recognition agreements, which have implications for substantive agreements, affiliated unions are expected to take into account the general level of terms and conditions that are already agreed with the company and to take all possible steps to avoid undermining them.

Unions and Europe

British unions, acting primarily through the TUC and the ETUC, recognise that the evolution of the EU poses immense challenges for trade unions and trade unionists. For the unions, the essential challenge of EU policy is to make a reality of Europe's social dimension, so that worker and citizen interests are taken into account within the EU, as well as those of business. The TUC is participating with the ETUC to develop economic and social policies aimed at maximising prosperity and economic security for working people in the Union's member states (TUC 1991b; 1996b).

Achievements

Trade unions at both national and European level claim to have achieved a number of their goals on behalf of their members, through European legislation and the courts. These include:

- advances in health and safety legislation and equal treatment between men and women on pay and retirement age
- new rights to maternity leave for women and removal of the upper limit on compensation in sex discrimination cases
- improved rights for part-time workers to claim unfair dismissal and redundancy payments and rights to written particulars
- protection of workers' terms and conditions when businesses change hands
- protection for young workers – although some rights will not apply to British young people until 2000
- introduction of the Working Time Directive
- introduction of the European Works Council Directive which, despite the former Conservative government's opt-out, now covers over 100 UK-based multinational companies and hundreds more based elsewhere in Europe but with subsidiaries in the UK
- introduction of the Posting of Workers Directive, under which pay and working conditions applying in an EU country will be extended to workers working there under contracts from other member states
- an agreement between the social partners on parental leave
- discussions between the social partners relating to part-time, temporary and fixed-term contract workers.

Further, the European Commission has produced a new Social Action Programme (SAP) in which the TUC worked closely with the European Parliament to negotiate the addition of:

- the right to information and consultation in national undertakings employing more than 50 workers
- the right to continued vocational training
- equal treatment for third country workers
- inclusion of a labour clause in public works contracts
- measures to strengthen legal guarantees for trade union freedoms and collective bargaining
- the right to a minimum income
- legislation on poverty, social exclusion and housing
- measures to combat racism and xenophobia.

The TUC's General Council also supports the ETUC's wish to generate more impetus behind the SAP, especially against those employers and governments wanting to block its momentum.

Employment, social and economic policy

The TUC considers that there can be no greater priority than reducing unemployment throughout the EU, which has risen to some 18 million. In its view, the problems associated with unemployment need to be tackled at the European level. The TUC therefore supported the Swedish government's proposal that an Employment Chapter be included in the Treaty of Amsterdam 1997. This was subsequently agreed at Amsterdam and employment strategy is now to be co-ordinated amongst member states of the EU. Its provisions are aimed at:

- enabling men and women to attain a secure livelihood through freely chosen productive employment
- preventing long-term unemployment and social exclusion
- ensuring that demand grows at an adequate rate to ensure sustainable growth
- promoting flexibility by providing workers and job seekers with the skills to adapt to a constantly changing economy.

Other decisions taken at the intergovernmental conference at Amsterdam in 1997 included:

- agreeing a human rights declaration, outlawing discrimination on the basis of gender, race, religion, sexual orientation and age
- guaranteeing free movement of persons throughout the EU, except the UK and Ireland who keep their national border controls
- co-operating over immigration, visas, political asylum, civil and judicial issues and harmonising divorce laws

- agreeing a stability pact regulating participating states' budgetary deficits once a single currency is introduced
- integrating the Social Chapter into the Treaty of Amsterdam, following the UK's agreement to sign it
- co-ordinating common foreign and defence policy through senior civil servants, not politicians
- providing more powers and a simplified co-decision-making role for the European Parliament.

On labour market policy, the TUC strongly supports the rolling review of governments' economic policies which began at Essen in 1994. This includes:

- complementing the employers' wish to see greater flexibility at work with new protections for workers, especially those working atypically
- making education and training a priority in the workplace
- reorganising and reducing working time to ensure that economic recovery is more employment-intensive
- reappraising the effectiveness of EU structural funds in terms of employment generation
- focusing employment programmes on those sections of the population where help is particularly needed
- strengthening job placement services to encourage labour market mobility throughout the EU.

Action on unemployment at European level is also focused on the proposal of the President of the European Commission for a Confidence Pact for Employment. This involves discussions between the social partners (ETUC and UNICE), European Commission, member states, European Parliament and Social and Economic Committee. The aim is to create more effective macro-economic policies including:

- stimulating public and private investment and using European funds to this end
- using private sector profits to raise currently low levels of investment in member states
- reducing real interest rates
- establishing wage-bargaining policies seeking a more equitable balance between wages and profits, whilst recognising the productivity gains being achieved by employees in many sectors of the economy.

The TUC and European unions also want increased provision for education and training for workers and investment in innovation and research.

Economic and monetary union (EMU)

The TUC and ETUC believe that the basic objectives of EMU must be to promote sustainable growth, full employment and stable prices. They want economic policies leading to greater convergence amongst member states in terms of industrial performance, job creation and living standards. Policy on EMU is illustrated in Exhibit 25.

Exhibit 25 **ETUC policy on EMU**

- to strengthen regional policy in the EU and transfer resources to regions in economic difficulty
- to ensure that a new European central bank is made democratically accountable and that the social partners are regularly consulted through an advisory committee
- to use European institutions to create a European industrial relations area as part of the social dimension
- to make member states not complying with agreed economic and employment objectives lose EU financial assistance.

Thus the decision whether or not to take part in EMU is of major importance for the UK economy, trade unions and trade unionists. It will have a lasting effect on the economy, living standards and the collective bargaining framework. With the continuing globalisation of the economy, and relentless moves towards commercial integration, the unions see the advantages of EMU as including:

- lower-risk premiums on cross-border investment
- comparability of prices within the Euro area
- ending uncertainties and the destabilising speculation that is linked to exchange rate variability
- the ability to influence European and global monetary policy
- lower transaction costs on trade and travel.

On the other hand, the potential disadvantages of EMU are:

- the end of exchange rate adjustments as a means of adapting to variations in economic performance amongst countries within the Euro area
- any reduction in influence over domestic monetary policy
- the costs of changing over to the single currency
- any effect on the UK/US dollar rates which are relatively more important for the UK than for other EU countries.

In encouraging debate and dialogue in the UK about the EMU issue, the TUC is speaking to the CBI, Bank of England, consumers and others, in order to work towards a national consensus. The TUC is also seeking real economic convergence, in employment, GDP, productivity and competitiveness – as opposed to nominal convergence in budget deficits, public debt and rates of inflation. 'If EMU goes ahead with the required number of countries, the General Council [of the TUC] believes that the balance of advantage is in joining' (Trades Union Congress 1996b: page 15).

Institutional reform

The ETUC seeks a number of measures to make EU institutions more democratic and accountable. These include:

- creating an enhanced law-making role for the European Parliament
- giving the European Parliament authority to move towards political union, in association with national governments;
- giving the European Parliament power to elect the president of the European Commission.

The ETUC's proposals for amendments to the European treaties are illustrated in Exhibit 26.

Exhibit 26 **Proposed amendments to the Community treaties by the ETUC**

Amendments are proposed:

- ensuring that social and employment policies are a basic EU activity
- giving ethnic minorities and third-world country nationals equal rights
- defining the undercutting of some terms and conditions of employment as unfair competition
- restricting the exclusion from qualified majority voting to fiscal provisions only
- extending qualified majority voting to:

  – job creation and employment protection
  – employment law
  – working conditions
  – equality of treatment
  – initial and continuing training
  – social security and welfare
  – health and safety at work
  – trade union law and collective bargaining
  – information and consultation of workers
  – working environment
  – the environment

- strengthening regional policy.

THE LAW AND TRADE UNION MEMBERSHIP

The law now provides a series of statutory rights for trade union members (see Chapters 3 and 4). The first set of rights, to join and organise trade unions (the right to associate), emerged slowly and took place in two phases. Phase one removed statutory criminal prohibitions, with the state allowing workers and unions to use 'self-help' measures to achieve 'voluntary' employer recognition for collective bargaining purposes. Phase two was the creation of positive legal rights for trade unionists against employers. Workers in Britain now have the right to join an independent trade union and not to be dismissed, or have action short of dismissal taken against them, because of their trade union membership. Such actions by employers are automatically unfair in law and where individuals think these rights have been infringed, they may make a complaint to an industrial tribunal.

The law also provides protections for those who do not want to join a trade union or a particular union (the right of dissociation). This makes it automatically unfair for employers to dismiss individuals where they refuse to belong to a union. This is a relatively new right which, apart from the period of the IRA 1971, has been built into public policy since the early 1980s (see Chapter 7). The strategy pursued has been to remove the legal props to the closed shop, built into the unfair dismissals legislation under the TULRA 1974 and 1976, and to provide a right for employees not to be union members, even where there is no closed shop arrangement. These rights are also enforceable through ITs, with the right of appeal to the EAT. Obviously, strengthening the right not to join a union can be done only at the expense of weakening the right to become a union member and the ways these rights are reconciled vary from country to country (von Prondynski 1987).

The legal relationship of unions to their members

A third and extended group of statutory rights provided to trade union members is to take part in trade union activities and trade union decision-making and to restrain certain trade union actions which are unlawful (intra-union rights). Traditionally, the 'freedom' for members to participate in union activities, and for unions to operate within boundaries of the law, was provided in the union rule book. These common law rights still exist and can be enforced in the courts, under the common law, where individuals consider that the rule book is not being applied by the union or its officials. Indeed, the CRTUM has powers to grant assistance to trade union members who complain that their union has failed to observe the requirements of the union rule book (Commissioner for the Rights of Trade Union Members 1988-96; see below). However, the statutory rights of trade unionists in relation to their unions have been extended in recent years and these are summarised below.

Industrial action ballots

Union members have the right to participate in industrial action ballots when a union is contemplating, authorising or endorsing industrial action and it would be lawful for the union to organise such action, if the statutory requirements of the ballot are satisfied. The law also gives union members the right to apply to the courts, with the assistance of the CRTUM, for an order restraining a union from inducing them to take any kind of industrial action in the absence of a properly conducted ballot. Where appropriate, the courts will make an order requiring the union to take steps to withdraw any authorisation or endorsement of the action, and to leave its members in no doubt that it has been withdrawn. If the court order is not obeyed, anyone who sought the order can return to the court, asking that the union be declared in contempt of court. Unions in contempt of court can be fined and refusal to pay fines can lead to the sequestration of union assets (Department of Employment 1990; see also Chapters 4 and 11).

Union elections

Union members have the right to elect by secret ballot all members of the principal executive committee of their union, at least once every five years. Unions must keep a register of their members' names and addresses and ensure that the entries on the register are accurate and reasonably up to date. Registers can be inspected by an independent scrutineer, where this is felt to be appropriate. The distribution, counting and storage of voting papers must be undertaken by someone independent of the process. All candidates seeking election must be given the opportunity to prepare an election address and have it distributed at no cost to themselves. Elections must be under independent scrutiny, with the scrutineer being responsible for supervising the election and producing a report. If a union fails to comply with these statutory requirements, members can make a complaint to the CO or to the courts. The CO's procedures are less formal than those of the courts but court proceedings may be assisted by the CRTUM (see below).

Union political funds and political fund review ballots

Members of unions have the right to vote, by secret ballot, if their union intends to set up a political fund – and then in political fund review ballots, at least once every 10 years. If a union with a political fund fails to hold a review ballot after 10 years, its authority to spend money on political objects automatically lapses. The rules for conducting political fund ballots must be approved as rules of the union and be approved by the CO. The CO gives approval only where: every member is entitled to vote; there is a postal ballot; and the ballot is subject to independent scrutiny. Where unions fail to comply with the balloting rules approved by the CO, members may complain to the CO or the courts. Union members also have the right to complain, to the CO or to the courts, if a union unlawfully spends money from its general funds on 'political objects'.

Misuse of union funds

Union members have the right to prevent the unlawful use of their union's funds or property. These include the right to seek a court order against union trustees in order to prevent them applying, or permitting the application of, union funds to any unlawful purpose. They also have the right to inspect their union's accounting records, accompanied by an accountant. Further, there is the right to prevent a union's funds or property being used to indemnify anyone for fines or other penalties imposed on them for any criminal offence or for contempt of court. Unions must also take all reasonable steps to provide their members, within eight weeks of sending the annual return to the CO, with a statement covering: income and expenditure; income represented by membership fees; salary and benefits paid to senior officers and the executive committee; and the report of the auditor(s) on the return.

Union membership registers

Union members have the right to ensure that their union maintains a membership register. Unions must allow any members who have given reasonable notice to check, free of charge, at a reasonable time, whether they are included in the register. They must also supply members with a copy of their register entry on request. Any complaints on these matters are dealt with by either the CO or the courts.

Unjustifiable discipline

Union members have the right not to be disciplined, by being expelled, fined or deprived of membership benefits by their union, where that discipline is unjustifiable. Discipline is unjustifiable in law where the individual's conduct is concerned with any of the reasons illustrated in Exhibit 27. Individuals who believe that they have been unjustifiably disciplined by their union may make a complaint to an industrial tribunal. If, after conciliation with ACAS, the tribunal finds that the complaint of unjustifiable discipline is well founded, it makes a declaration to that effect. An application for compensation may also be made to the EAT if the union does not lift the penalty imposed, with the award being 'just and equitable in all the circumstances'.

Exhibit 27 **Unjustifiable union discipline**

It is unjustifiable for a union to discipline its members where they:

- fail to take part in or support any strike or other industrial action;
- show opposition to or lack of support for the above;
- fail to break, for any purpose connected with the above, any obligation imposed by a contract of employment;
- encourage or assist other individuals honouring their contracts of employment;
- assert that the union or its officials has broken, or is proposing to break, any requirement imposed by the union rule book or the law;

- encourage or assist other individuals in making, defending or vindicating such assertions;
- fail to agree to or withdraw from an agreement with an employer for the deduction of union dues;
- resign from the union, refuse to join another union, belong to another union or propose to do so;
- work or propose to work with members of another union or non-union members;
- work or propose to work for an employer who employs non-union members or members of another union;
- consult or seek advice from the CRTUM or the CO;
- refuse to comply with any penalties imposed by the union following unjustifiable disciplinary action;
- propose to do any of the above.

Enforcing union membership rights

The bodies with the responsibility for enforcing the rights of trade members are the courts, CO, ITs and, most particularly, the CRTUM. The role of the CO, for example, is to deal with complaints by union members that trade unions have failed to comply with one or more of the provisions which impose the duty on trade unions to hold secret postal ballots for electing members of their principal executive committees and to maintain an accurate register of their members. In 1996, for example, a typical year, the CO dealt with only 15 decisions of this sort and there was only one outstanding claim at the end of the year (Certification Office 1997).

Table 9 **Applications to the CRTUM for assistance regarding the statutory rights of union members 1996–97**

Statutory right	Number of applications	Outcome
Trustees permitted unlawful application of union property	1	not assisted
Failure to allow access to union's accounting records	3	not assisted
Failure to comply with statutory requirements regarding elections to office	6	not assisted

The role of the CRTUM is much wider. The Commissioner provides material assistance to union members who are contemplating taking legal proceedings against their union in any complaint coming within his statutory remit. He also has the authority to grant assistance to union members who claim that their union has breached its rule book in certain matters.

Table 9 analyses the assistance provided by the Commissioner in the first category of applications, in 1996-97, and shows that he received only 10 applications, with assistance being provided in none of the cases.

Table 10 **Applications to the CRTUM for assistance in union rule book issues 1996–97**

Rule book issue	Number of applications	Outcome
Trustees permitted unlawful application of union property	1	not assisted
Failure to allow access to union's accounting records	3	not assisted
Failure to comply with statutory requirements regarding elections to office	6	not assisted
Appointment, election of a person or removal of person from union office	7	2 assisted
Disciplinary proceedings by union	7	not assisted
Balloting of members	8	not assisted
Application of union's property/funds	5	2 assisted
Constitution or proceedings of committees/conferences	20	3 assisted

Table 10 shows the number of applications for assistance received by the CRTUM in which union members complained that their union had failed to observe the requirements of their rule book. Of the 57 applications received, only seven were assisted by the Commissioner.

The workload of the Commissioner is not therefore very heavy. Summing up the situation in 1996-97, the Commissioner granted only seven applications out of 74 complaints. Four of these seven cases were resolved successfully, one receiving a favourable court order and the other three being resolved without the need for legal proceedings to be commenced. The three remaining cases were ongoing in spring 1997. Thirty applications were found to be outside the scope of the Commissioner and one applicant did not progress his application further. At the end of the year 1996-97, seven applications were under consideration by the Commissioner. The remaining 29 applications, though within the scope of the Commissioner's power to grant assistance, were not assisted (Commissioner for the Rights of Trade Union Members 1997).

UNION RECOGNITION

Recognition of trade unions by employers, for the purposes of collective bargaining on terms and conditions of employment, is a critical stage in the development of employee relations within an organisation. The act of recognition demonstrates a decisive level of acceptance by management of the union role in employee relations and represents a fundamental change in the nature of the employment relationship between employers and employees. It shifts from one based on unilateral management prerogatives, individualist employment practices and unitary personnel management principles to one based on joint regulation, collectivism and pluralism, in those areas covered by procedural agreements between the employer and the union(s) (see Chapter 3).

Table 11 shows the extent of union recognition in Britain, as a proportion of all establishments, for 1980, 1984 and 1990. From these figures, it is clear that whilst union recognition generally declined in the decade 1980-90, it is still more likely amongst:

- manual rather than non-manual workers
- manufacturing rather than service establishments
- public sector rather than private sector workers.

There is also a correlation between union recognition and size of establishment, with larger establishments being more likely than smaller ones to recognise trade unions. In periods of high unemployment, however, obtaining recognition from employers is increasingly a problem for the unions. As the General Secretary of the TUC asserted at its annual congress in 1991: 'Recognition and getting it is probably the single most urgent issue for us all' (TUC 1991c: page 294). Congress therefore reaffirmed its commitment 'to reaching new laws to help unions and members attain recognition from reluctant and hostile employers' (page 282). Discussion in this section focuses largely on union recognition in medium to large private sector establishments. It does, however, have implications for parts of the public sector, where, with the decentralising of management decisions and responsibilities – in hospital trusts, civil service agencies and the educational sector – new recognition issues are arising between the employers and unions.

Multi-union recognition

Multi-union recognition is the norm in British employee relations. This is because of the large number of trade unions in Britain, its trade union structure and its history of employee relations. These factors result in distinctive patterns of employee representation and bargaining structures in establishments where trade unions are recognised. Besides multi-union recognition, other features of employee relations where unions are recognised include multiple bargaining units and separate unions for manual and non-manual workers. In 1990, the WIRS estimates that:

Table 11 **Union recognition in Britain 1980, 1984 and 1990**

	Percentage of all establishments								
	Manufacturing			Services			Public sector		
	1980	1984	1990	1980	1984	1990	1980	1984	1990
Manual workers	65	55	44	33	38	31	76	91	78
Non-manual workers	27	26	23	28	30	26	91	98	84
All workers	65	56	44	41	44	36	94	99	87

Source: Millward *et al* 1992

- 2.5 unions, on average, were recognised in all establishments with recognised unions
- about a third of establishments with recognised manual unions had two or more unions
- over 50 per cent of establishments with recognised non-manual unions had two or more unions.

It also estimates that almost 60 per cent of establishments in the private sector had two or more bargaining units in 1990, with about a half of all unionised workplaces having 'manual-only' unions and some two-thirds 'non-manual-only' unions (Millward *et al* 1992).

Union recognition in Britain is largely a voluntary process. There is no statutory obligation on employers, at the time of writing, to recognise trade unions for collective bargaining purposes, even where there are high levels of union membership within an establishment or part of it. In the USA, in contrast, the National Labor Relations Act 1935 – as amended by the Taft-Hartley Act 1947 – provides a series of rights for American workers. These include the rights: to join unions and organise for collective bargaining purposes; to vote whether or not to be represented by a union by means of a secret ballot, enforced by the National Labor Relations Board; and to be protected from 'unfair labor practices', on the part of employers, which might interfere with their rights regarding trade union organisation (Kochan 1980). This results in more proactive employee relations policies by American employers than in Britain, leading to either union avoidance strategies or pre-emptive union recognition strategies, even though union recognition in the USA is the lowest in OECD countries. (Kochan *et al* 1984). New Labour in its 1997 election manifesto, however, pledged itself to provide enforced recognition in the UK, where a majority of a relevant workforce vote in a ballot for it.

The demand for recognition in Britain is usually a union-driven process. Recognition claims are made where a union, or a group of unions, with members within an establishment, approaches an employer to negotiate what is called a 'recognition and negotiating procedure' or, more simply, a 'recognition agreement'. In essence, a recognition agreement is one between an employer and the signatory union(s) which provides representational rights for a specified group of employees, through the agency of the union(s), in a defined bargaining unit, on agreed matters. This suggests, in all but a minority of cases, that British employers deal reactively with recognition claims made by trade unions, rather than initiating recognition agreements themselves. The employer then has to decide whether to reject, consider or accept a recognition claim on its merits. This is done on the basis of what management perceives to be in the best interests of the company and its employees.

In deciding whether to move towards a recognition agreement with the union(s), employers take a number of factors into account. These include: union strength and effectiveness, including their labour market position; employee attitudes and preferences; and employer policies and objectives. The risks of recognition and non-recognition are normally evaluated by management too, including the need to avoid industrial action, inter-union conflict, fragmented bargaining units and the loss of employer initiative in employee relations decision-making (Institute of Personnel Management 1977). Where, on balance, an employer decides to concede a union claim for recognition – and to negotiate an agreement – a number of decisions need to be taken between the parties in the interests of stable employee relations.

Determining the bargaining level

A crucial issue to be decided is the level at which collective bargaining is to take place. This is normally at employer level in single-site companies or, in multi-plant companies, at either central or site level. The factors influencing this decision include: what, if any, other bargaining arrangements already exist within the company; what comparative advantage management and unions see in bargaining at a particular level; the size and distribution of the potential bargaining group; the extent of union membership and potential membership; the organisational structure; the company's financial control system; and corporate personnel policies (see Chapter 9).

Determining the bargaining unit

Bargaining units are fundamental to collective bargaining and precise definition of a bargaining unit is important for a number of reasons. The bargaining unit:

- establishes rights of collective representation for individual employees in the unit
- defines the area in which procedural and substantive agreements negotiated between the employer and the union(s) apply
- enables employees to know with whom they are grouped for negotiating purposes.

In general, employers want bargaining units appropriate to their organisational structures and employment policies, whilst avoiding workforce fragmentation, and unions want bargaining units based on their recruitment policies and patterns of membership.

A number of factors affect the determination of bargaining units. These are typically grouped into three categories (Commission on Industrial Relations 1974: page 22):

> *(a) Factors relating to the characteristics of the work group*
> job skills and content; payment systems; other common conditions of employment; the training and experience of employees; qualifications and professionalism; and physical working conditions
>
> *(b) Factors introduced by the presence of trade union membership and collective bargaining arrangements*
> employee preferences of association; general employee wishes towards collective bargaining; the maintenance of existing collective bargaining arrangements which are working well; and membership of unions or staff associations
>
> *(c) Factors based on management organisation and areas of decision-making*
> the presence of procedures unilaterally operated by management; management structure; promotion patterns; geographical location; and recruitment source.

Bargaining units, in short, have to be appropriate to the situation in each case. This includes the circumstances of the workgroups concerned, existing collective bargaining arrangements and the needs of efficient management.

The key issue to be resolved in determining recognition claims is that of identifying the 'core group' of employees for recognition purposes, with the above factors being taken into account in doing this. The core group of employees is the one with strong common interests, around which a possible bargaining unit can be formed. For bargaining units to be stable and viable in the long term, it is essential that they are based on the common interests of the employees covered by the collective bargaining arrangement. The core group is central in determining bargaining unit issues, since each unit needs to be based on at least one core group with sufficiently strong common interests to support effective collective bargaining procedures.

Four questions have to be addressed when a core group, or groups, is being considered for inclusion in a bargaining unit. These are its potential in terms of:

- organisational coverage
- geographical coverage
- vertical coverage
- horizontal coverage.

The first two questions are commonly linked together, as are the second two. This means that once a core group is identified, it can be extended by including additional groups of employees within it, in one or more of the four directions listed above. In this way, bargaining units can be designated that cover as wide a common interest group as possible. This avoids creating too many small bargaining groups, which can result in fragmented negotiations and treating related groups of employees inconsistently.

Determining union bargaining agents

Employers normally prefer negotiating with a single union, rather than with several. Apart from the special case of 'single-union' recognition, however, which is discussed below, the majority of bargaining units contain more than one union within them. Two main factors influence the efficacy of the bargaining agents in union recognition claims: employee support for the unions, and the unions' effectiveness as negotiating bodies. Potential employee support can be assessed in terms of: actual union membership within the proposed unit; the number of employees supporting the union(s) claiming recognition; and the number who would be prepared to join the union(s) if recognition is agreed. Union effectiveness is the ability of the unions to organise members, maintain membership and represent members in dealings with the employer. Whilst some employers deal with staff associations, especially for some groups of non-manual workers, most, with few exceptions, prefer negotiating with *bona fide* unions. Union effectiveness can be assessed in terms of their: financial viability; experienced officials; research and legal expertise; and negotiating record.

Drafting the agreement

The types of clauses contained in a recognition agreement, negotiated with trade unions, are illustrated in Exhibit 28.

Exhibit 28 Clauses in recognition agreements

These include:

- names of the employer and the bargaining agent(s)
- a description of the bargaining unit and any sub-units
- the terms and conditions that are negotiable
- union membership and non-membership
- the numbers of, constituencies of and facilities for union representatives
- the negotiating procedures and procedures for handling grievances and avoiding disputes
- other provisions
- provisions for varying and terminating the agreement.

Single-union recognition

Single-union recognition is where a company recognises only one union for collective bargaining and related purposes. In some traditional collective bargaining arrangements, companies may recognise only one union per bargaining unit. But single-union recognition, in the sense that it is used here, provides for only one union bargaining agent, covering all employees with representational rights in the company. This practice is associated with what are called 'new-style' collective agreements or 'new-style' bargaining (see Chapters 3 and 9), although the newness of such activities is, in reality, questionable.

Management and single-unionism

The major difference between the process of single-union recognition and that of multi-union recognition is that it is management and commercially driven, not union driven, although the unions involved in single-union deals would dispute this. One of the first recorded single-union recognition agreements was between Toshiba Consumer Products (UK) and the EEPTU, at Plymouth in April 1981 (Bassett 1986). This agreement arose out of the closure of Rank Toshiba Ltd in 1980 and was negotiated when the new company was established as a single-site operation assembling colour television sets (Rico 1987). Since then, the numbers of such agreements have increased, but the number of firms and employees covered by them is still relatively small compared with those covered by traditional collective bargaining practices.

It is generally recognised that where managements negotiate and consult with trade unions, they often prefer to deal with one union rather than with many. The advantages of this include: having one representational channel for all employees through which all discussions are focused; avoiding inter-union competition and inter-union disputes within the workplace; and simplifying the bargaining structure within which the parties operate. Over and above this, some managements claim that single-union recognition is beneficial where a company is aiming at teamwork, quality and flexibility amongst its workforce – as in 'hi-tech', 'greenfield' site companies. In these circumstances, single-union recognition, with its emphases on harmonised terms and conditions of employment and a committed workforce, is seen as facilitating a common purpose within the company and good working relations between the company and its workers.

In the case of a greenfield site, the process of selecting an appropriate union by the employer is rooted in the management dictum: 'Talk to every union that could conceivably have an interest in representing your employees and then make a decision as to which union best fits . . . Those not selected will respect that decision' (Wickens 1987: page 133). Management's recognition objective is a clear one: to negotiate with one union, on terms, conditions and procedural issues, for all workers in the bargaining unit. This necessitates early discussions with the various unions wishing to represent the bargaining group, whether or not they already have members within the bargaining unit, with management emphasising that it alone will take the final decision as to which union will be invited to sign the draft recognition agreement.

That decision takes account of a number of factors. One is the attitudes and experience of the local union officials, who are normally invited to present their union's case for recognition, each arguing why their union is likely to give the 'best deal' to the company – the so-called 'beauty contest'. Even before this, it is customary for the company to investigate the backgrounds and policies of the unions, both locally and nationally, to 'make an assessment of the "comfort" factor which ranks very highly in the decision-making process' (Wickens 1987: page 134). These factors are likely to include the national and local politics of each union, the reputations of the local union officers and the unions' employee relations records. Information for this is gathered from local companies, employers' associations and media sources. In this respect, the experiences of employers with single-union recognition arrangements is particularly useful, as are those of companies that have not gone down this path – and the reasons why.

Another factor to consider is which union is likely to be the most acceptable to the employees within the bargaining group. Some judgement has to be made by the company about the potential willingness of employees to join the selected union. There are a number of indicators here: existing levels of membership; the respective membership bases of the competing unions; how these relate to the bargaining group; and the degree of occupational homogeneity within the bargaining unit. In some cases, the company surveys its employees, using a secret ballot to assess their preferred union and choice of bargaining agent.

Unions and single-unionism

Union attitudes to single-union recognition are ambivalent. In some sectors, single-union recognition has always been the norm; for example, in retailing and in parts of the white-collar Civil Service. In other cases – union recognition on greenfield sites – it is generally accepted that there are advantages in recognising the sense of having the entire workforce, in one establishment, in a single union in a single bargaining unit. On the other hand, there is hostility amongst some unions to the practice, incorporated in most single-union, new-style agreements, of including so called 'no-strike' or 'final offer' arbitration arrangements (Burrows 1986). These, it is claimed, remove the basic democratic rights of trade unions and their members to take legitimate industrial action against employers, when they deem this to be necessary, and they should be resisted.

The other concern that unions have with single-union agreements is to do with infringing the recruiting and negotiating freedoms of other unions with membership interests in the bargaining unit. According to the TUC (1988: page 9), single-union agreements cause particular differences amongst unions where they:

(a) exclude other unions who may have some membership in the unit covered by the agreement; or exclude unions which previously held recognition or bargaining rights;
(b) exclude other unions who, while having no members in the unit concerned, have recognition agreements in other UK units operated by the same employer;
(c) represent an intrusion by one union into areas considered to be the province of an industrial union(s), or the exclusion by an industrial union of unions representing particular occupations;
(d) are agreed by one union, where another has been previously campaigning for membership perhaps over a long period;
(e) lead unions to compete with each other for employers' approval which encourages dilution of trade union standards and procedures.

It is these factors which led the TUC to amend its rules on inter-union regulations in 1988 (see above).

Derecognition

Though it is still a relatively rare employee relations occurrence, derecognition is nevertheless practised by some employers. It takes place where an employer partially or fully withdraws union negotiating rights from the union(s) in a particular bargaining unit, by giving notice of the intention to terminate an existing recognition agreement. Full derecognition is where negotiating rights for a whole bargaining group are withdrawn – as was the case for school teachers in 1987, when the Burnham Committee was abolished by the government who replaced it with an interim pay advisory committee (Farnham 1993). In other cases, full derecognition takes place, as amongst white-collar staff in some insurance companies, where there is lack of support for the union or staff association amongst the staff concerned. Partial derecognition takes place where the employer unilaterally withdraws the number or coverage of the negotiating groups, and/or union negotiating rights, but at least one recognised union, and one bargaining unit, remains in the establishment or enterprise.

Claydon's analysis (1989) of derecognition is more sophisticated. He analyses derecognition in terms of a matrix and distinguishes between breadth and depth of derecognition. Breadth of derecognition can be 'general', 'grade-specific' or 'plant-specific'. There are five types of depth of derecognition:

- 'partial', where the union retains some bargaining rights
- as 'a bargaining agent', where the union retains only rights to consultation and representation
- 'collective', where the union can represent only members in individual grievances
- 'complete'
- 'deunionisation', where union membership is discouraged.

The most common forms of derecognition appear to be collective 'grade-specific' and complete 'grade-specific'.

The reasons given by Claydon for derecognition include: external pressures; ownership, management and reorganisation; company objectives; and union organisation and industrial relations history – with corporate objectives probably lying at the heart of union derecognition. According to Claydon (page 219) it is 'greater pay flexibility, more flexible working practices, and heightened commitment', especially amongst managerial and staff grades, that are the main employer goals associated with union derecognition.

ASSIGNMENTS

(a) Read Millward *et al* (1992: pages 57-77). (i) Identify union membership trends in Britain 1984-90 and (ii) examine the factors explaining these trends. How do these trends relate to your own organisation?

(b) Examine the latest Annual Report of the CO and explain the legal rules relating to union mergers and amalgamations. Report and comment on recent amalgamations and mergers in Britain and their implications for employee relations.

(c) From the TUC's last Annual Report, identify three key issues of concern to the TUC during this period and indicate how the TUC is attempting to address these issues.

(d) What are the main features of multi-unionism in Britain identified by the Workplace Industrial Relations Survey in 1990 (Millward *et al* 1992: pages 77-85)? What sort of problems associated with multi-unionism occur in your organisation?

(e) Read the Webbs (1913: Part II – Chapter V). Analyse and comment on the role of 'the Standard Rate' as a trade union rule. How significant is the concept of the 'standard rate' for trade union negotiators today?

(f) Read the TUC (1991a: pages 21-28) and analyse the new bargaining agenda developments which it highlights. What are the conditions which are necessary for this agenda to be effective at employer level? How relevant are they within your organisation?

(g) Read the TUC (1992a: pages 30-47). What are the employee relations implications of the case studies outlined in the report? Comment on the survey of quality initiatives provided in Chapter 8.

(h) Examine the view put forward by Anderman (1992: page 248) that:

> The right to dissociate currently embodied in UK legislation has been introduced in recent years as part of a wider legislative programme designed to promote individualism at the expense of established collective structures . . . it calls into question the legitimacy of trade unions as collectivities enhancing the freedom of their members as individuals by the use of collective institutions.

(i) An employer is in dispute with the union representing the technical staff who are taking strike action over a pay claim. One of the strike leaders, who has both a full-time and part-time contract, has been informed by her departmental manager – on the instruction of the chief executive – that he is not to renew her part-time contract. This is due for renewal at the beginning of next month for a further one-year period. What do you do? And why?

(j) Provide some examples of individual conduct that the law would regard as reasons for unjustifiable union discipline, in the case of a lawful trade dispute. What would be some of the employee relations implications of such conduct for (1) management and (2) the union(s) in such cases?

(k) Read the latest Annual Report of the CRTUM. What sorts of applications did she receive during the past year and what were the outcomes?

(l) Read Kochan (1980) and outline the main provisions for union recognition in the USA under the Wagner Act 1935, as amended. How might such a set of legal arrangements be applied to Britain?

(m) Outline the steps to be taken by the employer in responding to a union recognition claim by factory workers in a non-union company, operating on a single site, with 250 employees in the factory, 150 administrative and supervisory staff and 50 technical staff. The union claims 'over 40 per cent membership' amongst the factory workers, '25 per cent' of administrative and clerical staff and 'substantial support' amongst the technicians.

(n) Read Wickens (1987: pages 127-61). Examine how the companies discussed in this chapter went about getting single-union agreements and why. What distinguishes the approach to management-union relations outlined in this chapter from (1) non-union companies and (2) companies with multi-union representation?

(o) Read Burrows (1986: pages 52-62) and examine and evaluate trade union attitudes to single-union deals.

(p) Read Clayton (1989: pages 214-22) and examine the reasons why employers use union derecognition strategies.

(q) An employer recognises a single trade union in a negotiating unit comprising its supervisory and shop floor staff. Management wishes to withdraw recognition arrangements for the supervisors and to put them on personal contracts and performance related pay. Outline a strategy how this might be done and examine some of its implications for employee relations in the company.

REFERENCES

ANDERMAN, S. 1992. *Labour Law*. London: Butterworth.

BAIN, G. 1970. *The Growth of White Collar Unionism*. London: Oxford University Press.

BASSETT, P. 1986. *Strike Free: New industrial relations in Britain*. Basingstoke: Macmillan.

BURROWS, G. 1986. *No-Strike Agreements and Pendulum Arbitration*. London: Institute of Personnel Management.

CERTIFICATION OFFICE. 1992. *Annual Report of the Certification Officer 1991*. London: HMSO.

CERTIFICATION OFFICE. 1997. *Annual Report of the Certification Officer 1996*. London: HMSO.

CLAYDON, T. 1989. 'Union derecognition in Britain in the 1980s'. *British Journal of Industrial Relations*. 27(2).

COMMISSION ON INDUSTRIAL RELATIONS. 1974. *Trade Union Recognition: CIR Experience*. London: HMSO.

COMMISSIONER FOR THE RIGHTS OF TRADE UNION MEMBERS 1988-97. *Annual Reports*. London: Central Office of Information.

CULLY, M. *and* WOODLAND, S. 1996. 'Trade union membership and recognition: an analysis of data from the 1985 Labour Force Survey'. *Labour Market Trends*. May, 104 (5).

DANIEL, W. 1987. *Workplace Industrial Relations and Technical Change*. London: Policy Studies Institute.

DEPARTMENT OF EMPLOYMENT. 1990. *Code of Practice on Trade Union Ballots on Industrial Action*. London: Central Office of Information.

FARNHAM, D. 1993. 'Human resources management and employee relations'. In Farnham, D. and Horton, S. (eds) 1993, *Managing the New Public Services*, Basingstoke: Macmillan.

FARNHAM, D. *and* HORTON, S. (eds) 1996a. *Managing the New Public Services*. Basingstoke: Macmillan.

FARNHAM, D. *and* HORTON, S. 1996b. *Managing People in the Public Services*. Basingstoke: Macmillan.

FLANDERS, *A. 1961. 'Trade unions in the sixties'. In Flanders, A. 1970, Management and Unions*, London: Faber and Faber.

FLANDERS, A. 1968a. 'Collective bargaining: a theoretical analysis'. In FLANDERS, A. 1970, *Management and Unions*, London: Faber and Faber.

FLANDERS, A. 1968b. 'What are trade unions for?' In Flanders, A. 1970, *Management and Unions*, London: Faber and Faber.

GENNARD, J. 1990. *The History of the National Graphical Association*. London: Unwin Hyman.

GMB and UCW 1991. *A New Agenda: Bargaining for prosperity in the 1990s*. London: GMB/UCW.

HYMAN, R. 1975. *Industrial Relations*. Basingstoke: Macmillan.

INSTITUTE OF PERSONNEL MANAGEMENT. 1977. *Trade Union Recognition*. London: IPM.

JACOBI, O., KELLER, B. *and* MUELLER-JENTSCH, W. 1992. 'Germany: codetermining the future'. In Ferner, A. and Hyman, R. (eds) 1992, *Industrial Relations in the New Europe*, Oxford: Blackwell.

KOCHAN, T. 1980. *Collective Bargaining and Industrial Relations*. Illinois: Irwin.

KOCHAN, T., MCKERSIE, R. *and* CAPELLI, P. 1984. 'Strategic choice and industrial relations theory'. *Industrial Relations*. 23(1).

LABOUR PARTY 1997. *New Labour: Because Britain Deserves Better*. London: Labour Party.

MILLWARD, N., STEVENS, M., SMART, D. *and* HAWES, W. 1992. *Workplace Industrial Relations in Transition*. Aldershot: Dartmouth.

RICO, L. 1987. 'The new industrial relations: British electricians' new-style agreements'. *Industrial and Labor Relations Review*. 41(1), October.

STOREY, J. 1992. *Developments in the Management of Human Resources*. Oxford: Blackwell.

TRADES UNION CONGRESS 1966. *Trade Unionism*. London: TUC.

TRADES UNION CONGRESS. 1974. *Trade Union Strategy*. London: TUC.

TRADES UNION CONGRESS. 1981-90. *Annual Reports*. London: TUC.

TRADES UNION CONGRESS. 1988. *Meeting the Challenge*. London: TUC.

TRADES UNION CONGRESS. 1991a. *Collective Bargaining Strategy for the 1990s*. London: TUC.

TRADES UNION CONGRESS. 1991b. *Unions and Europe in the 1990s*. London: TUC.

TRADES UNION CONGRESS. 1991c. *Annual Report*. London: TUC.

TRADES UNION CONGRESS. 1992a. *The Quality Challenge*. London: TUC.

TRADES UNION CONGRESS. 1992b. *Quality Work Assured*. London: TUC.

TRADES UNION CONGRESS. 1994. *Human Resource Management: A trade union response*. London: TUC.

TRADES UNION CONGRESS. 1995. *General Council Report for 1995*. London: TUC.

TRADES UNION CONGRESS. 1996a. *Partners in Progress: New steps for the new unionism*. London: TUC.

TRADES UNION CONGRESS .1996b. *The European Union: Trade union goals*. London: TUC. London: TUC.

VON PRONDYNSKI, F. 1987. *Freedom of Association and Industrial Relations*. Dublin: Mansell.

WEBB, S. *and* WEBB, B. 1913. *Industrial Democracy*. NY: Longmans.

WICKENS, P. 1987. *The Road to Nissan*. Basingstoke: Macmillan.

9 Collective bargaining and joint consultation

Voluntary collective bargaining is still a major employee relations process in Britain (see Chapters 1, 3 and 7). As an employee relations strategy it was adopted by 51 per cent of the private manufacturing employers and 78 per cent of the public sector employers covered by the WIRS 1990. Although union recognition has declined in private maufacturing since then, to 49 per cent of establishments in 1995, it remains high in the public sector, where recognition was 88 per cent in public administration, 83 per cent in education and 64 per cent in the health sector in the same year (Cully and Woodland 1996). It is largely in agriculture and private sector services that collective bargaining is underrepresented – 13 per cent in agriculture, 14 per cent in hotels and restaurants and 23 per cent in the wholesale and retail trade. The coverage of collective bargaining reflects patterns of union membership and union recognition within establishments. In the private sector, for example, the characteristics of workplaces particularly associated with collective bargaining include:

- high union density
- larger enterprises
- predominantly manual or predominantly non-manual workforces.

Conversely, the WIRS 1990 concludes, 'part-time workers are less likely to be covered by collective bargaining because they are more difficult for trade unions to organise' (Millward *et al* 1992: page 93).

As an employee relations process, collective bargaining settles, by voluntary negotiations between representatives of employers and trade unions, the market and managerial relations between employers and employees. In other countries, however, such as in Europe and the USA, it is legally regulated, and collective agreements are legally enforceable between the parties. Collective bargaining is the major method used by trade unions in pursuing the employment goals of their members (see Chapter 8). In 1981, the International Labour Office (ILO 1986: pages 1-2) adopted Convention 154 which provides an operational definition of collective bargaining. This defines it as all negotiations between employers (or employers' organisations) and workers' organisations for the purposes of determining terms and conditions of employment and/or regulating relations between them. The ILO adds that 'not the least important objective of collective bargaining is that of avoiding violence as a means of resolving problems [between employers and employees].'

Although there are a number of different models of joint consultation, it too is a voluntary process and, where unions are recognised, it normally involves managerial and union representatives. By seeking to exclude matters subject to negotiation, joint consultation complements collective bargaining, rather than replacing it, by focusing on the common interests of the parties at employer and/or workplace levels, not their divergent ones. In this way, it provides a joint forum where management and unions can exchange views frankly on matters of mutual concern, such as health and safety, welfare, training, efficiency, quality and information. Unlike collective bargaining, joint consultation is not a power process but an information and communication exchange channel, where management can brief the unions about matters not subject to negotiation or about other issues prior to negotiation. Similarly, the unions can raise issues on which they wish to be informed by management. Whilst taking account of union views on these matters, however, management retains the power and authority to take the final decision on any issues under discussion. In this way, management protects the right to manage on non-negotiable matters and the unions are disassociated from unpopular decisions which they oppose.

THE ECONOMICS OF COLLECTIVE BARGAINING

In free labour markets, the price or wage of labour is established, in the short term, where the market between buyers and sellers is in equilibrium (Chapter 1). This is the market wage where the amount of labour demanded by the employers is equal to the amount supplied by workers. In practice, real life labour market characteristics are inconsistent with the perfectly competitive, free market model. This is because of (Adnett 1989):

- the heterogeneity of workers and jobs, resulting in persistent wage differentials amongst the workforce
- imperfect and costly information, making it difficult for firms and workers to be fully aware of labour market conditions
- the high costs involved in labour turnover for firms and job changing for workers
- the existence of imperfectly competitive product markets
- the behaviour of trade unions as wage bargainers with employers.

There is also the debate about 'segmented' labour markets. Those using this analysis argue that open labour markets are found only in the secondary labour market, characterised by labour-intensive, low-technology, low-paid industries. In the primary labour market, which is characterised by well-paid, high-status, secure jobs, firms operate structured internal labour markets (ILMs) which are often non-unionised. These structured ILMs are largely independent of competitive forces in the wider labour market. This requires firms to finance their own internal training programmes, partly because of the technological demands of jobs, thus encouraging them to reduce their labour turnover (Doeringer and Piore 1971). Because of these factors, the wages structure reflects custom and practice, rather than worker productivity or external market forces. It is social cohesion, rather than efficiency, which underlies the relative wage rigidity and seniority determined pay scales of ILMs (Doeringer 1986).

What, then, is the function of trade unions in the labour market? Basically, it is to offset the relative disadvantage in market bargaining power that workers have as individuals when negotiating wages and conditions of employment with employers. The employer is in a strong labour market position, if it negotiates separate wages deals with each of its workers individually, because it can undercut wages, especially in conditions of unemployment. The employer does this by recruiting only those workers willing to take the lowest wage offered. By joining the union, employees try to even up the wage bargaining disparity between themselves and the employer, thus remedying their labour market disadvantage.

Once it is recognised as a wage bargaining agent by the employer, the union aims to gain improvements in its members' terms and conditions of employment. It does this through its wages claims. Union wage claims are based on one or more of the following grounds:

- the rate of inflation
- the profitability of the enterprise
- increases in the labour productivity of its members
- inter-occupational wage comparabilities
- labour market shortages.

One way in which the union can achieve its wages objectives is by restricting the supply of labour to those who either are union members or who join the union once they are employed. If the employer can hire cheaper non-union labour, then the union will find it very difficult to protect the existing wage levels and conditions of work of its members. The classical method used by unions was to restrict labour supply through 'the device of the restriction of numbers' (the apprenticeship system) and the closed shop (Dunn and Gennard 1984). Current legislation, however, makes it very difficult for employers and unions to negotiate closed shop agreements – whether of the pre-entry or post-entry type.

Figure 12 **The union effect on wage rates and employment**

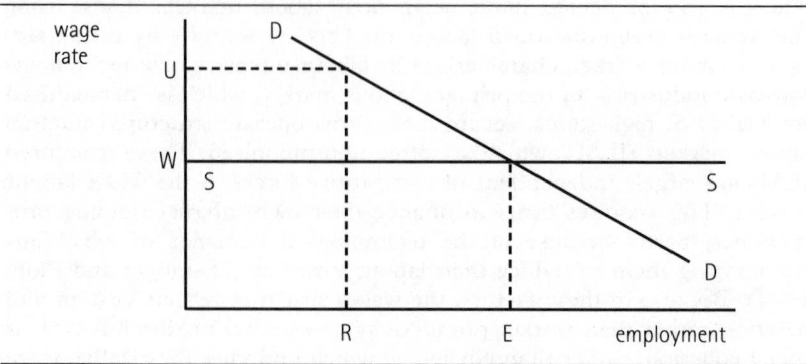

The union effect on wage rates and employment, through collective bargaining, is outlined in Figure 12. In the absence of a union, the firm, operating in a free labour market, faces a downward sloping labour demand curve DD and a horizontal labour supply curve SS, since labour supply is fixed in the short term. This results in a market wage of W and an employment level of E. By restricting labour supply to the firm to amount R, the union can increase the market wage to U, thus trading off lower employment for higher wages for its members. How far the union goes in this direction depends on the preferences and tastes of the union leadership and its members. It can try to maximise either the per capita income of those in employment or the total income of its members. What its wages policy is depends on the distribution of power and the structure of decision-making within the union.

Union wage bargaining power varies across firms and industries. In addition, the more inelastic labour demand is, in a firm or an industry, the larger is the wage differential for the workers. Since the demand for labour is a derived demand, which depends on the demand for a firm's output, there are differences in the wage rewards between firms and industries operating in different product markets. In industries in 'soft' markets, with little domestic or foreign competition, firms are likely to make substantial profits in buoyant market conditions, with the unions and their members benefiting from this.

In highly competitive industries with 'hard' markets, by contrast, if the union raises wages above the market level, firms will be driven out of business. It is possible to raise wages above the market level only where the union organises the whole industry. The result of this will be that firms will pass on wage increases, negotiated by the union for its members, to consumers in the form of higher product prices.

Union wage differentials can also arise from unpleasant conditions of work. Where unions operate in firms and industries with rising productivity, due to management-led changes in working practices, and this results in unpleasant working conditions, they try to negotiate compensating wage increases for their members. As a result, the employer obtains higher productivity, shareholders gain higher profits and union members are compensated for worsened conditions of employment. This practice is called productivity bargaining.

THE NATURE OF COLLECTIVE BARGAINING

It was the Webbs (1913) who provided the first detailed analysis of collective bargaining. They identify collective bargaining as one method by which unions enforce the common rules of the trade (see Chapter 8). They put forward the classical view of trade unions as primarily wage bargaining agents, whose role is to offset the inequalities of individual bargaining between employers and workers in the labour market. For Flanders (1968), collective bargaining is a power-centred rather than an economic process, with unions using their power to penetrate the management function by acting as institutions of 'job regulation' on any matter affecting the employment interests of their members (see Chapter 8). Dubin (1954), a sociologist, sees collective bargaining primarily as the industrial counterpart to political democracy, which provides a source of social stability, social order and social change in industry and society.

Kahn-Freund's (1954) penetrating analysis of collective bargaining, from a socio-legal perspective, argues that it is associated with the evolution of social norms to regulate social conflict in industry. The emergence of collective bargaining depends on the extent and forms of legal intervention by the state. For Marxists, collective bargaining is the process by which the working class, through experiencing industrial action, trade union militancy and employer exploitation, becomes politicised. Unions are the means not only of protecting the employment interests of their members but also furthering the class struggle between the wage earning 'proletariat' and profit seeking capitalists (Hyman 1975).

Bargaining: contract, law and governance

Chamberlain and Kuhn (1965) provide one of the most comprehensive and persuasive analyses of collective bargaining, by identifying three views of the process. These are 'the marketing concept', 'the governmental concept' and the 'industrial relations concept'. In outline, in the marketing concept, collective agreements act as a 'contract' between the parties to employee relations. In the governmental concept, they are a system of 'law-making', applied and adjudicated through collective bargaining. And in the industrial relations concept, collective agreements provide a method of 'industrial governance', whereby corporate decision-making focuses on 'jointly decided directives'.

The wage-work bargain

The marketing concept views collective bargaining as an exchange relationship. It is a means of contracting for the sale of labour, between employer and employee, through the agency of the union. The collective agreement acts as a contract for the buying and selling process which is strictly and definably limited, for a specified period. This view of collective bargaining is equivalent to that of the Webbs and is based on the assumption that the bargaining inequality in the labour market, between employer and employee, oppresses individual workers and needs to be remedied. Whether or not the substantive agreements arrived at establish an equality of bargaining power is irrelevant. What is important is the strict interpretation and application of the collective agreement. Its terms represent the bargain struck and its clauses are to be honoured for the period that it runs. In disputes over the contractual obligations of the parties, recourse may be made to the relevant procedural arrangements between the parties.

Industrial jurisprudence

The governmental concept of collective bargaining views it as a constitutional system in industry. It is a political relationship, in which the union shares industrial sovereignty with management over the workers and, as their representative, uses that power in their interests. The industrial constitution, written by management and union representatives, has legislative, executive and judicial elements. The legislative branch consists of the joint management-union committees which make and interpret agreements. Executive authority and the right to initiate decisions are vested in management, but within the framework of the industrial 'legislation' determined by the parties. Management has the right to manage, plan product development, change working methods and create personnel policy but it must act within the established 'rules'. Where differences between the parties cannot be resolved by negotiation, the judicial element of the industrial constitution is used. This involves the use of procedures to settle differences between the parties and, ultimately, the intervention of third parties to determine the issue, if necessary.

According to Chamberlain and Kuhn, the ethical principle underlying the governmental approach to collective bargaining is 'the sharing of industrial sovereignty'. It has two facets (page 124):

> In the first place, it involves a sharing by management with the union of power over those who are governed, the employees. In the second place, it involves a joint defense of the autonomy of the government established to exercise such power, a defense primarily against interference by the state. Both stem from a desire to control one's own affairs.

The sharing of power between management and union means that only employment rules which are mutually acceptable, and have the consent of employees, can be legitimised and enforced. Sovereignty is held jointly by management and unions in the collective bargaining process, resulting in participation by the union in job control. On the other side, sovereignty is also concerned with limiting the control of those, outside the employee relations constitution, who might wish to interfere in the autonomous collective bargaining process.

Chamberlain and Kuhn go on to distinguish between the 'constitutional law of industry' and its 'common law'. In the former, the collective agreement establishes the terms of the employer-employee relationship and individual cases are governed by these terms. In the firm's common law, developed through joint procedures for settling grievances and differences of interpretation of agreements, there are no written standards of control. 'It is the mutual recognition of the requirements of morality and the needs of operation which provides the basis of decision and ultimately the norms of action' (page 128). And these are often rooted in the social customs and unwritten conventions of the enterprise.

Industrial governance

The third concept of collective bargaining, the industrial relations concept, is a functional relationship. It is where the union joins with company officials in reaching decisions on matters in which both have vital interests. A system of industrial governance follows out of a system of industrial jurisprudence. The presence of the union allows the workers, through their representatives, to participate in the determination of policies guiding and ruling their working lives. Indeed, 'collective bargaining by its very nature involves union representatives in decision-making roles' (page 130). Since the nature of the bargaining process is appropriate to its own industrial setting, collective bargaining is a method of conducting industrial relations, using procedures for making joint decisions on all matters affecting labour.

The ethical principle underlying the concept of collective bargaining as a process of industrial governance is that those who are integral to the conduct of an enterprise should have a voice in making those decisions which are of most concern to them. This is the 'principle of mutuality' and is a correlate of political democracy. According to Brandeis (1934):

> collective bargaining is today the means of establishing industrial democracy – the means of providing for workers in industry the sense of work, of freedom, and of participation that democratic government promises them as citizens.

This view of collective bargaining implies that authority over workers requires their consent. And defining authority within the enterprise involves areas of joint decision-making through collective agreement. As conceptions of the corporate decisions affecting worker interests expand, so does the area of joint agreement. 'And as the area of joint concern expands, so too does the participation of the union in the management of the enterprise' (page 135). Ultimately, collective bargaining becomes a system of management.

Bargaining as a developmental process

These three views of collective bargaining are not mutually exclusive. They can be seen as stages in the development of the collective bargaining process and of the bargaining relationship between an employer and a union. As the scope of collective bargaining extends, there is a shift along the spectrum from the marketing, to the jurisprudential, to the industrial governance concepts. Similarly, as the scope of collective bargaining shrinks, there is a shift back towards the marketing concept.

These three approaches to collective bargaining represent different conceptions of what the bargaining process is about and they express normative judgements about it. Each stresses a different guiding principle and each influences the actions taken by the parties. For example, under the marketing concept, withholding data or distorting facts may be a legitimate negotiating tactic by the parties. Under the governmental concept, it may be difficult to determine whether specific data should be accessible to both parties, or confidential to one. Under the industrial relations concept, all relevant data become necessary to make informed, joint decisions.

The distinctions amongst these three approaches are not just academic ones but practical. The marketing approach emphasises the existence of alternative choices in any employer-union relationship, however limited these are. The governmental and industrial relations approaches emphasise the continuity of a given relationship and regard collective bargaining as a continuous process. Which approach is stressed is determined by the views adopted by the parties as to the nature of the bargaining process, the importance they place on particular bargaining outcomes and the balance of bargaining power between them.

NEGOTIATING BEHAVIOUR

A seminal but complex analysis of negotiating behaviour in the collective bargaining process is provided by Walton and McKersie (1965). They distinguish four sub-processes of negotiating activity, each with its own function for the parties to negotiation, its own patterns of behaviour and its own instrumental tactics. These are: distributive bargaining; integrative bargaining; attitudinal structuring; and intra-organisational bargaining. The originality of their study lies in its synthesis of the interaction and interrelationship amongst these four sub-processes.

The distributive bargaining model

Distributive bargaining is a conflict-resolving process, involving competitive bargaining behaviour between the negotiators. It is aimed at influencing the division of limited resources between them. It is central to management-union negotiations and is usually regarded as the dominant activity in their relationship. Distributive bargaining involves a 'win-lose' situation for the parties. In a wage negotiation, for example, what the management side wins, the union side loses. And what the management side concedes, the union side gains. In game theory, it is a 'fixed-sum' pay-off, with each side giving up something to achieve a compromise agreement.

In distributive bargaining, the collective bargaining agenda consists of 'issues' or areas of common concern in which the objectives of the parties are in conflict. Since distributive bargaining is the process by which each party attempts to maximise its own share of fixed, limited resources, the following sorts of issues are determined by it:

- wage levels
- conditions of employment
- working arrangements
- staffing levels
- union security
- employee job rights
- discipline
- lay-offs.

But there is also a degree of mutual dependency between the parties. This is because settling conflict between them enables each side to benefit from the relationship. Both sides need to continue their relationship, rather than terminate it.

The bargaining range of the parties is bounded by upper and lower limits. At some upper limit of wage costs, the employer is forced to cease trading. At some lower limit, it loses the ability to retain its workforce. For any settlement point chosen by the negotiators, within this bargaining range, there are two possible outcomes. The parties may agree or disagree. Yet what negotiators demand, and what they actually expect, depends on their preferences or 'subjective utilities' for possible settlements. These also depend on their preferences or 'subjective disutilities' for avoiding strikes – and the potential costs of these. Negotiators have to evaluate various possible settlements by assigning probabilities to them. Their target and resistance points, in the bargaining range, reflect assessments of these utilities, probabilities and expected outcomes.

The integrative bargaining model

Integrative bargaining is a problem-solving process in which the negotiators seek a solution to a common employee relations problem. It takes place when the nature of the problem permits solutions which benefit both parties, or at least do not require equal sacrifices by both of them. It is the process by which the parties attempt to increase the size of the joint gain between them, without regard to the division of resources. The resolution of the problem, by negotiation, represents a 'win-win' situation for the parties. In productivity bargaining, for example, where management and the union try to get lower unit costs of production, through more efficient working practices, the gains in cost savings are shared. This results in more profits for the company, higher wages for the workforce and lower prices for the customers. In game theory, this is a 'positive sum' game, with benefits to both sets of negotiators.

The integrative collective bargaining agenda focuses on 'problems', rather than issues. These contain possibilities of greater or lesser amounts of value to both parties. Walton and McKersie argue that integrative bargaining potential is more normally found in qualitative rather than monetary employee relations issues. These include:

- providing individual job security, whilst increasing management flexibility
- preserving jobs, whilst raising enterprise efficiency
- expanding employment benefits, whilst limiting the employer's costs
- facilitating union security, whilst providing management control, through closed shop or 'agency' shop agreements.

The integrative bargaining model comprises four main stages: identifying the problem; searching for alternative solutions and their consequences;

ordering preferential solutions; and selecting a course of action. The conditions facilitating collective bargaining problem-solving depend on a number of factors. These include:

- the motivation of the parties
- access to information by the parties
- their having the communication skills to exchange this information

a supportive and trusting climate between them.

The tactics used by negotiators for optimising integrative bargaining outcomes focus on developing and inducing these conditions between the parties.

Mixed bargaining

It is rare, in practice, for the collective bargaining agenda not to include items which can be pursued only through some combination of distributive and integrative bargaining. Management-union negotiations present few pure-conflict situations and few problems allowing the parties total mutual gain. This results in 'mixed bargaining' which is a complex combination of the two processes, involving a variable sum, variable pay-off structure. Distributive bargaining assumes little or no variability in the sum available to the parties, whilst integrative bargaining assumes no difficulty in allocating shares between them. Mixed bargaining confronts both of these possibilities simultaneously, recognising that they are interdependent. It involves complex bargaining strategies and presents the parties with difficulties in identifying the preferred strategy. As Walton and McKersie write (page 179):

> The point . . . is that as bargaining comes to a showdown, what is purely integrative bargaining or what is beginning to move toward distributive bargaining becomes difficult to separate. Both sides are trying to converge on a point, but at the same time they are trying to protect their own self-interests.

The attitudinal structuring model

According to Walton and McKersie, an additional function of negotiating is that of influencing the relationships between the parties. These attitudes include friendliness or hostility, trust, respect, the motivational orientation towards each other – especially regarding competition or co-operation between them – and beliefs about each other's legitimacy. Negotiators take account of personal interaction in negotiations to produce attitudinal changes between them. Attitudinal structuring is a socio-emotional process used by negotiators to attain desired relationship patterns between themselves and to change attitudes during negotiations.

Walton and McKersie construct a model of the social-psychological forces affecting bargaining relationships. These include:

- the structural determinants of behaviour
- attitudinal structuring activities
- emergent relationship patterns
- the consequences of these patterns.

They then develop a model of the attitudinal change process using two theories: cognitive balance theory and reinforcement theory.

The essence of cognitive balance theory is that individuals prefer consistency or balance amongst their cognitions, rather than dissonance. There is a psychological cost in holding discrepant cognitions. By introducing a discrepant cognition into another's awareness, the negotiator creates forces aimed at modifying existing cognitions, inducing a change in the target attitude and producing a change in negotiating behaviour.

Reinforcement theory assumes that people behave in ways which are rewarded, whilst avoiding behaviour which is punished. Negotiators therefore use rewards and punishments to shape the other party's behaviour. Where that party adopts co-operative patterns of behaviour, which are rewarded by his or her opposite number, it tends to develop more positive attitudes consistent with the new behaviour. In this case, a change in the target behaviour results in changes in negotiating attitudes.

The intra-organisational bargaining model

Intra-organisational bargaining is the process that takes place within the management side and union side, prior to and during negotiations. It seeks to resolve the conflicts over objectives, strategies and tactics within each bargaining organisation and to achieve internal consensus within them. Walton and McKersie analyse these conflicts in terms of the relationships between the chief negotiators and the groups they represent.

In examining the nature of internal conflict within bargaining organisations, Walton and McKersie focus on 'boundary role conflict' and 'factional conflict'. Boundary conflict results from the forces pulling chief negotiators in opposite directions; those forces arising from the internal expectations of their own groups and those arising from the other side's expectations during negotiations. Factional conflict arises from differences over negotiating objectives or the means of achieving them. The conditions under which internal conflict is likely to be most pronounced are where there are different preferences and feasibility estimates within the bargaining organisation. These, in turn, arise out of differences in underlying motivations, perceptual factors and emotional states of its constituents.

In response to boundary and factional conflicts, chief negotiators use a variety of behavioural techniques aimed at bringing the expectations of their constituent groups into line with their own. The problem arises from gaps between the expectations of the negotiators' groups and the negotiators' projections about the outcome and their judgements about the best way to bargain. 'The problem is resolved if expectations are brought into alignment with achievement, either *before the fact* of settlement or *afterward*, or if *perceived* achievement is brought into alignment with expectations' (Walton and McKersie 1965: page 303).

Chief negotiators have to make strategic choices about whether to modify, ignore or comply with the substantive and behavioural expectations of their groups, applying appropriate 'tactical assignments' to them:

- They may attempt to modify the aspirations of their group, ignoring their behavioural expectations. This is the most active strategy for achieving intra-organisational consensus.
- They may attempt to modify their group's aspirations, but less directly, by managing to comply with their behavioural expectations. This is a moderately active strategy.
- They may ignore, rather than change, their group's aspirations, whilst complying with their behavioural expectations, which is a passive strategy.

Synthesising the sub-processes

In synthesising the four sub-processes of negotiation, Walton and McKersie identify the 'commitment pattern' as the key aspect of distributive bargaining: 'openness in communication' in integrative bargaining; 'trust' in attitudinal structuring; and 'internal control' within the bargaining organisation in intra-organisational bargaining. Strategic and tactical issues arise, however, in the synthesising process. For example, whilst an 'early and firm commitment strategy' is preferable in distributive bargaining, it frustrates integrative bargaining, is likely to be negative for attitudinal structuring and could frustrate the other party's aim of achieving internal consensus in his or her bargaining organisation.

Similarly, a high degree of open communication is preferable for integrative bargaining and is consistent with efforts to improve relationships between the parties. However, anything but openness is required for distributive bargaining. It can also be problematic for intra-organisational bargaining, where negotiators often keep their organisations in the dark about bargaining developments or exaggerate their bargaining achievements.

Trust is a key element affecting attitudinal structuring. It plays a limited but essential role in distributive bargaining, has a more central role in integrative bargaining and facilitates intra-organisational bargaining. 'The fact is that trust appears to be an unmixed asset in [all] negotiations. There is little to commend a policy of distrust [in any respect]' (Walton and McKersie 1965: page 358). The amount of 'internal control' influences how negotiators attempt to resolve intra-organisational bargaining within the bargaining organisation: the more the control, the more the chief negotiator is able to persuade the group to adopt his or her views. However, whilst control is important for purposive attitudinal structuring, it has advantages and disadvantages for both distributive and integrative bargaining.

BARGAINING POWER

Bargaining power is a central and important concept in collective bargaining. As Fox and Flanders (1969: page 250) comment: 'Power is the crucial variable determining the outcome [of collective bargaining] . . . [though] only when the group is able to mobilise sufficient power . . . does [employee relations] conflict become manifest.' Various theories have been proposed to explain bargaining power and its impact on negotiating outcomes.

One group of theories analyses how bargaining power is generated or created by the participants. The writers examining the 'causes' of bargaining power include Hoxie (1921), Pen (1952), Hicks (1932) and Dunlop (1950). Hoxie, for example, discusses the factors giving unions bargaining strength. Pen suggests a model of bargaining which incorporates the relative satisfactions of the parties in the bargaining process. He also considers how time brings about changes in the balance of power as economic conditions and public opinion shift. Hicks, an economist, sees wage bargaining power in terms of the levels of sacrifice made by the parties, to achieve specific advantage for themselves and those they represent. For Dunlop, bargaining power is determined primarily by the preferences of employers and workers, market conditions, negotiating skills and the ability to coerce the other party.

Atkinson (1980) argues that certain propositions can be derived from what these theorists have hypothesised about the generation of bargaining power. These are:

- What creates bargaining power can be appraised in terms of subjective assessments by individuals involved in the bargaining process.
- Each side can guess the bargaining preferences and bargaining power of the other side.
- There are normally a number of elements creating bargaining power.
- The volatile elements in creating bargaining power may be positive or negative. Positive elements provide inducements to adopt certain bargaining positions, whilst negative elements are the costs or disadvantages likely to be incurred by negotiators in not adopting certain bargaining positions.
- Bargaining power is dynamic and not static.

The second group of theories analysing bargaining power examines the consequences or the 'effects' of that power in bargaining relationships. Phelps Brown (1966: page 331), for example, estimates the differences made by collective bargaining to wage movements and identifies 'a positive association between those movements and collective bargaining'. Schelling (1963) suggests that bargaining power is, in the last analysis, the strength of the negotiator's position in the 'non-bluff' situation. And Stevens (1963: page 81) defines bargaining power as either 'power which is fully inherent in the original (pretactical play) pay-off matrix' or power which 'is (in part) tactically contrived by "moves" which rig the game'.

According to Atkinson (1980: page 11) the propositions following from these analyses of the effects of bargaining power are:

- The scarcer the resource in contention – and the greater the desire of the parties to possess it – the greater the importance of the strengths of the positions from which they make their demands.
- Bargaining power determines the position that can be adopted by each party, after all bluff has failed.
- The credibility of a negotiating position depends on whether the other side perceives that power to be real and that it will be used in support of a bargaining commitment.
- It is not total bargaining power that is important in the negotiating process but the '*area of imbalance*' between the two sides in the bargaining relationship.

Assessing bargaining power

A useful model for assessing bargaining power is provided by Atkinson. He links the definition of bargaining power provided by Chamberlain and Kuhn (1965: page 170) with the bargaining model provided by Levinson (1966). Chamberlain and Kuhn define bargaining power as the ability to secure another's agreement on one's own terms. A union's bargaining power, for example, is management's willingness to agree to the union's terms, with that willingness, in turn, depending 'on the cost of disagreeing with the union terms, relative to the cost of agreeing to them'. This definition assumes that negotiators adopt the course of action *least* likely to hurt them and the side they represent.

Your party's 'bargaining power', according to Atkinson, is indicated by *disadvantages to your opponent of disagreeing with your proposal* relative to *disadvantages to your opponent of agreeing with your proposal.* Conversely, their bargaining power is indicated by *the disadvantages to you of disagreeing* with their proposal relative to *the disadvantages to you of agreeing with their proposal.*

Both the disadvantages of disagreement and the disadvantages of agreement need to be examined in terms of the costs of the disadvantages to the party and the *likelihood* of the *costs* being incurred. Atkinson suggests that the costs for each element representing a disadvantage may be rated from 1 (a very low cost) to 10 (a very high cost). Similarly, the likelihood of the cost being incurred for each element may range from 0.1 (where the element has little chance of becoming a cost) to 1.0 (where the element is certain of becoming a cost).

Combining the costs and likelihoods for each element gives a total weighting for the disadvantages of disagreeing and of agreeing with a bargaining proposal. Where agreement with the proposal incurs more weighting (costs) than disagreement does, bargaining power rests with *the party to whom that proposal is made* (for that proposal alone). Where agreement with the proposal incurs *less* weighting (costs) than disagreement does, bargaining power rests with *the party making the proposal.*

Applying the bargaining power model: an example

A hypothetical example of how the above model can be used to assess bargaining power is shown in Figure 13. In this case, the model is being used to provide guidance to the management negotiators, in determining their immediate response to the annual wage claim of the unions representing the manual workers in their company. The basic question facing management is where bargaining power rests and why.

Let us examine a situation where the unions are claiming an across-the-board wage increase of 7 per cent and a shortening of the working week from 37.5 hours to 35 hours. The factors to be taken into account by management in making their response include: inflation is 4 per cent and falling; the going rate for local wage increases is 2-3 per cent; unemployment locally is low but rising; and demand for the company's products is rising. The unions have balloted, and received support, for a 'work to rule' if the wage claim is not satisfied.

Figure 13 **An illustrative use of the bargaining power model**

Disadvantages to management of disagreeing with the unions' claim

Element	Cost	Likelihood	Total
work to rule	8	1.0	8.0
lost orders	8	0.9	7.2
some workers might leave firm	7	0.4	2.8
			18.0

Disadvantages to management of agreeing with the unions' claim

Element	Cost	Likelihood	Total
increased unit costs of production	10	1.0	10.0
settlement higher than 'going rate'	7	1.0	7.0
could set a precedent	8	0.5	4.0
			21.0

In this example, agreement by management with the unions' bargaining proposal is likely to incur more weighting (or costs) to management than disagreement. This indicates that bargaining power rests with management for this proposal. In this case, however, the balance of power is relatively marginal. This illustrates both the strengths and weaknesses of this approach to assessing bargaining power. On the one hand, when individuals make such assessments:

- they are clearly subjective

- reassessments are necessary as bargaining proceeds, in the light of new information
- it is difficult to quantify 'bargaining power'.

On the other hand, this approach:

- identifies the elements contributing to bargaining power in different situations
- provides a basis for analysing a bargaining position
- helps to formulate a bargaining strategy and prepare a case.

EMPLOYER BARGAINING STRATEGY

In deciding to recognise trade unions for collective bargaining purposes, employers also have to determine a strategy as regards the bargaining level on which they will negotiate with the unions (see Chapter 8). Post-recognition, a reassessment of bargaining levels may also be necessary. A number of strategic choices of bargaining levels is available: multi-employer, single employer and enterprise bargaining or a combination of these levels (see Chapter 3). The level or levels at which collective bargaining takes place is a vital management task and a crucial element of an employer's bargaining strategy. As Towers (1992: page iii) concludes, it has implications for the process of bargaining and the distribution of power between the parties. 'It affects the content of collective agreements and has important "knock-on" effects for the role and status of the personnel function and trade unions.' The bargaining level is also significant in the control of labour costs and for national economic policy objectives.

Bargaining trends

Table 12 shows the most important bargaining level for determining the most recent pay increase for manual and non-manual employees in private manufacturing, the private services and the public sector in 1984 and 1990. It is limited to those employers that bargained with unions in these sectors and relates only to the most important pay-bargaining level. In many instances pay-bargaining for these groups of employees took place at more than one level, whilst in some cases non-wage issues were also determined at the 'most important' pay-bargaining level. Despite its limitations, however, Table 12 indicates some important trends in pay-bargaining levels since the mid-1980s.

The most striking feature of Table 12 is the predominance of multi-employer-level pay-bargaining in the public sector. This was true for both manual and non-manual bargaining groups, even though there was a slight decline in the proportion of non-manual employees covered by it in 1990, compared with 1984. There were declines in the importance of multi-employer-level pay-bargaining for both manual and non-manual employees in the private services between 1984 and 1990, though its importance

Table 12 **Most important bargaining level for most recent pay increase in manufacturing, private services and public services, 1984 and 1990**

per cent

	Manual employees		Non-manual employees	
	1984	1990	1984	1990
Manufacturing				
multi-employer	41	37	20	33
single employer	21	19	36	24
enterprise	38	44	44	43
Private services				
multi-employer	56	35	38	20
single employer	33	52	52	76
enterprise	11	13	10	4
Public sector				
multi-employer	81	81	86	84
single employer	18	18	13	16
enterprise	1	1	1	–

Source: Millward *et al* 1992

appeared to grow amongst non-manual employees in private manufacturing.

By 1990, single-employer-level pay-bargaining was the major feature of the private sector services, for both manual and non-manual employees. Correspondingly, between 1984 and 1990, the importance of single-employer-level pay-bargaining had declined in private manufacturing. This was accompanied by the growth in importance of enterprise-level pay-bargaining for manual employees in private manufacturing between 1984 and 1990 and by the relatively high proportion of non-manual employees in this sector who were covered by enterprise-level pay agreements in both 1984 and 1990.

The decline in multi-employer-level pay-bargaining in the private sector is part of a long-term trend which can be traced back to the 1950s and which accelerated in the early 1980s (Confederation of British Industry 1988). Even where multi-employer bargaining persists, its content progressively excludes pay. The trend towards decentralised pay-bargaining within private sector organisations accelerated from the late 1970s. Indeed, the CBI survey reports that in 1986 nearly 90 per cent of all employees in establishments with collective bargaining had their basic pay negotiated at company or establishment level. However, the situation is complicated by the fact that some employers seek an optimum balance between centralised and decentralised bargaining arrangements (Kinnie 1987), whilst others retain central or corporate control within which local pay bargainers operate (Marginson 1986).

A definitive updating of this data will have to await the outcomes of the next Workplace Industrial Relations Survey, planned to take place during 1997. But more recent data provided by the Labour Force Survey indicates current patterns of union recognition and bargaining across the entire workforce in Britain (Cully and Woodland 1996). This suggests that whilst enormous diversity in the extent and patterns of recognition and collective bargaining amongst different parts of the private sector remains the norm, the public sector continues to be characterised by much greater uniformity and homogeneity (Farnham and Horton 1996).

Towers (1992) highlights a number of factors explaining the trend towards decentralised pay-bargaining levels. These include:

- trade union weakness
- corporate decentralisation preceding decentralised bargaining
- the growth of performance-related pay
- the pressures for employers to link worker productivity with appropriate pay increases.

Palmer (1990: page 27) suggests that the shift towards pay decentralisation has been heavily influenced by the need to recruit, motivate and retain employees of the right calibre to ensure business success. Employers also seem to want the freedom not only to determine pay rates and pay increases locally but also to introduce new pay strategies, including profit-sharing, merit pay and pay bonuses, more suited to their own business strategies. 'For many organisations, pay policy has become a critical element of their strategic business planning.'

Multi-employer bargaining

Multi-employer bargaining, sometimes called industry-wide or national bargaining, is where minimum terms and conditions of employment are negotiated for all employers that are party to the 'national agreement'. Multi-employer bargaining normally requires the constituent employers to belong to the appropriate employers' association (see Chapter 2). The advantages and disadvantages to employers of multi-employer bargaining are outlined in Exhibits 29 and 30 below.

Exhibit 29 **Advantages of multi-employer bargaining**

These include the following:

- it concentrates employer and union employee relations resources
- it leaves local management to concentrate on other business issues
- it provides equitable treatment of employees by all employers in the sector, covered by national bargaining
- it prevents employers playing each other off in the wage-bargaining process.

Exhibit 30 **Disadvantages of multi-employer bargaining**

These include the following:

- it reduces the ability of individual employers to negotiate according to local circumstances
- it leads employers to pay something for nothing locally
- it forces some employers to pay more than they can afford
- it can lead to employees' expecting that national pay increases will be applied to local pay rates, irrespective of effort, whilst some employers will want to pay less than what is negotiated nationally
- it ignores local labour markets, worker productivity and employee performance
- it concentrates union bargaining power and negotiating skills.

Single-employer bargaining

Single-employer or company bargaining is where all terms and conditions are negotiated at employer level, in either single-site or multi-site organisations. The advantages and disadvantages of single employer bargaining to employers are outlined in Exhibits 31 and 32.

Exhibit 31 **Advantages of single-employer bargaining**

These include the following:

- it provides uniform terms and conditions across the company for similar jobs
- it provides stable pay differentials amongst different bargaining groups within the company
- it provides a common approach for handling grievances and resolving disputes in the company
- it concentrates the bargaining power of management and the negotiating skills of management
- it provides greater predictability of labour costs for management
- it avoids wage 'leap-frogging' and minimises wage parity claims across the company.

Exhibit 32 **Disadvantages of single-employer bargaining**

These include the following:

- it is inflexible and makes it difficult to accommodate differences in production systems, product markets, labour markets and technologies within a centralised bargaining system
- it raises the level of management decision-making, reducing local management and employee commitment to these decisions
- it requires very effective in-company communications

- it can lead to over-formalisation of employee relations, be slow to respond to change and be too inflexible
- it can be expensive because of the need to maintain a centralised employee relations system
- it may be difficult to integrate new businesses within the employee relations system.

Enterprise bargaining

Enterprise or plant bargaining is where terms and conditions are negotiated between management and union representatives locally, not at corporate level. Enterprise bargaining is either *autonomous* or *co-ordinated.* Autonomous enterprise bargaining is where each plant has the authority to settle all terms and conditions locally. Co-ordinated enterprise bargaining is where negotiations are conducted at plant level within limits set by the centre. The advantages and disadvantages of enterprise bargaining to employers are outlined in Exhibits 33 and 34.

Exhibit 33 **Advantages of enterprise bargaining**

These include the following:

- it provides shorter lines of communication and speeds the resolution of disputes
- it increases the authority of local management by providing clear responsibility for employee relations
- it increases management ability to respond flexibly to employee relations by introducing pay, conditions and incentives, geared to local conditions
- it increases the commitment of employees through locally determined agreements;
- it dissociates union bargaining power.

Exhibit 34 **Disadvantages of enterprise bargaining**

These include the following:

- it requires management planning and negotiating skills which may not exist at plant level
- it increases the danger of claims for 'wages parity' by the unions
- it requires total pay decentralisation, otherwise it is difficult to maintain differentials
- it complicates labour cost control.

Two-tier bargaining

Two-tier bargaining is where some elements of the reward package are determined at one level, whilst others are determined at another, lower level.

In some cases, multi-employer agreements settle minimum pay rates or minimum earnings nationally and company agreements supplement them by providing the means for determining actual earnings, including pay flexibility, at employer level. In this way, employers combine the stability of framework agreements at industry level with maximum flexibility for individual employers, who are party to national agreements, at corporate level. Such arrangements are claimed to stabilise wage costs at industry level, whilst remaining sensitive to variations in regional and local labour markets.

In other cases, two-tier bargaining takes place within single-employer bargaining arrangements. Here basic conditions of employment can be settled at corporate centre, with pay – especially performance pay – being determined at establishment or plant level. This enables employers to obtain the best of two worlds. Even where decentralised bargaining takes place, coordination at corporate level may be retained through 'the budgetary control mechanism, where labour cost targets are often specified in line with broader targets or rates of return on sales and capital employed' (Purcell 1987: page 55).

Factors affecting bargaining levels

Determining the appropriate bargaining level is a complex task for employers and management, especially those with multi-plant operations and complex business structures. A study by ACAS (1983) suggests that certain structural and organisational factors are key determinants of an organisation's collective bargaining structure, especially bargaining levels. These factors include: the firm's product market; its forms of work organisation; the technology used; its geographic location; its business structure; the union structure; and the payment system.

An analysis by Palmer (1990) which seeks to help employers identify the type of bargaining structure best suited to their own needs, discusses the internal factors, external factors and bargaining topics likely to affect an employer's decision in determining the optimum bargaining level. The internal factors include:

- company organisation (such as decision-making levels, degrees of diversity and plans for expansion)
- management style and management strengths
- plant characteristics (such as size, technology and degrees of interdependence)
- job categories and relationships (such as wage policy, payment systems and bargaining reference groups).

The external factors are:

- union organisation (such as representation, power and membership levels)
- the industry structure (such as market competition, national collective agreements and trading relationships).

The bargaining topics likely to affect decisions on bargaining levels include: the terms and conditions which are negotiable; the procedural agreements which exist; and whether arbitration is used for resolving disputes between the employer and the unions.

General indicators of multi-employer bargaining being preferred by employers are industries having: a large number of small companies; competitive product markets; high levels of trade union membership; high labour costs relative to other costs; and geographical concentration of the sector. Single-employer bargaining is likely in companies with: single product businesses; stable product markets; a centralised corporate structure; and strong trade union organisation. Enterprise bargaining is likely in companies with: multi-product businesses; unstable product markets; multi-divisional structures; and weak trade union organisation locally.

THE NEGOTIATING PROCESS

John Dunlop, a major theoretician of employee relations, and an outstanding mediator, argues that there have been two main approved institutional arrangements for resolving conflicts of interest amongst groups and organisations in Western societies for over 200 years. These are 'the give and take of the market place and government regulatory mechanisms established by the political process' (Dunlop 1984: page 3). He sees negotiating as a positive, alternative mode of conflict resolution between competing groups, such as employers and unions, which has made inroads into both the market and governmental distributive processes. Negotiating provides benefits to both sides, involves compromise, avoids uncertainty and is flexible in its approach. Moreover, even if collective bargaining does not entirely displace market forces, he argues, the differences between negotiators in 'pure bargaining skills and power' may 'result in somewhat different terms and conditions of employment over time than would arise through markets or under governmental dictation' (page 6).

Based on his experience and research, Dunlop provides a 10-point basic framework for analysing the negotiating process:

- It takes agreement within each negotiating group to reach a settlement between them.
- Initial proposals are typically large, compared with eventual settlements.
- Both sides need to make concessions in order to move towards an agreement.
- A deadline is an essential feature of most negotiating.
- The end stages of negotiating are particularly delicate, with private discussions often being used to close the gap between the parties.
- Negotiating is influenced by whether it involves the final, intermediate or first stages of the conflict resolution process.
- Negotiating and overt conflict may take place simultaneously, with the conflict serving as a tool for getting agreement.

- Getting agreement does not flourish in public.
- Negotiated settlements need procedures to administer or interpret the final agreement.
- Personalities and their interactions can affect negotiating outcomes.

An overview

The purpose of negotiating in employee relations is to resolve any conflicts of interest or conflicts of right between employers and trade unions, through both sides modifying their original demands to achieve mutually acceptable compromises between them. The issues may relate to terms and conditions of employment, non-wage matters or combinations of these. A number of stages are discernible in the negotiating process: objective-setting; preparing; bargaining; and implementing.

Objective-setting

To enable movement to take place between the bargaining parties in the negotiating process, each side has to establish a realistic spectrum or set of bargaining objectives. As shown in Figure 14, these consist of an 'ideal settlement point' [ISP], a 'realistic settlement point' [RSP] and a 'fall-back point' [FBP]. The ISP is what the negotiators would ideally *like to achieve* through negotiation, if possible. The RSP is what they *intend to achieve*, whilst the FBP is what they *must achieve* at the very minimum, and without which no settlement can result. The bargaining range of each side lies between its ISP and its FBP, with final settlement taking place between each of the parties' FBPs. Where the FBPs of the two sides do not overlap, there is a 'bargaining gap' between them and, unless there is a modification of their bargaining objectives, no negotiated compromise is possible.

Figure 14 **Hypothetical wage-bargaining objectives for management and unions**

Management Side	ISP *		RSP *		FBP *			
	3	4	5	6	7	8	9	per cent wage rise
Union Side		* FBP		* RSP		* ISP		

Preparing

Identifying, collecting and deciding how to use relevant information across the bargaining table are key elements in preparing for negotiating. Information relates to a number of areas including: facts, precedents, personalities, power and issues. Decisions have to be taken by the bargaining teams about what information is to be disclosed to the other side, when it is to be disclosed and what is to be withheld. In this sense, 'knowledge' or information is power and it can provide a cutting edge in the negotiating process if it is used tactically and authoritatively by either or both sides. Information is normally provided to support and justify the propositions made by each party, as well as to challenge each other's propositions. Bargaining conventions dictate that initial negotiating propositions focus on each party's ISP, with neither side revealing its full strength initially.

Preparing also involves each team deciding who is to be the lead negotiator, who is to take records at the meetings and who is to observe. The leader's role is to conduct the negotiation for the bargaining team. The leader does most of the talking, makes proposals, trades concessions and calls adjournments. Recorders take notes, ask questions, summarise situations and generally keep negotiations on track, especially when the going gets tough. Recorders support the lead negotiator but never 'take over' the main negotiating role. Observers 'read' negotiations. They do not normally say much but analyse the negotiations, pick up the subtleties and moods of the participants and provide inputs of new information and ideas during adjournments, as appropriate.

Bargaining

Bargaining involves a number of phases which are described in more detail below. Atkinson (1980) identifies four phases: clarifying the other side's position; structuring the expectations of the other side; getting movement; and closure. Kennedy and his colleagues (1984) propose three similar phases to Atkinson, once the parties have determined their bargaining objectives. These are: 'arguing'; 'proposing'; and 'exchanging' and 'agreeing'. They also identify three sub-phases. These are: 'signalling' within the arguing phase; 'packaging' within the proposing phase; and 'closing' within the exchanging and agreeing phase. What differentiates each phase from the other is the skills and activities appropriate to them. However these phases are defined and delineated, they provide a 'negotiating landscape' within which negotiators direct their resources, skills and knowledge, structure their behaviour and act out their roles, according to the situations facing them.

Implementing

This is the process by which both parties are responsible for carrying out the decisions and outcomes determined by the parties jointly. Final decisions need to be recorded, put in writing and signed by both sides. This avoids further conflict over interpreting what has actually been agreed between the negotiators!

Arguing

In this initial phase of bargaining, each side makes its opening statements and the arguments underpinning them. Both parties normally reveal only their ISPs and are reluctant to concede anything to the other side in terms of information or clues to their real negotiating objectives. The underlying aim of the negotiators is to justify the positions of their own sides, to maximise the information obtained about the other side's RSP and to reveal the minimum information about their own. There is intense listening on both sides, questioning for clarification and challenging the other side to justify its negotiating stance. Each side remains non-committal about the other party's proposals, whilst testing its commitment to its case. There is mutual seeking of information but little exchanging takes place at this phase. This is because arguments cannot be negotiated; they only set the contexts and parameters of each side's opening positions.

The process of 'signalling', identified by Kennedy and his colleagues (1984: page 62), is where qualifications are 'placed on a statement of a position.' The initial statements of the parties are absolute ones. For example, 'We'll never agree to that'; 'Your offer is totally unacceptable to our members'; or 'Your proposal is nonsense.' Signalling provides the parties with the opportunity to move towards each other in the early stages of negotiation, after the initial stone-walling responses of both sides. Examples of signalling by one of the parties could be: 'Well, we could discuss that point' (meaning that it is negotiable) or 'We would find it very difficult to agree to that' (meaning that it is not impossible to do so). Skilled negotiators reward signalling behaviour where possible. It moves the parties away from their opening gambits and creates the possibilities for concessions later. To be productive, signalling needs to be reciprocated. It is important to reward signals, not obstinacy. This is done by responding positively to the other side with phrases such as: 'We're always prepared to consider reasonable proposals.'

Proposing

A proposition in the negotiating process is an offer, or a claim, made by one of the parties to the other, moving it away from its original position. Initial proposals tend to be tentative and are non-committal. They aim at reassuring the other party and at marking out the parameters within which exchanges can take place between them and agreement can finally be reached. Proposals become more specific as negotiations proceed, thus providing a means for moving towards real bargaining or concrete exchanges between the parties later. Propositions are conditional, never absolute. They are stated in the following way: 'If you are prepared to do "A", then we will consider doing "B".' Generally, negotiators open with realistic proposals and move only slowly towards each other. Choosing the opening position therefore is crucial.

Propositions are normally firm on generalities, such as 'We are determined to settle this issue quickly.' But they are flexible on specifics, such as 'We propose an offer of X.' The party receiving a proposal needs to listen to it carefully and not to reject it out of hand, so that it can respond and provide a counter-proposal. Opening conditions are normally large, whilst opening concessions are normally small. However, since negotiators learn their craft through experience, and about each other through observation, these influence the ways in which they structure their proposals, respond to initiatives and act out their negotiating roles.

'Packaging' is the term used by Kennedy and his colleagues to describe the bridging that is made between the opening movements of the parties and their shifting into final agreement. 'It is, effectively, the activity which draws up the agenda for the bargaining session' (Kennedy *et al* 1984: page 89). Packaging aims to facilitate convergence between the parties, from where they are, after the arguing and proposing phases have taken place, to where they can finally agree a settlement. This entails:

- identifying the other party's reservations about coming to an agreement, its negotiating objectives and its bargaining priorities
- considering its possible 'signalled' concessions
- each side's reviewing its own negotiating objectives, bearing in mind its ISP, RSP and FBP, and those of the other side.

This enables each side to determine whether there is enough movement between them to produce a package and how it can modify it or adapt it to meet some of the other side's reservations.

Each side has to consider:

- the concessions it wants
- the room it has for manoeuvre
- the concessions it is prepared to signal in the package
- what it wants in return.

This enables each party to tell the other what 'package' is on offer, thus providing a negotiating platform, including the readiness to trade concessions, which prepares the ground for exchanges between them. These exchanges of concessions follow the general rule of not giving anything away without getting something back in return. The pattern is: 'If you move on that issue, then we will move on this one.' In trading concessions, each party needs to value them in terms of their perceived value to the other party. This means evaluating the worth of a concession to the other party, its cost to your side and what is wanted in exchange for it.

Exchanging and agreeing

This is the most crucial phase of the bargaining process. Unless the parties are able to make final exchanges and concessions between them, bargaining reaches an impasse and a failure to agree is recorded. The key to reaching a successful agreement is for each of the parties to come up with positive propositions, which remain linked but are conditional on movement by the other side. The sorts of statements made by the parties are: 'If your side agrees to A, then we will agree to B.' By continuing to put conditions on what they are prepared to exchange, negotiators ensure that they do not concede anything without getting something back in return.

Linking all the issues ensures that every item in the package is listed by both sides. This means that when either party raises an issue, it can be dealt with in the context of the package as a whole. This provides the negotiators with some degree of flexibility and leverage. They also have the opportunity to link each concession to corresponding concessions on other items, as they move towards final agreement. All the items are negotiated conditionally upon the package as a whole being agreed. Keeping items linked makes them available for trading and exchange, as bargaining proceeds to its concluding stages. The more items that there are to exchange, the stronger the bargaining positions of the negotiators. The process of linking facilitates moves on one issue with trade-offs for something else. In this way, single items in the negotiating package are not picked off in a piecemeal way. And the negotiators are provided with more room for manoeuvre, providing that the linking amongst the items is realistic.

Closing a negotiation requires judgement. If the parties are unable to close their bargaining activity, their continued negotiating can result in further concessions that collectively may be costly to each side. One way of closing is for one side to make a 'final' concession to the other, preferably on a minor issue. A second way is by summarising what has been agreed to date, stressing the concessions which have been made and emphasising the benefits of agreeing to what is on offer. A third way is through an adjournment. This enables the other side to have time to consider what is on 'final' offer. Fourth, one side can present the other with an ultimatum. This states, in effect, that unless what is on offer is accepted, a failure to agree will result. Finally, the choice of alternatives may be given to the other side. This enables it to consider which alternative is preferable, whilst not changing what is actually on offer.

Once final agreement has been reached, it must be listed in detail and recorded in writing. Both sides must be absolutely clear what has been agreed, with all relevant points being listed, clarified and explained as necessary. Where there is any disagreement on any item, negotiations must continue until agreement is reached. In short, what has been agreed has to be clearly summarised, accurately recorded and finally signed by both parties.

COLLECTIVE AGREEMENTS

Collective agreements are the outcome of collective bargaining, determined between employer and union representatives. Being bilateral employment rules, they differ from company rules and employer policy statements, which are unilateral in origin. The collective nature of these rules is also reflected in the fact that the terms and conditions of employment, and employee relations procedures, incorporated in collective agreements, apply to groups of workers covered by them. Substantive agreements cover any kind of payments and a wide range of working conditions. Procedural agreements spell out the steps by which employee relations processes are to be carried out.

These include: machinery for negotiation, consultation and arbitration; negotiating, handling grievances and resolving disputes; discipline and dismissal; and facilities for trade union representatives.

The formulation of collective agreements

Good practice suggests that formal, written collective agreements are now the norm in employee relations. Although over-formality is not conducive to good employee relations, written agreements are preferred by employers and unions for a number of reasons:

- They focus attention on problem areas and lead to joint policies bringing about agreed solutions.
- Written agreements create order in employee relations and facilitate change. They overcome, for example, the problems involved where either management or union negotiators move on for one reason or another.
- They provide continuity in employee relations, enabling decisions to be determined in the light of past practice, precedent and accepted norms.

In some cases, agreements are drafted by management, with the final details being considered and agreed by the parties jointly. In other cases, unions take the initiative and management respond to what is proposed. In yet other cases, the development of agreements is best handled by a joint working party.

The legal status of collective agreements

A collective agreement is defined in law as any agreement or arrangement made by or on behalf of one or more trade unions and one or more employers or employers' associations, relating to one or more of the matters listed in the TULRCA 1992. These are (section 178):

(a) terms and conditions of employment, or the physical conditions in which any workers are required to work;
(b) engagement or non-engagement, or termination or suspension of employment or the duties of employment, of one or more workers;
(c) allocation of work or the duties of employment between workers or groups of workers;
(d) matters of discipline;
(e) a worker's membership or non-membership of a trade union;
(f) facilities for officials of trade unions; and
(g) machinery for negotiation or consultation, and other procedures, relating to any of the above matters, including the recognition by employers or employers' associations of the right of a trade union to represent workers in such negotiation or consultation or in the carrying out of such procedures.

The distinctive feature of British collective agreements is that they are not legally enforceable between the employers and unions negotiating them. As the TULRCA 1992 states (section 179): 'a collective agreement shall be conclusively presumed not to be a legally enforceable contract', unless it is in writing and contains a provision stating that it is intended to be enforceable. Unlike in many other countries, collective agreements in Britain do not have a 'contractual function' between the parties making them, they are 'binding in honour' only. But they do have a 'normative function'. This means that the terms, conditions and rules determined by them become incorporated into individual contracts of employment, expressly or sometimes by implication.

The non-enforceability of collective agreements was underlined by the *Ford Motor Company v. AUEF and TGWU* case in 1969. The company brought a legal action alleging breach of contract against the unions, on the grounds that they had supported their members' strike action in breach of agreed collective bargaining procedures. The High Court decided that the unions were not liable because their collective agreements with the employer were not intended to be legally enforceable contracts. The Court argued that, as experienced negotiators, management and unions had no intention of creating legal enforceability, so there was no contract between them – only 'an unenforceable gentleman's agreement'. This judgement was not taken to appeal, and although the Industrial Relations Act 1971 presumed all collective agreements to be legally binding unless the parties declared them otherwise, almost every collective agreement between 1971 and 1974 contained a clause stating that 'this is not a legally enforceable agreement' (Weekes *et al* 1975).

The customary way of securing the normative function of collective agreements is to incorporate their provisions into the personal contracts of employment of each worker. Whilst in some countries collective agreements have an automatic effect upon employment contracts, in Britain they do not. The best way for the employment contract to incorporate the collective terms relating to pay, conditions and benefits is to incorporate them expressly. The most useful vehicle for doing this is the written statement of particulars given to employees within two months of starting employment where the employees work eight or more hours a week. A problem with trying to incorporate the terms of a collective agreement as implied terms is that the normal rules of contract law determine that nothing can be implied into a contract affecting any matter covered by an express term. Thus personal contracts of employment cannot be overridden by collective agreements.

The incorporation of procedural clauses of collective agreements into individual contracts is less clear-cut and more problematic. Procedures dealing with individual employee rights, such as those relating to grievances and disciplinary matters, provide little problem. For example, the Employment Protection (Consolidation) Act 1978 requires employers to set out matters relating to discipline and grievances in the note accompanying a worker's written particulars in a way that envisages these procedures being incorporated into individual contracts of employment. There is more doubt about procedures concerned with workers' collective action, such as no-strike clauses, restrictions on industrial action until the procedure to avoid disputes is exhausted or other collective procedures.

One problem with these procedures is that they sometimes involve questions of policy. In the case of *British Leyland v. McQuilken* [1978], for example, the employer had made an agreement with the union that, in the closing down of a department, all employees would be interviewed for retraining or redundancy. McQuilken was not interviewed because management changed its policy but he was told he could transfer to another place or be retrained. He claimed a redundancy payment and went to an industrial tribunal. The tribunal declared the refusal to implement the agreement to be constructive dismissal. On appeal, the EAT rejected this on the grounds that the terms of the agreement between the employer and the union did not alter McQuilken's individual contract of employment. 'That agreement was a long-term plan, dealing with policy rather than with the rights of individual employees.'

Types of agreement

There are a variety of types of collective agreements. Collective bargaining is an infinitely flexible process of employee relations and the format of collective agreements reflects this. So far, earlier discussions have focused primarily on what may be described as fairly standardised approaches to the content of substantive and procedural agreement (see Chapter 3). This section is more selective in its approach and focuses on some of the 'newer' types, and less common forms, of collective agreement such as 'technology agreements', 'new-style agreements', 'flexibility agreements' and 'partnership agreements'.

Technology agreements

Technological change is endemic to the work process (see Chapter 6). Since the 1980s especially, micro-electronic and related technologies have been continuously applied to a range of industries, occupations and sectors, with non-manual employment being particularly affected by these changes. Although research shows that it is common for these changes to be imposed unilaterally by management, largely without consultation with staff (Daniels 1987), in some cases attempts have been made to negotiate the introduction of 'new technology' and new working methods between management and unions. This is done to facilitate the introduction of new equipment, train people to use it and reduce the anxieties associated with change, thus providing benefits to the employer and to employees in conditions of uncertainty. Such agreements are sometimes referred to as 'technology agreements'.

A number of negotiating issues arise with the introduction of new technology, each of which has procedural and substantive implications for employee relations. The negotiating issues include: job contraction; job content; job control; and health and safety at work (Winterton and Winterton 1985). Job contraction is synonymous with new technology, and potential job losses account for many of the fears felt amongst employees when new technology is being introduced into organisations. Job content, too, can be adversely affected either by the de-skilling of the work of employees or by dehumanising it, as a result of technological change. The impact of new technology on individual job control is twofold. First, it can result in workers having less discretion in the ways in which their jobs are performed. Second, where technology creates less-skilled work, job control shifts from workers to management, since these operations are easier for management to direct. Also, although new technology reduces some physical hazards at work, there is also evidence of its potentially damaging effects where it results in irregular shift work, social isolation or physical strain, such as repetitive strain injury.

The sorts of procedural issues arising from the introduction of new technology cover include its impact on: existing procedures and bargaining arrangements; employee training; and the monitoring and operation of new technology. Existing procedures likely to be affected by technological innovation are: union recognition; grievances and disputes; discipline; redeployment and redundancy; and the level at which bargaining takes place. Employee training is an important aspect of introducing new technology, and procedures need to be determined regarding both the job training needs of employees and the employee relations training needs of union representatives. Two main procedural mechanisms are used to monitor new technology: either joint management-union study teams or outside consultants.

The sorts of substantive issues arising from the introduction of new technology arrangements cover a number of matters, including: how the savings generated from productivity increases are to be shared between management and workers; how any job losses are to be managed; the impact of changes on terms and conditions of employment; and their impact on health and safety. The benefits of increased productivity can be shared in a number of ways. These include: higher wages; shorter working periods; early retirement; and additional leave. Where job losses result, these can be achieved by a variety of means including: natural wastage; redeployment; voluntary redundancy; or compulsory redundancy, with the relevant terms with being negotiated and agreed between the parties.

Procedural provisions may need to be made to improve the quality of working life after the introduction of new technology. These can take the form of: additional breaks; job rotation; job enrichment; and job design. The problems associated with the health and safety hazards connected with new technology need to be addressed. Such provisions can cover such matters as eye strain, shift working, the implications of robotics and any psychological hazards arising from the work environment. Introducing new technology can also affect equality of opportunity at work in matters such as job grading, promotion, patterns of work and job retraining. Procedural adjustments need to be made here too.

New-style agreements

New-style agreements (NSAs) contain a number of procedural elements distinguishing them from standardised or more traditional procedural arrangements. As Burrows (1986) indicates, a major feature of NSAs is that their negotiating and disputes procedures are based on the mutually accepted 'rights' of the parties, expressed in the recognition agreement. The intention is to resolve any differences of interest on substantive issues between the parties by negotiation, with pendulum arbitration providing a resolution of these issues where differences persist.

The general principles underlying NSAs aim to reinforce the harmony of interests between the company, the signatory union and its employees. Employees are not required to join the union but are encouraged to do so. NSAs frequently stress the need for quality, teamwork and flexibility in the work process, for avoiding unnecessary industrial action which disrupts production and for open and direct communications between the company and its employees. Only one union is recognised for the purposes of negotiation, consultation and information-giving to staff. And all these processes are normally carried on within a 'company council' consisting of management and employee representatives. Employee representatives are elected by a secret ballot of all the workforce, with the balloting process being supervised by the local full-time union officer. Company and union often provide joint training for these representatives to enable them to carry out their duties satisfactorily and effectively.

The negotiating procedure for determining new substantive issues within NSAs normally incorporates two underlying principles. The first is that during negotiations – and during conciliation and arbitration – there is to be no recourse to industrial action. Second, management and the union often affirm their commitment to resolving issues within the company but, where there are any remaining differences between them, if they fail to agree, these are resolved through binding conciliation or arbitration. Arbitrators are required to make a decision, based on the 'final offer' of one or other of the sides. There is no 'split' decision. Pendulum arbitration of this sort, it is argued, not only encourages realistic bargaining positions by each of the parties but also provides a means of peacefully resolving persisting disputes of interest between the company and its workforce.

Individual grievances and collective issues of 'rights', in contrast, are resolved through the grievance procedure and procedure to avoid disputes respectively. The latter states that there is to be no industrial action, whilst the issue is in procedure. Where such matters are not resolved 'in house', they may be referred to ACAS or another third party who may conciliate or arbitrate, with the terms of reference being agreed by the parties, within the time limits set for determining the issue.

Procedures also frequently exist for ensuring the fullest use of human resources and labour flexibility in the single-union company. These include agreed changes in working practices likely to affect productivity and staffing levels, and can involve the use of appropriate industrial engineering and human resource planning techniques. Finally, to ensure labour flexibility and organisational change, provisions are made for training and retraining the workforce for future human resource requirements.

Flexibility agreements

Collective agreements aimed at changing entrenched working practices, and removing job demarcations, by introducing labour flexibility in firms, have been a common feature of employee relations since the 1980s. In its assessment of the scope and nature of some of these flexibility agreements, Industrial Relations Review and Report (1992a, 1992b) concludes that there are limits to the usefulness of such agreements in introducing flexible working practices. Whilst the companies investigated no longer faced 'who does what' disputes, they questioned the extent to which the total interchangeability of labour is desirable. Further, in technologically sophisticated environments, in particular, it appeared to be uneconomic to train the whole workforce in complex skills which are used by only small numbers of employees.

Of the four organisations examined, two – Mobil Coryton and Babcock Energy – changed working practices at times of financial difficulty. The other two – Toshiba Consumer Products and the Co-operative Wholesale Society (CWS) at Deeside – introduced new working practices on greenfield sites but also against a background of economic difficulties. These studies focused on six aspects of flexibility deals: flexibility developments; flexibility and labour force size and composition; the extent to which flexibility had progressed; training needs and their implications; the collective bargaining effects; and the impact of flexibility on corporate performance.

The flexibility agreements at Toshiba and Mobil established the principle of a total end to demarcation so that these companies did not feel any need for any substantial changes in working practices subsequently. In the CWS, broad flexibility measures were expanded to a single group of employees who combined both production and maintenance skills. At Babcock, the initial flexibility agreement listed specific changes in required working practices. This was followed by a later agreement on broad flexibility, with further changes focusing on individual issues.

The flexibility deals at Mobil and Babcock contributed to labour force reductions, with substantial hiving-off of some job activities to subcontractors. Toshiba, in contrast, being a greenfield site operation, did not use much contract labour but, in adapting to product market fluctuations, varied its use of temporary staff to maintain the stability of its permanent workforce.

At Babcock, the principle was established that multi-skilled craftworkers would not have the specialist skills required in a complex industry. Its agreement was based on the need to train workers in 'secondary' skills. At Mobil and Toshiba, the flexibility agreements were based on the principle of multi-skilling, so reducing the risks of demarcation disputes. In practice, however, some employee specialisation was essential, especially in conditions of technological sophistication. In these companies, production-maintenance flexibility was limited to production workers doing minor maintenance on the plant for which they were responsible. Flexibility seemed to have progressed furthest at the CWS but even here it was not economic to provide all employees with all the skills required within the workplace. In general, it seems that these flexibility deals increased the breadth of workforce skills, but not their depth.

In all four companies, it appeared that flexibility provisions meant that new workers required certain skills training. Both Babcock and Toshiba operated their own apprenticeship schemes, whilst Mobil had wound its scheme down. This enabled Mobil to direct some of its resources at a skills training centre in a local town. It also provided opportunity for the workforces of its subcontractors to become adequately skilled.

At both Toshiba and the CWS, the employee relations structures remained as they had been. Toshiba had one of the earliest single-union agreements and the CWS combined its consultative and collective bargaining machinery. Babcock did not consider that introducing labour flexibility had a great effect on union influence. However, because of contracting out and union mergers, a smaller number of unions was recognised than had been the case some 10 years earlier. At Mobil, on the other hand, culture change was seen as laying the groundwork for targeting employee relations practices at individual employees and their performance. This, it was envisaged, might lead to a change in the role of trade unions in the future.

In terms of the impact of labour flexibility on corporate performance, all four case studies found it difficult to separate the effects of introducing labour flexibility from those of other company innovations. All the companies felt that labour flexibility had contributed to organisational well-being, especially in producing acceptable labour productivity levels. Mobil and the CWS added that an employee relations climate free of demarcation disputes was a direct result of changed working practices.

Partnership agreements

These are a relatively new type of collective agreement. They generally emphasise three inter-related elements:

- the development of mutually acceptable pay review formulae
- the establishment of single status for all employees
- co-operation between management and union(s) as an obligation within the partnership arrangements.

Pay review formulae can incorporate a number of elements. These include changes in the retail price index, the employer's position in relevant pay markets and the employer's financial and operational performance, which can provide a profit-related pay element in the pay package. The main features of pay review formulae are that they are open, rational and mutually agreed in advance by the employer and the union(s), normally for an agreed period. This enables all parties – including employees – to understand the principles upon which pay is based.

Single status for all employees in partnership agreements is commonly rooted in three main principles:

- that since all employees contribute to customer or client satisfaction, they should all have good terms and conditions of employment
- that change is best introduced through discussion and agreement with all those involved
- that any additional costs because of single status can be offset by improved customer provision.

Single status programmes typically incorporate the following sorts of procedural and substantive provisions: single table negotiating and consultative arrangements; standard working hours; monthly pay; an integrated pay structure; expectations about productivity improvements and job flexibility; and job security arrangements, sometimes including a 'no compulsory redundancy' agreement.

The mutuality and co-operation expected between management and union(s) in partnership agreements is normally set out in the general principles of their procedural arrangements. A good example of this is provided in the partnership agreement negotiated between Welsh Water and the Signatory Unions (1991: page 15). This states that both the company and the recognised unions agree that it is in the best interests of employees and the company to maintain constructive and co-operative relationships at all times. The principles underpinning this agreement are:

- Promoting openness on problems and issues of mutual concern.
- Valuing good communications both to employees and trade unions.
- Consulting and involving employees and their representatives at an early stage of formulating proposals for change.
- Ensuring that the focal point of dealing with employee issues is as near to the workplace as possible, and that any problems are resolved wherever possible through informal discussion at the lowest possible organisational level.
- Conducting formal consultation and negotiations on a joint basis covering all employees, wherever it is practical and relevant to do so.
- Devoting formal consultative meetings to matters of concern and relevance to all employees and the business.

The institutional arrangements for facilitating the partnership approach to employee relations and partnership agreements is often a company council. This is a representative body consisting of employer and union representatives which has a number of functions. These normally include: acting as a negotiating forum; acting as a consultative forum; establishing sub-committees and working parties; facilitating the resolution of grievances and disputes; and promoting the agreed principles of employee relations between the employer and the union(s).

JOINT CONSULTATION

Joint consultation is a complex process. It has a long history which can be traced back at least to the recommendations of the Whitley Committee in

1917-18. Its influence as an employee relations process has fluctuated widely however: decline in the interwar years; resurgence during the second world war; decline again during the 1950s and 1960s; further resurgence in the 1970s and early 1980s; and renewed decline in the late 1980s and early 1990s (Millward and Stevens 1986; Millward *et al* 1992). As Hibbet (1991: page 664) comments: 'Consultation based on formal committee structures appears to have reduced somewhat . . . In recent years companies appear to have concentrated on expanding employee involvement arrangements other than formal consultation', with employees being consulted individually or in small groups. Whatever its history and present importance, however, there are four different models of joint consultation (see also Chapter 3):

- the non-union model
- the marginal model
- the competitive model
- the adjunct model.

These models need to be borne in mind, if the structures and content of joint consultation are to be understood and evaluated.

Factors influencing joint consultation

Marchington (1989) identifies four main factors influencing the development of joint consultative machinery within organisations. These are:

- management philosophy
- union organisation and worker resistance
- trust and co-operative relations
- the external environment.

Most joint consultative arrangements are initiated by management, therefore the model of consultation that is adopted within an organisation reflects the management's dominant employee relations philosophy and its basic intentions in managing people. Management's underlying purpose in supporting the non-union, marginal and competitive models of joint consultation, for example, is to weaken trade unions and to maintain power by opposing or even confronting the unions. In contrast, in adopting the adjunct model of joint consultation, management does so with the expectation that this will result in co-operation with the unions and their incorporation in the employee relations process, rather than in conflict and discord with them.

Related to this is the strength of union organisation and the willingness of workers to resist management plans for setting up and running joint consultative arrangements on management's terms alone. Again the non-union, marginal and competitive models are more likely to be established where unionism is weak or where worker organisation is channelled into staff associations, 'house' unions or company-based 'works councils'. Where joint consultation is used to undermine trade unionism or to bypass it, unless this is resisted by the unions and their members, union representatives are in effect marginalised or excluded from the consultative process. As Cressey and MacInnes (1984) point out, with the power balance favouring managements, it is management that determines what items to take to joint consultative committees, the form of discussion within them and the outcomes arising from them.

In adjunct joint consultation, union representatives are more likely to have joint ownership of the consultative machinery and the right to refer issues to the negotiating machinery. This increases their commitment to the consultative process. Moreover, as Marchington and Armstrong (1983) indicate, where shop stewards are well organised, they value joint consultation. But where they are poorly organised, they are generally neutral or negative about it.

It is also argued that high trust between management and union representatives is an important ingredient in 'good industrial relations' (Purcell 1981). High trust is more likely to be part of adjunct joint consultation than it is in other consultative arrangements. However, high trust, where it exists, is more common in soft product market conditions than in hard ones. As Marchington (1989: page 397) concludes: 'If employers are attempting to prevent or marginalise unions, a tight economic climate makes consultation less necessary since the unions are further weakened, and the time for involvement is less available.' Conversely, where the adjunct model is adopted, economic recession might well induce both sides to continue maintaining good working relationships together, within both the consultative and the negotiating machinery. This is likely to ensure that high trust is sustained between the parties, even in difficult external circumstances.

Finally, the level of decision-making within an organisation also has an impact on the efficacy of joint consultation. Where management decision-making is largely centralised, this is unlikely to give much authority to local consultative committees. This fits the marginal or competitive models of joint consultation. In contrast, where management decision-making is devolved, or at different levels within an organisation, this is more likely to provide the consultative process with added authority. This fits the adjunct model of joint consultation, especially where the consultative machinery is linked hierarchically throughout the organisation.

Constitutional arrangements

The constitutional arrangements for setting up and operating joint consultative committees (JCCs) vary widely. Where joint consultation is entirely management driven, such as in the non-union, marginal and competitive models, the constitutional arrangements for JCCs are obviously determined by management decision alone. It is management that decides the terms of reference, membership, structures, frequency of meetings and the agenda of such committees. The underlying purpose of such committees is to keep them firmly under management control, either by excluding the union presence (the non-union model) or by weakening union influence (the competitive and marginal models). The terms of reference of these types of JCCs are normally unitary in purpose, whilst membership on the 'staff' side is usually drawn from employee representatives, rather than from union representatives. Sometimes these employee representatives are elected by their constituents, in other cases they are appointed by management. These JCCs are located largely at site level and rarely have links higher up the organisation. The frequency of meetings varies but is likely to lie within the range of monthly, quarterly or half-yearly meetings. The agenda of these sorts of JCCs is likely to be soft, with management using them largely as downward information-providing bodies, rather than as opportunities for asking employees about their views on workplace matters and listening to them before decisions.

Adjunct JCCs are formally constituted bodies, at site and/or corporate level, established through negotiations between management and union representatives. They are normally the result of formal joint consultation agreements. And it is the joint responsibility of both management and unions to ensure that the consultative arrangements, established within the procedure, comply with their terms of reference and the constitution embodied within the agreement.

Adjunct consultation

Joint consultation is at its most advanced when it is of the adjunct variety. The sorts of arrangements set out for adjunct JCCs are outlined below.

Aims

The underlying purpose of adjunct joint consultation is to establish arrangements that involve the signatory unions in the consultative process between management and the employees covered by the joint consultation agreement. In this sense, adjunct consultation is normally concerned with those matters of mutual concern to management and employees that are not covered by the negotiating procedures. Matters may be discussed within the consultative machinery, prior to negotiation, and be referred to the negotiating machinery subsequently. Adjunct consultation is a problem-solving, two-way information exchange process between the parties rather than a bargaining or a 'top-down' process.

Adjunct consultation enables management, employees and the unions to consider and, as far as is practicable, to resolve the problems facing them. In this sense it may be considered as an integrative process. Joint consultation thereby increases the effectiveness of the organisation's operations to the mutual benefit of both the employer and its employees. JCC systems of this type are thus ways of improving staff morale, reducing tensions between management and employees, increasing job satisfaction and raising employee productivity.

Perkins (1986: page 44) sees the underpinning aims of effective joint consultation as being fourfold:

- Joint consultation ensures continuity of structure, enabling it to be used as a method of communication on all matters of concern to management and employees.
- Used correctly, it reinforces the trust and goodwill existing between management, employees and unions.
- It provides problem-solving procedures between management and employee representatives, although these are only meaningful if they precede final decisions.
- It allows employees to raise their own issues and grievances, to receive management's views and to instigate action where appropriate.

Effectively constituted and properly managed joint consultation, in short, enables employees, through their union representatives, to discuss and consider matters of mutual concern to them and management, thus allowing them to influence management proposals before final decisions are taken.

Functions

Exhibit 35 The functions of JCCs

These can include discussions on:

- productivity, efficiency and quality
- safety at work
- education and training
- working conditions such as leave, holiday arrangements, working hours, absenteeism, meal breaks, transport and catering facilities
- the health and welfare of employees
- the welfare of retired employees
- staffing levels
- new equipment.

The primary function of local JCCs at plant, site or works level is to provide regular and recognised opportunities for the joint consideration, by management and employee representatives, of all issues affecting them which are not covered by joint negotiating machinery. They are also recognised channels of communication between the parties to any matter put on the JCC agenda by either management or employee representatives. Examples of the functions of JCCs are provided in Exhibit 35 but these are neither exclusive nor exhaustive, and some JCCs have narrower functions than those listed.

Membership, structure and rules

Adjunct JCCs are based on the principle that shop stewards or other trade union members represent employees within the consultative system. Such representatives, however, act on behalf of all their constituents, regardless of whether or not they are union members. The number of union representatives usually takes account of the number and types of employees working in the plant, site or workplace. Management representatives, in turn, are selected by senior management, again in accordance with the joint consultation agreement.

Many JCCs only operate locally, but in multi-plant or multi-site organisations arrangements are sometimes made to coordinate the consultative machinery throughout the organisation, by means of vertically linked consultative committees. JCCs at organisational level have union members drawn from locally based consultative committees. But these trade unionists are not usually elected directly by the employees within the plants. They are drawn from amongst the shop stewards on the lower-level committees. In some cases, full-time union officers take on the role of employee representatives at corporate level. Management representatives, as is normally the case, are appointed to such committees by senior management.

The rules of JCCs are found in the constitutions determined by the joint consultation agreement. Terms of reference, for example, are essential to establish what subjects are matters for consultation and what subjects are negotiable. Guidance is given on the objectives of the consultative procedure and the means by which these are to be affected. Examples of JCC rules are illustrated in Exhibit 36.

Exhibit 36 **Examples of JCC rules**

These include:

- title of the JCC
- parties to the agreement
- preamble
- aims of the JCC
- means of achieving the aims
- functions
- definitions
- membership
- retirement of members
- casual members
- substitutes
- co-options
- periods of office
- secretariat
- meetings
- quorum
- decisions and recommendations
- agenda
- minutes
- variation or termination of the agreement.

The agenda is often the most important part of JCC meetings and its contents reflect whether or not the committee is really working. Agendas and other relevant papers must be circulated well in advance, except where meetings are held at short notice, if the JCC is to operate effectively. It is the nature of joint consultation meetings that agendas tend to reflect management topics, especially at local level, so every effort must be made to get employee representatives to submit their own items for discussion.

Resolving conflicts

It is normally the right of a signatory union, or of a group of signatory unions, or of management, to require a matter to be dealt with through the negotiating procedure, rather than the consultative machinery, where it thinks this is appropriate. Further, if a JCC fails to resolve any disagreement on a matter on which it is competent to take a decision, this matter is normally dealt with in the formal negotiating procedure. Finally, where a JCC exercises its advisory or consultative functions in ways likely to affect any other JCC within an organisation, it usually transmits its recommendation on that matter to the JCC concerned.

ASSIGNMENTS

(a) What are the advantages and disadvantages to employers of collective bargaining as a method of determining terms and conditions of employment and for regulating relations between employers and employees?

(b) What is the case for and against legally enforceable collective agreements? What are the main implications for employers, unions and employees where 'collective contracts' are negotiated?

(c) Read Adnett (1989: Chapter 2). What are the main features of the neoclassical model of the labour market and that of the structural model? How do these models relate to the labour markets in which your organisation operates?

(d) Read Kahn-Freund (1954) in Flanders, A. (1969: pages 59-85). Comment on his analysis of how 'intergroup' conflicts between employers and unions are regulated through collective bargaining in Britain, Europe and the USA. How does he account for the differences amongst the bargaining systems?

(e) Read Chamberlain and Kuhn (1965: pages 162-90). How do they conceptualise bargaining power? How useful is their analysis for practical bargaining purposes?

(f) Read Walton and McKersie (1965: Chapter VII, pages 222-80). Examine the nature of attitudinal structuring and why it is an important sub-process in collective bargaining. What tactics can be used by negotiators to change the attitudes of their opposite numbers in the bargaining process, applying the concepts of either 'balance theory' or 'reinforcement theory'?

(g) Use the bargaining power model to assess the relative balance of power in your organisation, when either the union presented its last wage and conditions claim to your employer or management made its last wage proposal to the union. Did the bargaining outcome fit with your analysis?

(h) Read Towers (1992: pages 7-11). What does he identify as the reasons for employers withdrawing from multi-employer bargaining, what are the experiences of decentralised bargaining for employers and what are the wider organisational effects of it?
(i) Identify the organisational conditions – such as product markets, labour markets, technology, business structure and so on – where (1) multi-employer (2) single employer and (3) enterprise bargaining is most favourable to employer interests.
(j) What are the advantages and disadvantages to unions of (1) multi-employer-level bargaining? (2) single-employer-level bargaining? (3) enterprise-level bargaining? Under what conditions are each of the above levels most favourable to union negotiators?
(k) The unions representing white-collar staff in your organisation have presented management with their annual pay claim. This is for a 5 per cent across-the-board wage increase, a reduction in weekly hours of 20 minutes and improved sickness benefits for their members. Identify the sort of information that management would need to collect in this situation, where it might be collected and how it might be used in the negotiating process.
(l) Read Atkinson (1980: pages 137-54). What are some of the main tactics used by negotiators to get movement by their opponents in the latter stages of negotiating? Alternatively, what are some of the tactics used to get closure (pages 155-80)?
(m) Bring in a set of procedural and/or substantive collective agreements of your organisation to the group you are studying with and make a presentation of the main content and features of these agreements.
(n) Read Burrows (1986: pages 72-92) and comment on the content and practicalities of the single-union deal signed by Nissan (UK) and the AEU.
(o) Read Industrial Relations Services Employment Trends No. 505 (Industrial Relations Review and Report, February 1992: pages 11-15). Analyse and report on the flexibility package concluded at Rolls-Royce Motor Cars.
(p) Provide a report on the joint consultative arrangements in your organisation. How effective are they from a management point of view? What is a typical list of agenda items?
(q) Draft a constitution for a JCC.

REFERENCES

ADNETT, J. 1989. *Labour Market Policy*. London: Longman.

ADVISORY, CONCILIATION AND ARBITRATION SERVICE. 1983. *Collective Bargaining in Britain: Its extent and scope*. London: ACAS.

ATKINSON, G. 1980. *The Effective Negotiator*. Newbury: Negotiating Systems Publications.

BRANDEIS, L. 1934. *The Curse of Bigness*. Quoted in Chamberlain, N. and Kuhn, J. 1965, *Collective Bargaining*, NY: McGraw-Hill.

British Leyland UK Ltd v. *McQuilken* [1978] IRLR 245.

BURROWS, G. 1986. *No-Strike Agreements and Pendulum Arbitration*. London: IPM.

CHAMBERLAIN, N. *and* KUHN, J. 1965. *Collective Bargaining*. NY: McGraw-Hill.

CONFEDERATION OF BRITISH INDUSTRY 1988. *The Structure and Processes of Pay Determination in the Private Sector: 1979-1986*. London: CBI.

CRESSEY, P. *and* MACINNES, J. 1984. *The Relationship between Economic Recession and Industrial Democracy*. Glasgow: Centre for Research in Industrial Democracy and Participation, University of Glasgow.

CULLY, M. *and* WOODLAND, S. 1996. 'Trade union membership and recognition: an analysis of data from the 1985 Labour Force Survey'. *Labour Market Trends*. May, 104 (5).

DANIEL, W. 1987. *Workplace Industrial Relations and Technical Change*. London: Pinter.

DOERINGER, P. 1986. 'Internal labor markets and non-competing groups'. *American Economic Review*. 76(2).

DOERINGER, P. *and* PIORE, M. 1971. *Internal Labor Markets and Manpower Analysis*. Massachusetts: Lexington.

DUBIN, R. 1954. 'Constructive aspects of industrial conflict'. In Kornhauser, A., Dubin, R. and Ross, A. (eds) 1954, *Industrial Conflict*, NY: McGraw-Hill.

DUNLOP, J. 1950. *Wage Determination under Collective Bargaining*. NY: Macmillan.

DUNLOP, J. 1984. *Dispute Resolution*. London: Auburn.

DUNN, S. *and* GENNARD, J. 1984. *The Closed Shop in British Industry*. London: Macmillan.

FARNHAM, D. *and* HORTON, S. 1996. *Managing People in the Public Services*. London: Macmillan.

FARNHAM, D. *and* PIMLOTT, J. 1995. *Understanding Industrial Relations*. London: Cassell.

FLANDERS, A. 1968. 'Collective bargaining: a theoretical analysis'. In Flanders, A. 1970, *Management and Unions*, London: Faber and Faber.

FLANDERS, A. (ed.) 1969. *Collective Bargaining: Selected Readings*. London: Penguin.

Ford Motor Co. v. *AUEF and TGWU* [1969] 2 QB 303.

FOX, A. *and* FLANDERS, A. 1969. 'Collective bargaining: from Donovan to Durkheim'. In Flanders, A. 1970, *Management and Unions*. London: Faber and Faber.

HIBBERT, A. 1991. 'Employee involvement: a recent survey'. *Employment Gazette*. December.

HICKS, J. 1932. *Theory of Wages*. NY: Macmillan.

HOXIE, R. 1921. *Trade Unionism in the United States*. NY: Appleton.

HYMAN, R. 1975. *Industrial Relations*. London: Macmillan.

INDUSTRIAL RELATIONS REVIEW AND REPORT 1992a. *Industrial Relations Services Employment Trends*. 505, February.

INDUSTRIAL RELATIONS REVIEW AND REPORT 1992b. *Industrial Relations*

Services Employment Trends. 512, May.
INTERNATIONAL LABOUR OFFICE 1986. *Collective Bargaining*. Geneva: ILO.
KAHN-FREUND, O. 1954. 'Intergroup conflicts and their settlement'. *British Journal of Sociology*. 5(3).
KENNEDY, G., BENSON, J. *and* MCMILLAN, J. 1984. *Managing Negotiations*. London: Business Books.
KINNIE, N. 1987. 'Bargaining within the enterprise: centralized or decentralized?' *Journal of Management Studies*. 214(5).
LEVINSON, H. 1966. *Wage Determination under Collective Bargaining*. NY: Wiley.
MARCHINGTON, M. 1989. 'Joint consultation in practice'. In Sisson, K. (ed.) 1989, *Personnel Management in Britain*, Oxford: Blackwell.
MARCHINGTON, M. *and* ARMSTRONG, R. 1983. 'Shop steward organisation and joint consultation'. *Personnel Review*. 12(1).
MARGINSON, P. 1986. 'How centralized is the management of industrial relations?' *Personnel Management*. October.
MILLWARD, N. *and* STEVENS, M. 1986. *British Workplace Industrial Relations 1980-1984*. Aldershot: Gower.
MILLWARD, N., STEVENS, M., SMART, D. *and* HAWES, W. 1992. *Workplace Industrial Relations in Transition*. Aldershot: Dartmouth.
PALMER, S. 1990. *Determining Pay: A guide to the issues*. London: IPM.
PEN, J. 1952. 'A general theory of bargaining'. *American Economic Review*. 42.
PERKINS, G. (ed.) 1986. *Employee Communications in the Public Sector*. London: IPM.
PHELPS BROWN, H. 1966. 'The influence of trade unions and collective bargaining on pay levels and real wages'. In McCarthy, W. 1987, *Trade Unions: Selected readings*, London: Penguin.
PURCELL, J. 1981. *Good Industrial Relations*. London: Macmillan.
PURCELL, J. 1989. 'How to manage decentralized bargaining'. *Personnel Management*. May.
SCHELLING, T. 1963. *The Strategy of Conflict*. London: University Press.
STEVENS, C. 1963. *Strategy and Collective Bargaining Negotiation*. NY: McGraw-Hill.
TOWERS, B. 1992. *Issues in People Management No. 2: Choosing Bargaining Levels – UK experience and implications*. London: IPM.
TRADE UNION AND LABOUR RELATIONS (CONSOLIDATION) ACT 1992.
WALTON, R. *and* MCKERSIE, R. 1965. *A Behavioral Theory of Labor Negotiations*. NY: McGraw-Hill.
WEBB, S. *and* WEBB, B. 1913. *Industrial Democracy*. NY: Longman.
WEEKES, B., MELLISH, M., DICKENS, L. *and* LLOYD, J. 1975. *Industrial Relations and the Limits of the Law*. Oxford : Blackwell.
WINTERTON, J. *and* WINTERTON, R. 1985. *New Technology: The bargaining issues*. Nottingham: Universities of Leeds and Nottingham in association with the IPM.

10 Non-union patterns of employee relations

Collective bargaining, as an employee relations strategy, is based on a policy of union incorporation in employment decision-making with employers (see Chapters 2, 3, 9). It is a joint approach to employee relations and depends on employees being organised into independent trade unions, the unions being recognised by the employer for negotiating purposes and a fair balance of power existing between the two sides in the bargaining relationship. Individualist, human resources management (HRM) approaches to managing people and the employment relationship, in contrast, have grown in importance and scope in recent years (Millward *et al* 1992) and are not generally based on trade union organisation, though they may operate in parallel with unionism, and have been used by some employers since the mid-1980s. They tend to be employer-driven and unitary in their employee relations emphases. They are normally task- or job-centred, aimed at individual employees and based on a management policy of employee commitment. An alternative more pluralist, but still a non-union, approach to involving employees in their organisations were the attempts and experiments in worker participation, involving employee representatives in strategic decision-taking with senior management at corporate level, in the public sector in Britain during the late 1970s, with varying degrees of success (Ferner 1988). Unlike in western Europe, where employees often have legal rights to representation on company boards, such as in Denmark, Germany and the Netherlands, and in works councils or works committees (Incomes Data Services 1991), there is no statutory, or even voluntary, provision for worker participation in management in Britain. Indeed, worker participation remains a controversial and contentious issue amongst companies, employers and managers in Britain.

EMPLOYEE INVOLVEMENT PRACTICES

Companies in Britain with over 250 employees are required to state in their annual reports, as a result of the Employment Act 1982, now incorporated within the TULRCA 1992, what action they have taken to promote 'employee involvement' practices within their organisations. They have to describe what steps they have taken to introduce, maintain or develop employee involvement arrangements in the following areas:

- information and communication between management and employees
- economic awareness of their businesses
- financial participation by employees in the companies employing them

- consultative arrangements.

Information and communication systems are the means by which employers provide systematic information on matters of concern to employees. Economic awareness schemes are aimed at achieving a common understanding by employees of the economic and financial factors affecting the performance of the company employing them. Financial participation is aimed at encouraging the involvement of employees in their company's financial performance, through employee share schemes or other means. Consultation, in the sense that it is used here, normally refers to 'informal consultative arrangements'. These are the processes through which employers provide regular channels of communication, between management and individuals or with small groups of employees, so that the views of employees can be taken into account by management when it takes decisions likely to affect employee interests at work.

Employee commitment

Employee commitment is at the heart of employee involvement programmes. Although 'commitment' and 'involvement' are different concepts, they are closely linked, since both are concerned with how employers can encourage employees to identify with a company's business interests through a variety of communication processes, employee relations activities and corporate policies. Employee commitment, in outline, is the extent to which employees identify with the organisation's work ethic, co-operate with its goals and objectives and contribute to corporate performance. Employee involvement, in contrast, is the term normally used to denote the processes set up within an organisation to enable its employees to become involved in decisions largely affecting the ways in which their work is done.

The argument, from the employer's point of view, for trying to win a high level of employee commitment to work, jobs and the company, in contrast with merely seeking instrumental compliance by employees to management decisions, is based on a number of assumptions. These include the claims that employees who are committed:

- devote their energies to working for the employer rather than for their own private interests
- favour the company in which they are employed rather than other companies
- give additional time and effort to the company when this is needed
- give priority to corporate values and employer interests when these seem to be in conflict with those of external bodies such as trade unions or professional associations.

The degree to which employees are committed to their work, job and employer can be inferred from their feelings, attitudes, behaviour and actions whilst at work. According to White (1987), employee commitment denotes three kinds of feelings or behaviour relating to the company in which an individual is employed. First, employees believe in and accept the goals, values and ethos of their employer. Second, employees are willing to work beyond what is normally expected under their contracts of employment: there is an extended 'psychological contract' between employer and employee. Third, there is a desire by employees to maintain membership of the organisation, rather than to leave it. Further, because commitment is voluntary and personal, it cannot be imposed by management, it cannot be initiated by others but it can be withdrawn by those offering it, if they decide to do so.

A number of factors appears to influence employee commitment. These include:

- gender and marital status
- education and length of service
- personality
- individual needs
- the dominant societal culture.

It also seems that underlying employer attempts at increasing employee commitment is the assumption that it improves organisational performance. Employee commitment is claimed to relate to corporate performance in three ways (White 1987: page 13). These are:

> First, strong commitment to work in general is likely to result in conscientious and self-directed application to work, regular attendance, minimal disciplinary supervision, and a high level of effort.
>
> Second, . . . strong commitment to a specific job will also result in a high level of effort insofar as good performance is related to self-esteem, including ambition and career plans . . .
>
> Third, commitment to the organisation . . . includes the intention to stay, and is associated with turnover. As might be expected, commitment normally also becomes weaker as the event of leaving draws nearer. It is difficult to assess which is cause and which the effect but there is a definite link between a fall in expressed commitment and turnover. This, of course, adds to the costs of production when it necessitates recruitment, training and supervision.

The concept of employee commitment is clearly a complex one and is associated with several objectives, but the commitment of employees at work certainly affects a variety of organisational variables. These include: absenteeism, turnover, effort and the quality of performance within organisations. It therefore has a number of implications for personnel and corporate policies. These include:

- generating early commitment amongst new employees
- designing strategies for improving commitment
- maintaining the reciprocity between the rewards received and the contribution being made by employees

- reducing turnover by increasing commitment
- developing participative strategies for introducing new technology
- implementing appropriate personnel policies, sometimes in association with employee representatives.

Employee involvement

The term 'employee involvement' first began to appear in management literature in the late 1970s. After its National Conference in 1978, the CBI published its first set of guidelines on employee involvement (CBI 1979). These were aimed at promoting the voluntary development of employee involvement practices within companies. What the CBI was talking about, at that time, was an open style of management, operated by managers with the necessary skills, self-confidence and 'pride in their jobs', so as to facilitate appropriate communication and consultation arrangements with employees. This approach, it was believed, would help managers achieve the consent which they needed to put their decisions into action. It would also, it was anticipated, bring about 'collaboration and involvement in the common purpose of the company and the mutual interest which all employees have in the success of the business' (CBI 1979: page 4).

The objectives of such a strategy were to achieve a more competitive and efficient British industry, through improved employer-employee relationships, by ensuring that decision-making took place with the understanding and acceptance of the employees concerned. 'In this way, companies can reduce conflict by fostering co-operation and making the most of the individual employee's contribution' (page 6). The CBI suggested that arrangements for involving employees could therefore be directed at:

- promoting understanding of their contribution to wealth creation in their companies
- promoting employee involvement in job content and job purpose
- ensuring employees were aware of the reasons for management decisions
- ensuring employees were aware of the business situation of their enterprises
- informing employees of their company's future objectives and plans.

The CBI went on to say that it was very easy 'to get hung up on words' (CBI 1979: page 3). However:

> We have decided to use the word 'involvement' in order to avoid the emotional and political overtones of other words. There has, however, been so much talk and political argument about 'industrial democracy', 'participation', 'consultation' and 'a participative style of management' that we are in danger of missing the woods for the trees.

The CBI's stance, it was claimed, was based on its long-standing policy that employee involvement was best developed voluntarily, not though legislation, and in accordance with the circumstances of the industry and the company concerned. There was no universal blueprint for employee involvement practices.

Other CBI statements on employee involvement builds on its earlier position and the recent experiences of its members. It believes that employee involvement (CBI 1990: page 7):

- is a range of processes designed to engage the support, understanding and optimum contribution of all employees in an organisation and their commitment to its objectives
- assists an organisation to give the best possible service to customers and clients in the most cost-effective way
- entails providing employees with the opportunity to influence and where appropriate, take part in decision-making on matters which affect them
- is an intrinsic part of good management practice and is therefore not confined to relationships with employee representatives
- can be developed only voluntarily and in ways suited to the activities, structure, and history of an organisation.

The CBI goes on to argue that employee involvement promotes business success. It does this by: fostering trust and a shared commitment to an organisation's objectives; demonstrating respect for individual employees; and enabling employees to get maximum job satisfaction. There is a range of means for generating management-led employee involvement practices. These include: two-way communications between management and employees; regular consultation; devolving decision-making to the lowest possible levels; training in communication skills; financial participation; harmonising terms and conditions of employment; and seeking individual contributions aimed at 'continuous improvement' in the organisation.

The CBI's position has not altered over the years. In one of its most recent policy statements, the CBI (1997: page 11) continues to emphasise the need for companies to drive 'business-led improvements in employee involvement and motivation':

> Successful companies need high levels of motivation and commitment. These can only be achieved through high-quality workplace communication and involvement and well designed remuneration policies which give employees a stake in the prosperity of the company.
>
> The approach to these goals must be driven by business in line with individual companies' specific needs. So business opposes *legislative imposition of specific forms of employee relations.* The challenge is for business to develop and widely adopt best practice adapted to their own particular needs.

INFORMATION AND COMMUNICATION

Information provision involves any process used by management for communicating with employees on issues affecting the organisation and employee interests at work. The information provided may be passed on in writing, orally or visually, with combinations of these methods normally being used. In ACAS's view (ACAS 1989), successful workplace communication enables organisations to function effectively and employees to be properly informed about corporate developments. Done effectively, it helps (page 4):

- employees perform better and become more committed to their company's success
- managers perform better and make better decisions
- create greater trust between managers, trade unions and employees
- reduce misunderstandings
- increase employees' job satisfaction.

Both the CBI (1977) and the IPM (1981) support the view that information provision should focus on the five 'Ps'. These are:

- progress
- profitability
- plans
- policies
- people.

Progress refers to information about the success of the organisation in achieving its corporate goals and targets. It covers three categories of information: markets; costs; and the working environment. The sort of information that can be provided by management in this area is outlined in Exhibit 37.

Exhibit 37 **Examples of information on company progress**

These include:

- Markets
  - sales
  - market share
  - trading position
  - state of the order book
  - contracts gained or lost
- Costs
  - return on capital
  - labour costs per unit of output
  - inflation
  - raw material and input prices
  - productivity
  - quality
  - waste measures
  - number of employees
- Working environment
  - accident and safety records

The importance of profitability to a company can be demonstrated by providing relevant financial information to its employees. This often incorporates the company balance sheet, statements of income and expenditure and more specific information relating to 'value added', how the company is financed and how its income is spent. This information needs, as far as possible, to be free from accounting jargon and to encourage greater awareness by employees of the sources of corporate income, investment and expenditure and their impact on business activity and the firm's future prospects.

As far as company plans are concerned, employees are normally most interested in the ones affecting them directly, particularly those relating to expansions, closures, relocations and reorganisations. The information provided here normally includes details on:

- investment
- relocations and reorganisations
- amalgamations and redeployments
- expansion
- training
- human resources issues.

A company's policies, especially on human resourcing, employee relations and training, need to be explained to all employees, along with the reasons for them. These cover areas such as pay, conditions, holidays, sickness benefits, pensions and employee relations procedures. As these policies are updated, they can be disseminated to employees so that they are kept continuously informed on all matters affecting their job and employment interests.

Information about people covers such matters as:

- appointments
- resignations
- retirements
- promotions
- vacancies
- awards.

Other more personal information relating to births, deaths and marriages and to sporting and social events is also sometimes communicated to employees. This is done to facilitate employee awareness of what is happening amongst colleagues and to encourage group maintenance at the workplace.

Communicating in writing

There is a wide variety of methods by which management can provide written information to employees. The following forms of written communication are the ones most commonly used by managements in organisations.

Notice boards

These are a cheap and easy way of getting instant, current messages across to employees. They can provide information clearly, accurately and positively, although if the notice board is in a bad position, no one may read the notices provided. Notice boards may also get cluttered, information may get lost and it may be presented in an unattractive and unimaginative way. On the other hand, information may be read by one individual and passed on to others orally.

Letters to employees

These are useful for presenting information on a single, important topic. They can be sent to an employee's home, put in pay packets or circulated internally. Internal memos are a variant of these but they focus on specific issues so that they are not confused with management directives or employer instructions.

Bulletins and briefing notes

These are used to update employees, especially middle and junior managers, on important matters. They need to be up to date and well-informed, taking account of the latest information and details available from senior management.

Newsletters

Newsletters provide the lower tiers of formal written communications in organisations and are useful means for enabling junior managers to inform their staff of issues relevant to them. They are most successful where they are used as an informal adjunct to the 'company' newspaper or house journal. Means need to be provided for retrieving such information and updating it when necessary.

House journals

Well-produced house journals, steering a neutral course between employer and employee interests, can provide a useful, regular communication medium within organisations. Unfortunately, they are expensive to produce and distribute, they need professional journalistic direction and their content can be so bland that they fail to attract the interest of their potential readership. A well-designed, well-edited and well-produced house journal, however, can be a very effective means for enabling management to provide employees with relevant organisational information and for employees to have their say about in-house matters which concern them.

Employee handbooks

These are an important and often neglected source of one-off communication from management to employees. And through continuous updating, they allow a lot of basic information to be provided to employees over time. The sorts of information covered include:

- the history and background of the organisation
- its products or services
- its objectives, structures and methods of operating
- the main employment conditions and benefits to employees
- the principal rules of the organisation.

Employee reports

It is increasingly common for larger companies to provide an annual report to all their employees. The annual report is an ideal place for bringing together all the information provided to employees over the year, in an up-to-date form. It normally includes financial information, general information about sales, investment and employment, future trends and other relevant indicators of 'corporate health and wealth'. Annual employee reports need to be attractively presented, free from jargon and readable. In this way, employees are more likely to become aware of how they contribute to organisational performance and effectiveness. They are better able to understand the company's sources of income, investment and expenditure. And, with information presented to employees in a systematic, fair and easily understood manner, greater trust can be engendered between management and its workforce.

Communicating interactively

There are a number of options available to management for communicating orally with employees. These 'interactive' methods normally enable two-way communication to take place between management and employees. The method used depends on the size of the group being communicated with, what is being communicated and to whom it is being communicated. Used effectively, they enable genuine feedback to be generated between management and workforce and trust and openness to be reinforced between them.

Meetings

These include departmental meetings and mass meetings. The departmental meeting represents a step towards the briefing group system, which is examined below. Departmental meetings represent the bottom end of the communication chain and they are the basic means of enabling departmental managers to pass on information to staff from higher management, as well as of taking up points and issues raised by members of their own departments. Such meetings are often fairly informal, although they are likely to have pre-circulated agendas and agreed rules for conducting business. They also tend to be held fairly frequently and therefore may provide a useful forum for enabling departmental heads to meet staff regularly and for staff to put their points of view to management, and the issues of immediate concern to them, as they arise.

Mass meetings are more formal, set-piece occasions. They enable members of senior management to address all staff at a given location, on specific issues. They are not normally held very frequently and the opportunity for interaction between management and employees is more limited than for departmental meetings. However, with skilful use of 'question and answer' sessions, exchanges can take place and the usefulness of the meetings can become enhanced as a result of this. Because of their size, however, such meetings require professional planning if they are to be successful. Speakers need to be sufficiently briefed, well prepared and clearly structured in their presentations, using appropriate visual aids and learning technologies to get their messages across.

Briefing or discussion groups

These have been popularised by a number of organisations and management interest groups, especially the Industrial Society, since the 1970s (Garnett 1983). In essence, a briefing group system seeks to bring down the levels of oral communication, between management and workforce, below those of departmental or unit meetings, into workgroups. There are a variety of types of briefing groups but a 'briefing group system' is defined by the Industrial Society (1970) as:

> A group which is called together regularly and consistently in order that the decisions, policies and the reasons for them, both at company and departmental levels, may be explained to other people. Those briefed communicate in turn to their own briefing group so that information is systematically passed down the management line, in a number of interlocking steps . . . The objective of a briefing group system is to convey understanding of a communication to every employee through face to face contact with his or her supervisor.

The benefits claimed of briefing groups are that they enable supervisors to take on the role of workgroup communicators. They also provide for face-to-face communication amongst people who know each other well. They are likely, therefore, to be informal and to allow genuine two-way communication to take place within them.

The size of briefing groups varies from about 4 to 18 members who meet for up to half an hour monthly or bi-monthly, under the leadership of their supervisor. Typically, these groups focus on the five 'Ps', outlined above. The two most important elements in creating and sustaining effective briefing group systems are the commitment of senior management and the training of group leaders. Supervisors, in particular, have to be made aware that operating the briefing group system is part of their job, and not an optional extra to be ignored during periods of pressure. Equally, every effort needs to be made to ensure that briefing group leaders receive appropriate training in running their groups, and in understanding the aims and objectives of the system, so that the groups can operate effectively.

Conferences and seminars

These are meetings of selected or specified employees who come together to study, discuss and examine a particular problem. Emphasis is placed on questioning and group discussion. For example, when major organisational changes are envisaged, full-day conferences or seminars are a useful means of creating communication channels between senior management and those likely to be affected by the changes. Conferences and seminars can be in-house or off-premises, with the latter being particularly useful where management wants to encourage an informal atmosphere. For successful results and outcomes, conferences and seminars need to be organised in accordance with a number of accepted guidelines. These include:

- the meeting should be of manageable size to ensure informality and the flow of ideas
- it should last at least one day
- management presentations should be short, snappy and to the point
- delegates should be encouraged to ask questions, put their views and work collaboratively
- all ideas provided should be followed up, analysed and acted upon.

Quality circles

A quality circle is a group of people within an organisation who meet together on a regular basis to identify, analyse and solve problems on quality, productivity or other aspects of daily working life, using problem-solving techniques. Membership of such groups, which usually have 4 to 12 members, is normally voluntary and members are commonly from the same work area or do similar job tasks and activities. The reasons for introducing quality circles into organisations are to develop employees, to facilitate communications, to improve quality, to increase competitiveness and to make cost savings. Having met together, quality circles then present solutions to management and are usually involved in implementing and monitoring them.

Where quality circles are used effectively, it has been shown that they develop individuals, provide personal progression for circle members, improve managerial leadership, promote teamwork and contribute to quality improvements (Russell and Dale 1989). Appropriate attitudes, skills and behaviour by managers are essential if quality circles are to succeed, grow and develop. Top management commitment is crucial for the effectiveness of quality circles. This means management willingness to listen and respond positively to quality circle presentations, to implement their outcomes and to monitor implementation. Middle and supervisory managers, however, can be obstacles to the success of quality circles, where they fear loss of managerial control. One way in which this problem is addressed is by creating such things as quality circle leaders, facilitators and steering groups. But it is also sometimes necessary to establish a 'parallel' organisational structure, one concerned with production and the other with change. In other words, quality circles can exist as parallel structures in organisations, in tandem with the operating hierarchy, and be mainly concerned with facilitating change.

Apart from some misgivings about the members of quality circles being selected rather than elected, many trade unionists are not opposed to quality circles in principle. Their main concern is that quality circles may be manipulated by some managements to undermine the rôle of trade union representatives in the workplace and they therefore could lead to a weakening of the union function and even to union derecognition. Yet some quality circles have workplace representatives as their leaders, whilst one piece of research contends that most of the issues dealt with by quality circles have few employee relations implications (Bradley and Hill 1987). Another approach used to mitigate trade union anxieties about quality circles is the creation of a joint management–union steering group at the outset. By involving both parties from the beginning, the initiators of quality circles can be clear about the intentions, objectives and expectations of quality circles from the start. They are then better able to create the conditions conducive to trust and openness amongst management, workers and union representatives.

Health and safety committees

Joint management–worker or management–union health and safety committees provide useful, interactive channels for information and communication between employers and employees at workplace level. Improving health and safety in the workplace is an integrative activity in which both employers and employees have a common concern. Unhealthy working conditions and accidents at work cause considerable hardship to individuals, create additional expense for organisations and damage the reputations of employers. Positive health and safety measures, to which all employees can contribute, are a vital part of management's responsibility. Joint committees on health and safety are a valuable medium for management–worker dialogue and can ensure that the highest standards of health and safety are established and maintained within the enterprise. Effective joint committees can help to produce healthy and safe working environments by:

- ensuring that there are regular inspections in the workplace
- monitoring health and safety records
- analysing records and statistics
- making sure that appropriate training takes place
- keeping in touch with new developments
- seeing that legislation is implemented
- stimulating health and safety awareness
- providing specialist advice within the workplace.

Where they are active and properly constituted bodies, joint health and safety committees benefit the employer, employees and, where they are recognised, the trade unions.

Attitude surveys

Structured, regular attitude surveys within organisations provide a systematic means for managements to investigate the opinions and views of employees on issues of specific relevance to both employer and workers and to get valuable feedback on them. Attitude surveys are undertaken for various reasons including:

- diagnosing organisational problems
- assessing the effects of organisational change
- measuring employee attitudes prior to and subsequent to a programme of change
- providing feedback on management policies, actions and plans
- identifying matters of collective concern to employees.

Suggestion schemes

These are used to encourage employees to put forward ideas about improving methods of working, cutting costs, increasing productivity or modifying any aspect of the work environment which might benefit the organisation and/or its workforce. Financial or other rewards are normally provided to individuals whose ideas are accepted and put into operation by the employer. Special forms or suggestion boxes are provided by the employer and publicity can be given through the house journal, posters and employee pay packets.

Training

Training is an important form of communication. It can help employees understand the information given to them and encourage them to play a fuller part in the ways an employer conducts its affairs. Training is needed because information about corporate performance or management activities sometimes involves specialist terminology and data that are difficult to interpret. Well-designed training courses are a useful way of giving employees factual information about their employment. Training events can provide explanations of what is happening in the organisation, and opportunities for questions to be put to management and answers to be given on issues raised by course members. Training in communication skills is also important for those who have to communicate. It can enable managers to:

- become more aware of the importance of effective workplace communications
- understand their roles and responsibilities as communicators
- improve their ability to communicate.

Such training is particularly important for supervisors who have a critical communication role but may have limited experience in doing it well.

Communicating visually

Some organisations have taken communications a step further by linking them to sophistication aids like films and videos. They have done this because:

- linking the spoken word with the visual gets messages across more effectively
- it ensures consistency in the information that gets across
- some employees prefer such an approach.

Films are useful for getting information over to large groups. Unfortunately, they are expensive and the medium is rather inflexible, because films soon get out of date and parts of them cannot be updated. Videos, on the other hand, are gaining in popularity. This is because of their advantages of providing 'in-house' productions, flexibility and relatively low cost. The ease of preparing videos allows them to be kept up to date, whilst the use of playback facilities ensures that the message to be transmitted can be got across very effectively. Some organisations are using videos to enable their senior managers to give 'corporate updates' and top-level communications to staff, on periodic but regular bases.

FINANCIAL PARTICIPATION

Financial participation is a form of employee involvement which, like all other forms of employee involvement, is employer-driven, unitary in its emphasis and normally centred on individuals. The approach is used by companies to encourage employees to identify more closely with their firm's aims and objectives and to promote the idea that their common interest lies in maximising corporate profits. It is hoped that employees will see the advantages of co-operation, flexibility and teamwork and the disutility of conflict and the pursuit of uncoordinated self-interest at work (Ridley 1992). The main types of financial participation schemes used by employers in Britain are profit-sharing, profit-related pay, employee share ownership and gainsharing, all of which, by definition, are limited to private sector businesses. This approach to seeking employee commitment has to some extent been encouraged by legislation since the early 1980s. This has arisen, in part at least, because, in the view of successive governments, financial participation breaks down the 'them and us' attitudes between management and employees in the private sector. As such, it is thought likely to bring about a greater identity of interest between the two parties at enterprise level.

Profit-sharing

It is a widespread view that there is an inexorable trend towards profit-sharing in Britain, the EU, Japan and the USA. Yet Japanese bonus payments –

which are paid only in larger firms – vary very little over time and increase in line with earnings. In Germany, where almost all employees are covered by financial participation arrangements as a result of the Capital Formation Act, the legislation requires employers to make a fixed financial contribution to a form of savings for employees, chosen by them, but not necessarily in their own companies. Even in the USA, regarded by some as the home of profit-sharing, only some 16 per cent of full-time employees are covered by actual profit-sharing arrangements. The vast majority of schemes in the USA provide deferred payments which are usually invested on behalf of the employees in savings plans for their retirement (Incomes Data Services 1992).

'Pure' profit-sharing is paid to employees at management's discretion. It is the 'residue' profit allocated for payment to employees, after the company's obligations to its shareholders have been fulfilled. It is left entirely to management to decide:

- the proportion of total profit to be used for profit-sharing
- the amount to be allocated to individual employees (and the rationale for this)
- the frequency of such bonus payments.

Profit-sharing, then, is a periodic bonus paid by an employer, out of corporate profits, which is added to the employee's basic pay. Experience suggests, however, that problems arise for management when they use periodic profit-sharing bonuses as a substitute for a competitive wage. Flanders and his colleagues (1968) found, for example, in their study of the John Lewis Partnership, that there was a much higher level of staff dissatisfaction with basic pay than with profit-sharing. In other words, profit-sharing is only likely to work where employees have reasonable pay levels, good conditions of employment and confidence in management's basic approach to employee relations. It is no remedy for bad employee relations.

A significant feature of profit-sharing is the way in which payouts average around 5 to 6 per cent of annual salary over time. According to Matthews (1989), where profit-sharing bonuses become too large or too small, they are often terminated by the company and their replacement schemes normally pitch their bonuses at around the 5 per cent level. Difficulties arise where, because of trading difficulties, bonuses fall to zero. Yet the durability of some schemes is surprising. This is normally where there is an ideological commitment to them by the management and owners, who continue to support the scheme, however poorly the company is performing financially.

To some extent, the introduction of profit-sharing is optimised when the market conditions facing companies are tight. Tying profit-sharing arrangements to the overall performance of the company or enterprise carries a strong message of collective responsibility for corporate efficiency during difficult times. There are clear advantages in introducing a scheme when initial costs are low, with the likelihood that payments will improve in the future. On the other hand, problems are created by continually rising payments, especially if the scheme is presented as an incentive. By the very nature of incentives, they fluctuate each year. But if profits are maintained at a constant level, or are on a rising curve, the expectation is that profit-sharing payments will remain as they are or will increase too.

Profit-related pay

There has been a growth in profit-related pay in recent years (Millward *et al* 1992). The introduction of profit-related pay into the corporate sector was stimulated by the Finance Act 1987. After an initial surge, schemes tailed off, but interest in them revived after the Finance Act 1991. This Act doubled the tax relief on such schemes and model rules were published to help employers implement them. The sudden rush of schemes was also stimulated by the major accountancy firms that provided clients with formula-based schemes to avoid paying tax on elements of basic pay.

Part of government thinking about the introduction of profit-related pay is the assumption that financial participation by employees in the economic success of their firms encourages loyalty to their employer and support for the profit motive. But it is also linked with the aim of getting firms to substitute a variable profit bonus for basic pay. An implication of this is that paying flexible wages encourages firms to retain their employees in difficult economic times and to reward them when times are good.

Employee share ownership

There is also growing interest by both employers and government in employee share ownership (ESO). There are three main types of ESO:

- *Approved Deferred Share Trust (ADST) schemes*. In these, profits are put in a trust fund which acquires shares in the employing company for employees. These shares are then allotted to participating employees according to a set formula. Employees must retain the shares for a specified period to avoid tax liability.
- *Save as You Earn (SAYE) share option schemes*. These schemes are where employees can buy their employer's shares from the proceeds of a SAYE savings contract. Employees then accumulate savings over a five or seven year period and use them to purchase shares at a predetermined price. There is no liability to income tax, although capital gains tax is payable.
- *Discretionary or executive share option schemes*. These are, by definition, limited to company executives. They are used both to reward executive employees and to reinforce their loyalty to their company.

Other types of share ownership scheme are found in partly employee-owned firms like the National Freight Corporation (NFC). NFC, an internationally based company, was formed when the National Freight Consortium was privatised in the early 1980s. It was floated on the Stock Exchange in 1989 and more than 90 per cent of its employees are now shareholders, although they own only about 20 per cent of the company's equity. To protect the principles on which the company was established, employee shareholders have a double vote on all issues. This is provided that they collectively hold more than 10 per cent of the equity. The employee ownership philosophy of the company enables the NFC to use it as a marketing tool. Each individual employee is in contact with customers, which is a good sales pitch. In addition, employee ownership helps maintain a strong corporate identity which might otherwise be lost.

Gainsharing

The main distinguishing feature of gainsharing is that it is a group incentive payment linked to productivity, based on a formula which in turn is linked to past performance. Also, unlike some other financial participation schemes, it can involve trade unions in the way it operates. The thinking behind gainsharing is the desire of management to promote a team philosophy amongst employees by rewarding them collectively for improvements in performance. Gainsharing is most commonly found in the USA but a prominent example in Britain is at British Steel. This scheme was developed in the early 1980s and took the form of a quarterly pay bonus, based on the ratio of added value to employment costs, together with more sophisticated measures such as quality of output and delivery to time.

One of the most common gainsharing schemes is the Scanlon Plan. One version is based on the ratio of labour costs to total production value, with negotiators agreeing on a normal ratio so that any savings are distributed to employees on a monthly basis. Management's profit from the plan is derived from increased sales with no corresponding increases in costs. The plan allows for revisions to be made to the basic formula where there are changes in product prices or increases in basic pay. Schemes can also be revised where capital investment takes place which obviously raises productivity without additional employee effort.

Another approach is that of 'added value', a concept developed by A. W. Rucker, again in the USA. Added value is defined as the difference between sales revenue and the cost of goods and services bought in. It represents, in effect, the 'wealth' created by a company. Rucker showed that labour costs, expressed as a proportion of added value, remain stable over long periods. It can thus provide a measure of productivity. The weakness of the Rucker scheme – and of the Scanlon Plan – is that the ratios used may be affected by factors that have little to do with the productivity of employees. Technological changes, or changes in prices or product mix, may affect sales revenue without affecting wage costs.

Gainsharing appears to be a better motivator than profit-sharing – although they are not mutually exclusive. It is particularly attractive where labour costs are a high proportion of total costs. And gainsharing schemes can be geared to improvements in quality, delivery and the cost of waste. They are also more flexible than profit-sharing. On the other hand, gainsharing can inhibit change, its formulae can be difficult for employees to understand and such schemes require a lot of monitoring and communication on the part of management and supervisors. Gainsharing also assumes that employees actually influence performance measures, whereas in many organisations they do not.

TOTAL QUALITY MANAGEMENT

Total quality management (TQM) has become a major issue for many companies in Britain in recent years. Yet the term is often used imprecisely, loosely and without defining what 'total quality' actually is. The 'management of quality' in Britain is not a new concept but, with the move away from the traditional role of quality inspection, there has been a tendency to label all approaches to quality management as total quality. This is inaccurate and fails to take account of the complex origins of TQM, the diversity of TQM practices and the links it has with employer attempts to obtain employee commitment and to structure employee involvement initiatives in organisations (Marchington *et al* 1992).

Origins and variations

The origins of TQM can be traced back to the search by Japanese companies for quality improvements in the 1950s. By the 1960s, ideas on quality improvement combined the pioneering works of Deming (1986) and Juran (1989) with the concepts of statistical process control and teamwork. It was around this time that the first quality circles were introduced in Japan. Both Deming and Juran argued that quality control should be conducted as an integral part of management control, with 'continuous improvement' as the ultimate goal. In asserting that 'quality is free', Crosby (1978) argued that, in expressing their concerns with quality issues, managements are also dealing with people situations. His approach was closely linked with those of Deming and Juran but stated, in essence, that quality starts with sets of attitudes for which management has the major responsibility. But changing attitudes within organisations, at all levels, takes time and needs to be managed on a long-term, proactive basis. The development of quality control into total quality control (TQC) emerged from these debates, with TQC becoming known as TQM by the late 1980s.

TQM is distinguished from quality circles in a number of ways. According to Wilkinson and his colleagues (1992), quality circles have five main characteristics that contrast with TQM. They are voluntary groups, 'bolted on' to organisations, acting 'bottom-up' and operating at departmental or unit level. Their aim is to improve employee relations. TQM, on the other hand, is compulsory, an integrated quality system, 'top-down' and company-wide. Its underlying purpose is quality improvement. Nevertheless, TQM has implications for employee relations. Employees take greater responsibility for quality, are accountable for its achievement and work in teams. In addition, TQM is supposed to place greater emphasis on employee self-control, personal autonomy and individual creativity. The active co-operation of employees is expected, rather than just their compliance with management policy decisions and the employment contract. However, since TQM comprises both production and employee relations elements, it 'highlights tensions between, on the one hand, following clearly laid-down instructions whilst, on the other, encouraging employee influence over the management process' (Wilkinson *et al* 1992: page 6).

The British Quality Association provides three definitions of TQM. The first focuses on its soft, qualitative characteristics: customer orientation, culture excellence, removal of performance barriers, training, competitive edge and employee participation. The second emphasises its hard, operations management aspects: systematically measuring and controlling work, setting performance standards and using statistical control procedures to assess quality. The third definition incorporates a mixture of hard and soft approaches to TQM and consists of three features: an obsession with quality, the need for a scientific approach to total quality and the view that all employees are part of the same team.

In Britain, TQM focuses on variants of the hard and mixed approaches. Oakland (1989), for example, views TQM as improving business effectiveness, flexibility and competitiveness and meeting customer requirements both inside and outside the organisation. He sees TQM as a triangle and a chain – indicating the interdependence of customer-supplier links throughout the organisation – with the three points of the triangle representing management commitment, statistical process control and teamworking. Dale and Plunkett (1990: page 6), whilst focusing on the statistical and operational characteristics of TQM, also link it with employee relations arguing that the 'key features of TQM are employee involvement and development and a teamwork approach to dealing with improvement activities'. Collard (1989) regards TQM as a management discipline aimed at preventing problems from occurring in organisations by creating attitudes and controls that make problem prevention possible. For him, improved quality need not lead to increased costs. Indeed, costs are likely to fall because of a decline in failure rates and reduced costs of detection.

The basic elements of TQM

A useful general definition of TQM is provided by the Institute of Management Services (1992: page 5). It emphasises that TQM is not simply a system for achieving zero defects in the products or services provided by a company but that it also involves people. In its view, TQM is:

> A strategy for improving business performance through the commitment and involvement of all employees to fully satisfying agreed customer requirements, at the optimum overall cost, through the continuous improvement of the products and services, business processes and people involved.

TQM, in short, is focused on achieving business success through satisfying customer needs. This is facilitated by involving every employee within the organisation in achieving this end and by expecting employees to see others, both internal and external to the organisation, as customers for their services.

There is no 'blue print' for developing, implementing and evaluating a TQM programme within an organisation. It is contingent upon organisational circumstances, management preferences and the resources available. However, a number of common elements can be identified by examining the literature on TQM. These are:

- the emphasis on continuous improvement
- the need for commitment from top management
- the issue of attitudinal change
- the impact of TQM on the organisation as a whole.

There are also human resource implications arising from TQM, such as training, development and the creation of appropriate organisational structures. These are examined in the next section.

Since the focus of TQM is continuous improvement aimed at satisfying customer needs and providing value for money, at optimum cost to the organisation, this requires that everyone in an organisation that has introduced TQM should become involved. This includes:

- using a defined process of delivering quality
- continuously identifying opportunities for improvement
- delivering improvement through structured problem-solving techniques.

People also have to use error prevention mechanisms, practise corrective feedback mechanisms and apply key business processes, across the whole organisation, rather than within individual functions alone. The idea of continuous improvement means that people have to understand and identify any quality problems early on, at all levels in the organisation, and accept their responsibility for doing this. Continuous improvement is based on continuous measurement and evaluation, with this taking place both within the organisation and externally with clients or customers.

For TQM to be successful, its proponents argue that it needs effective leadership and long-term commitment by management – with managers acting as role models, leading and empowering change within their organisations. This needs to be supported by a culture of 'learning together', with guidance and support for the learning process being provided by management. TQM also incorporates clearly defined business objectives, communicated by managers and understood and owned by all employees. It is also management's task to encourage and empower every employee to adopt appropriate ownership behaviour (Hakes 1991). This includes ownership of outputs, customer problems and improvement actions. Most importantly, TQM focuses on success through people. This involves invoking solutions by consensus, providing education and training opportunities based on user needs, and facilitating teamwork and effective intra-organisational communications.

This means that top management has a major responsibility to continuously reinforce a TQM programme through its example as a group.

Whether in meetings, newsletters or in-house journals, management has to demonstrate its complete commitment to total quality. In this sense, some writers assert that changing management attitudes is the key to developing successful TQM and that this must start at the very top of an organisation. To show this commitment, it is argued, top management should make sure that everybody, from top to bottom in the enterprise, is clear about its long-term goals and objectives. This affects styles of management, communication systems and the way things are done within the organisation.

The issue of attitude change is critical in introducing, maintaining and implementing TQM programmes. Because of the consequences of TQM, it requires a complete change of attitudes, expectations and the prevailing culture in an organisation. These consequences may include: reductions in staffing, for example amongst inspectors and those administering complaints procedures; lack of staff knowledge of the techniques used in TQM, such as new statistical and control techniques; and anxieties about the implications of change. TQM also involves more participative management styles, with middle management having less control over the supervisory and quality processes. Further, changes in management style, with greater devolution of management responsibilities, are often seen as a threat by middle managers. The need for attitude change is not confined to managers, however – it is required of all the workforce – but it applies particularly to management.

As an organisationally based process, TQM focuses on the best use of resources for the total organisation, organisational flexibility and responsiveness to change. It is also concerned with customer/supplier relationships which embrace not only external and internal customers but also external and internal suppliers. It is concerned, in short, with all those people who are bound together in long-term business relationships inside and outside the organisation. Other aspects of the TQM process include: measuring performance in terms of agreed customer requirements, customer satisfaction and process efficiency; anticipating customer needs; and delivering products and services which 'delight' customers. This requires identifying and adopting best working practices, as well as monitoring continuous improvement.

Some human resources implications

There are three main sets of human resource implications arising from the introduction of a TQM programme. These comprise:

- the need for management leadership to facilitate employee motivation
- training and development implications
- the creation of an appropriate organisational structure to facilitate TQM.

A major feature of introducing TQM into any organisation is often the need to change corporate culture into one that is more people-oriented. This entails leadership at all levels, opportunities for employee empowerment and the development of relevant skills within the workforce. Managers act as motivators, stimulating employees to accept responsibility for satisfying the agreed needs of their customers, whilst also encouraging employees to become committed to total quality. Meetings need to run effectively, team-building skills need to be facilitated and communication skills need to be developed. Another aspect of motivation is providing recognition, rewards and performance feedback to the employees concerned.

Training for TQM aims to develop self-motivated, self-reliant employees and enable them to achieve both their personal goals and those of the organisation, whilst satisfying the requirements of their customers. It commonly focuses on:

- the top-down cascading of ideas and information
- workgroup training, with managers leading the training of their teams
- relating the training content to the team's actual work.

The content of TQM training includes quality delivery, quality improvement and quality management. There is also the need to develop interpersonal skills amongst people within the workplace, such as teambuilding, motivating, leadership and communicating skills.

Collard (1989) is both descriptive and prescriptive about the training needs arising from TQM. He claims that a total quality training programme combines three elements:

- management skills training
- training in quality management techniques, such as in the use of appropriate statistical techniques
- corporate culture development.

He also identifies four levels of training for: top management; middle management; task group leaders; and facilitators. The development of group leadership, group working and communication and presentation skills for managers, for example, is seen as being particularly important. These include competency in: chairing meetings; developing the skills of group members; and developing appropriate leadership styles. Other behavioural skills that need to be developed include: problem-solving techniques; presentation techniques; and brainstorming. In Collard's view, organisations need to develop company-specific training programmes, not off-the-shelf packages. These should incorporate the concept of continuous development, with total quality training 'occurring regularly for all levels, not just at the beginning of the programme. The training should seek to extend and develop understanding of the basic techniques' (page 138).

Developing an appropriate organisational structure and a quality function includes a number of measures, such as:

- providing a quality support organisation to help management develop a strategy to implement the total quality process

- co-ordinating the application of quality management
- tracking the cost of quality.

It is also necessary to co-ordinate quality management systems and integrate health, safety and customer considerations into products, services and business processes. This is important in order to ensure effective communication structures and to facilitate employee involvement and co-operation in each case.

WORKER PARTICIPATION

Throughout this book the emphasis has been on how the potential conflicts arising from the pay–work bargain are managed in an advanced capitalist economy like that of Britain. There are four policy choices available to managements in determining their employee relations strategies, including how work relations are structured, how work is organised and what emphasis they should adopt in managing people at work. These policy choices are (see also Chapter 2):

- worker subordination (effected through managerial prerogative)
- union incorporation (effected through collective bargaining and formal joint consultation)
- employee commitment (effected through employee involvement practices)
- worker participation (effected through worker directors, board level representation and enterprise committees).

These management policy thrusts are not necessarily mutually exclusive: they can operate in parallel within the same organisation, with different policies being used for different groups of employees. The traditional management policy in Britain for much of the nineteenth century was worker subordination. During the first three-quarters of the twentieth century, union incorporation became the dominant policy model, particularly when this was supported by the state during the years of the employee relations consensus (see Chapter 7). More recently, since the mid-1980s, with increasing product competition, rising unemployment and growing market deregulation, employee commitment has become a favoured policy choice for increasing numbers of employers. Worker participation, however, has not been either a management policy issue or a major political one in Britain since the late 1970s, when the report of the Bullock Committee of inquiry into industrial democracy was published (Department of Trade 1977). This is largely because of hostility to it by successive Conservative governments and the changed balance of power in the labour market and workplace favouring employers and management.

Approaches to worker participation

Worker participation is any employee relations process that enables employees to share in the making of enterprise or corporate decisions. In Britain, managements and management organisations generally argue that worker participation is best operated at the individual or small group level. This is most usefully done, it is contended, by providing opportunities for individuals and small groups to 'participate' in the ways their jobs are organised, in quality circles, in the ownership and profits of the company employing them, in TQM initiatives at departmental and corporate levels and in the communication, information and consultative channels of their employer. This type of 'worker participation', which is management-defined and employer-centred, can be best described as task and work-based participation, aimed at individual employees. It is low-level participation, soft on power and management-driven, and is essentially a managerial definition of the term 'worker participation'.

In Britain, trade unions, in contrast, claim that the best method of advancing worker participation at work is collective bargaining. In this view, collective bargaining becomes less a method of sharing in the making of managerial decisions than a method of promoting 'industrial democracy' in the workplace and at employer level. Democracy, in essence, means providing the opportunity to influence the making of decisions by individuals and groups whose vital interests are affected by these decisions. The concept of industrial democracy, therefore, envisages employees having the right to exert influence over those decisions most affecting their daily working lives. These include the economic, social and personnel aspects of the workplace and of the enterprise employing them. Industrial democracy, it is argued, calls for real worker participation in the decision-making process, through the agency of trade unions. Conversely, it implies a sharing of the right to manage in those areas involving employee representatives. In this sense, industrial democracy is high-level, power-centred, and union and worker-driven. It is for this reason that British employers are hostile to such a concept of 'worker participation in management' or what the unions describe as industrial democracy.

It is arguable, however, that industrial democracy goes beyond traditional collective bargaining. Collective bargaining is a power relationship and is a process of interest group representation in certain limited areas of personnel decision-making. It is an assertion of power, or of countervailing power, in a procedural framework negotiated between management and union representatives. The emphasis is on resolving conflicts of interest between the parties, with the outcomes of collective bargaining being determined by the relative balance of negotiating power between them. Collective bargaining becomes industrial democracy only where the negotiating agenda is widened beyond that of the pay–work bargain – the 'managerial concept' of collective bargaining (see Chapter 9) – and where an integrative or co-operative approach to the management–union relationship is adopted by both parties.

Marsden (1978) views industrial democracy as a contest over collective control within enterprises. It takes a variety of forms resulting from the struggle for control and from power shifts between the competing parties – employer and employees, and management and unions. The outcomes of this struggle depend on the level and scope of participation exercised and the ways in which effective worker participation is determined. In effect, worker participation can take place at enterprise or corporate level. But since participation at corporate level challenges the right to manage more than it does at enterprise or work-group level, it is even more strongly resisted by management and management interest groups than at other levels.

There are two routes, in effect, through which industrial democracy/worker participation can be advanced. One is by the 'bottom-up' process of local initiatives driven by workers and their trade unions. This aims to develop participative working relationships with employers and management. In Britain, the voluntary, bottom-up route, led by shop stewards, has been the preferred method for trade unions and their members. This strategy is likely to be successful in well-organised enterprises and industries, with strongly based trade unions, in conditions of full employment. It is less likely to achieve results where there are high unemployment, hostile employers and weak trade unions. Moreover, since the bottom-up model is based on adversarial employee relations, it is difficult to reconcile with the objective of creating consensus within the enterprise and integrative management–union relationships.

The other route to worker participation is the 'top-down' process of supportive public policy, with legal enactment or centrally determined 'framework' collective agreements between employer and trade union confederations. This, in contrast, has been the preferred approach in most of western Europe since the end of the second world war. Works councils at plant level, co-determination at board level and other sets of participatory rights for workers have been the product of political struggle and political representation at government level. Unlike the bottom-up model, the top-down model is based on the idea of social partnership between employers and unions and management and workers. It is rooted in providing a set of legal rights and responsibilities for the parties to employee relations, based either on statute law or on legally enforceable collective contracts. This model of worker participation aims to create identity and harmony of interest between management and workers, in order to increase the enterprise's potential for wealth creation and to weaken the likelihood of industrial conflict. It also seeks to institutionalise co-operative and trusting working relations between employers and employees, at both the workplace and corporate level.

Participation in the workplace

Formal systems of worker participation in the workplace are at their most advanced in western Europe. Most EU member states, and some countries in post-communist central and eastern Europe such as Bulgaria, the Czech

Republic and Hungary (Farnham 1997), have some form of statutory provision or agreed systems for facilitating worker participation at workplace level. The precise mechanisms vary according to each country's legal framework for employee relations, the relative strengths of employers and unions, the coherence and unity of the trade union movement and the dominant culture of employee relations (Ferner and Hyman 1992). The Netherlands and Germany, for example, have highly legalistic systems, with extensive and detailed powers for worker representatives. In Denmark and Italy, by contrast, worker participation is built into central collective agreements. It is these which provide broadly defined obligations for employers and employees in determining their participation arrangements.

Legal systems

The most institutionalised system of worker participation at workplace level is provided in Germany. Here industrial democracy or worker participation is embodied in the concept of co-determination (see Chapter 3). This is based on the principle of co-decision-taking between management and elected worker representatives on a number of issues considered to be vital to each party. At the level of the workplace, this is done through the institution of 'works councils', although since the Works Constitution Act 1972, workers are represented not only at plant level but also at company level. The most important participation rights of German works councils are outlined in Figure 15. These cover a wide range of issues and give German workers some measure of joint control in areas affecting their conditions of employment, working practices and workplace organisation. Assessments of the effectiveness of German works councils vary. Berghahn and Karsten (1989) argue that works councils have strengthened the position of workers in the enterprise. Jacobi and his colleagues (1992: page 243), on the other hand, claim that: 'in general, works councils' participation rights are strong in relation to social policy; weaker in the case of personnel issues; and weaker still in financial and economic matters.'

In the Netherlands, the dominant form of worker representation at enterprise level is through the statutory system of works councils. These must be established by employers in any enterprise employing at least 100 employees or at least 35 employees working more than one-third of normal working hours. They are employee-constituted bodies, elected by all the employees within an enterprise who have at least six months' service. The size of the works councils varies according to the size of the enterprise and all employees can stand for election providing they have at least one year's service with the employer. Works councillors have protection against dismissal, time off with pay to attend works councils meetings and time off with pay for relevant training. But they are also bound by the requirements of confidentiality and must not disclose their employer's business or trading secrets, even when their periods of office as works councillors have finished (Incomes Data Services 1992a).

Works councils in the Netherlands are obliged to meet with management

Figure 15 **Main participation rights of German works councils**

Rights	Social matters	Personnel matters	Economic matters
Co-determination	working time holidays payment system piecework work organisation	staff files selection training	social plan
Veto		recruitment redeployment wage groupings dismissal	
Consultation and information	labour protection accidents	HR planning appeals	major plans new plant job content

at least six times a year. They have rights of information, consultation and veto. Employers, for example, are required to provide works councils with all the information reasonably required for them to carry out their tasks (Visser 1992). This information includes:

- the legal constitution of the employer
- its annual accounts
- reports on the general conduct of the business
- at least once annually, a report on employment trends in the enterprise and its social policy.

The main issues on which employers are required to consult works councils are:

- transfers of control of the enterprise
- acquisitions and joint ventures
- closures or relocations
- changes in the enterprise's activities
- the recruitment of employees
- the commissioning of expert advice by the employer.

The agreement of the works council is also required where the employer seeks to amend provisions relating to:

- hours and holidays
- job evaluation schemes
- pensions or profit-sharing
- health and safety at work
- grievance procedures
- rules relating to recruitment, dismissal, promotion, training and appraisal.

Systems of statutory works councils are also established in other European states such as in Belgium, France, Greece, Portugal and Spain. They vary in their legal and constitutional details (Ferner and Hyman 1992) but they all basically provide sets of legal rights and duties for employers, works councils and elected employee representatives at enterprise level. In some cases, such as in Belgium and France, works councils are paralleled by other representative bodies at enterprise level. In Belgium and France, for example, in addition to statutory works councils there are 'trade union delegations', which are made up of elected trade union representatives and have collective bargaining functions. In Belgium, trade union delegations are not statutory bodies but are established by central collective agreements between employer and union confederations. In France, in contrast, trade union delegations are regulated by law, which provides their members with paid time off work to carry out their duties, with protections against dismissal – during their periods of office – and with consultative and negotiating rights.

In most cases, apart from those of the Netherlands, Italy and Portugal, there is also a statutory duty on employers to establish plant-based health and safety committees. These complement works councils and their main functions are to elect employee safety representatives and to ensure that issues relating to the health and safety of employees are discussed regularly with management. They are also legally required to oversee health and safety issues, improve working conditions and ensure that employers comply with relevant health and safety legislation.

Voluntary systems

In Denmark, employee representation at workplace level is based on a voluntary, corporatist approach and is largely through union-based shop stewards and 'co-operation committees', established through centralised, framework collective agreements. There is, for example, a long tradition of shop steward representation of employees in Denmark and agreed provisions for their election, status and role within the workplace. Central and industry-wide agreements define their functions, prescribe their activities and regulate their employee relations duties. In essence, shop stewards are direct links between management and employees on issues relating to workplace terms and conditions. They are also a focal point through which local grievances are articulated, channelled and resolved. In larger organisations, with many shop stewards, they establish joint union delegations and union 'clubs' incorporating several different unions. In acting within the authority of framework and national agreements, Danish shop stewards are expected to act with restraint and to help maintain good working relations and joint co-operation within the workplace between management and employees.

The principle of employee relations co-operation in Denmark is extended through the creation of co-operation committees at workplace level. Their aim is to promote industrial harmony, business competitiveness and employee job satisfaction in the workplace. The Co-operation Agreement, between the Danish Employers' Confederation and the Federation of Trade Unions, stresses the importance of active participation by employees and their union representatives in the arranging and organising of their daily working lives. It also facilitates the setting-up of co-operation committees in enterprises with more than 35 employees. These consist of managers, senior personnel who are not union members, directly elected employees and shop stewards.

The rights and duties of co-operation committees, under the Co-operation Agreement, are (Incomes Data Services 1992a: page 29):

- Establishing principles for the work environment and human relations, as well as the principles for the personnel policy pursued by the enterprise . . .
- Establishing the principles of training and retraining for employees who are to work with new technology.
- Establishing principles for the in-house compilation, storage and use of personnel data.
- Exchanging views and considering proposals for guide-lines on the planning of production and work, and the implementation of major changes in the enterprise.
- Assessing the technical, financial, staffing, educational and environmental consequences of the introduction of new technology and major changes to existing technology.
- Informing employees about proposals for incentive systems of payment . . . Also informing employees about the possibility of setting up funds for educational and social security purposes.

Co-operation committees are not empowered, however, to deal with matters covered by collective bargaining. But employers are required to inform employees of their firm's financial position, its prospects and any major changes likely to occur in the future.

Employee relations in Italy are in a state of considerable fluidity and instability (Ferner and Hyman 1992) but, in workplace relations, employee participation remains based on union organisation, not on works council legislation. Collective agreements remain the principal source of workers' rights to information and consultation, whilst the Workers' Statute 1970 confers a number of rights on the most representative unions at enterprise level. The principal national agreements, for example, generally include provisions outlining the information and consultation rights of trade unions. At company level, firms with over 200 employees must provide information to trade union representatives on significant changes to the production process or work organisation and on planned large-scale transfers of employees. Where there are over 350 employees, information must be provided about investment and the employment and environmental implications of new working operations or an extension of existing operations.

Under the Workers' Statute 1970, employees have the right to set up representative bodies for dealings with management within the enterprise, provided that such bodies are initiated by the employees, the employer has over 16 employees and the bodies are under the auspices of the most representative trade unions. Trade union representatives have the right to represent members in the workplace and to be involved in bargaining. They are entitled to time off work to undertake their duties, to unpaid leave of absence for other union duties and not to be dismissed by the employer, except for serious misconduct.

Board-level participation

Statutory worker participation arrangements providing for employee representation on company boards exist in Denmark, the Netherlands and Germany. This representation is normally facilitated through the device of two-tier board structures, consisting of an upper-tier 'supervisory' board and a lower-tier 'management' board. Supervisory boards determine overall company policy and must be consulted on important corporate decisions, whilst management boards are concerned with day-to-day operations and issues. Employee representatives sit on the supervisory board.

In Denmark, the law provides for employee representatives on the supervisory boards of all limited liability companies and companies limited by guarantee. They have the same rights and duties as other board members. The supervisory board must ensure that employees are given information about the company's circumstances, including finances, employment and production plans. The arrangements in the Netherlands have existed since 1971. They require all public limited companies with more than 100 workers to establish a supervisory board with employee representatives. The most advanced system of board-level co-determination is in Germany, where there are three models of board-level participation. In joint stock and limited liability companies and limited partnerships with more than 2,000 employees, the supervisory board consists of equal numbers of employee and shareholder representatives, with the size of the board varying according to company size. Enterprises with more than 1,000 employees in the coal, iron and steel industries have supervisory boards consisting of an equal number of employee and shareholder representatives. In companies with between 500 and 2,000 employees, one-third of the members of the supervisory board must be employee representatives. As in the other countries, employee board members have the same rights and duties as shareholder members (Lane 1989).

In France, there is no statutory system of employee representation at board level. However, under a decree of October 1986, companies may provide for a number of employee representatives on the board of directors, with renewable periods of office of up to six years. Additionally, the Auroux laws provide rights for employees to express their views on the content, conditions and organisation of work. These rights are essentially collective and the legislation stipulates that agreements on employees' rights should be concluded between employers and unions where companies employ 50 or more employees and have trade union delegates. Nevertheless, individuals may go straight to members of management with opinions or problems, without having to go through the normal employee representation channels (Goetschy and Rozenblatt 1992).

ASSIGNMENTS

(a) By what criteria would you assess whether or not your organisation operates an 'employee commitment' strategy? You might consider your analysis under headings – which are neither exclusive nor exhaustive – such as: jobs; workgroups; departments; other units of organisation; products/services; type of organisation; functional roles within the organisation; corporate values; or work in general.

(b) Identify and critically evaluate the methods of information provision used by management in your organisation.

(c) Read Millward *et al* (1992: pages 165-72) and identify the major trends in employee communication highlighted by the WIRS survey.

(d) As head of department, provide a draft agenda for your next departmental meeting. What sort of preparation will you have to do to make the meeting a success?

(e) Prepare a position paper for your chief executive outlining the case for introducing (or revising) a briefing group system in your organisation.

(f) Present a report on the structure, operation and effectiveness of quality circles in your organisation.

(g) What would be the pros and cons of introducing a profit-sharing scheme in your company?

(h) Read Marchington and his colleagues (1992: pages 33-42). Report on the impact of employee involvement practices on employees, managers and trade union representatives, as outlined in this research.

(i) Read either Collard (1989), or Dale and Plunkett (1990), or Hakes (1991), or Oakland (1989) and make a presentation on the elements of TQM as examined by one of these authors.

(j) To what extent has 'total quality' been introduced in your organisation? Report on the issues, problems and human resource implications arising from this.

(k) Read Ferner and Hyman (1992) and provide a report on one European system of industrial relations analysed in this book. Indicate how this system differs from that of Britain.

(l) What are the cases for and against employee representation on company boards as happens in other parts of the EU? On what grounds do British employer groups oppose this type of worker participation?

(m) Read Lane (1989: pages 224-48) and provide a comparison of the patterns of industrial democracy in Germany, France and Britain.

REFERENCES

ADVISORY, CONCILIATION AND ARBITRATION SERVICE. 1989. *Workplace Communication*. London: ACAS.

BERGHAHN, V. *and* KARSTEN, D. 1989. *Industrial Relations in West Germany*. London: Berg.

BRADLEY, K. *and* HILL, S. 1987. 'Quality circles and management interests'.

Industrial Relations Journal. 26(1), Winter.
COLLARD, R. 1989. *Total Quality: Success through people*. London: IPM.
CONFEDERATION OF BRITISH INDUSTRY. 1977. *Communication with People at Work*. London: CBI.
CONFEDERATION OF BRITISH INDUSTRY. 1979. *Guidelines for Action on Employee Involvement*. London: CBI.
CONFEDERATION OF BRITISH INDUSTRY. 1990. *Employee Involvement – Shaping the Future*. London: CBI.
CONFEDERATION OF BRITISH INDUSTRY. 1997. *Prospering in the Global Economy*. London: CBI.
CROSBY, P. 1978. *Quality is Free*. NY: McGraw-Hill.
DALE, B. *and* PLUNKETT, J. 1990. *Managing Quality*. London: Allen.
DEMING, W. 1986. *Out of Crisis*. Cambridge, Mass.: MIT.
DEPARTMENT OF TRADE 1977. *Report of the Committee of Inquiry on Industrial Democracy*. London: HMSO.
FARNHAM, D. 1997. 'The role of trade unions in economic and social transition in central and eastern Europe since 1989: a review and assessment'. In Montanheiro, L. and Nevenska, N. (eds) 1997, *Private and Public Partnership: Learning for Growth*, Sheffield: PRU.
FERNER, A. 1988. *Governments, Managers and Industrial Relations*. Oxford: Blackwell.
FERNER, A. *and* HYMAN, R. 1992. *Industrial Relations in the New Europe*. Oxford: Blackwell.
FLANDERS, A., WOODWOOD, J. *and* POMERANTZ, R. (1968). *Experiment in Industrial Democracy*. London: Faber.
GARNETT, J. 1983. *The Manager's Responsibility for Communication*. London: Industrial Society.
GOETSCHY, J. *and* ROZENBLATT, P. 1992. 'France: the industrial relations system at a turning point?' In Ferner, A. and Hyman, R., *Industrial Relations in the New Europe*, Oxford: Blackwell.
HAKES, C. (ed.) 1991. *Total Quality Management*. London: Chapman and Hall.
HIBBERT, A. 1991. 'Employee involvement: a recent survey'. *Employment Gazette*. December.
INCOMES DATA SERVICES. 1992a. *Industrial Relations*. London: IPM.
INCOMES DATA SERVICES. 1992. *IDS Focus: Sharing Profits*. 64, September.
INDUSTRIAL SOCIETY. 1970. *Systematic Communication by Briefing Groups*. London: Industrial Society.
INSTITUTE OF PERSONNEL MANAGEMENT. 1981. *Communication in Practice*. London: IPM.
JACOBI, I., KELLER, B. *and* MUELLER-JENTSCH, W. 1992. 'Germany: codetermining the future?' In Ferner, A. and Hyman, R. 1992, *Industrial Relations in the New Europe*, Oxford: Blackwell.
JURAN, J. 1989. *Juran on Leadership for Quality*. NY: Free Press.
LANE, C. 1989. *Management and Labour in Europe*. Aldershot: Edward Elgar.
MARCHINGTON, M., GOODMAN, J., WILKINSON, A. *and* ACKERS, P. 1992.

New Developments in Employee Involvement. London: Employment Department.

MARSDEN, D. 1978. *Industrial Democracy and Industrial Control in West Germany, France and Great Britain*. London: Department of Employment.

MATTHEWS, D. 1989. 'The British experience of profit sharing'. *Economic History Review*. November.

OAKLAND, J. 1989. *Total Quality Management*. London: Heinemann.

MILLWARD, N. *and* STEVENS, M. 1986. *British Workplace Industrial Relations 1980-1984*. Aldershot: Gower.

MILLWARD, N., STEVENS, M., SMART, D. *and* HAWES, W. (1992). *Workplace Industrial Relations in Transition*. Aldershot: Dartmouth.

PERKINS, G. (ed.) 1986. *Employee Communications in the Public Sector*. London: IPM.

PURCELL, J. 1981. *Good Industrial Relations*. London: Macmillan.

RIDLEY, T. 1992. *Motivating and Rewarding Employees – Some Aspects of Theory and Practice: Work Research Paper 51*. London: ACAS.

RUSSELL, S. *and* DALE, B. 1989. *Quality Circles – a Broader Perspective: Work Research Unit Occasional Paper 43*. London: ACAS.

VISSER, J. 1992. 'The Netherlands: the end of an era and the end of a system'. In Ferner, A. and Hyman, R. 1992, *Industrial Relations in the New Europe*, Oxford: Blackwell.

WHITE, G. 1987. *Employee Commitment: Work Research Unit Occasional Paper 38*. London: ACAS.

WILKINSON, A., MARCHINGTON, M., GOODMAN, J. *and* ACKERS, P. 1992. 'Total quality management and employee involvement'. *Human Resource Management Journal*. 2(4).

11 Industrial action

Industrial action or a 'trade dispute' takes place whenever employers and employees, and/or the organisations representing them, are unable to resolve their differences peacefully and constitutionally in determining, regulating or terminating the pay-work bargain. In law, a trade dispute means any dispute between 'employers and workers, or between workers and workers, which is connected with one or more of the following matters' (TULRCA 1992: section 218):

(a) terms and conditions of employment, or the physical conditions in which any workers are required to work;
(b) engagement or non-engagement, or termination or suspension of employment or the duties of employment, of one or more workers;
(c) allocation of work or the duties of employment between workers or groups of workers;
(d) matters of discipline;
(e) the membership or non-membership of a trade union on the part of a worker;
(f) facilities for officials of trade unions; and
(g) machinery for negotiation or consultation, and other procedures, relating to any of the foregoing matters, including the recognition by employers or employers' associations of the right of a trade union to represent workers in any such negotiation or consultation or in the carrying out of such procedures.

Where a trade dispute takes place, this results in a temporary breakdown of the employment relationship between employer and employee, the imposition of industrial sanctions by either or both parties (or their agents) against the other and the emergence of industrial conflict between them.

Kornhauser and his colleagues summarise the nature of industrial conflict neatly and succinctly (1954: page 13). They describe it as: 'the total range of behavior and attitudes that express opposition and divergent orientations between individual owners and managers on the one hand and working people and their organisations on the other hand'. In taking any kind of industrial action against one another, the parties to employee relations are using their economic and social power to try to coerce the other party into conceding an employment decision – whether over wages, conditions, job security or working arrangements – which cannot be resolved by negotiation, compromise or third-party intervention. Industrial action and the use of industrial sanctions, therefore, involve the application of naked force by one or more of the parties to employee relations against the other. This undermines good working relations between them, imposes financial costs on them and might even threaten the social order, if matters were to get out of control.

Because of this, the state takes an active role in regulating industrial conflict. If the state cannot achieve industrial peace by persuasion, argument or third-party intervention, it provides certain legal backstops to contain and constrain what it defines to be legitimate industrial action. These are aimed at protecting those damaged by industrial action, keeping the sanctions within acceptable constitutional bounds and discouraging what the state defines as politically destabilising employee relations conflict (see Chapters 3, 4, 7 and 8).

THE FUNCTIONS AND FORMS OF INDUSTRIAL SANCTIONS

The taking of industrial sanctions, by any of the parties to employee relations, represents the breakdown of trust, co-operation and goodwill between them. Industrial sanctions, therefore, tend to be the means of last resort used by the parties in attempting to resolve their differences arising from the pay–work bargain. When employers, employees or their agents take industrial sanctions against one another, it is because they believe that it is only by imposing their unilateral power on the other side that they can achieve their employee relations goals.

The aim of industrial sanctions is to weaken the other side's resolve in opposing what is on offer at the bargaining table. If the employees are not unionised, then the employer's ability to impose its unilateral decisions on them is less likely to be resisted, because they have no countervailing collective power to use against management. If the employees are unionised, however, the employer is obliged to take account of the employees' collective power, and its potential impact on the outcome of the conflict, in taking its decision. It also has to listen to what is being proposed by the union leaders on behalf of their members.

Similarly, in deciding whether to take industrial sanctions against their employer, employees and their union leaders have to take account of the likely outcome in terms of costs to them, whether a successful outcome to the action is possible and the consequences of the action for employee relations in the future. In all trade disputes, the potential for coercive power between employer and employees, or between management and unions, is a crucial determinant of the propensity to apply industrial sanctions, the form that the sanctions might take and their likely outcomes on the conflict between the parties.

Theories of industrial conflict

There are three main competing sets of theories seeking to explain the nature of industrial conflict between employers and employees and between management and unions (Farnham and Pimlott 1995). These are:

- structural or Marxist theory
- unitary or 'human relations' theory
- functionalist theory.

In outline, Marxist theory sees industrial conflict between employers and employees as inevitable and deep-rooted, since it emerges out of the class and power relations within capitalist societies. Human relations theory sees industrial conflict as anti-social, dysfunctional and disruptive of enterprise harmony and effectiveness. Functionalist theory sees industrial conflict as having positive benefits for the parties to employee relations, as long as it is channelled into appropriate institutional mechanisms and resolved accordingly.

Marxist theory

Marxist theory views industrial conflict as rooted in the economic structures of capitalist societies. It is a theory of social change and, although there are a number of schools of Marxian scholarship, Marxism is essentially a method of analysing power relationships in society. It assumes:

- that the capitalist mode of production is but one stage in the development of human society
- that class conflict is the catalytic source of change within capitalism
- that out of the dialectical conflict between the social classes, with opposed economic interests, social change takes place, leading eventually to the socialist state.

As Allen (1976: page 21) writes:

> When reality is viewed dialectically it is seen as a process involving interdependent parts which interact on each other. When reality is also viewed materialistically it is seen as phenomena predominantly influenced by economic factors. The dialectical relationship between economic factors, therefore, provides the prime motivation for change. This briefly is what Marxism in the first instance is about.

In the bourgeois capitalist state, the competing class interests are between those of profit-seeking capitalists and the wage-earning proletariat. The struggle for economic hegemony between them is deemed to be inevitable, irrevocable and irreconcilable. Industrial conflict between employer and employee, and between management and union, is merely a reflection of the dominant class interests within capitalism and is synonymous with class conflict. As such, employee relations conflict, between those buying labour in the market place and those selling it, is seen as a permanent feature of capitalism (Hyman 1975). Industrial conflict, in its various forms, in short, arises out of economic contradictions within the capitalist mode of production and is a means for advancing and fighting the class struggle and the class war. The protagonists are those owning and representing private capital and those supplying their skills for wages in the labour market. In an economic system driven by market forces, private ownership of the means of production and profit-seeking, mutual accommodation between capital and labour is impossible and continuous class conflict between them is inevitable.

Human relations theory

The unitary or human relations theory of industrial conflict is at the opposite end of the theoretical spectrum. This set of theories holds, in essence, that conflict at work between employer and employee is dysfunctional, that trade unions cause industrial conflict and that industrial conflict in any form is a corroding and disruptive social influence in the workplace and the wider society. The ideas and concepts associated with what is sometimes misleadingly called the 'Human Relations School' were first gestated and publicised by American industrial sociologists such as Mayo (1946), Roethlisberger (1946) and Warner and Low (1947). Their ideas were further refined and developed by the more sophisticated 'neo-human relations' theorists such as McGregor (1960) and Argyris (1964). The main implications of their analyses are that conflict at work is unnatural, subversive and destabilising and, as it cannot be suppressed, it should be eradicated by enlightened management policies and participative styles of management.

All of Mayo's research was carried out with the permission and collaboration of management. For Mayo, management embodies the central purposes of society and, with this initial orientation, he never considered the possibility that organisations might contain conflicting interest groups, such as management, workers and unions, as distinct from different attitudes or 'logics'. For him, industrial conflict was a social disease, whilst the promotion of organisational equilibrium, or a state of 'social health', should be management's prime aim and objective. The issue that Roethlisberger sought to address was (1946: page 112): 'how can a comfortable working equilibrium be maintained between the various groups in an industrial enterprise such that no group . . . will separate itself out in opposition to the remainder?' Warner and Low (1947) had similarly overwhelmingly negative connotations of industrial conflict. The subjective bias in their writing towards stability, harmony and social integration within organisations meant that they saw conflict exclusively as a dissociative and disintegrative phenomenon, although they conceded that 'frictional' conflicts could arise from personality differences, poor management and bad communications. Industrial conflict, by this view, is a pathological social condition, upsetting the 'normal' state of organisational equilibrium, and must be avoided at all costs.

Functionalist theory

The functionalist theory of industrial conflict, in contrast, sees conflict as inevitable in any human situation. Individuals group together in society for associative purposes – such as in politics and employee relations – and intergroup conflicts arise which, if resolved, result in new behavioural norms, thus eliminating the sources of dissatisfaction amongst the groups involved. Moreover, as Coser (1956: page 31) writes: 'Far from being necessarily dysfunctional, a certain degree of conflict is an essential element in group formation and the persistence of group life.' In employee relations, this means that conflict creates links between employers, management and unions. It modifies the norms for readjusting these relationships, leads each party to match the other's structures and organisation and makes possible a reassessment of their relative power in achieving consensus or agreement amongst themselves. In this way, industrial conflict serves as a social balancing mechanism maintaining and consolidating the instrumental relationships amongst employers, employees and unions.

For functionalists, industrial conflict is therefore generated by the divergent interests of the parties in the employment relationship. With industrial enterprises being the dominant institutions of modern society, 'where few command and many obey', Dahrendorf (1959: pages 250-53) takes issue with the scientific management and human relations views that the 'true interests' of management and workers are identical. He asserts that:

> Taylor's exclusive emphasis on the community of interests among all participants of the enterprise is plainly insufficient for the explanation of certain phenomena, such as strikes, and that it is therefore necessary to assume a conflict of latent interests in the enterprise emerging from the differential distribution of authority.

The significance of the functionalist theory of industrial conflict for employee relations is the need for the parties to the pay–work bargain to accept the inevitability of potential conflict between them, to institutionalise it and to resolve it through appropriate constitutional mechanisms. Only then is it likely that either or both parties will resort to unilateral force, and the use of industrial sanctions, to achieve their employee relations goals. This will happen only after these institutional arrangements have broken down. Furthermore, the application of industrial sanctions by any of the parties to employee relations is possible only within the limits of the law.

Manifestations of industrial conflict

In practice, industrial conflict takes a variety of forms. Writers such as Kornhauser and his colleagues (1954) and Hyman (1989) distinguish between industrial conflict that is individual and unorganised and that which is collective and organised. Individual and unorganised conflict, for example, takes place at the personal and interpersonal levels. It involves certain types of worker behaviour and managerial behaviour and manifests itself in a variety of ways, as outlined in Figure 16. The essence of unorganised industrial conflict is that it is unpredictable, is not directed into conflict-resolving channels and is difficult to manage.

Examples of how collective and organised industrial conflict manifest themselves are provided in Figure 17. These relate to management–union conflict and are more formalised types of industrial conflict. Although strikes are often considered to be the main manifestation of organised conflict, it is clear from Exhibit 39 that collective industrial conflict is not limited to strike activity alone. Nor does collective conflict manifest itself only in the workplace. It also takes place in the socio-political spheres through elections, lobbying, public relations activities and educational propaganda by both employers and unions.

Figure 16 **Manifestations of individual and unorganised industrial conflict**

Worker behaviour	Management behaviour
absenteeism	autocratic supervision
withholding effort	tight discipline
time-wasting	harassment of workers
industrial sabotage	discrimination at work
labour turnover	demoting individuals
complaints	one-sided propaganda
rule-breaking	speeding up work
low morale	anti-union propaganda
'griping' against management	'slagging off' the workforce

PATTERNS OF STRIKE ACTIVITY IN THE UK

Strike activity is not an easy term to define and the official statistics of the United Kingdom (UK), collected by the Department for Education and Employment (DfEE) (formerly the Employment Department, Department of Employment and earlier still the Ministry of Labour) cover only what are described as 'stoppages of work'. Technically, a stoppage of work is any trade dispute between employers and workers, or workers and workers, which is connected with terms and conditions of employment. The official statistics exclude disputes not resulting in stoppages of work, such as working to rule or going slow, and stoppages involving fewer than 10 workers or those lasting one day or less, except where the total number of working days lost is greater than 100. The statistics also include lockouts by employers and unlawful strikes. But they do not distinguish between: strikes and lockouts; 'lawful' and 'unlawful' stoppages; and, since 1981, 'official' and 'unofficial' disputes.

Figure 17 **Manifestations of collective and organised industrial conflict**

In the workplace	In society
restrictions of output	political lobbying
going slow	union political affiliations
working to contract	corporate political donations
removal of overtime	political demonstrations
strikes and lockouts	using the media
closing down plants	educational propaganda

In practice, a strike is any stoppage of work, or withdrawal of labour, initiated by workers, whilst lockouts are stoppages of work initiated by employers who prevent their employees working, by refusing entry to the workplace. A lawful strike is one undertaken in accordance with the legal requirements of the TULRCA 1992, as amended. To be lawful, strikes must be between workers and their direct employer, must relate to matters covered in section 218 of the Act and can take place only after a properly conducted strike ballot has been held, thus providing legal immunities to the strike leaders and the union(s) involved. Unlawful strikes are not protected by legal immunities and can result in injunctions and fines being awarded against the unions. An official dispute, or more properly a 'constitutional' one, is where strike action occurs which is in accordance with agreed negotiating procedures between the employer and the union(s). Unofficial or 'unconstitutional' disputes, in contrast, are in breach of agreed procedures for avoiding disputes.

Another meaning sometimes given to an 'official' dispute is one which is supported by the union(s) and is in accordance with union rules. 'Official' disputes of this sort normally involve the payment of strike benefits to the workers taking industrial action. Similarly, the term 'unofficial' disputes can also refer to industrial action not normally in accordance with union rules where the unions pay no benefits to the striking workers.

Strike statistics

In analysing stoppages of work annually, the DfEE uses three measures of strike activity. These are: the number of working days lost; the number of workers involved in stoppages of work; and the number of stoppages.

Working days lost

The number of working days lost is the total time lost as a result of trade disputes in the basic working week, over a given period, usually a year. Overtime and weekend working are excluded, with allowances being made for public and known annual holidays and for absences from work due to sickness and unauthorised leave. Where strikes last less than the basic working day, the hours lost are converted to full-day equivalents. Similarly, days lost by part-time workers are also converted to full-day equivalents. In disputes where employers dismiss their employees and subsequently reinstate them, the total working days lost include the days lost by the workers during the period of dismissal.

Workers involved

The number of workers involved in stoppages of work are those individuals directly and indirectly involved at the establishment where the dispute occurs. Workers indirectly involved are those who are not themselves party to the dispute but are laid off because of it. Workers at the other sites who are indirectly affected are not counted. This is because of the difficulty of deciding the extent to which a particular employer's reduction in output or services is due to the effects of a strike elsewhere or to some other cause. Workers involved in more than one stoppage during the year are counted for each stoppage in which they take part. Part-time workers are counted as whole units.

Number of stoppages

This records the total number of stoppages, lasting more than one day, over the year. Because of recording difficulties, the number of working days lost per year is normally regarded as a better indicator of the impact of trade disputes than the number of recorded stoppages.

Stoppages of work

A time series of stoppages of work in the UK for the period 1971-95 is shown in Table 13 (Sweeney and Davies 1996). A number of conclusions may be inferred from it. First, the number of working days lost per year varied widely over this 25-year period, with relatively high figures for some years – such as 1972, 1979 and 1984 – and some low ones, especially since 1985, followed by a dramatic fall in working days lost between 1991 and 1995. The unusually high number of working days lost in certain years was due, in the main, to large individual stoppages. In 1972, for example, a miners' strike over a national wage increase accounted for 10.7 million (45 per cent) of the 23.9 million working days lost for that year. Similarly, in 1979, a strike by engineering workers accounted for 16 million (54 per cent) of the 29.5 million working days lost in that year. And in 1984, the days lost in the miners' strike, in protest against pit closures, accounted for 22.4 million (83 per cent) of the 27.1 million working days lost during that year (Bird 1992a). It is important therefore to consider the size of the major stoppages in each period when making comparisons between individual years.

Second, the annual average number of working days lost per 1,000 employees declined substantially during the 1980s, compared with the 1970s. For the 10 years 1971-80, the annual average was 572 working days lost per 1,000 employees; for the 10 years 1981-90, it was 288 working days; and for the five years 1991-95, it was remarkably lower, at 24 working days. If the miners' dispute is discounted in 1984, then the annual average for the period 1981-90 falls to only 160 lost working days per 1,000 employees. The 1980s, and especially the 1990s, were clearly times of relatively low levels of industrial conflict in the UK compared with the 1960s and 1970s (Smith *et al* 1978).

Third, the average number of workers involved annually in stoppages of work for the five years 1971-75 was 1,375,000. This rose to 1,667,000 workers per year, on average, for the five years 1976-80, falling to 1,289,000 workers per year for the five years 1981-85. For the five years 1986-90, the annual average fell even more dramatically to 840,000 workers, whilst for the five years 1991-95 the annual average fell even further to 198,000 workers per year.

Fourth, the number of recorded stoppages during the 1970s averaged around 2,300 per year. During the 1980s, they fell to a little over a thousand stoppages per year on average and, for the five years 1986-90, to an average of about 840 stoppages per year. For the years 1991-95, the average fell substantially to 255 stoppages per year.

Table 13 **Stoppages of work in progress: the UK 1971-95**

Year	Working days lost ('000s)	Working days lost per 1,000 employees	Workers involved ('000s)	Stoppages
1971	13,551	612	1,178	2,263
1972	23,909	1,080	1,734	2,530
1973	7,197	317	1,528	2,902
1974	14,750	647	1,626	2,946
1975	6,012	265	809	2,332
1976	3,284	146	668	2,034
1977	10,142	448	1,666	2,737
1978	9,405	413	1,041	2,498
1979	29,474	1,273	4,608	2,125
1980	11,964	521	843	1,348
1981	4,266	195	1,513	1,344
1982	5,313	248	2,103	1,538
1983	3,754	178	574	1,364
1984	27,135	1,278	1,464	1,221
1985	6,402	229	791	903
1986	1,920	90	720	1,074
1987	3,546	164	887	1,016
1988	3,702	166	790	781
1989	4,128	182	727	701
1990	1,903	83	298	630
1991	761	34	176	369
1992	528	24	148	253
1993	649	30	385	211
1994	278	13	107	205
1995	415	19	174	235

Source: Employment Department

The causes of industrial action

Ever since the nineteenth century, government has recorded information on the principal causes of industrial stoppages in the UK. Government officials review all the available information from employers, conciliation officers and newspaper reports and then identify what is stated by the parties to be the main reason for each strike. Table 14 shows that the dominant issue in the strikes occurring in the UK during the period 1925-90 was pay. Over this 65-year period, pay was cited as the main reason for over two-thirds (68 per cent) of the working days lost. Although the relative importance of pay issues declined progressively up until the immediate postwar period (1945-54), it subsequently recovered in the 20 years after 1955. During the 1980s, pay once again declined in relative importance but still remained the most important single cause of working days lost annually, at around 58 per cent of the total.

Table 14 **Number and percentage of working days lost over pay: the UK 1925-90**

Period	Number (000s)	Over pay (000s)	Over pay per cent
1925–34	200,935	175,751	87.5
1935–44	18,956	11,405	60.2
1945–54	20,694	10,293	49.7
1955–64	38,910	27,586	70.9
1965–74	90,164	74,217	82.3
1980–90	78,118	45,309	58.0

Source: Department of Employment and Employment Department

The pay issues causing disputes between employers, employees and unions are wide ranging. They include union demands for:

- increases in wage rates or bonuses
- the restoration of pay differentials
- special rates for particular jobs or for the conditions in which the work is performed
- guaranteed earnings.

Pay disputes also commonly occur over reductions in earnings, changes in payment systems and the grading or regrading of jobs. Other pay issues that have been identified as likely to cause disputes between managements and workers include conflicts over cash allowances, holiday pay and fringe benefits.

Table 15 provides a detailed analysis of the percentage of working days lost by principal cause of dispute, for all industries in the UK, for the years 1980-5. Again, stoppages over pay accounted for most of the working days lost in every year, except for 1984, 1985 and 1993, when redundancy issues predominated, whilst in 1992 pay and redundancy issues were in joint first place. In 1991, whilst pay was the major issue causing disputes (41 per cent of the total), redundancy was a close second (33 per cent). It is also noticeable that in 1988 and 1994 about a third of all working days lost were caused by issues relating to staffing and the allocation of work.

International comparisons

From the analysis provided so far, it is clear that the number of working days lost, the number of workers involved and the number of recorded stoppages in the UK vary annually and over time, due to a variety of complex economic and related factors. It is also clear that the principal causes of trade

Table 15 **Working days lost in the UK by cause of dispute 1980–95**

Year	Cause – percentage of total						
	Pay	Hours	Redun-dancy	Trade union matters	Conditions of work	Staffing	Dismissal/ discipline
1980	89	1	3	2	1	2	2
1981	62	5	15	7	1	4	6
1982	66	5	16	2	1	6	3
1983	58	3	17	2	4	8	8
1984	8	0	87	1	0	2	1
1985	25	3	67	1	1	2	2
1986	59	3	15	3	3	13	4
1987	82	2	5	1	2	5	4
1988	51	0	7	4	1	33	3
1989	80	8	4	2	1	4	1
1990	58	25	2	2	3	8	3
1991	41	2	33	1	9	8	7
1992	37	0	37	2	9	10	5
1993	23	5	60	1	0	10	1
1994	58	3	5	0	0	30	4
1995	49	7	17	1	1	21	4

Source: Employment Department

disputes in the UK vary over time too. To obtain a balanced overview of the UK's 'strike rate', or its numbers of working days lost per 1,000 employees, comparisons can be made with the strike rates in 19 other advanced capitalist countries, out of the 24 that are members of the Organisation for Economic Cooperation and Development (OECD). This is done for all industries and services in Table 16, for the period 1982-86, although some care must be exercised in interpreting the data, due to differences in the methods used for selecting and compiling data on industrial disputes in the countries represented. Also, since there are considerable variations between years in the incidence of working days lost, with some years being heavily influenced by a small number of very large stoppages, international comparisons based on the average for a number of years are more useful than annual comparisons alone, as shown in Table 16.

First, it can be seen from Table 16 that there are quite wide differences in the strike rates between each of these countries within given periods and between different periods of time. For the whole period 1982-5, for example, eight countries – Greece, Spain, Italy, Canada, New Zealand, Finland, Australia and Ireland – had consistently higher strike rates than the UK. Similarly, in the period 1982-86, the UK ranked eighth out of the 20 countries, whilst in the period 1987-95, it ranked eleventh (Sweeney and Davies 1997). According to Bird (1992b), the UK's average of 130 lost working days per 1,000 employees for the period 1987-91 is approximately one-eighth of a working day lost per employee or about one working hour per

Table 16 **Industrial disputes in OECD countries: working days lost per 1,000 employees, all industries and services 1982–95**

Country	Averages	
	1982–86	1987–95
UK	420	81
Denmark	250	43
France	80	102
Germany	50	12
Greece	560	3,641
Ireland	450	172
Italy	700	249
Netherlands	20	24
Portugal	150	57
Spain	520	534
Japan	10	4
USA	120	62
Canada	490	292
Austria	–	4
Finland	530	321
Norway	170	102
Sweden	60	94
Switzerland	–	–
Australia	280	176
New Zealand	550	242

Note: the averages for Greece, Italy, Portugal and Japan are based on incomplete data

Source: Employment Gazette and Labour Market Trends

week. This represents a 70 per cent decrease in the UK strike rate for the years 1987-91, compared with the previous five-year period. This decrease was greater than for all the other OECD countries, except Denmark (80 per cent), Norway (80 per cent) and Germany (90 per cent).

Second, some countries have consistently high strike rates and others relatively low ones. Greece, Spain and Italy are in the former category. Switzerland, Austria and Japan – with less than five lost days per 1,000 employees – and the Netherlands and Germany, with an average of between 12 and 24 lost days per 1,000 employees for the period 1987-5, are in the latter category. Countries like the UK, the USA and Portugal lie in the middle range of strike activity.

Third, there was a general downward trend in the incidence of working days lost per 1,000 employees in OECD countries for the whole period 1982-5, with strike rates being generally higher for the period 1982-86 than for the years 1987-95. This is apart from Greece, Spain and Sweden, where strike rates rose in the late 1980s. In the case of Greece, there were general strikes in both 1987 and 1990 and these account for its relatively large numbers of working days lost per 1,000 employees for the period 1987-91.

Table 17 **Industrial disputes in OECD countries: working days lost per 1,000 employees in strike-prone industries 1982-91**

Country	Averages		
	1982–86	1987–91	1982–91
UK	980	240	610
Denmark	560	90	330
France	150	80	120
Germany	100	10	50
Greece	920	5,360	4,470
Ireland	510	350	430
Italy	280	440	360
The Netherlands	40	40	40
Portugal	270	110	200
Spain	520	770	650
Japan	20	10	10
USA	310	210	260
Canada	940	760	850
Austria	–	–	–
Finland	760	180	470
Norway	300	30	170
Sweden	10	170	90
Switzerland	–	–	–
Australia	610	530	570
New Zealand	2,740	520	890

Note: the averages for Greece, Italy, Portugal and Japan are based on incomplete data

Source: Employment Department

One feature of trade disputes is the variation in strike activity amongst different industrial sectors. Some industries are particularly strike prone such as mining and quarrying, manufacturing, construction, and transport and communication (see below). This variation, and the contrasting industrial structures of different countries, in part explains why some countries have relatively high or low rates of strike activity compared with others. To help reduce this effect, Table 17 compares the working days lost per 1,000 employees in these four strike-prone sectors in 20 of the OECD's 24 member states, for the period 1982-91. Overall, for the period 1982-91, the incidence of working days lost per 1,000 employees in these strike-prone industries was between one-and-a-half times to twice as high as for all industries and services (Table 16), although it was three times as high in the USA. Nevertheless, like all industries and services, these strike-prone ones also experienced a general decrease in strike rates over this period.

INFLUENCES ON INDUSTRIAL ACTION

Employee relations are not conducted in a vacuum (see Chapters 1, 4 and 6). They take place in specific economic, institutional and political contexts. It is these broad categories of factors which have been identified by scholars as the main ones influencing industrial action, patterns of strike activity and the outcomes of industrial conflict between employers and unions. There is, however, no general theory of strikes or industrial action. As Jackson (1987: page 149) concludes: 'Strikes are enormously complex and are themselves a classification of a variety of different kinds of activity under one head.' Each strike is undertaken 'for different reasons at different times and has a different meaning for different participants'. Because strikes are the most obvious form and most quantified type of industrial action, this section, like the previous one, focuses, albeit selectively, on the main factors influencing strike activity rather than other manifestations of industrial conflict.

Economic factors

A number of studies use economic variables to explain strikes or stoppages of work. These include: inter-industry comparisons; unemployment; and the business cycle.

Inter-industry comparisons

An early comparative study of the major variations in strike incidence amongst different industries, in 11 countries, was undertaken by Kerr and Siegel (1954). Their focus was on why industrial conflict was prevalent in some industries and absent in others. Previous studies had concentrated on labour market and product market factors, management and union policies, procedures for adjusting disputes and the influence of dominant personalities on industrial conflict. Kerr and Siegel showed that these factors did not explain why some industries are strike prone in many parts of the world and others are not. Their central explanation of strike propensities (see Figure 18) was in the location of workers in society, with the nature of their jobs acting as a secondary influence. Isolated masses of workers, insulated from society at large, were identified as being most likely to take strike action, frequently and bitterly, especially when employed on unpleasant tasks. Individuals and groups who are integrated into the general community, on the other hand, through a multiplicity of associations, were identified to be least likely to strike.

Figure 18 **General pattern of strike propensities**

Propensity to strike	Industry
high	mining seafaring and docks
medium high	lumber textiles
medium	chemicals printing leather manufacturing construction food
medium low	clothing gas, water and electricity services
low	railways agriculture trade

Source: Kerr and Siegel (1954)

A more recent, detailed study of variations of inter-industry strike activity in the UK was undertaken by the Department of Employment for the period from the mid-1960s to the mid-1970s (Smith *et al* 1978). It had six main conclusions:

- There were very considerable differences between industries in terms of their propensity to strike, with five industries – coalmining, docks, car assembly, shipbuilding, and iron and steel – accounting for at least a quarter of stoppages and a third of the days lost.
- Stoppages were overwhelmingly a manual worker phenomenon, although stoppages amongst non-manual workers were increasing.
- On average, over the period 1966-73, almost three-quarters of stoppages, accounting for over a half of the working days lost, involved members of

only one union. Furthermore, six unions, accounting for about half of total union membership, were involved in about 80 per cent of stoppages.

- Strike activity was concentrated in a very small number of plants, with the incidence of strikes rising strongly with plant size.
- There were regional differences in strike proneness, over a considerable period of time.
- High average earnings, high labour intensity and large average establishment size were associated with relatively high strike frequency, and high strike incidence, whilst a high proportion of female employees was associated with low strike proneness.

Unemployment

Another key economic variable claimed to be linked with patterns of industrial action is unemployment. Hibbs (1976), for example, looked at data for 10 countries between 1950 and 1969 and argues that there is a negative relationship between unemployment and strike activity (ie as unemployment falls, strike activity rises). He concludes that the inverse relationship between industrial conflict and unemployment demonstrates considerable sophistication by workers and unions in their use of the strike weapon, since they seek to capitalise on the strategic advantages provided to them by tight labour markets. Furthermore, strikes are responses by workers to movements in real wages, rather than money wages. With unemployment low, workers have the opportunity to seek alternative jobs which might offer higher rates of pay. But as the cost of labour mobility is high, they will first try to increase their wages in their present jobs, by striking if necessary. It is also argued that both unions and their members are more able to withstand stoppages of work during the periods of prosperity. Their financial resources are relatively buoyant then, and the costs incurred in striking tend to be lower than in periods of recession.

Creigh and Makeham (1982), in contrast, suggest a positive relationship between unemployment and strike activity (ie as unemployment rises, strike activity rises). Their study examined data relating to 15 countries between 1975 and 1979 and focuses on the role of employers in trade disputes. They argue that during periods of high unemployment employers may be less willing to resist industrial action or to take countervailing steps to avoid the disruption caused by strikes. Consequently, where strikes occur during periods of high unemployment, they are likely to last longer. However, with unemployment inversely related to levels of economic activity, an employer's strike costs, in terms of lost production, are likely to increase as unemployment falls. So employers tend to avoid strike action in these conditions. Indeed, during periods of prosperity, employers are able to pass on increased costs to their customers. Low unemployment may increase worker demands for high pay rises but it also induces employers to raise their pay offers to them.

A third set of writers claim that there is no correlation, either negative or positive, between unemployment and strike activity (Knight 1972; Shorey 1976; Smith *et al* 1978). Clearly, the relationship between the two is a complex one. But to date, a definitive general relationship between unemployment rates and measures of strike activity, either at industry level or nationally, does not appear to have been demonstrated.

The business cycle

It has long been recognised that there are cycles of strikes and that they are possibly related to the business cycle. Rees (1952) identifies a pronounced positive correlation between them, with strikes increasing in frequency during periods of prosperity and diminishing in frequency during recessions. The timing of the relationship appears to be such that strikes typically turn down before business activity reaches a peak and turn up some time after recovery has begun. Rees's explanation is based on the assumption that the strike weapon has become the strategic tool of well-organised 'business unions', rather than the spontaneous protest of aggrieved workers, and that union strategy is the driving force in the situation.

According to Rees, the strike peak represents a maximum divergence of expectations between unions and employers. As the business cycle rises, unions are influenced by the wage increases of other unions, increases in the cost of living and buoyant labour market. Employers, in contrast, seek higher sales, higher profits and new markets. They are, therefore, likely to resist wage demands for which the unions are prepared to fight and this can result in union strike action. The issues of special interest to employers, normally preceding the peak of the business cycle, are rises in the number of business failures, falls in investment and declines in orders. The issue of special concern to the unions is future employment prospects. As the business cycle peaks, the more pessimistic expectations may be shared by some union leaders and strikes fall off. The lag in strikes at the troughs of business cycles represents a 'wait and see' policy by union leaders. They want to be sure that the revival is genuine before risking their members' jobs.

Institutional factors

These are another set of factors that are claimed to influence industrial action. Those supporting the institutional approach explain particular aspects and patterns of industrial conflict by reference to the institutions of conflict resolution, especially that of collective bargaining. The Donovan Commission (1968), for example, sought to explain the number of unofficial strikes in Britain in the 1960s in terms of the inadequacies of multi-employer collective bargaining machinery (see Chapter 7). The Commission identified the growing gap between industry-wide pay rates and actual earnings at the workplace and argued that existing procedural agreements were failing to cope adequately with the resolution of disputes between managements and workgroups within the workplace. The Commission went on to recommend the reform of company and factory-level collective bargaining machinery. This was to be based on comprehensive company-wide agreements aimed at regulating pay, grievances, discipline and redundancy and providing facilities for shop stewards within the firm.

The idea that collective bargaining helps to identify, regularise and institutionalise industrial conflict is based on a number of assumptions:

- It is argued that collective bargaining regulates conflict between employers and employees by keeping it within acceptable bounds, providing a forum for resolving it and legitimising the joint decisions made between the representatives of the two sides.
- When there is a dispute, collective bargaining enables management and unions to pause, think and reflect upon the consequences of their actions before taking industrial sanctions against each other.
- Collective bargaining absorbs energies that might otherwise be directed into more destructive channels of industrial or social conflict.
- Collective bargaining, in providing a forum for communication between management and unions, facilitates not only improved working relations between them but also peaceful change in society generally.

Collective bargaining is predicated, however, on the premises that employers recognise and accept the nature of industrial conflict, that they agree to institutionalise it and that there are appropriate agents of worker representation.

A seminal study is that of Ross and Hartman (1960) who examined the patterns of industrial conflict in 15 countries between 1900 and 1956. Although their methodology and their findings have been challenged subsequently (Eldridge 1968; Ingham 1974; Edwards 1981), Ross and Hartman's analysis is important for two main reasons. First, their research provides a useful framework for analysing industrial conflict. Second, they have been instrumental in influencing further studies on the institutionalisation of industrial conflict and its implications for the parties to employee relations (Kassolow 1969; Clegg 1976).

Ross and Hartman's central thesis is the 'withering away of the strike'. They argue that there was a general reduction in strike activity over the period they studied. The reasons given for this were: employers had developed more sophisticated policies for dealing with employees; the labour movement was forsaking strike action in favour of political action; and the state had become more prominent as an employer. In fact, strike activity did not wither away but started to grow in the 1960s and 1970s, although, as indicated above, it diminished again in the 1980s. Whilst it has been difficult to identify consistent trends across different countries since they wrote, their thesis is persuasive for the period they reviewed.

It is important to recognise the differing employee relations contexts of the 1960s, 1970s and 1980s. In Britain at least, the 20 years after the publication of Ross and Hartman's work were characterised by full employment, Keynesianism and a large public sector. The years since the late 1970s, in contrast, have featured deregulated labour markets, supply-side economic policies and a smaller public sector. These factors most certainly affected the institutions of employee relations and the willingness of the parties to become involved in industrial action. It is not surprising, in the circumstances, that industrial action was particularly centred on the public sector during the 1980s, as it was subjected to compulsory competitive tendering, privatisation and new styles of personnel management (Farnham 1993).

The second main theme of Ross and Hartman's study is the identification of distinctive patterns of industrial conflict and the linking of them to different employee relations systems. They identified five categories of employee relations, each with its own forms of strike activity. These were: two northern European patterns; a Mediterranean-Asian pattern; a North American pattern; and three special cases – Australia, Finland and South Africa. The first northern European pattern incorporated Denmark, the Netherlands, Germany and the UK. These were characterised by a nominal propensity to strike, with strikes of low or moderate duration. The second north European grouping of Norway and Sweden featured infrequent but long strikes. The Mediterranean-Asian pattern, comprising France, Italy, Japan and India, had high participation in strikes but these were of short duration. Finally, the North American pattern of the USA and Canada had a moderately high propensity to strike and the disputes were of relatively long duration.

In comparing different employee relations systems, Ross and Hartman identified five key features, which were claimed to be associated with distinctive patterns of strikes, and these are summarised in Figure 19. Denmark, the Netherlands, Germany and the UK were characterised by mature trade unions, stable union memberships and subdued union leadership conflicts. There was a wide acceptance of trade unions by employers and centralised collective bargaining. These countries had important Labour parties, and whilst governments rarely intervened to regulate terms and conditions of employment, they did intervene in the resolution of industrial disputes. Norway and Sweden shared many of the above characteristics but had less active government intervention in management-union relations.

The Mediterranean-Asian countries, in contrast, had relatively young trade union movements, low union membership and continual union leadership conflicts. Collective bargaining was weak, left-wing parties were divided and there was considerable government intervention in industry. In North America, there was an old trade union movement, with a stable membership and little factionalism. Unions were increasingly accepted by employers, collective bargaining was decentralised and terms and conditions were largely determined privately. There was not a successful Labour party.

Political factors

Political power is seen by some scholars as a major variable determining long-term patterns of strikes and industrial action. Korpi and Shalev (1979: page 181) argue, for example, that where labour movements are organised effectively and co-ordinated politically, they try to achieve their goals not only through collective bargaining but also through political rather than strike action. On the other hand, where labour movements are fragmented, are politically weak and have little nor no political influence, strikes are likely to

Figure 19 **Principal features of comparative employee relations systems**

1 Organisational stability of the labour movement
- 1.1 age of labour movement
- 1.2 stability of membership

2 Leadership conflicts in the labour movement
- 2.1 factionalism and rivalry
- 2.2 strength of communism in the unions

3 State of management–union relations
- 3.3 degree of union acceptance by employers
- 3.4 consolidation of bargaining structure

4 Labour political activity
- 4.1 a Labour party as a leading political party
- 4.2 Labour governments

5 Role of the state
- 5.1 extent of government activity in defining terms of employment
- 5.2 dispute settlement procedures

Source: Ross (1959)

remain high. Thus in Scandinavian countries and Austria, which have well-organised union movements and where democratic socialist political parties have been in power for many years, strikes are rarely used to pursue union goals and objectives. In countries like the USA, Canada and Ireland, on the other hand, where labour movements are less well organised and socialist parties are weak or non-existent, strikes are more common.

> In these instances, conflicts between buyers and sellers of labour power continue to be manifested primarily within the employment contract, something which is no longer the case elsewhere. The long duration of strikes in these countries has contributed to give them very high relative volumes of strikes (man-days idle) in the postwar period.

In countries like Britain, Belgium and Denmark, the relationship between the political activities of their labour movements and strike activity is claimed to be more complex. Up until the late 1970s in Britain, for example, whilst the Labour Party gained periods of political power, its control of and its long-term impact on the political system were relatively insecure. Labour governments were therefore unable to manage class conflict through 'political exchange' for any long period of time. Consequently, Britain's postwar strike record was similar to that of the prewar period and the strike weapon, as a union tactic, failed to wither away. In postwar Belgium, despite labour's involvement in government, strike mobilisation was as high as it had been in the prewar period. In Denmark, although organised labour had periodic influence in Danish governments in the years up till the late 1970s, its power was less stable than in the rest of Scandinavia. According to Korpi and Shalev (1979: page 182): 'This instability may well have contributed to the continuing wave-like incidence of industrial conflict in postwar Denmark, at what is nevertheless a relatively low level by international standards.'

Another political analysis of strike activity is provided by Shorter and Tilley (1974), They argue, first, that trade unions have a crucial role in channelling worker dissatisfaction into strike action and, second, that strikes have political aims which do not simply express economic interests. Where trade unions do not have political power through representation in the political system, strikes are used to put direct pressure on governments to change their existing policies or to initiate new ones. In this sense, strikes are an expression of class conflict between workers and their organisations and the political authorities, with 'strike waves' often coinciding with periodic political crises as they have done in France and Italy.

In Shorter and Tilley's analysis, strike activity prior to the second world war was of a similar intensity throughout western Europe. After the war, however, patterns differed. In countries such as those in Scandinavia, where labour gained political power, strike activity declined. Where labour failed to gain political power, such as in France and Italy, strikes continued at relatively high levels and expressed the political aspirations and expectations of the working class. The USA, in contrast, was seen as a special case, because strike activity did not wither away as it had done in northern Europe. This has been explained in terms of the failure of successive Federal governments to substantially protect workers' interests through interventionist political reforms. As a result, North American 'labor unions' drew a sharp dividing line between free collective bargaining, used to protect their members' job interests, including the use of strike action if necessary, and *ad hoc* 'interest-coalition' politics used to advance union political action.

MANAGING INDUSTRIAL ACTION

Nowadays industrial action in Britain is normally initiated by trade unions. Industrial action initiated by employers, such as lockouts, is very rare, although to what extent plant closures, transfers of businesses and large-scale redundancies are regarded by trade unions and their members as covert forms of 'industrial action' by management is a matter of debate. This section, therefore, concentrates on the main issues to be considered by employers when they face organised industrial action from trade unions. These involve both legal and non-legal issues, although the suitability of any management response depends on the nature of the dispute, the estimated costs of pursuing any particular course of action and the balance of bargaining power between the two sides (Martin 1992).

Preparing for industrial action

Every trade dispute is unique. The type of action threatened by the trade unions, the extent and scope of the expected action and the nature of the issue in dispute, all affect the ways in which management is likely to respond and plan its own counter-actions to the situation. Once it seems likely that industrial action is being planned by trade unions and their members, management has to prepare and consider its possible responses. There are four key points:

- *Assess the scale of the problem.* Management needs to identify the scope of the dispute, estimate its possible support amongst the workforce and assess the potential difficulties and costs of resolving it. This includes considering the likelihood of a settlement in the short term.
- *Make contingency plans.* In doing so, management has a number of decisions to take: how any work is to be covered during the dispute; how adequate health and safety standards are to be maintained; and how any relevant property of the employer, such as keys, vehicles or other equipment, is to be returned to management before industrial action takes place.
- *Extend the communication systems.* Over and above existing communication channels, new communication systems may be necessary whilst the dispute is in progress. This is to ensure: effective management co-ordination of the dispute; publicity to employees and the press; and open channels of communication with the unions and their members.
- *Plan actions in response.* This should include considering what sort of warnings are to be given to employees, unions and customers about the legal and non-legal implications of the dispute.

Some of the key points needing to be considered by management, prior to industrial action being taken, are summarised in Exhibit 38.

Exhibit 38 **Key points for management in preparing for industrial action**

These include:

- make plans before industrial action takes place
- assess the effects the action will have
- remember that industrial action is normally in breach of the contract of employment
- ensure that strikers do not get paid during the dispute
- bear in mind that picketing must be peaceful and at the employees' place of work
- do not use the disciplinary procedure in response to industrial action
- the law on industrial action is normally invoked by the employer
- laying off employees without pay is only lawful where there is a term in the contract that allows it
- keep in touch with those co-ordinating management action and seek advice where necessary
- remember that management and employees have to work together after the dispute is settled

The legal issues

The main legal issues arising from industrial action which employers have to consider are: legal immunities, balloting, and picketing.

Legal immunities

Where employees take industrial action, they are normally in breach of their contracts of employment. Also, when trade unions, their officials or others organise industrial action, they are calling for breaches of, or interferences with, the performance of employment contracts. They may also be interfering with the ability of employers to fulfil commercial contracts. Since it is unlawful, under the common law, to induce individuals to break or interfere with a contract, the legal device of statutory immunities – most commonly called 'trade union' or 'legal immunities' – enables unions and individuals organising industrial action to do so without being sued in the courts (see Chapters 4, 7, 8). Legal immunities do not, however, protect individual strikers, or those taking action short of a strike, from being dismissed, or from having legal proceedings taken against them by their employer, because they have broken their employment contracts.

For unions and strike leaders to be protected by legal immunities, the following conditions are necessary. First, there must be a trade dispute and a properly conducted industrial action ballot. Second, the action must not: be secondary action, which does not involve the primary or direct employer; promote a closed shop; or support employees dismissed whilst taking unofficial industrial action. Further, the action must not involve unlawful picketing.

Legal immunities only apply where a union or its officials are acting 'in contemplation or furtherance of a trade dispute' (the 'golden formula'). In law, a trade dispute must be: (1) between workers and their own employer; and (2) wholly or mainly about employment-related matters. This legal definition does not cover actions:

- between groups of workers or inter-union disputes
- between workers and employers other than their own
- between a union and an employer where none of its workforce is in dispute with it
- not 'wholly or mainly' due to employment-related matters
- relating to matters taking place overseas.

Where legal immunities do not apply, employers (and customers and suppliers) that are damaged by the industrial action may take civil proceedings in the courts against the union or the individuals concerned. They have to show that:

- an unlawful act has been done or is threatened
- a contract to which they are a party has been or will be broken or interfered with
- they are likely to suffer loss because of it.

Unless legal immunities apply, a union is held responsible for any acts that are done, authorised or endorsed by its principal executive committee, general secretary, president or any other committee of the union. To avoid legal liability, a union or its agents must repudiate the act as soon as is reasonably practicable, after it has come to their notice. They must give written notice of the repudiation to the committee or individuals concerned. And they must do their best to give written notice of the fact and date of the repudiation to every member involved in the action and to the employer.

Where legal immunities do not apply, those damaged may seek an injunction from the courts. This may be issued on an interim basis, pending a full hearing of the case. The courts also have the authority to require any union found in breach of the law to take such steps to ensure that:

- there is no further inducement to take or continue the action
- no further action is taken after the injunction is granted.

If an injunction is not obeyed, the employer may return to court and ask that those concerned be declared in contempt of court. Any party found in contempt may be fined or have other penalties issued against it. Unions may be deprived of their assets, through the sequestration of their funds. This means that union funds are placed under the control of a person, appointed by the court, who may pay any fines or legal costs incurred as a result of the court's proceedings. It is also possible for employers (and others) to claim damages for any losses resulting from the unprotected industrial action. There are, however, upper limits on these damages in any proceedings and these are according to the size of union membership.

Balloting

Where a union calls on its members to take part in or to continue industrial action, it must hold a properly conducted secret ballot to maintain its legal immunity. And unless all the relevant statutory requirements are satisfied, the ballot does not preserve this immunity. The ballot must always be held before a union calls for or otherwise organises industrial action. Those entitled to vote are all the union members whom the union reasonably believes are, at the time of the ballot, to be called upon to take industrial action. There must normally be a postal ballot. The ballot paper must contain a question requiring the voters to indicate that they are prepared to take part in the action. The law also requires that the following statement must appear on every voting paper: 'If you take part in a strike or other industrial action, you may be in breach of your contract of employment' (Employment Department 1990: page 11).

Unions are required to give the employer seven days' notice of the intention to hold a ballot, the date of the ballot and a description of the employees who will vote. Not later than three days before the ballot paper is sent to any union member, the employer must be provided with a sample of the voting paper or, where there is more than one, of each voting paper. Majority support must be obtained in response to the question(s) asked. Votes must be accurately and fairly recorded and an independent scrutineer must be appointed, whose name must be on the ballot paper. As soon as is reasonably practicable after the ballot, the employer must be informed of the result and the scrutineer must make a report. Written notice must be given to the employer, specifying the employees who are to be induced to take industrial action, or to continue it, before the action commences.

Picketing

To be protected in law, pickets must comply with the basic rules embodied in the law. This is to ensure that picketing is organised lawfully and in accordance with good practice. According to the Employment Department (1992: page 5), the law requires that picketing may only:

(i) be undertaken in contemplation or furtherance of a trade dispute;
(ii) be carried out by a person attending at or near his own place of work; a trade union official, in addition to attending at or near his own place of work, may also attend at or near the place of work of a member of his trade union whom he is accompanying on the picket line and whom he represents.

Furthermore, the only purpose involved must be peacefully to obtain or communicate information or peacefully to persuade individuals to work or not to work. Picketing which is not peaceful and leads to violence, intimidation, obstruction or molestation is likely to involve offences under the criminal law.

Responding to employees

An employer's response to industrial action is normally aimed at preventing the action or, if this fails, achieving a return to work on acceptable terms as early as possible, whilst at the same time avoiding an escalation of the dispute. For these purposes, employers need to develop action plans which are coherent, flexible and effective. Considered responses need to be given to employees individually and to their unions.

Responses to individual employees are normally preceded by a written warning to them, by either a personal letter or a general circular, with some means by which they can acknowledge its receipt. Ideally, this communication should make clear the nature of the employer's response to the proposed action and it should provide sufficient time for the employees to change their minds. Since employees refusing to take industrial action cannot be 'unjustifiably disciplined' by their unions, employers sometimes include information to this effect in the warning letters sent to individuals before and during industrial action.

When deciding how to respond to industrial action, employers need to answer two key questions (Local Authorities Conditions Advisory Board 1991: page 13). These are:

- Has the action led to a breach of the terms of the individual's contract?
- How important is any breach that may have occurred?

Where a strike is involved, this is a fundamental breach of the employment contract, since the employees are refusing to do the work required of them, even though work is available. Action short of a strike is not so straightforward. It depends on the form of action and its effects. With go-slows, work-to-rules or bans on voluntary overtime, there appear to be no breaches of contractual terms. Where overtime is customary, however, and the ban is severely disruptive to the employer, it may be possible to argue that this has breached an implied term of the employment contract.

The nature and extent of the breach of contract, therefore, are major factors in determining an employer's responses to industrial action by some or all of its workforce. A summary of the possible responses available to employers faced by industrial action is provided in Exhibit 39. In adopting any of these actions, employers have to bear in mind the legal implications of what they are doing and any likely reactions by employees to the employer's initiatives. When employers are taking strike action, for example, there is no legal obligation on the employer to pay them, since they are not ready and willing to work under the terms of their contracts. In other cases, such as when employers propose taking disciplinary action against employees for breach of contract, the situation is less clear-cut, and indeed there are disadvantages to doing this. For example, the stage at which disciplinary action is invoked depends on the relevant procedure. Furthermore, the individual employee may not take any notice of formal warnings and then the employer may be forced to take further disciplinary action without really wanting to.

Similarly, there are important statutory provisions regarding dismissal for industrial action. These provide that employees dismissed whilst taking part in industrial action will not be able to make a complaint to an industrial tribunal unless:

- at the date of the dismissal one or more of the employees also taking industrial action was not dismissed
- one or more of the other employees dismissed for taking part in the action was subsequently offered re-engagement within three months of their date of dismissal, and these employees were employed at the same establishment as the employee claiming dismissal.

Where, however, the call to take industrial action has been repudiated by the trade union, no union member who is sacked, whilst continuing to take action, is able to claim unfair dismissal, even if there has been selective dismissal or re-engagement.

Exhibit 39 **Possible responses by employers to industrial action**

These include:

- deducting pay for strike action
- deducting pay for action short of a strike
- refusing partial performance of the contract
- sending employees home
- suspending with pay
- suspending without pay
- using the disciplinary procedure
- locking-out
- summary dismissal
- taking civil action against individual employees.

An employer failing to follow these statutory provisions will not automatically have any dismissals declared unfair by an industrial tribunal, since dismissals for taking strike action are normally considered fair. But where a union has not repudiated the action and an employer dismisses selectively from amongst those taking part in the dispute, it has to be shown that it was reasonable to do so in the circumstances. Similarly, where an employer re-engages selectively, the dismissal of other employees may not necessarily be declared unfair. The question is whether it was reasonable to re-engage some but not others. In practice, however, employers normally re-engage all sacked strikers once a dispute is settled, provided that their jobs remain after the dispute has ended.

The general effect of industrial action on conditions of employment is clear-cut as far as strike action is concerned. Employees not available for work cannot expect to receive any employment benefits. For example, the employer is under no obligation to provide occupational sick pay should an employee fall sick during strike action. However, if an employee has taken annual leave and strike action starts during this period, then in the absence of evidence to the contrary, that individual should be deemed to be on leave, not on strike. Similarly, employees who are on sick leave before industrial action starts should be assumed to be on sick leave, providing that the necessary certification is produced. Also, the operation of the Health and Safety at Work Act 1974 is not suspended during a period of industrial action and employers continue to owe a duty to any employees remaining at work and to others. The employer may need to come to an arrangement with employee representatives to ensure that essential safety measures are carried out before the strike action takes effect.

Responding to trade unions

An employer's responses to the trade unions, when a trade dispute is either threatened or is taking place, tends to centre on the issue of whether or not to take legal action against the union(s) involved. What the employer does is as much a matter of management judgement as it is of legal technicalities. The central issues are:

- What will be the likely long-term effects on relations between the employer and the union(s) if legal action is initiated by the employer?
- What will be the likely outcome on the dispute of legal intervention by the courts?

The key legal issue is that successful legal action by an employer against trade unions in the courts depends on a union losing its legal immunities when it and its members take part in what is deemed to be 'unlawful' or 'unprotected' industrial action (see pages 387-8 above; also, Chapter 4). Legally, employers need to determine in the first instance whether (Employment Department 1992):

- a trade dispute is taking place
- the 'golden formula' applies (ie that the action is 'in contemplation or furtherance of a trade dispute')
- a proper industrial action ballot has been conducted
- the action is authorised by the relevant trade union(s)
- the action is primary, not secondary
- picketing is peaceful and in accordance with the Employment Department's code of practice.

The normal civil law remedies are available to employers when unlawful industrial action takes place or is threatened. Proceedings against individual employees are rare but liability for civil claims extends beyond those taking part in industrial action. Those organising the action may also be liable, including the union officials and the union, except where they are protected by legal immunities. But legal immunities only have the effect of protecting employees as union members, not as individual employees who have no immunity for the act of breaking their individual contracts of employment.

The immediate civil remedy is an injunction. This is a court order seeking to stop the industrial action and is normally granted only if the court decides that such action is unlikely to be shown to have immunity on the full hearing of the case. An injunction is a holding measure, until a full trial decides the matter properly. An injunction is usually sought as a way of immediately preventing the action from taking place, since a full trial is only possible some time after the intended action has been carried out. The courts are generally ready to grant injunctions to employers, providing that the proposed action might not have immunity. They do this by taking account of the 'balance of convenience' between the parties. This means that judges tend to favour the party that is likely to suffer the most, if the injunction is not granted. Normally, this is deemed to be the employer. However, the courts also consider the likelihood of the union establishing at full trial that legal immunity does apply and they give the union the opportunity to put its side of the case, before granting an injunction.

Many employers, in practice, are very reluctant to use the law to resolve industrial disputes because of the detrimental long-term effects it can have on employee relations. Much depends on the damage being done by industrial action. Moreover, an injunction may be disregarded by the union or individuals concerned and then the employer has to consider whether to institute contempt of court proceedings against the union. These may lead to fines, damages or other penalties against the union. Employers, therefore, need to give very careful consideration to the consequences of invoking the law in an industrial dispute, before making a definitive decision to proceed with it.

The return to work

Once a settlement has been reached between management and unions, a full return to normal working as soon as possible is essential. Where action has been short of a strike, there is no great difficulty. With strikes, a phased return may have to be arranged. The formal terms of the return may have to be negotiated at the time of settlement and employers should try to seek reciprocal arrangements with trade unions on the terms of the return to work. But written agreements do not always reflect all aspects of the employment relationship. For example, as far as is possible, employers should ensure that there is no victimisation of union members who did not take part in the industrial action. This might mean advising employees of their rights of appeal under trade union rules and the law, such as the right not to have 'unjustifiable discipline' taken against them.

It is normally important to restore the pre-existing employee relations climate, so that the return to work can take place without any recriminations on either side. On the employer's side, this means the job or career structures of employees should not be prejudiced by the fact that they took industrial action. The employer has to decide whether disciplinary warnings arising from misconduct during the industrial action should be kept on record or deleted. It also needs to decide what effect any break in continuous service is to have on employee benefits and conditions of employment. Employees who have been dismissed and subsequently re-engaged are normally re-appointed on the same terms and conditions, provided their posts still exist. Overall, then, employers and management have a prime role in ensuring that the return to work proceeds smoothly, fairly and in accordance with what has been formally agreed with the trade unions.

ASSIGNMENTS

(a) Read Dahrendorf (1959: pages 241-79). What is his theory of industrial conflict and what are its implications for the managing of employee relations? Also read Jackson (1987: pages 155-84) and compare his explanations of industrial conflict with that of Dahrendorf's analysis.

(b) Report and comment on any forms of individual and unorganised conflict in your organisation.

(c) Describe and analyse a strike with which you are familiar. Get your material either from a situation that you have directly experienced yourself or from the literature of employee relations, newspaper reports, television documentaries or individuals who have actually been involved in a dispute.

(d) Read the latest annual report on industrial stoppages in the Employment Gazette. What were the trends for the past year? What were the principal causes? And what were the duration and size of stoppages?

(e) Read Smith *et al* (1978: pages 84-90). What are their main conclusions about the nature of strike activity in Britain for the period of review (1966-75)? To what extent do you think that their analysis is still relevant today?

(f) Read Clegg (1976). What is his explanation of strike proneness?

(g) What guidance does the Employment Department's (1992) code of practice on picketing provide relating to numbers of pickets on picket lines and the organisation of picketing? What is the legal status of the code?

(i) Your organisation has been informed by the unions of their intention to take strike action as a result of a properly conducted industrial action ballot. Consider the responses you will advise the employer to take in the circumstances and draft a letter to the employees concerned warning them, individually, of the employer's intended responses.

(j) An organisation has informed the unions of its intentions of closing its manufacturing plant, and of instituting compulsory redundancies, if they do not accept lay-offs and a reduction in the terms of the present lay-off agreement. The unions are now in dispute with the company, having taken a properly conducted industrial action ballot. The company has proposed rotating lay-offs for its staff for six months, with access to independent arbitration, a 10 per cent cut in employee benefits and a profit-sharing scheme. This has been rejected by the unions and the 400 staff have been dismissed by the management and replaced by a new workforce. (1) What is the legal position? (2) What advice would you give to senior management at this stage of the dispute?

REFERENCES

ALLEN, V. 1976. 'Marxism and the personnel manager'. *Personnel Management*. December.

ARGYRIS, C. 1964. *Integrating the Individual and the Organization*. Chichester: Wiley.

BIRD, D. 1992a. 'Industrial stoppages in 1991'. *Employment Gazette*. May.

BIRD, D. 1992b. 'International comparisons on industrial disputes'. *Employment Gazette*. December.

CLEGG, H. 1976. *Trade Unionism under Collective Bargaining*. Oxford: Blackwell.

COSER, L. 1956. *The Functions of Social Conflict*. London: Routledge and Kegan Paul.

CREIGH, S. *and* MAKEHAM, D. 1982. 'Strike incidence in industrial countries: an analysis'. *Australian Bulletin of Labour*. 8(3).

DAHRENDORF, R. 1959. *Class and Class Conflict in Industrial Society*. London: Routledge and Kegan Paul.

DONOVAN, LORD. 1968. *Royal Commission on Trade Unions and Employers' Associations*. London: HMSO.

EDWARDS, P. 1981. *Strikes in the USA*, 1871-1974. Oxford: Blackwell.

ELDRIDGE, J. 1968. *Industrial Disputes*. Routledge and Kegan Paul.

EMPLOYMENT DEPARTMENT. 1990. *Trade Union Ballots on Industrial Action*. London: COI.

EMPLOYMENT DEPARTMENT. 1992. *Code of Practice on Picketing*. London: COI.

FARNHAM, D. 1993. 'Human resources management and employee relations'. In Farnham, D. and Horton, S. (eds) 1993, *Managing the New Public Services*, Basingstoke: Macmillan.

FARNHAM, D. 1996. 'New Labour, the new unions and the new labour market'. *Parliamentary Affairs*. 49(4), October.

FARNHAM, D. and Pimlott, J. 1995. *Understanding Industrial Relations*. London: Cassell.

HIBBS, D. 1976. 'Industrial conflict in advanced industrial countries'. *Political Science Review*. 70(4).

HYMAN, R. 1975. *Industrial Relations*. London: Macmillan.

HYMAN, R. 1989. *Strikes*. Basingstoke: Macmillan.

INGHAM, G. 1974. *Strikes and Industrial Conflict*. London: Macmillan.

JACKSON, M. 1987. *Strikes*. Brighton: Wheatsheaf.

KASSOLOW, E. 1969. *Trade Unions and Industrial Relations*. NY: Random House.

KERR, C. *and* SIEGEL, A. 1954. 'The interindustry propensity to strike – an international comparison'. In Kornhauser, A., Dubin, R. and Ross, A. (eds), *Industrial Conflict*,. NY: McGraw-Hill.

KNIGHT, K. 1972. 'Strikes and wage inflation in British manufacturing industry 1950-1968'. *Bulletin of the Oxford Institute of Economics and Statistics*. 34(3).

KORNHAUSER, A., DUBIN, R. *and* ROSS, A. (eds) 1954. *Industrial Conflict*. NY: McGraw-Hill.

KORPI, W. *and* SHALEV, M. 1979. 'Strikes, industrial relations and class conflicts in capitalist societies'. *British Journal of Sociology*. 30(2).

LOCAL AUTHORITIES CONDITIONS OF SERVICE ADVISORY BOARD. 1991. *Employers' Responses to Industrial Action*. London: LACSAB.

MCGREGOR, D. 1960. *The Human Side of Enterprise*. NY: McGraw-Hill.

MARTIN, R. 1992. *Bargaining Power*. Oxford: Clarendon.

MAYO, E. 1946. *The Social Problems of an Industrial Civilization*. London: Routledge.

REES, A. 1952. 'Industrial conflict and business fluctuations'. *Journal of Political Economy*. 60(5).

ROETHLISBERGER, F. 1946. *Management and Morale*. Cambridge, Mass.: Harvard University Press.

ROSS, A. 1959. 'Changing patterns of industrial conflict'. In Somers, G. (ed.), *Proceedings of the 12th Annual Meeting of the Industrial Relations Research Association*.

ROSS, A. *and* HARTMAN, P. 1960. *Changing Patterns of Industrial Conflict*. NY: Wiley.

SHOREY, J. 1976. 'An interindustry analysis of strike frequency'. *Economica*. 43, no. 172.

SHORTER, E. *and* TILLEY, C. 1974. *Strikes in France 1830-1968*. Cambridge: CUP.

SMITH, C., CLIFTON, R., MAKEHAM, P., CREIGH, S. *and* BURN, R. 1978. *Strikes in Britain*. London: Department of Employment.

SWEENEY, K. *and* DAVIES, J. 1996. 'Labour disputes in 1995'. *Labour Market Trends*. June, 104 (6).

SWEENEY, K. *and* DAVIES, J. 1997. 'International comparisons of labour disputes in 1995'. *Labour Market Trends*. April, 105 (4).

WARNER, W. *and* LOW, J. 1947. *The Social System of the Modern Factory*. New Haven: Yale University Press.

Author index

Subject index